Lymphomas 1

Cancer Treatment and Research

WILLIAM L. MCGUIRE, *series editor*

Volume 4

1. R.B. Livingston, ed., Lung Cancer 1. 1980. ISBN 90-247-2394-9.
2. G.B. Humphrey, L.P. Dehner, G.B. Grindey and R.T. Acton, eds., Pediatric Oncology 1. ISBN 90-247-2408-2.
3. J.J. DeCosse and P. Sherlock, eds., Gastrointestinal Cancer 1. 1981. ISBN 90-247-2461-9.

series ISBN 90-247-2426-0.

Lymphomas 1

including Hodgkin's disease

edited by

JOHN M. BENNETT
University of Rochester Cancer Center

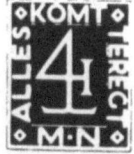

1981

MARTINUS NIJHOFF PUBLISHERS
THE HAGUE / BOSTON / LONDON

Distributors:

for the United States and Canada

Kluwer Boston, Inc.
190 Old Derby Street
Hingham, MA 02043
USA

for all other countries

Kluwer Academic Publishers Group
Distribution Center
P.O. Box 322
3300 AH Dordrecht
The Netherlands

Library of Congress Cataloging in Publication Data   ⊂ｌₚ

Main entry under title:

Lymphomas.

  (Cancer treatment and research; v. 4)
  Includes index.
  1. Hodgkin's disease. 2. Lymphoma. I. Bennett, John M., 1933– . II. Series.
RC644.L9   616.99′446   81-9633
AACR2

ISBN-13: 978-94-009-8281-9   e-ISBN-13: 978-94-009-8279-6
DOI: 10.1007/978-94-009-8279-6

Contents

Contents

Cancer Treatment and Research

Foreword

Where do you begin to look for a recent, authoritative article on the diagnosis or management of a particular malignancy? The few general oncology textbooks are generally out of date. Single papers in specialized journals are informative but seldom comprehensive; these are more often preliminary reports on a very limited number of patients. Certain general journals frequently publish good in-depth reviews of cancer topics, and published symposium lectures are often the best overviews available. Unfortunately, these reviews and supplements appear sporadically, and the reader can never be sure when a topic of special interest will be covered.

Cancer Treatment and Research is a series of authoritative volumes which aim to meet this need. It is an attempt to establish a critical mass of oncology literature covering virtually all oncology topics, revised frequently to keep the coverage up to date, easily available on a single library shelf or by a single personal subscription.

We have approached the problem in the following fashion. First, by dividing the oncology literature into specific subdivisions such as lung cancer, genitourinary cancer, pediatric oncology, etc. Second, by asking eminent authorities in each of these areas to edit a volume on the specific topic on an annual or biannual basis. Each topic and tumor type is covered in a volume appearing frequently and predictably, discussing current diagnosis, staging, markers, all forms of treatment modalities, basic biology, and more.

In Cancer Treatment and Research, we have an outstanding group of editors, each having made a major commitment to bring to this new series the very best literature in his or her field. Martinus Nijhoff Publishers has made an equally major commitment to the rapid publication of high quality books, and world-wide distribution.

Where can you go to find quickly a recent authoritative article on any major oncology problem? We hope that Cancer Treatment and Research provides an answer.

WILLIAM L. McGUIRE
Series Editor

Preface

This first volume of the series on lymphomas provides a concise and complex pathophysiology, staging and therapy of these diseases. Since it is the intent of the publisher to provide an ongoing series with volumes appearing at approximately two-year intervals, this issue emphasizes only the most important aspects essential for physicians involved in the care of patients with Hodgkin's disease and non-Hodgkin's lymphomas (NHL).

In any multiple authored volume the choice of the individual contributors is often very difficult. Rather than going far afield, I have selected individuals with whom I have had a close professional relationship, whose judgments I have considered to be most reasonable, and who have commanded the respect of their peers.

Despite the enormous progress that has been made in our understanding of the pathology of the lymphomas, controversy rather than concordance continues to reign. Attempting to predict the future is not an easy task, but my choice of Dr. Barbara Tindle as the responsible pathologist appears to be a wise one. Trained by Dr. Robert Lukes, Dr. Tindle has been in the forefront of the advances in the cytoimmunologic classification of the non-Hodgkin's lymphomas (Lukes-Collins; Kiel classification), and those diseases that mimic lymphoma, such as immunoblastic lymphadenopathy. Both the section on Hodgkin's disease and NHL are supplemented by outstanding photographs, providing an excellent syllabus for pathologists and clinicians. Even with the wide acceptance of the Rye modification of the Lukes-Butler classification for Hodgkin's disease, the ability to reproduce accurately the various pathologic subtypes by American pathologists has been only moderately successful (around 65% concordance against an expert Pathology Panel). Dr. Tindle provides insight into the problems encountered in Hodgkin's disease, particularly in the cellular phase of nodular sclerosis and the nodular variant of the lymphocyte predominant form.

In the NHL category, Dr. Tindle acknowledges the success of the Rappaport classification in identifying prognostic categories, particularly in adults.

The classification has had great relevance in identifying two prognostic groups: nodular, poorly differentiated lymphocytic lymphoma, and diffuse histiocytic lymphoma. Both of these cell types are readily recognized by most pathologists. Utilizing these terms, several groups have described the indolent nature of the former and the aggressive behavior of the latter type with its potential for cure with specific radiation or chemotherapy. She then develops the thesis of the immunologic nature of the NHLs with convincing evidence for a 'B' cell origin for nodular lymphomas, i.e. truly 'follicular' in origin and the failure to confirm a histiocytic origin for the majority of the histiocytic lymphomas. Whether the immunologic classification of NHL will replace the Rappaport classification will depend on two important factors. The first is the ability to reproduce the various cytological subtypes (small cleaved, larged cleaved, large noncleaved, etc.), and the second will be to demonstrate that response rates to therapy and survival data can be established and reproduced by several cooperating groups and cancer centers.

Once the diagnosis is established, a careful and detailed clinical, laboratory, and radiographic evaluation of patients with lymphomas is mandatory. Dr. Richard Stein has had considerable experience, based on material at the University of Chicago, on staging of patients, and has summarized his approach with a well written chapter. He emphasizes the higher incidence of extra nodal involvement in NHL, leading to the usefulness of bone marrow biopsy and liver biopsy in 'downstaging' patients and avoiding staging laparotomies. Even though computerized axial tomography (CAT) has improved dramatically our ability to locate areas of involvement previously not detected (retrocrural nodes, peripancreatic, celiac, periportal, mesenteric nodes), staging laparotomy continues to be the rule rather than the exception for Hodgkin's disease clinical stages IA, IIA, IIB, and IIIA, and for a modest number of NHL patients who remain with localized disease after appropriate workup (fewer than 10%).

The radiologic approach to staging has become an extremely important aspect to the total evaluation of patients with lymphomas. Too often the clinician utilized the radiographic services without considering the radiologist as a full member of the diagnostic physician team. With the availability of isotopic scans for assessing node, spleen and liver status, ultrasound for abdominal masses, lymphangiography, and CAT scanning, the question of accuracy (sensitivity and specificity) of each test for each organ in question, and overall cost for the procedures compared to the real yield of additional useful clinical information, needs to be addressed. Dr. Derek Hamlin examines critically each of the available radiologic tests and provides an excellent set of graphic representations of positive studies. He provides an appropriate comparison between lymphangiogram, ultrasound, and CAT scans for intra abdominal disease.

Drs. Zagars and Rubin have provided a remarkably succinct, yet detailed review of the principles of radiation therapy as applied to the malignant lymphomas. The world's literature has been reviewed carefully and tabulated by clinical and pathologic stage, wherever possible. The concept of extended field irradiaion for Hodgkin's disease and more limited radiation for NHL, is explored and then defended well. The relatively new applications of low dose consolidation radiation in Hodgkin's disease, and total body irradiation in stage III lymphocytic lymphoma are placed in proper perspective.

In most clinical or pathologic staging settings in Hodgkin's disease, the addition of potentially curative chemotherapy (usually a 4-drug combination) to curative radiation has not produced the anticipated improvement in survival at 5 or 7 years. In some situations the disease free interval has been dramatically improved (IIIA, for example), but 'salvage' chemotherapy restores the balance for those patients who fail with radiation alone. To compromise by lowering the known tumoricidal dose of radiation or by reducing the number of cycles of chemotherapy that has proven to be curative in advanced disease, appears to be unreasonable except in carefully controlled clinical trials.

Whereas radiation therapy became a proven modality for control of the earlier stages of the malignant lymphomas in the late 1960s, it required an additional 5–10 years before chemotherapy was demonstrated to be equally effective in advanced disease. Dr. John Glick, whose training and background included involvement with the lymphoma clinical trials at both Stanford University, and the National Cancer Institute, and currently, as chairperson of the Hematology Committee of the Eastern Cooperative Oncology Group, develops the fascinating story of the change from single agent treatment to combination therapy in both Hodgkin's disease and NHL. The result has been the achievement of 50% long-term remissions (consistent with cure) of greater than 5 years in Hodgkin's disease, clinical stages IIIB, IVA, and IVB. In NHL the percentage of complete remissions has increased to over 50% with 'cures' in approximately 30% of patients with unfavorable histologies.

With the dramatic improvement in survival of patients with malignant lymphomas has come the unfortunate realization that there are long-term side effects from both radiation and chemotherapy, but of particular concern where both modalities are employed in the same patient. The most critical of these complications are the development of second malignancies, including epithelial cancers and acute leukemias (mostly myeloid). The exact incidence is not known, but some projections place the figure at 5–6 cases for every 100 patients cured. Therefore, the greatest care should be taken not to give both modalities in full courses when one is either sufficient for cure in the majority of patients or can result in the reinduction of a long term remission in a significant percentage of those who fail primary therapy.

In summary, all of the authors have presented their material in a manner that is equally suitable for the specialist involved in that particular area as well as for the general practitioner desirous of improving his (or her) field of knowledge on lymphoma diagnosis and management. The common goal of a continued improvement in overall survival in the malignant lymphomas, associated with acceptable cost and morbidity, demands the multidisciplinary approach that this volume attempts to present.

List of Contributors

GLICK, John H., Hospital of the University of Pennsylvania, 3400 Spruce Street, Philadelphia, PA 19104, U.S.A.

HAMLIN, Derek J., Department of Radiology, University of Florida College of Medicine, Gainesville, FL 32610, U.S.A.

RUBIN, Philip, Radiation Oncology, University of Rochester Cancer Center, Rochester, NY 14642, U.S.A.

STEIN, Richard S., Vanderbilt University School of Medicine, Nashville, TN 37232, U.S.A.

TINDLE, Barbara H., University of Vermont, Medical Alumni Building, Burlington, VT 05405, U.S.A.

ZAGARS, Gunar, Radiation Oncology, University of Rochester Cancer Center, Rochester, NY 14642, U.S.A.

1. Pathology of Lymphomas, Including Hodgkin's Disease

Malignant lymphomas, as neoplasms of lymph nodes and other lymphoid tissues, present challenges to the pathologist first in the recognition of a neoplastic process, and secondly, in the subclassification of the process when a definite diagnosis of lymphoma has been established. Lymphomas are classified broadly as Hodgkin's disease and non-Hodgkin lymphomas. While difficulty in subclassification is encountered in both major categories, the problems are greater in dealing with the terminologies proposed for the non-Hodgkin lymphomas. Added to the problem of diagnosis is the current knowledge that some prelymphomatous lesions are recognizable, and the pathologist has the task of distinguishing between abnormal or unusual reactive processes and frank neoplasia. This chapter approaches these problems separately as Hodgkin's disease, non-Hodgkin lymphomas, and prelymphomatous lesions.

The recognition of histological variation of lymphomas has caused less of a dilemma than the finding of ideal words to describe heterogeneous groups of lesions. Neoplasia of lymph nodes has been recorded at least since 1832 when Thomas Hodgkin described extraordinary lymphoid proliferation with massive lymphadenopathy and splenomegaly in a small number of cases [1]. A distinction between Hodgkin's disease and non-Hodgkin lymphomas was proposed as early as 1913 [2, 3], but the idea that lymphoma could or should be subgrouped, however, was not universally accepted for decades [4–8]; and the relationship between Hodgkin's disease and the non-Hodgkin lymphomas has not yet been clearly resolved.

The distinction of Hodgkin's disease from the non-Hodgkin lymphomas is generally accepted as the recognition of the Reed-Sternberg cell in a proper setting for Hodgkin's disease. This is not to say that the distinction of Hodgkin's disease from non-Hodgkin lymphoma or from reactive lesions is always easy, but the Reed-Sternberg cell as a guideline in diagnosis has been important and useful.

The subclassification of Hodgkin's disease has gone through two major

J.M. Bennett (ed.), Lymphomas 1, 1-127. All rights reserved.
Copyright © 1981 Martinus Nijhoff Publishers, The Hague/Boston/London.

phases, the first of which was based on the report of Jackson and Parker in 1944 [9]. The second and current phase has proved useful to pathologists and clinicians since a modification of the proposal of Lukes and Butler was accepted by the participants of the symposium on Obstacles to the Control of Hodgkin's Disease held in Rye, New York in 1966 [10]. The criteria for the various categories of Hodgkin's disease as proposed by Lukes and Butler are clear and readily followed by experienced pathologists. The rarer subtypes, which include lymphocyte predominant Hodgkin's disease and lymphocyte depleted types, cause problems in diagnosis more often in that they may not be recognized by less experienced pathologists, than in any real disagreement concerning histopathological criteria.

The non-Hodgkin lymphoma terminology is quite a different matter. Various attempts to subclassify the lesions have not yet reached a satisfactory conclusion. Early classifications related terminology to cell size as the major criterion [11–13], and the concept of neoplastic follicles was proposed in the early 1930s [14]. Subsequently, parameters of cell differentiation, as well as pattern of involvement, were reported [15]. However, while Rappaport's proposal that nodularity was an important issue [16], and this subsequently was found to be of clinical relevance [17], Rappaport suggested that the nodularity of lymphomas bore no relationship to the follicles of lymph nodes [16]. Until the late 1960s and early 1970s, classifications were based mainly on cytological and morphological features. Then investigators in the United States [18] and in Germany [19] proposed that lymphomas were related to specific cell types, notably to cells within the follicular centers of lymphoid tissue and in the interfollicular tissue. These proposals expanded with the increasing accumulation of immunological information that indicated functional parameters of various subclasses of lymphocytes. The immunological information has supported the premise that (1) most lymphomas are of B or T lymphocyte origin, (2) that some lymphomas have no easily detectable identity as to subtype, and (3) that very few lesions are recognizable as neoplasms of macrophages or histiocytes [20]. The clinical relevance of lymphoma terminology cannot be overemphasized, for clinicians and pathologists must have a common language for communication. Attempts have been made to evaluate large numbers of cases in order to correlate pathological and clinical data [21]. One goal of these studies is to establish a universally acceptable terminology. For the purposes of this chapter, Lukes' terminology will be used as the major refrence, reflecting the functional concepts of lymphoma classification [20].

Before presenting the pathology of the lymphomas, it is pertinent to emphasize the approach to lymphoma diagnosis.

1. APPROACH TO LYMPHOMA DIAGNOSIS

The approach to lymphoma diagnosis has two major objectives: (1) to prepare tissue ideally for histological diagnosis; (2) to perform variôus special procedures as aids to diagnosis, or to extend the present understanding of the pathogenesis of the disease. The approach to lymphoma diagnosis is reviewed briefly from both aspects.

1.1. Technical Aspects in Lymphoma Diagnosis

Lymphoma diagnosis may be difficult under the best of circumstances, and it is self-evident that histological interpretation in general depends on the pathologist being able to review optimally prepared materials. Unfortunately, there is not uniformity of tissue processing in all laboratories. Various factors which are involved in the preparation of ideal material include: (1) selection of the proper tissue for examination, (2) careful dissection to avoid crushing of the specimen, (3) proper fixation, (4) processing of the tissue to achieve sections which are intact, flat, thin, and (5) ideal staining for good contrast of nuclear and cytoplasmic detail. The preparation of ideal sections therefore depends on several persons: the clinician and/or surgeon who selects the tissue for biopsy; the surgeon who recalls the necessity of presenting unaltered tissue for examination; the pathologist who handles the specimen with great care; and the technologist who really understands the problems of processing and can avoid the many pitfalls which may be encountered in preparing lymphoid tissue for examination.

Lymphoid tissue is fragile. Lymphocytes are easily affected by local adverse conditions, and cellular distortion under a variety of circumstances may alter lymphocytes enough to cause confusion in diagnosis. A notable example of cellular alteration is that of lymphocytes in tissue which has been frozen. Small round lymphocytes, or 'well-differentiated lymphocytes', may appear to have irregular nuclei in such circumstances and erroneous diagnoses or confusion in the subclassification of lymphoma may occur. Necrosis is associated with altered cell detail. Immunoblasts in areas of necrosis may appear particularly pleomorphic. This feature may cause confusion in diagnosis between Hodgkin's disease and immunoblastic reactions, such as infectious mononucleosis, when the pleomorphic cells resemble Reed-Sternberg cells [22]. Various chemotherapeutic agents cause alteration of lymphocytes, especially small round cells, and precise subclassification of lymphomas may be difficult or impossible in the post-therapy state. These features are considered in the selection of lymph nodes for biopsy away from areas of potential necrosis, i.e. soft fluctulant nodes are bypassed for firmer masses; and biopsy is performed, when at all possible, prior to the institution of therapy.

Lymphoma may involve lymph nodes in a partial or focal manner. To decrease the need for rebiopsy because of an inadequate or non-diagnostic biopsy, it is important to select the most likely area of involvement. This generally means picking the largest lymph node for biopsy, not necessarily the most accessible one. The problem of dealing with non-diagnostic tissue obtained through dissection of small superficial masses by avoidance of biopsy of large masses, often for cosmetic reasons, is frustrating for all concerned and often leads to rebiopsy. The folly of excising superficial lymph nodes in the presence of large masses, has been emphasized [23].

Having selected a proper site for biopsy, great care must be used to avoid distortion of the tissue. Lymph nodes should be dissected away from surrounding connective tissue with minimal handling of the lymph node itself. For the most consistent results in lymphoma diagnosis, an intact lymph node should be presented to the pathologist. Percutaneous needle biopsy, while ideal for examination of many organs, particularly lung, liver, and bone marrow [24, 25], is not reliable for lymphoma diagnosis [26, 27]. Although diagnosis of lymphoma may be made on needle biopsy, diagnosis is essentially limited to the separation of Hodgkin's disease from non-Hodgkin lymphoma, and subclassification of either may be impossible [28]. Since *needle biopsy* would generally be followed by lymph node excision in cases of lymphoma, to allow for subclassification, we find the procedure is not of use in initial lymphoma diagnosis. The procedure may be useful for repeat biopsy in some established cases of lymphoma, especially Hodgkin's disease. One of the major pitfalls of this surgical technique is the mimicking of normal cells by lymphoma cells, a feature which emphasizes the need for review of the basic lymph node structure for appreciation of intact or obliterated architecture.

Tissue must be well-fixed in order to achieve optimal results. The particular fragility of lymphocytes which results in easy distortion of cells should be emphasized at all steps of the tissue processing. Details of common artifacts of fixation and processing are presented elsewhere [29]; however, several aspects of tissue handling deserve emphasis. Care to prevent drying of tissue is emphasized because a common mishap involves the transportation, examination and cutting of the tissue on a dry surface, i.e. paper or cloth towel. This situation can be avoided by transporting the tissue from the surgery area to the laboratory quickly and in a moist state. We ask that the specimen be sent to the laboratory unfixed and in a small sterile receptable containing physiological saline to keep the tissue moist.

The thickness of the section submitted for processing is important and depends on the specific fixative used. Several excellent fixatives are used routinely; pathologists have individual preferences for the types of fixatives used in their own laboratories. The major point is that whatever the fixative, it be used properly [29]. It is important that tissue be sliced thin enough to allow for full penetration of the fixative. Fixation is the single most important feature in proper tissue evaluation. While other artifacts of processing can be handled, poor fixation is an end result which may lead to necessary rebiopsy.

Tissue must be cut thin for proper fixation, and sections must be thin for proper evaluation. A good rule for thickness of sections is that they be 'one cell' thick, or about the size of a small lymphocyte, i.e. 4 µm. The pathologist is at a disadvantage when he cannot view cells as single tissues for lymphoma diagnosis lies largely with cytologic interpretation. Sections in which two or three cells overlie each other may be impossible to evaluate.

Improper staining, while not the crucial problem in interpretation, nevertheless is very important. Good contrast of nuclear and cytoplasmic stains allows for easier diagnosis. Erroneous diagnosis may occur if the cytologic features of a process cannot be appreciated.

There is no substitute for ideal tissue preparation, and proper diagnosis depends on the demonstration of clear histological and cytological detail. Students of pathology are urged, during their training programs, to make diagnosis on the basis of routine histological sections whenever possible and to avoid using special studies as crutches for diagnosis. We have found this approach to be reasonable to a point, since we believe lymphoma diagnosis is basically a cytological diagnosis. In the past decade, however, there has been a firm challenge to the premise that routine sections alone are enough for establishing lymphoma diagnoses. As a matter of fact, lymphoma diagnoses are generally made on well-prepared, and routinely processed and stained tissue sections. However, exciting advances in immunology and cytogenetics, together with new observations of cytochemical reactions, and the greater use of electron microscopy have added important dimensions to our interpretations of lymphoma. Cognizance of multiple parameters commonly employed for the study of lymphoproliferative disorders is important. Major techniques currently employed in lymphoma diagnoses are discussed briefly.

1.2. Multiparameter Approach to Lymphoma Diagnosis

Lymphoma classification primarily rests on the identification of distinctive cell types, and most tissues can be definitely categorized in ideally prepared tissue sections. The subclassification of the lymphomas is supported by special studies including cytochemical, immunochemical, immunological (lymphocyte transformation, specific antisera, and surface markers), cell kinetics, chromosome analysis, and ultrastructure (Table 1).

Ultrastructural studies usually do not play a crucial part in lymphoma diagnosis, although interesting findings have been demonstrated, and the fine detail of various cell types can be appreciated at the ultrastructural level. The spectrum of nuclear irregularity of neoplastic T cells as demonstrated by transmission electron microscopy has been reported in several studies and include illustration of the convoluted lymphocyte [30], Sézary's cells and

Table 1. Special studies in lymphoma diagnosis.

Cell type	Histopathology Cytology	Cytochemistry Immunochemistry *	Immunology	Other
Any cell type	Light microscopy Electron microscopy Tissue imprints			Enzymes ** Cytokinetics Cytogenetics
B lymphocytes		Methyl green Pyronin is of help but is not diagnostic Cytoplasmic Ig ***	Surface Ig Antisera HBLA	
T lymphocytes		Acid phosphatase	E rosette test Antisera HTLA	
Macrophages		Non-specific esterase Cytoplasmic lysosome	EA rosette test	

* Immunoperoxidase technique; ** i.e. terminal deoxynucleotidyl transferase; *** immunoglobulin
HBLA = human B lymphocyte antisera; HTLA = human T lymphocyte antisera

mycosis fungoides cells [31, 32], and the large lobated T cell [33]. The peculiar nuclear irregularity of lymphoepithelioid lymphoma cells (lymphocytes) by light microscopy was reported [34], and we observed the phenomenon of T cell nuclear irregularity by electron microscopy in those cases. Nuclear detail of T cell neoplasms is reported to be distinguishable from that of B cell lesions [35]; and, when present, the plasmacytoid features (well-developed granular endoplasmic reticulin with dilated cisternae) indicate a B cell origin [35]. Ultrastructure studies have demonstrated correlation between follicular center cells in reactive and in neoplastic settings [36].

Scanning electronmicroscopic studies of malignant lymphomas have also demonstrated interesting findings, and indicate potential applications of this method in lymphoma diagnosis [37]. However, the technique, so far, has not contributed significantly to the diagnosis of lymphoma [38].

Cytochemical studies, while usually not specific, in general, nevertheless, by mode of staining in certain cells, lend support to specific subclassification of lymphomas by identification of cell types. Non-specific stains include periodic acid Schiff (PAS) [39], methyl green pyronin (MGP) [40], and acid phosphatase (AP) [41].

The PAS stain is useful in separating out certain subtypes of acute lymphocytic leukemia from granulocytic leukemia. Although in the diagnosis of leukemia its most frequent use is related to review of bone marrow and peripheral blood smears, PAS positivity may be detected in imprints of lymph nodes in which there is an otherwise unclassified process on routinely prepared tissue sections. Thus the diagnosis of acute lymphocytic leukemia may be made on the basis of tissue imprints in the unusual circumstance in which the presentation of the disease is associated with lymphadenopathy of other tissue masses such as skin lesions. In the characterization of plasma-cytic-lymphocytic lymphomas, cytoplasmic and nuclear inclusions may be vividly demonstrated by the PAS stain. The PAS stain is a good stain for demonstrating reticulin and thus is ideal for the examination of spleen and lymph node sections, and for evaluation of the character of tissue involvement in infiltrative processes such as lymphoma. It is particularly useful in the demonstration of the extraordinary proliferation of small caliber vessels in pre-lymphomatous lesions such as immunoblastic lymphadenopathy.

The MGP stain is important in lymphoma diagnosis. As a stain for RNA, it is not specific for identification of cell type per se, but it is useful for demonstrating the spectrum of lymphocyte transformation in tissue, particularly of B cell proliferations since there is abundant RNA in transformed B lymphocytes. This feature makes the stain useful in the differential diagnosis of 'undifferentiated' lymphomas in tissue sections. Thus Burkitt lymphoma, which is a B cell lesion with intensely pyroninophilic cytoplasm, may be easily distinguished from the convoluted cell lymphoma, which is a T cell proliferation composed of cells with a scant amount of low density cytoplasm having little if any pyroninophilia. Similarly, B immunoblasts have intensely pyroninophilic cytoplasm in contrast to the T immunoblast with its pale, lightly pyroninophilic cytoplasm. This stain allows for easy evaluation of the number of plasma cells in tissue and allows for rapid identification of large bizarre cells such as Reed-Sternberg cells when they include huge inclusion-like nucleoli.

Acid phosphatase has been demonstrated as a marker for some T cell subpopulations when focal intense positivity is observed close to the nuclear membrane [42–44]. Acid phosphatase is also a marker for hairy cell leukemia in that the 'hairy cells' are resistant to tartrate and remain acid phosphatase positive after treatment with tartrate. Other lymphocyte lines, as a rule, are tartrate sensitive [45]. Alkaline phosphatase may be a distinctive marker for certain B cell neoplasms [46].

Non-specific esterase (NSE) and fluoride sensitive esterase are markers for histiocytes-monocytes. The alpha-naphthol butyrate method identifies active macrophages and typical monocytes which are positive with the stain and are sensitive to fluoride [47]. The naphthol AS-D acetate (NASDA) method allows identification of granulocytes and monocytes, the granulocytes being resistant to fluoride and the monocytes being sensitive to fluoride [48]. The NSE method is a supporting study for the identification of lymphomas of true histiocytes or macrophages.

Sudan black (SB), chloroacetate esterase (CAE) and peroxidase (PEX) methods [47, 49, 50] identify granulocyte differentiation in tissue (CAE) and in imprint preparations (CAE, SB, PEX). These stains are important in lymphoma diagnosis in that granulocytic sarcoma, or chloromas, may involve lymph node and other tissues without evidence for bone marrow involvement, and may be confused with lymphomas, particularly 'undifferentiated' lymphomas. The CAE method, because it works well in tissue sections, is useful in this diagnostic problem when other evidence for a granulocytic proliferation is not apparent (including the presence of eosinophilic myelocytes, and/or a leukemic pattern of lymph node involvement).

Oil red 0 has been reported as a characteristic positive stain in Burkitt lymphoma [51]. This is not a specific finding, but is useful in the interpretation of lesions observed in imprint preparations and in frozen sections in cases of Burkitt and Burkitt-like lymphomas.

Surface markers: The advent of immunologic marker techniques brough a new dimension to lymphoma classification. While most lymphomas can be classified cytologically in well-prepared tissue sections [52, 53], their B cell, T cell, or macrophage natures have been confirmed by a number of techniques [54–70]. Several key methods are easy to perform in most laboratories, while others are probably better in investigative laboratories.

B cells are demonstrated by surface immunoglobulins using polyvalent antisera for general classification of B cell neoplasms; specific antisera are used to detect monoclonicity and to allow for subclassification. The limitations of this immunofluorescence technique relate to (1) lack of a permanent specimen, (2) inconsistencies in interpretation when the studies are not performed often and by well-trained personnel, and (3) confusion between lymphocytes and monocytes-granulocytes because all of these cell series have Fc receptors. Despite the difficulties, and difference of interpretation in different laboratories [71, 72], surface marker methods remain the major means for detecting B cell neoplasms. A discussion of the details for performance of the procedures is reported elsewhere [73].

T cell neoplasms are demonstrated best by spontaneous lymphocyte rosetting by sheep red blood cells (E rosettes) [57, 62–64]. Recently distinctive T cell subsets have been identified [74–79].

Subpopulations of T cells and of B cells mark with EAC (IgM complement receptor) rosette formation [80]. However, hematopoietic cell lines and monocytes also possess complement receptors [81].

Histiocyte-monocytes are demonstrated by EA (IgG-Fc receptor) rosettes [80], but this procedure is not useful in all laboratories [82].

Additional immunological markers which have been used for B and T cell identification include specific T lymphocyte antisera (HTLA) and B lymphocyte antisera (HBLA); however, access to the antisera is limited, and the studies are carried out in only a few laboratories [83–87].

Immunochemical markers: An immunoperoxidase method for demonstrating cytoplasmic as well as surface immunoglobulin [88, 89] adds to the study of lymphomas particularly because it allows for a permanent record which can be reviewed and studied as desired. In addition, fixed tissues may be retrieved from paraffin blocks which have been long filed for evaluation of cytoplasmic immunoglobulin and for cytoplasmic lysosome.

In vitro lymphocyte transformation [90, 91] has added considerable information regarding lymphocyte kinetics and was important in the conceptualization of lymphomas as neoplasms of the immune system [18].

Cytokinetics adds still another dimension to the interpretation of lymphomas [92–94]. These techniques, which include cytofluorometry and microfluorometry, identify large and small cell populations, distinguish cells with aneuploidy from those which are diploid and essentially identifies cell subpopulations in lymphomas.

These techniques are an exciting addition to the exploration of the cell behavior and aim to demonstrate correlation between visualized tumor cytology and DNA content of the tumor cells.

Cytogenetics: A variety of chromosome abnormalities have been identified in the lymphomas [95–97]. Abnormalities of chromosome 14 are frequent in non-Hodgkin lymphomas and in immunodeficiency disease [98, 99]. A particular translocation between chromosome 8 and 14 has been identified in Burkitt's lymphoma [100]. However, specific markers have not proved useful in the diagnosis of lymphoma as have been demonstrated in myeloproliferative disease, i.e. Philadelphia chromosome as a consistent finding in chronic granulocytic leukemia. Neverthless, identification of chromosome abnormalities may be of considerable importance in monitoring of lymphoma for identification of recurrent disease, and in the monitoring of prelymphomatous lesions in which abnormal chromosomes are identified.

Terminal deoxynucleotidyl transferase (TdT): TdT is an intracellular protein/enzyme found in primitive lymphocytes in thymus and in bone marrow [101–103]. The detection of this enzyme in leukemias and lymphomas may aid in differential diagnosis. However, since it is present in both T and B cell lines (primitive T cells and pre-B cells), it is not useful for correlation with cytologic interpretation. It may, however, be an important prognostic indicator, i.e. TdT positive cells may be associated with a better prognosis than TdT negative cells [104, 105]. Techniques for detecting TdT positivity include enzyme assay and immunochemical methods [103].

Special studies for support of lymphoma diagnosis are useful for correlation with the histology-cytology of lymphomas, and have in themselves contributed immensely to our current understanding of these neoplasms. The current classifications of lymphomas incorporate the proposal that lymphomas are expressions of 'blocked' or 'switched-on' lymphocyte transformation [53]; the hypothesis must be tested with a variety of tools including those noted above as well as more sophisticated methods which are beyond the scope of this chapter. Essentially, this chapter is devoted to the description of lymphoma, including major groups and subgroups.

2. HODGKIN'S DISEASE

Hodgkin's disease, while included in the classification of lymphoma, has been an enigma in regards to its basic nature. For decades, the controversy continued as to whether the lesion was basically an inflammatory process or was neoplastic [106–109]. Recent epidemiological studies [110, 111] which suggest that clustering of cases occurs, add to the concept that the disease may be transmissable between human contacts even if the process itself does not fulfill the criteria for an inflammatory process. Reports of familial disease add to the intrigue of this disease [112, 113]. Currently the evidence favors a neoplastic etiology for Hodgkin's disease, the Reed-Sternberg cell being identified as the neoplastic component in a process which for most of the subtypes is composed largely of inflammatory elements. This is indeed a strange neoplasm in which the recognized neoplastic (cell) component is far outweighed in volume (in all but possibly the reticular type) by the presumed inflammatory milieu. It is strange too that the diagnostic tumor cell is very likely an end stage polyploid cell which is incapable of division [114]. The fact that the Reed-Sternberg cell is a polyploid cell and therefore undergoes nuclear division without cell division is peculiar for a 'cancer' cell, since by definition, 'cancer' is an uncontrolled cellular proliferation. Polyploidy in tumor cells is not unique. In Hodgkin's disease, however, the polyploid cell is the only recognizable neoplastic cell, whereas in other neoplasms no matter how pleomorphic, the polyploid cell is only a part of the spectrum of recognizable neoplastic elements. Despite the rigid criteria for diagnosis [115], it has become apparent that the Reed-Sternberg cell is, after all, one of a spectrum of cells in this disease process. As indicated by some investigators [114], the mononuclear cell is the proliferating cell, even if it is considered to be non-diagnostic in itself. The observation that Hodgkin's cells demonstrate aneuploidy has been supported, and the neoplastic nature of Hodgkin's disease has been further emphasized by reports in which distinctive marker chromosomes indicate a clonal proliferation [97, 116, 117].

The debate of whether Hodgkin's disease is inflammatory or neoplastic having faded, there remains the problem of understanding the basic nature of the disease, particularly the lymphocyte component which plays such an important part in the terminology as well as the nature of the Reed-Sternberg cell itself. The presence of the Reed-Sternberg cell in a lesion is generally accepted by pathologists as a necessary criterion for the diagnosis of Hodgkin's disease; the roles of the additional components which include lymphocytes, histiocytes, plasma cells, eosinophils, and fibroblasts, are not clear.

While the pathogenesis of non-Hodgkin lymphomas may relate to uncontrolled proliferation of certain lymphocyte types, or to blocks in lymphocyte transformation [53], the hypotheses for the pathogenesis of Hodgkin's disease are not so easily stated. One hypothesis for the basic mechanism in Hodgkin's disease suggests that transformation of T lymphocytes may, by way of some viral agent, lead to cell mediated autoimmunity with exhaustion of T cell compartments, and finally to neoplasia [118]. The suggestion that Hodgkin's disease may follow viral infection has not been substantiated, but during the past decade considerable attempts have been made to establish a relationship between Epstein-Barr virus and Hodgkin's disease [119–121]. Recently, cases of Hodgkin's disease following vaccination have been reported [122]. It seems clear that individuals with Hodgkin's disease have altered immune systems which may be expressed in various ways including increased susceptibility to infection, anergy, inability to reject skin grafts, defective lymphocyte transformation [123–129], and lymphopenia with a decrease in T lymphocytes [130–133].

The small lymphocytes in Hodgkin's disease lesions are probably of T cell type [134, 135], but the character of the Reed-Sternberg cell remains a matter of controversy. While the small T lymphocyte no doubt plays some major role in the mechanism of Hodgkin's disease, the current discussions of the Reed-Sternberg cell center on arguments for lymphocyte (B or T) versus macrophage origin [136].

The diagnosis of Hodgkin's disease depends on the observation of Reed-Sternberg cells in one of several histopathological settings or cellular backgrounds. The subclassification depends on the recognition of distinctive cellular backgrounds as the setting for particular Reed-Sternberg cell variants. In 1963, Lukes suggested a revision of the Jackson and Parker classification of Hodgkin's disease [137]. Subsequently, this proposal was expanded to a classical paper by Lukes, Butler and Hicks [138]. This proposal was accepted in modified form at the Symposium on Hodgkin's disease in Rye, New York [10] and reaffirmed at the Ann Arbor staging conference five years later [139]. The modification of the subclassifications to include four instead of six groups, as initially proposed by Lukes, was based on the anticipated clinical relevance of the subgroups.

The probable significance of the lymphocytic component in Hodgkin's disease as an indicator for prognosis was recognized in 1936 [140], and subsequent classifications reemphasized this point [9, 137]. It has been suggested that the lymphocytes and Reed-Sterberg cells have an inverse relationship in this disease process [115], and, that when lymphocytes predominate in the lesion, and Reed-Sternberg cells are in small number, the findings indicate indolent disease and reflect the host's ability to cope with the neoplastic process. Thus, as a rule, lymphocyte predominant Hodgkin's disease implies a much less ominous diagnosis than does the terminology (lymphocyte depletion), which reflects a smaller component of lymphocytes and easily detectable diagnostic Reed-Sternberg cells. The Reed-Sternberg cell component, nevertheless, is the major consideration in any lesion in this disease, and more emphasis is given in subclassification to the number of easily detected Reed-Sternberg cells than to the lympocyte component. The term 'mixed cellularity type' has been considered a worse lesion because of the greater paucity of small lymphocytes and the ease in detection of diagnostic Reed-Sternberg cells. Staging procedures have indicated the greater likelihood of more advanced disease in this subtype, as compared to lymphocyte predominant disease, the latter often being detected in Stage I. In Hodgkin's disease of the lymphocyte depleted (reticular) type, the ratio of small lymphocytes to Reed-Sternberg cells essentially is the reverse of that in the lymphocyte predominant type. While current modes of therapy have been associated with a dramatic response and overall better survival in all histological subgroups, nevertheless, pathologists and clinicians remain concerned with identifying specific subgroups in evaluation of afflicted individuals [141].

The Reed-Sternberg itself has been the object of discussion and debate since its recognition. The earliest reports indicate its ready identity in tissue sections [107, 142–144], and at least one of the early observers [107] in her distinguished drawings and text, while noting the presence of the peculiar multinucleated or polyploid giant cells in Hodgkin's disease, did not explicitly state that the cell was unique to that disease. As further observations have shown, the Reed-Sternberg cell, while necessary for the diagnosis of Hodgkin's disease, is not pathognomonic for that disease and may be observed in other processes [141]. Reed-Sternberg cells, or excellent facsimiles, are observed in other processes [145], most notably in immunoblastic proliferations and especially in exuberant immunoblastic reactions such as infectious mononucleosis [22, 146].

The diagnosis of Hodgkin's disease, while depending on the presence of diagnostic Reed-Sternberg cells in a proper setting, can be very troublesome when the 'proper setting' is not recognized. We have found a frequent problem in the diagnosis to occur when the pathologist does not recognize that a spectrum of transformed lymphocytes or immunoblasts are not part of the usual cellular milieu for Hodgkin's disease. The reason for this phenomenon is not clear, and it is disturbing in view of the proposal that the Reed-Sternberg cell itself may be a transformed lymphocyte or immunoblast [22]. Nevertheless, it is apparent from the review of hundreds of cases of Hodgkin's disease that the lesions are characterized by small lymphocytes and large bizarre cells, and that there is no obvious spectrum of lymphocyte transformation with a gradation of cell size and nuclear characteristics between the two in routine histologic sections. The exception to this observation is the similarity of some lacunar cell variants, in nodular sclerosing Hodgkin's disease, to T immunoblasts.

2.1. The Reed-Sternberg Cell

The Reed-Sternberg cell is recognized in tissue sections and in smears and imprints by its huge size (20-50 μm) and large inclusion-like nucleoli (4-5 μm). The cell varies in size, but in well-prepared material, it is easily identified at a medium magnification (160×) because of its large size in relation to the surrounding small lymphocytes. The classical or typical cell is binucleate or multinucleated with each nucleus containing a large nucleolus. This actually is artifactual because the cells are polyploid, as can be confirmed when the same cells are reviewed in sequential histologic sections. At different planes in section, a single cell will show an array of nuclear configurations. Nevertheless, the characteristic binucleated or multinucleated cell must be identified for diagnosis. In most proliferations a number of large mononuclear cells with large single nucleoli are observed. It has been suggested that the mononuclear variants are the proliferating cells in Hodgkin's disease [114]; and pathologists have been cautioned to avoid using the mononuclear cells as a basis for diagnosis because of the possible confusion with other lesions [115]. Reed-Sternberg cell variants have been described for the various subtypes of Hodgkin's disease and will be described further under the histologic expressions of the disease. An array of Reed-Sternberg cell variants are illustrated in Figures 1, 2, 3, and 4.

The precise character of the Reed-Sternberg cell remains in doubt, although a number of investigators have studied the cell in routine histological sections and by ultrastructural methods, and in vitro, and have reached various conclusions. Until recently the major discussion concerning this cell was whether it was a reticulum cell or histiocyte, or a lymphocyte. The discussion goes further. If the cell is a lymphocyte, is it a B cell or a T cell? Proponents of the theory that Reed-Sternberg cells are lymphocytes of B cell origin indicate that the cells may produce immunoglobulin [147, 148]. Investigators have demonstrated immunoglobulin in the cytoplasm of Reed-Sternberg cells, yet evidence for immunoglobulin synthesis is not convincing in all studies. Demonstration of a polyclonal pattern of immunoglobulin, by immunoperoxidase methods, does not resolve the matter of the nature of the Reed-Sternberg cell as a B cell, since it is possible that the polyclonal staining pattern could indicate absorption of immunoglobulin by a damaged cell, or the material could be phagocytized. It has been suggested that the Reed-Sternberg cell might be a B cell, notwithstanding the polyclonal cytoplasmic staining [147], and it has been noted that in human disease there has been demonstration of two light chains by individual tumor cells [149, 150]. A few cases have been reported in which monoclonal immunoglobulin staining by the immunoperoxidase method supports the interpretation of the Reed-Sternberg cell as a B cell [147, 151]. Others who have demonstrated cytoplasmic immunoglobulin in Reed-Sternberg cells propose that the material is not synthesized by the abnormal giant cell [152-155].

While most of the proponents of a lymphocyte origin for the Reed-Sternberg cell suggest that the B cell is incriminated, several investigators propose that the Reed-Sternberg cell may be of T cell origin, since there is a T cell deficiency in Hogkin's disease [118, 156]. No direct proof has been offered, however, that the Reed-Sternberg cell is indeed a T cell.

It has even been proposed that a fused B/T cell phenomenon may occur to create the Reed-Sternberg cell [157].

The idea that the Reed-Sternberg cell may be a histiocyte is based largely on the results of studies of cultured cells [158]. However, cells in culture have not uniformly resembled Reed-Sternberg cells. Proliferating mononuclear cells in culture have been called Hodgkin's cells, a term whch has been confused with the diagnostic cells [159]. Kadin, who on the basis of early studies of cultured cells favored a lymphocyte origin of the Reed-Sternberg cell, later studied cell suspensions from Hodgkin's disease lesions and concluded that the abnormal cells were derived from macrophages [160–161].

While the continued debate over the origin of the Reed-Sternberg cell has been based largely on the observations of cultured cells and the results of functional studies of those cells, morphologists have also addressed this issue. A sequence of evolution from small lymphocytes to lacunar cell variants and/or diagnostic cells has been proposed [162]. Others have noted the resemblance of the diagnostic cell in Hodgkin's disease to pleomorphic immunoblasts observed in tissue sections in infectious mononucleosis and have suggested that this phenomenon may indicate that the Reed-Sternberg cell is a lymphocyte [22].

Leukoerythrophagocytosis has been reported in Reed-Sternberg cells [163], and emperipolesis, as a mechanism for cell entry into the tumor cells, has been suggested [164, 165]. The possibility that lymphocytes may actually enter the Reed-Sternberg cell and become trapped and destroyed, as proposed by one observer [164], is an exciting concept that raises new questions concerning the relationship of lymphocytes and Reed-Sternberg cells and their proportion to each other in different types of Hodgkin's disease. It is remarkable, however, that in reports of hundreds of cases of Hodgkin's disease, little mention has been made of what would be extraordinary phenomena in this disease process. It seems unlikely that such events, if common in this disease, would have been overlooked.

2.1.1. The Lymphocytes in Hodgkin's Disease. Interest has centered on the obvious component in the tissues of Hodgkin's disease, i.e. the Reed-Sternberg cell. More recently, questions have been raised concerning the nature of the small lymphocytes which are found in variable quantity in different subtypes of the disease, and the presence of which direct the terminology of Hodgkin's disease. As indicated above, the number of

Table 2. Major classifications of Hodgkin's disease and their interrelationships.

Reference	Histopathologic types

9	Paragranuloma		Granuloma		Sarcoma
138	*L & H nodular	*L & H diffuse	Mixed cellularity	Nodular sclerosis	**DF	Reticular
115, 139	Lymphocyte predominant		Mixed cellularity	Nodular sclerosis	Lymphocytic depletion

lymphocytes seems to be related to the number of diagnostic Reed-Sternberg cells in most cases. It has been suggested that, in view of the T lymphocyte deficiency in Hodgkin's disease, that the small lymphocyte in this process is a T cell. A number of studies have indicated an increase in T cell content in lymph nodes and spleen from patients with Hodgkin's disease [166–176]. Several investigators have demonstrated T-lymphocytes in close proximity to, or even attached to, Reed-Sternberg cells [166–168]. Peculiarities of the T cells in Hodgkin's disease have been noted with T lymphocytes possessing tumor-related antigens [169], as well as T lymphocytes, as detected in cell suspensions from Hodgkin's disease by E rosettes, which failed to respond to phytohemagglutinin [134].

The role of the small lymphocyte in Hodgkin's disease and its precise character remains unclear. In review of the lymphocyte subpopulations in tissue sections in Hodgkin's disease, the paucity of a spectrum of transformed lymphocytes or immunoblasts is apparent. The reason for this intriguing feature has yet to be stated, but the indication that this phenomenon may be related to the lack of *in vitro* lymphocyte transformation merits special attention. Major classifications of Hodgkin's disease are listed in Table 2.

2.2. Lymphocyte Predominant Hodgkin's Disease

The term 'lymphocyte predominant' is a useful term which implies clinical relevance in Hodgkin's disease [10, 135]. Lukes and Butler, however, emphasized a difference in pattern of lymph node involvement in this lesion, and suggested that nodularity or diffuseness of the lesion might be significant [10, 135]. Firm data supporting this premise that pattern is clinically significant has not been reported, and the distinction of nodular and diffuse forms is only exceptionally encountered in the recent literature [177, 178]. Since the pattern of involvement may create a problem in differential diagnosis, it is important for the pathologist to have a firm grasp of the histopathology of the lesions.

2.2.1. Nodular Type. The lymph node is usually completely involved, although occasionally the lymphomatous process involves part of the lymph node as an expanding mass which compresses uninvolved tissue in the subcapsular area (Figure 5). The lesion itself has a vaguely nodular appearance at low magnification, and this may in some cases be appreciated on gross examination. On gross examination the involved lymph node has a firm but not hard texture; the tissue is easily sliced (in contrast to the sometimes hard, even gritty, texture of the tissue in nodular sclerosing Hodgkin's disease). The tissue is generally uniformly tan on cut surface. Occasionally capsular fibrosis may raise a problem in differential diagnosis from nodular sclerosing Hodgkin's disease, but this may be attributed to capsular reactive changes in a slowly expanding lesion in the lymphocyte predominant type.

Microscopically, the tissue in this lesion is characterized by a profound proliferation of lymphocytes. Epithelioid histiocytes are present in variable number and may be prominent, but their number is generally minuscule in comparison to the small lymphocyte component. The epithelioid histiocytes are arranged in small clusters and singly throughout the lymph node sections, and, when particularly prominent, may cause confusion in diagnosis with other lesions, including non-Hodgkin lymphoma and reactive processes. When epithelioid histiocytes are prominent in the nodules, the differential diagnosis from sarcoid and from toxoplasmosis may be of concern.

Lymphocyte predominant Hodgkin's disease is characterized by a peculiar Reed-Stenberg cell, the L & H cell, so called because of the initially proposed term lymphocytic-histiocytic type of Hodgkin's disease [138]. This cell is not to be mistaken for the typical Reed-Sternberg cell which is necessary for the diagnosis of Hodgkin's disease. The L & H cell is a large cell, at least four to five times the size of the surrounding small lymphocytes (in the range of $16-20\,\mu m$), and it is easily detected even in the mixed milieu of small lymphocytes and reactive histiocytes, standing out from the latter because of its distinctive cytologic features. In the nodular expression of lymphocyte predominant Hodgkin's disease, the L & H cell is abundant in the nodules and may be scattered in the intervening tissue and in the subcapsular areas. The L & H cell is a large, fragile-appearing cell with a scant, if discernible, rim of pale cytoplasm which is minimally pyroninophilic. The nucleus occupies most of the cell, has a lobated contour, very fine chromatin, and tiny nucleoli (Figures 4 and 6). In many cells nucleoli are not detected in light microscopic sections. Occasionally L & H cells have prominent nucleoli, and in such instances if Reed-Sternberg cells are detected easily, the concern is for a more aggressive histologic type, i.e. mixed cellularity type Hodgkin's disease. L & H cells may comprise up to 10% of the cellular components in this lesion [115].

Diagnostic Reed-Sternberg cells are found with great difficulty in lymphocyte predominant Hodgkin's disease. Despite the tedium of searching for diagnostic cells in this distinctive lesion, it is important to search for them, in many sections in some cases, and to demonstrate the diagnostic cells before stating a diagnosis of Hodgkin's disease.

This lesion is associated with few inflammatory cells other than small lymphocytes and histiocytes. Plasma cells and eosinophils are rarely encountered. Fibrosis within the lymph node itself is rare, although occasionally some hilar fibrosis and capsular thickening may be encountered. Necrosis is not observed. Immunoblasts, as in other subtypes of Hodgkin's disease, are noticeably absent from the proliferation, and the large L & H cells and few diagnostic Reed-Sternberg cells stand out sharply in the background of small lymphocytes with little evidence for a spectrum of lymphocyte forms between the small and large cells.

The nodules of this lesion cause some difficulty in differentiation from those of non-Hodgkin lymphoma. It is helpful when presented with this problem to recall that the nodules of lymphocyte predominant Hodgkin's disease appear to represent the mounding effect of involvement of interfollicular tissue in lymph nodes, while the 'nodules' of non-Hodgkin lymphoma clearly represent lymphomatous follicular centers. The interfollicular involvement fits with the observation that Hodgkin's disease arises in the T cell or paracortical zones of lymph nodes [179]. The nodules in Hodgkin's disease of this type are vaguely demarcated structures which merge together and with the intervening tissue (Figure 7); follicles of non-Hodgkin lymphoma, even when merging, tend to maintain a distinct margin (Figure 8).

The critical point in diagnosis is to be able to recognize the cellular composition of the lesion, particularly the L & H cells as a distinctive feature. The major proliferation in this entity is obviously the small lymphocyte, but careful inspection of the small lymphocytes reveals the cells to have minimal nuclear irregularity. This feature causes confusion with the typically irregular-nucleus cell of poorly differentiated lymphocytic lymphoma, a non-Hodgkin lymphoma which commonly has a nodular expression.

2.2.2. Diffuse Type. This lesion may be very similar in cellular composition to its nodular counterpart, but it is characterized by a diffuse obliteration of lymph node architecture (Figures 9 and 10). The lesion creates a problem in diagnosis, as does the nodular variant, in differential diagnosis from reactive lesions. A problem of precise subclassification, between lymphocyte predominant Hodgkin's disease and mixed cellularity type, occurs when the lesion appears to be intermediate between the two subtypes with easily found diagnostic Reed-Sternberg cells and numerous L & H variants with large single nucleoli intermingled with the lymphocyte and epithelioid histiocyte populations. Plasma cells and eosinophils may be found in small numbers. Fibrosis is unusual, and necrosis does not occur. As a means of revolving the conflict of subclassification between lymphocyte predominant and mixed cellularity type Hodgkin's disease, we have used the criteria of easily detectable diagnostic Reed-Sternberg cells, together with more obvious populations of plasma cells and eosinophils, to classify the process as mixed cellularity type, even in the presence of a predominant background of small lymphocytes and epithelioid histiocytes. The weight of the diagnosis finally lies with the number of diagnostic Reed-Sternberg cells rather than with the lymphocyte component.

Like the nodular type of lymphocyte predominant Hodgkin's disease, the diffuse type is infrequently encountered, comprising from 6 to 15.5% of Hodgkin's disease cases [180–184].

2.3. Mixed Cellularity Type

This process may involve the lymph node in two ways: (1) as a diffuse process obliterating the normal architecture (Figure 11), or (2) in a focal manner which partially involves the lymph node mainly in interfollicular tissue and sparing reactive follicular centers (Figure 12). The diagnosis is readily established when the process is diffuse, Reed-Sternberg cells are abundant, and diagnostic cells are easily detected. Typical large binucleated and multinucleated cells are observed, as are large mononuclear variants. Lymphocytes are variable in number, but generally are decreased from those observed in reactive lymph nodes. Inflammatory cells are present in variable quantity and include epithelioid histiocytes, eosinophils, and plasma cells. As with other subtypes of Hodgkin's disease, a spectrum of transformed lymphocytes or immunoblasts is lacking in this lesion. Confusion in diagnosis occurs when a reactive lymph node is focally involved with Hodgkin's disease, and immunoblastic proliferation is present in uninvolved areas. Mixed cellularity type Hodgkin's disease is commonly characterized by tissue necrosis, but only occasionally is it associated with profound eosinophilia and even eosinophilic necrosis (Figure 13), with the areas of necrosis resembling those of allergic granulomas. We have found no correlation with hypersensitivity phenomena in the few cases in which there has been profound tissue eosinophilia, but some questions are worth asking: Does the patient have a hypersensitivity response to his/her tumor? Does the individual have two processes, one being Hodgkin's disease, the other being an unrelated allergic reaction? We have reviewed one case in which an extreme degree of eosinophilia, as well as eosinophilic necrosis with structures resembling Charcot-Leyden crystals, were present in a staging laparotomy specimen in a young woman. Peripheral eosinophilia has not corresponded to the profound tissue eosinophilia in these unusual cases of Hodgkin's disease, nor to that reported to be associated with allergic granulomatosis [185].

Scattered epithelioid histiocytes are an expected component in all subtypes of Hodgkin's disease, and their significance is not clear. Histiocyte aggregates associated with multinucleated giant cells of the Langhans type are worrisome in that the patient with Hodgkin's disease may be suspected to have a peculiar immune-type process or an inflammatory process [186, 187]. Studies by some investigators to evaluate this phenomenon revealed no significant findings which would indicate that the histiocyte component is necessarily associated with a second (inflammatory) process [188, 189]. Nevertheless, we continue to evaluate patients whose tissue pathology even remotely suggests a possibility of infection to insure that cancer therapy can be used to full advantage and that the patient is not jeopardized by undergoing treatment in the presence of infection.

Focal involvement of lymph nodes with Hodgkin's disease of mixed cellularity type is generally troublesome. The tumor foci lie in the interfollicular tissue, expanding this area, but are surrounded by reactive lymphoid tissue, including active follicular centers and reactive interfollicular tissue which may contain immunoblasts. While the lesion is usually recognized because of the eosinophil component and readily detected Reed-Sternberg cells, mixed cellularity type Hodgkin's disease represents a spectrum of histopathologic changes from lesions in which the background is close to the bordeline of lymphocyte depletion Hodgkin's disease. When focal Hodgkin's disease is associated with a prominent lymphocyte background, the differentiation from reactive lymph node hyperplasia may be difficult. In any equivocal cases, it is wise to suggest rebiopsy. Focal Hodgkin's disease of this type may represent extended disease, and rebiopsy of residual large lymph nodes will generally confirm the diagnosis if the disease is present [190].

Plasma cells are usually abundant in mixed cellularity type, and occasionally this includes a profound proliferation (Figure 14). As with any extraordinarily profound plasma cell proliferation, serum immunoglobulins may be of interest in such cases in the event of a second or dysglobulinemic process.

Mixed cellularity type by its name implies a mixed cellular background. While this fact is true, nevertheless, mixed cellularity type Hodgkin's disease spans the variation in histological pattern and composition between lymphocyte predominant type and lymphocyte depletion type. Lesions with a lymphocyte predominant background, but too readily found diagnostic Reed-Sternberg cells, are classified as mixed cellularity type. Those with lymphocyte depletion background, but mild to moderate fibrosis, are classified as mixed cellularity type. Lukes suggested that the term be used when the cellular milieu cannot be readily classified as one of the other subtypes [115].

Some observers, however, designate such lesions unclassifiable Hodgkin's disease, rather than use the term 'mixed cellularity type' as a catchall term [191]. Another lesion (described further in the chapter) which some of us include with mixed cellularity type Hodgkin's disease, is that in which lacunar cell variants are observed in great abundance, as in nodular sclerosing Hodgkin's disease, but without the sclerosing bands (Figure 15). While some observers refer to this lesion as mixed cellularity type with lacunar cells, others have preferred to use the term cellular phase nodular sclerosis Hodgkin's disease [182, 189, 191].

2.4. Lymphocyte Depletion Hodgkin's Disease

As the term implies, there is a tissue lymphopenia in this type of Hodgkin's disease. There is, as well, peripheral lymphopenia which may be the first detectable laboratory sign of the entity in individuals who present with typical signs and symptoms of progressive, debilitative disease [192, 193]. For clinical correlation, as proposed at the staging symposia in 1966 and 1971 [10, 115], the term lymphocyte depletion is used as an inclusive term. Lukes and Butler [10, 115] have suggested, however, that pathologists recognize that the terminology includes two distinct histological types. Both types are characterized by a paucity of small lymphocytes, but otherwise are remarkedly different in their histopathology. They share the common feature of having large bizarre cells, the so-called pleomorphic Reed-Sternberg cell variant (Figure 16). The cellularity is different in the two lesions, although both lesions may be represented in a single specimen or in different lymph nodes in the same individual. Like lymphocyte predominant Hodgkin's disease, this major subgroup of lymphocyte depletion type is an infrequent form of the disease [182–184].

2.4.1. Diffuse Fibrosis Type.
In this lesion, the lymph node architecture is obliterated, and partial involvement of lymph nodes is very unusual. Throughout the lymph node there is a disorderly array of fibrous tissue without collagen formation (Figure 17). Small lymphocytes are scattered throughout, but lymphocytes are in minute quantity in the typical case. Occasionally small lymphocyte foci may be observed. Variable numbers of plasma cells, eosinophils, and reactive histiocytes are present, but, except for histiocytes, which may be abundant, thee is a general paucity of inflammatory cells. Necrosis is occasionally observed in this lesion. Reed-Sternberg cells may be few in number, but they are generally easily detected in well-prepared sections, as they stand out in the hypocellular tissue (Figure 18). They are particularly easy to detect in methyl green pyronin stained sections which allows the huge nucleoli to be emphasized. In the spectrum of histologic findings, an abundance of amorphous material may encompass most of the process. Pleomorphic Reed-Sternberg cell variants may be

scattered in the sections, and occasionally niduses of such cells will be observed.

2.4.2. Reticular Type. Unlike the pale, hypocellular tissue observed in the histological examination of the diffuse fibrosis type of lymphocyte depletion Hodgkin's disease, the reticular type is very cellular and is characterized by a mass of cellular tissue composed of bizarre mononuclear and multinucleated or polyploid cells (Figure 19). If Reed-Sternberg cells were to demonstrate emperipolesis [164], or phagocytosis [163], these peculiar pleomorphic cell variants might be expected to do so. The reticular lesion is a rare type of Hodgkin's disease, the most uncommon in our experience. Lukes describes two types of reticular Hogkin's disease [115]. In one type, the cellularity includes diagnostic Reed-Sternberg cells in great abundance. In the second type, the pleomorphic cell type is so abundant that the process has been aptly described as sarcomatous. A problem in distinguishing subtypes of Hodgkin's disease occurs when the array of pleomorphic cells is confused with a proliferation of lacunar cells having large nucleoli. The differential diagnosis on a histological basis may be difficult between reticular Hodgkin's disease, histiocytic lymphoma (lymphoma of macrophages) and immunoblastic sarcoma. The background of reticular Hodgkin's disease is similar to that of the diffuse fibrosis type, with amorphous material and/or disorderly fibrosis. Inflammatory cells generally are not present in any great number. Necrosis is occasionally encountered.

2.5. Nodular Sclerosis

The diagnosis of this subtype of Hodgkin's disease depends on the recognition of a peculiar Reed-Sternberg variant and dense collagen bands arising from a thickened sclerotic lymph node capsule. The diagnosis presents little or minimal difficulty when the lesion presents in classical or typical form in lymph node (Figure 20). In the most easily recognized form, the lymph node architecture is largely obliterated. Follicular centers may remain; however, the sinusoidal and other interfollicular components are replaced by broad thick birefringent collagen bands which extend from a thickened capsule and surround cellular nodules which contain lacunar cells. The difficulties in diagnosis relate to the variable degree of sclerosis, which is observed in different lymph nodes and in the cellular variability of the cellular nodules containing the lacunar cells. Sclerosis varies from single thin bands, whch may be overlooked if the lymph node specimen is not adequately sampled, to marked sclerosis of the lymph node. Some observers have suggested that a severe degree of sclerosis is necessary for diagnosis of this lesion; however, Lukes has emphasized that sclerosis of varying degree, together with the characteristic lacunar cells, demonstrate the evolution of this strange process [115].

The lacunar cell is a Reed-Sternberg cell variant and typically is a large cell with abundant cytoplasm (in contrast to the L & H cell with its low nuclear: cytoplasmic ratio). The cytoplasm is of low density and usually stains a pale pink with the methyl greeen pyronin stain, reflecting its minimal content of polyribosomes [162]. The cytoplasm extends to the cell wall in tissue prepared in mercuric fixatives such as Zenker's fixative and B-5 fixative (Figure 21). The term 'lacunar cell' was proposed by Lukes because of the appearance of the cell in formalin-fixed tissue in which the cytoplasm is retracted toward the nucleus leaving a space or *lacuna* inside the cell wall (Figure 22). This phenomenon can cause confusion when it is not appreciated that the lacuna or space is within the Reed-Sternberg cell variant. Large cells in formalin-fixed tissue generally appear to lie in spaces. Thus, reactive multinucleated giant cells, megakaryocytes and other large cells may appear to lie within spaces in formalin-fixed tissue and be confused with lacunar cells. It has been suggested that the lacuna is created in this Reed-Sternberg cell variant in formalin-fixed tissue because the cell contains cytoplasmic fat which is leached away. Indeed, lacunar cells do stain with the Oil red 0 method for neutral fat [162]. The nucleus of this cell is multisegmented, often resembling that of neutrophils in configuration; however, the resemblance to neutrophils goes no further, for the lacunar cell is polyploid and the large nucleus has fine chromatin and discernible, although small, nucleoli. The confusion of lacunar cells and L & H cells has been mentioned. Another difficulty in diagnosis may occur when the lesion contains a large number of mononuclear lacunar cells in which large nuclei resemble those of transformed lymphocytes (T immunoblasts) with large pale rims of low-density cytoplasm (Figure 23), and the lesion may be misdiagnosed as T cell immunoblastic sarcoma. The cell, when recognized in a proper cellular environment, should cause little difficulty in diagnosis since typical multinucleated lacunar cells are always found in nodular scleorsing Hodgkin's disease.

The lacunar cell variants may fulfill the criteria for diagnostic Reed-Sternberg cells when the nucleolus is huge and inclusion-like (Figure 24). Diagnostic Reed-Sternberg cells of the non-lacunar variety may be difficult to identify in this lesion, but in review of multiple sections, they are almost always demonstrated. As with the other subtypes of Hodgkin's disease, caution should be used in diagnosis when diagnostic cells are not apparent in a lesion presumed to be nodular sclerosis because of otherwise characteristic cytologic features.

Necrosis is a fairly common finding in nodular sclerosing Hodgkin's disease and is usually of the non-eosinophilic type (Figure 25). Bizarre lacunar cell forms, particularly mononuclear forms, may be found in abundance around the areas of necrosis, as may diagnostic Reed-Sternberg cells. It is interesting that Reed-Sternberg cells and Reed-Sternberg-like cells are also found in close proximity to areas in necrosis in immunoblastic reactions such as infectious mononucleosis. The reason for this phenomenon is not clear. The mononuclear lacunar cell is often found in focal areas of early vascular proliferation and in close proximity to fine sclerotic bands. This feature is demonstrated as pale, apparently hypocellular areas in hematoxylin-eosin stained sections (Figure 26).

The characteristic collagen component in nodular sclerosis Hodgkin's disease varies from single thin bands to essentially complete sclerosis of the lymph node. Multiple sections may be necessary to locate cellular areas in which lacunar cells and Reed-Sternberg cells of the diagnostic type can be demonstrated. The collagen bands almost always extend from a thickened capsule of lymph node. This is an important point and helpful in distinguishing this type of Hogkin's disease from sclerotic reactive lesions. In the latter, the major sclerotic component usually extends from the lymph node hilus.

The nodules containing lacunar cells and diagnostic Reed-Sternberg cells and involved intervening tissue may resemble any of the cellular backgrounds for the other subtypes of Hodgkin's disease, including lymphocyte predominant, mixed cellularity type, and lymphocyte depletion types. Occasionally the Reed-Sternberg cell component in nodular sclerosis is so bizarre and admixed with lacunar cells that it suggests reticular type Hodgkin's disease. There is some indication that the cellular background in nodular sclerosis may be significant clinically. As indicated for the other subtypes of Hodgkin's disease, the paucity or abundance of diagnostic Reed-Sternberg cells is probably of clinical significance [194–197]. The mononuclear lacunar cell variants may resemble immunoblasts, but, as in other subtypes of Hodgkin's disease, a spectrum of immunoblasts is not a common feature of nodular sclerosis. Somewhat as a paradox, at least one report [162] illustrates the ultrastructure of various cells found in nodular sclerosing Hodgkin's disease, and the authors suggest a possible scheme for evolution of the lacunar cell and of the diagnostic Reed-Sternberg cell from small transformed lymphocytes. This concept increases the mystery of the lack of a spectrum of immunoblasts observed in routine histological sections.

2.6. Extranodal Hodgkin's Disease

Hodgkin's disease is essentially a lesion arising in lymph nodes. Reports of extranodal Hodgkin's disease almost invariably indicate that the 'extranodal' disease is always associated with primary lymph node disease [198–208]. One author has reported three cases of primary skin involvement [209], but in reports of skin involvement [206–209], gastrointestinal involvement [200–202], and central nervous system involvement [203–205] investigators have indicated that the extranodal sites are expressions of extended disease rather than primary foci. It is of interest to note that in a large series of cases in which skin involvement was emphasized, eight of the nine cases in which there was skin involvement were of the nodular sclerosing type [208]. As for primary skin involvement with Hodgkin's disease, the caution is raised that lesions may be confused with other neoplastic and non-neoplastic lesions. One of the most troublesome skin lesions in the differential diagnosis of Hodgkin's disease is the bizarre cellular proliferation of lymphomatoid papulosis [210].

Two types of extranodal disease have been described [198]. Disease may spread to contiguous organs, or it may disseminate to distant sites. Contiguous spread is presumably the result of tumor infiltration of tissues in close proximity to involved lymph nodes. Lung involvement in association with mediastinal disease may thus be explained; skin and bone are other likely sites for such spread. Disseminated disease has never been fully explained, although vascular invasion is a likely mechanism [211, 212]. Investigators reporting on this phenomenon suggest that vascular invasion will be found in about 10% of diagnostic lymph node biopsies in Hodgkin's disease. Fifty percent of the cases with involvement were interpreted as lymphocyte depletion type in patients with extensive disease [211]. A subsequent study by the same authors revealed the incidence of vascular invasion to be 5.9% in patients with stage I and II disease in which the histologic types included nodular sclerosis, mixed cellularity and lymphocyte depletion [212]. In vascular invasion, Reed-Stenberg cells and other bizarre appearing cells lie in the luminar of vessels and/or infiltrate vessel walls. Destruction of the vessel walls is often demonstrated. Elastic stains are particularly helpful in evaluating for this process, both in defining disruption of the structure of the vessel wall, and in identifying the location of abnormal cells [211].

As indicated above, Hodgkin's disease is primarily a disease of lymph nodes. While non-lymphoid organs are essentially never involved as primary sites of Hodgkin's disease, it is interesting that lymphoid tissues, other than lymph nodes, such as spleen, Waldeyer's ring, even thymus, are not commonly identified as sites of primary disease. Hodgkin's disease in thymus occurs perhaps more often than can be appreciated, since involved mediastinal tissue may hot have demonstrable lymph node or thymus structure. Nevertheless, we occasionally do observe thymus involved by Hodgkin's disease, usually nodular sclerosis type. Spleen is probably never involved as a primary site. It is more surprising that Waldeyer's ring is seldom involved as a primary focus [213].

2.7. Pathology of Staging

Staging for extent of disease has been important for establishing a baseline for treatment [214–217]; but it has served, as well, as a mode of understanding the disease process. Details of treatment in any case are based on the pathologic stage of the disease, yet it has been apparent from reviewing the results of many staging laparotomies that histology and stage of disease do bear some relation, and the histopathology of Hodgkin's disease subtypes remains important in the overall consideration of the individual's disease [141, 218]. The pathologist in examining tissues from staging procedures has several tasks. The tissue must be examined with careful scrutiny to assure recognition of focal involvement of lymph node, spleen, liver, and bone marrow, as well as involvement of any additional tissues which might be submitted for evaluation.

The identification of foci of Hodgkin's disease in lymph nodes from staging laparotomies may present difficulty when minute areas of involvement must be distinguished from the changes evoked by the pre-operative lymphangiogram. Generally, the lymphangiogram is performed within a few days prior to the laparotomy, and the changes in lymph node structure which are related to the procedure, while striking, generally do not cause confusion in interpretation. The lymph sinus system in such lymph nodes is dilated to give a 'Swiss cheese' appearance under the microscope (Figure 27); lipid laden macrophages and many huge multinucleated giant cells are present within the sinuses and often adhere to the vessel linings. Plasma cells are occasionally abundant, and eosinophils intermingle with small lymphocytes in the intersinusoidal septae. Reactive follicles may or may not be present. The more distal lymph nodes, pelvic and paraaortic, are commonly characterized by these features. When focal involvement with Hogkin's disease is present in such sections, the identity of the discrete lesion is readily achieved. In higher placed lymph nodes in the celiac area and at the porta hepatis, the demonstration of discrete lesions may present more difficulty when the neoplastic foci are small. In these 'high' areas, sinus dilatation is less pronounced and a more compact reaction in the peripheral areas of the lymph node sections is more difficult to distinguish from small foci of involvement by Hodgkin's disease. The rule for interpretation is, however, clear. Whether the focus of involvement is in lymph node or other organs, *a discrete lesion disrupting the organ's architecture must be identified.* The criteria for the cellular composition of the lesion in the extranodal site in these circumstances, however, are less rigid than for the initial diagnosis. Large abnormal cells must be demonstrated in a proper cellular background; as for the initial diagnosis; however, diagnostic Reed-Sternberg cells may not be found [115]. In the interpretation of extranodal Hodgkin's disease, large bizarre cells with single or multiple nuclei and large nucleoli, in the proper cellular setting as described for the initial diagnosis, fulfill the criteria for involvement in these sites.

Spleens involved with Hodgkin's disease are often enlarged, but spleen size does not relate to involvement or lack of involvement [219, 220]. As for lymph node involvement, a discrete lesion must be identified, although the precise cytologic criteria for the initial diagnosis may not be fulfilled. Splenic involvement occurs in the peripheral area of the Malpighian corpuscle, and the lesions are usually large enough to present no problem in interpretation of splenic involvement. Only rare cases of splenic involvement are observed as microscopic foci [219]; almost all splenic involvement is detectable or at least highly suspicious on careful examination of the gross specimen [221]. Careful examination of the spleen implies consecutive thin sectioning of the whole organ at small intervals, i.e. 3 to 4 mm. In the fresh state this may be very difficult to achieve unless a slicing apparatus is available. Sectioning at wider intervals (6–8 mm), allowing the tissue to fix for 30 minutes, and then resectioning for thinner sections, allows for optimum examination of the specimen. The examination of random sections without such careful gross inspection is inadequate evaluation.

Spleen is seldom involved in the absence of abdominal lymph node involvement; liver involvement is presumed not to occur in the absence of spleen involvement, with the exception of isolated case reports to the contrary [222, 223]. As for involvement by Hodgkin's in other sites, a discrete lesion must be demonstrated in the liver for diagnosis. The involvement is observed in the portal areas with invasion of the surrounding hepatic parenchyma. Involvement by Hodgkin's disease in the liver may cause consternation for the observer who does not recognize portal lympho-cyte infiltration as a usual finding in liver sections removed at staging laparotomy. Obviously, the interpretation of liver involvement in Hodgkin's disease is at best tenuous, because the random sampling of this huge organ, as for sampling of the bone marrow, does not allow for really complete examination.

At the time of staging laparotomy, it is customary to obtain a wedge biopsy of the iliac bone marrow. The review of large bone marrow sections achieved by this method allows for a better evaluation for tumor than do small random needle biopsies and aspirated bone marrow particle sections. A discrete lesion in bone marrow must be observed, as for other areas of extranodal involvement.

Figures 28, 29, and 30 illustrate extranodal involvement in Hodgkin's disease.

Peculiar histopathological findings in the staging of Hodgkin's disease have caused some confusion in interpretation. These findings namely include lymphocytic infiltration in the liver, and epithelioid granulomas in any or all of the laparotomy specimens. Lymphocytic infiltration in the portal triads of the liver is a common feature of laparotomy specimens. The infiltration varies in amount. When the initial diagnosis is lymphocyte predominant Hodgkin's disease, lymphocyte infiltration in the liver may cause great concern for hepatic involvement. Fortunately, lymphocyte predominant Hodgkin's disease presenting in Stage IV disease is unusual; nonetheless, the pathologist must take care to adhere carefully to the criteria for involve-ment [115]. Any area of involvement, including that of lymphocyte predominant type, would be found as a lesion with infiltration of the surrounding parenchyma. The non-neoplastic lymphocyte proliferation in the portal triads in the laparotomy specimens intermingles with the portal structures and remains confined within the triad (Figure 31). The presence of epithelioid granulomas is not considered diagnostic of Hodgkin's disease. This finding is fairly common in staging specimens in lymph node, spleen, liver and bone marrow. The significance is not clear, although some observers report a better prognosis in cases in which there is such a presence of the epithelioid cell proliferation [224, 225]. The histiocytes generally do not form well-defined granulomas and intermingle with the associated small lymphocytes.

Other histologic peculiarities associated with Hodgkin's disease, which are considered to be non-diagnostic and possibly related to the underlying immunological defects, include mesenchymal reaction observed in bone marrow and liver [226, 227]. Amyloidosis is a very rare phenomenon in untreated Hodgkin's disease. We have observed only one case in which amyloid deposition was present in the liver biopsy of a patient with Hodgkin's disease. Reports in the literature document a small number of cases of amyloidosis in Hodgkin's disease [228], but most reports present data from treated cases [229, 230].

In the bone marrow of patients with Hodgkin's disease, the degree of megakaryocytosis is often surprising and may mimic the megakaryocyte hyperplasia observed in patients with reactive lesions, especially granulomatous processes. Granulopoiesis is also increased along with megakaryopoiesis, while erythropoiesis is more often not noticeably increased in random bone marrow samples.

In addition to the challenges of establishing the presence or absence of Hodgkin's disease, and the recognition of non-specific findings in staging specimens, the pathologist is confronted with the problem of subclassification of lesions in the involved organs. The lesions in staging laparotomies usually mimic those of the initially biopsied lesions. However, in the instance of nodular sclerosing Hodgkin's disease, the definite subclassification may be apparent in involved laparotomy tissues when the initial biopsy was interpreted as mixed cellularity type. This situation usually occurs when the initial biopsy of a supraclavicular or low cervical lymph node shows a mixed cellular pattern with or without lacunar cells, but without the sclerosing component of nodular sclerosing Hodgkin's disease. Abdominal involvement in such cases may be characterized by the definite criteria for nodular sclerosis. Conversely, biopsies which provided the basis for nodular sclerosis may be associated with limited abdominal involvement in which the full criteria for that process are not fulfilled. It is important in the staging of Hodgkin's disease to recall that a diagnosis of nodular sclerosing Hodgkin's disease takes precedence in the subclassification [115]. Other than for purposes of identifying nodular sclerosis as the subclassification, the reporting of 'Hodgkin's disease involvement' in the laparotomy specimens is usually sufficient, the subclassification being based on the initial diagnostic biopsy. Marked differences in histology at different sites should be recorded.

2.8. Recurrent Hodgkin's Disease

Progression of Hodgkin's disease of favorable subtype to more ominous subtype has been documented [9, 10, 115, 231–233]. In review of a large number of lymph node biopsies over a period of many years, we have had the opportunity to review rare cases in which progress from favorable to unfavorable subtypes in untreated cases has been obvious. Currently, however, when early diagnosis and treatment is the usual sequence, few cases are observed in the untreated state. Information gained in review of recurrent Hodgkin's disease indicates that the histopathology of the initially diagnosed subtype is maintained when relapse occurs outside of previously irradiated fields, in patients who have not received systemic therapy [234]. In patients who have received systemic chemotherapy, histologic changes in involved tissues at relapse may be more difficult to evaluate, especially if there is a considerable mesenchymal reaction present which could have been related to therapy rather than the basic disease process.

2.9. Special Studies in Hodgkin's Disease

Hodgkin's disease can usually be diagnosed on the basis of well-prepared histologic sections stained with hematoxylin-eosin or Giemsa stains. Reed-Sternberg cells and Reed-Sternberg cell variants are usually easily demonstrated in such sections because of the size of these abnormal cells. We have found several other stains to be helpful in the evaluation of lymph nodes, with special application to Hodgkin's disease. The *methyl green pyronin* stain is used routinely in our preparation of lymph node sections because as a stain for RNA, it allows for easy detection of Reed-Sternberg cells in cases in which few abnormal cells are apparent, as in lymphocyte predominant type, and it aids in the overall assessment for the plasma cell component. As a good stain for mast cells, the methyl green pyronin stain provides another measure for evaluation of the background histology of the lesion in Hodgkin's disease. *Periodic acid Schiff* stained sections are helpful in the delineation of sclerosis in the diagnosis of nodular sclerosing Hodgkin's disease.

Reticulin or elastic stains are useful for evaluating for vascular invasion [211, 212]. Use of a *polarizing lens* for detection of fine collagen band formation is helpful in nodular sclerosing Hodgkin's disease. Electron microscopy, while of interest, does not add directly to the diagnosis of Hodgkin's disease, nor are surface marker studies of lymphocytes from cell suspensions of the involved tissue important as a diagnostic measure at this time. Lymph node imprints, while rarely a basis for diagnosis, in some cases allow for tentative diagnosis at the time of biopsy, when Reed-Sternberg cell variants are observed in the absence of an associated immunoblast proliferation (Figure 32).

We believe that aspiration cytology by itself has no place in the initial diagnosis of Hodgkin's disease. As a tool for assessing extension of disease, it may be helpful, and it may prove valuable as a measure complimenting the usual surgical biopsy [235]. The limitations of the procedure are the same as for imprint preparations in diagnosis; the manner of tissue involvement as demonstrated in biopsy sections is critical in histologic diagnosis and this demonstration is not possible on imprint or aspiration preparations.

3. NON-HODGKIN LYMPHOMAS

The attempts to revise classifications for the non-Hodgkin lymphomas have met with considerably more discussion, alas even contention, than were the modifications proposed for the terminology of Hodgkin's disease. While the biological aspects of Hodgkin's disease remain unclear, a communication mode between pathologists and between pathologists and clinicians has been firmly established for that lesion. For the non-Hodgkin lymphomas, the biological basis for the disease generally has become clear, but the vehicle for transmitting the information between concerned parties has faltered. Classifications based on morphology [11–16] have given way to concepts of function [18], but there has continued to be tremendous difficulty encountered in the attempts to establish an acceptable universal terminology. Current classifications which aim to correlate function and cytology have appeared to be in conflict with traditional classifications. However, mechanisms for neoplastic lymphoid proliferations have been studied by many investigators, and at least some of the more recently proposed categories of lymphomas appear to have clinical relevance.

Prior to the last decade, a lack of understanding of the biology of the lymphomas probably contributed to the difficulty of management, because the heterogeneous groups of lymphomas were not appreciated [236]. Certainly, the recognition that lymphomas of small lymphocytes came in many cell sizes, with different clinical presentations and prognostic implications, is an extremely important factor confirmed in recent publications of concepts of lymphomas as related to functional parameters. Lukes challenged the concept of lesions collectively called lymphosarcoma [237]. The term reticulum cell sarcoma likewise gave way to more meaningful terms [238], as emphasized when Gall in a marvelous essay on the multiplicity of the description of the term 'reticulum cell' [239] sped that term on its way to oblivion insofar as it related to lymphoma classification. The proposal that reticulum cell sarcoma is associated with fibril production by lymphoma cells [240] came under scrutiny when it was found that rare, if any, lymphomas involved fibril production [236].

In reviewing lymphoma classification, it is apparent that the same term does not mean the same lesion to every observer. As Lukes indicated over a decade ago [236], the use of general terms for small cell lymphomas (lymphosarcoma) and large cell lymphoma (reticulum cell sarcoma) included such broad categories of lesions that one author reporting on lymphosarcoma might mean a diffusely disseminated lesion of small lymphocytes with little mitotic activity; another individual using the same term might mean an aggressive tumor with high mitotic rate. That difficulty was not overcome in the refinement of terminology, for 'small' lymphocytes in indolent lesions, seen usually in adults as 'poorly differentiated lymphocytic lymphoma' were categorized together with aggressive lesions observed in a much younger age group (later subclassified by the same author as 'lymphoblastic' [241].

Reports for decades have indicated that lymphomas change from one cell type to another. Before the advent of common use of immunologic techniques for verification of cell types, Lukes proposed that lymphoma, while being monomorphous proliferations of cells, allow for mixtures of cells with different cytologic features which are expressions of one cell type [236]. An instance in which two such apparently different lesions occur, but are variable expressions of one cell type, is the transformation of small lymphocytes into large transformed lymphocytes in the so-called 'Richter's syndrome' [242, 243]. The relationship of lymphomas and leukemias is a matter largely of distribution, leukemia arising in bone marrow and lymphoma arising in lymph nodes or other lymphoid tissue, as a rule. Changes of cellular expression can cause confusion if the pathologist thinks solely in terms of distribution of the lesion, rather than considering the nature of the neoplastic cell as the major factor. The idea that lymphomas and leukemias are artificially separated, and in fact, reflect only different areas of involvement of what we now call the immune system, is an old concept [244].

Follicular lymphomas as B cell neoplasms is a new concept, but the recognitions of lymphomatous follicles goes back decades [14, 244–247]. The early reports of giant follicle hyperplasia proposed a benign state [248, 249]; however, neoplastic transformation of follicle was soon recognized. The prognostic significance of a follicular pattern in lymphoma was recognized in the early reports of the lesion [248, 249], and this has been reaffirmed [17]. Current information, however, indicates different prognoses for follicular lymphomas of *different* cell types [250–255], a factor which behooves the pathologist to pay close attention to the make-up of follicular lesions and to understand that lesions composed mainly of small follicular center cells behave better than do lesions in which small and large cells of the follicular center are intermingled. It has been reported that the degree of nodularity influences survival [254]. Rappaport discounted nodules as neoplastic follicles, but emphasized nodular and diffuse patterns of involvement, presumably for all cell types [16], and reset the stage for evaluating the clinical relevance of nodular lymphoma. Rappaport proposed that distinctions could be made between lymphoma nodules and reactive follicular centers [256], and these guidelines remain useful, but not absolute.

The premise that nodular lymphoma does not represent follicular lymphoma has been proven wrong. Essentially all 'nodular' lymphomas arise from follicular centers and are therefore of B cell type [257-259].

The classifications based on general categories, namely on cell size (lymphosarcoma and reticulum cell sarcoma with follicular lymphoma as a distinct entity), gave way to terminology [16] which retained the concept of cell size, modified the concept of follicularity, claimed its counterpart 'nodularity' and diffuseness as expressions of all cell types, and added the concept of cell differentiation. This terminology gained favor with pathologists and clinicians and became commonly referred to as 'The Rappaport Classification'. It proved useful for definition of subtypes as related to clinical staging and tumor responsiveness to therapy [260]. With the advent of the immunology revolution (or revelations) in the 1960s, the basis of support for new cytologic classifications again were in part dependent on pattern of involvement [18, 19].

To cope with changing terminology several times within one's lifetime is a cumbersome burden for the pathologist and clinician. As recently emphasized, 'nothing is really new, only newly described' [261]. Indeed, 'new' classifications have been appearing periodically since the lymphomas were first recognized, but the proliferation of recently 'new' classifications [18, 19, 262-265] causes great consternation for the pathologist attempting to (1) understand the lesion, and (2) communicate a meaningful interpretation. The problem becomes more complex as the pathologist is confronted with proposed modifications (of the modifications) of the 'new' terminologies [266-268] and the attempts to analyze various terminologies and to offer compromises and alternatives.

The goal of the attempt to find meaningful terminology in the classification of lymphomas is to relate types of disease to clinical management. Disagreement between institution pathologists and referee groups associated with large cooperative oncology groups add to the general aura of confusion in this area [269] and emphasizes the need for a clear working terminology.

While it would be most desirable to have a histologic basis for diagnosis, some investigators indicate that histology alone may not suffice for interpretation of the lymphomas.

Thus traditional classifications based on cell size mainly, with follicular lymphomas as a distinct entity, gave way to lymphoma based on cell size, cell differentiation, and pattern of nodularity and diffuseness. As the proposal that lymphocytes were represented by two major classes (B and T cells) gained strength [270], investigators who had already declared that different lymphomas related to different sites of origin [18, 19] found a firm basis for declaring lymphomas to be lesions of the immune system [270–272]. These new proposals seemed immunologically sound as evaluated by independent observers who correlated histology and surface markers. In one such study, the correlation between histology and surface markers was 97% for nodular lymphomas and 61% for diffuse lesions [273].

The proposal for B and T cell lymphomas has been further strengthened by evidence for homing patterns of B cells to follicular centers [259] and of T cells to specific 'T cell' sites such as skin [275].

Evaluation of disease is difficult to understand completely in the post-therapy state, but interesting patterns of disease have been observed in reviewing autopsy material. Patterns of disease during the course of lymphoma appear to have some consistency with (1) diffuse lesions remaining diffuse, and (2) nodular lymphomas showing change to diffuse patterns and from small cell to large cell type [276].

Three areas of major differences and concerns are apparent in comparing the Lukes' and Rappaport's classifications: (1) 'Histiocytes' of Rappaport are 'transformed lymphocytes' of Lukes and are found in a heterogeneous group of lesions which may have different prognostic significance [277–280]; (2) Poorly differentiated lymphomas of Rappaport are translated to small cleaved follicular center cells (B cells) of Lukes [18] and to convoluted lymphocytic lymphoma, or lymphoblastic lymphoma, of Rappaport [30, 241]; (3) Undifferentiated lymphoma of Rappaport gains prognostic significance in approach to treatment when B and T subtypes are considered. Burkitt [51, 281] and Burkitt-like lesions are the small noncleaved follicular cell lymphomas of Lukes; these are always B cells [282]; lymphoblastic or convoluted cell lymphomas are of T cell type [30, 283].

The incidence of cell types has been recorded, and it is apparent that B cells lesions (follicular center cell lymphomas) are more common than T cell lesions [283], and the lymphomas of the small cleaved cell of the follicular center are the most common type [283, 284].

Lymphomas have diffuse clinical presentations, yet there is some consistency to their pattern of involvement, i.e. convoluted lesions are prominent in the mediastinum; T cell lesions, i.e. Sezary's and mycosis fungoides, involve skin; histiocytic type are often extranodal. Sclerosing lymphomas often involve the retroperitoneum. Burkitt lymphomas often present in abdominal areas and particularly in gonads.

Patterns of involvement have been recognized, despite the problems of classification, but the new immunologic parameters add excitement and education in the struggle for diagnosis. As confusing as the maze of terminologies may seem, attempts of correlation between and translation of, major classifications seems possible [53, 268, 284].

Recently a study of hundreds of cases of lymphomas was conducted to evaluate and compare different classifications [21]. The final goals of the effort has been to produce a universally acceptable classification which is scientifically accurate, usable and reproducible by different observers, and clinically relevant.

Lymphomas currently may be illustrated in several ways: as nodular or follicular versus diffuse lesions [16, 18], as B cell versus T cell lesions [18, 19], as small cells versus large cells [161, 285], as well differentiated and poorly differentiated types [16], as lymphocytic and histiocytic types [16], and as aggressive versus non-aggressive [21]. Keeping in mind that B cell lymphomas may be 'nodular' (follicular) or diffuse, and that T cell lesions are diffuse, the pathology of the non-Hodgkin lymphomas is presented in the classification according to Lukes and Collins [18] and is presented as B cell lesions, T cell lesions, histiocyte (macrophage) lesions or as unclassified. Correlation with Rappaport's and other classifications are stated where it seems pertinent to the discussion. A comparison of some proposed classifications for non-Hodgkin lymphoma is shown in Table 3. Correlation of the Lukes, Rappaport and International Panel classifications are shown in Table 4.

3.1. B Cell Lymphomas

3.1.1. Diffuse Expressions. B cell lymphomas are expressed in either follicular or diffuse form, with a spectrum of patterns between those with discrete well-defined follicles extending throughout the whole lymph node (Figure 33), to complete obliteration of the lymph node architecture by a diffuse process (Figure 34). Descriptions such as 'partially nodular' and 'diffuse lymphoma with residual nodularity' are encountered in the literature. Nodularity is a term which is generally used in discussing the lymphomas, although it is clear that nodular lymphomas are follicular lymphomas; that is, tumors arising in follicular centers. In the attempt to remain consistent in relating the concept of lymphoma pathogenesis, we prefer to use the term follicular where it aptly applies. The expression of lymphomas which arise within follicular centers may be observed in follicular or diffuse form. The diffuse B cell lymphomas presumably arise outside of the follicle and are never expressed in a follicular pattern.

Lymphoma of small B lymphocytes: This lesion has been called well differentiated lymphocytic lymphoma by Rappaport and has been listed as a tumor of low aggressiveness. The lesion is a diffuse process. Although a few such lesions have been reported as 'nodular well differentiated lymphocytic lymphoma' [286], the rarity of the reported nodular cases has prompted some observers to question the interpretation, or to state that the rarity allows for the general classification of the lesion as essentially diffuse [287].

Table 3. Some (current) classifications * of non-Hodgkin's lymphomas.

Rappaport 1966 [256]	Rappaport 1978 [268]	Lukes 1979 [53]	International panel 1980 [21]
Nodular and/or diffuse	Nodular and/or diffuse	U cell (undefined)	Low grade
Lymphocytic WD	Lymphocytic WD	T cell	small lymphocyte
Lymphocytic WD	Lymphocytic PD	small lymphocyte	follicular, small cleaved cell
Mixed L & H	Mixed type	convoluted cell	follicular, small cleaved and large cell
Histiocytic	Histiocytic	cerebriform	
Undifferentiated	Undifferentiated	Sézary/mycosis fungoides	Intermediate grade
	non-Burkitt	lymphoepithelioid	follicular large cell
	Burkitt	immunoblastic sarcoma	diffuse small cleaved cell
	Lymphoblastic convoluted	B cell	diffuse mixed small and large cleaved cell
	and non-convoluted	small lymphocyte	diffuse large cell
		plasmacytic-lymphocytic	High grade
		immunoblastic sarcoma	immunoblastic
		follicular center cell	small non-cleaved
		cleaved, small, large	lymphoblastic
		non-cleaved, small, large	Miscellaneous
		Histiocyte	composite lymphoma
			mycosis fungoides
		Uncertain (Hodgkin's)	
		Unclassifiable (technical)	extramedullary plasmacytoma
			unclassifiable/other

WD = well differentiated;   PD = poorly differentiated;   L & H = lymphocytic and histiocytic
* Modifications and condensations of cited references.

Table 3 (continued)

British 1974 [262]	Dorfman 1974 [263]	WHO 1976 [265]	Lennert [316, p 92]
Grade 1	Follicular lymphomas		Low grade
Follicular	Follicular/diffuse		lymphocytic B and T
follicle cell	small lymphoid		lymphoplasmacytoid
small	mixed small and large		immunocytoma
mixed small, large	lymphoid		plasmacytic
large	large lymphoid		centrocytic
Diffuse	Diffuse	Nodular	centroblastic/centrocytic
lymphocytic PD	small lymphocytic	lymphosarcoma	High grade
lymphocytic intermediate	atypical small	prolymphocytic, cleaved	centroblastic
Grade 2 – diffuse	lymphocytic	non-cleaved	lymphoblastic
lymphocytic	lymphoblastic	Diffuse	B cell type
mixed	convoluted, non-convoluted	lymphosarcoma	T cell type
undifferentiated	large lymphoid	lymphoplasmacytic	unclassified
plasma cell	mixed small, large	prolymphocytic cleaved,	immunoblastic
true histiocyte	histiocytic	non-cleaved	B cell type
unclassified	Burkitt's	lymphoblastic, convoluted	T cell type
	mycosis fungoides	non-convoluted	
	undefined	immunoblastic	
		Burkitt's	

Table 4. Non-Hodgkin's lymphomas. Correlation of classifications.

Rappaport [238]	International panel [21]	Lukes [53]*
	Low grade	
Well differentiated lymphocytic	Small lymphocytic	Small lymphocyte B and T
		Plasmacytic-lymphocytic
Poorly differentiated lymphocytic nodular	Follicular small cleaved cell	Small cleaved follicular center cell
		Lymphoepithelioid
		Cerebriform cell
		Sézary, mycosis fungoides
Mixed nodular	Follicular small cleaved and large cell	Large cleaved follicular center cell
	Intermediate grade	
Histiocytic nodular	Follicular large cell	
Poorly differentiated lymphocytic diffuse	Diffuse small cleaved cell	
Mixed cell type diffuse	Diffuse mixed small and large cell	
Histiocytic diffuse	Diffuse large cell	
	High grade	
Histiocytic, immunoblastic type	Immunoblastic large cell	Immunoblastic sarcoma B and T
Lymphoblastic convoluted and non-convoluted	Lymphoblastic	Convoluted
Burkitt	Small non-cleaved cell	Small non-cleaved Burkitt and
Undifferentiated non-Burkitt		non-Burkitt
	Miscellaneous	

* Lukes includes lymphomas of low aggressiveness and of high aggressiveness.

The feature of diffuseness of this lesion fits with the concept that lymphomas of B cell nature arising outside the follicle are expected to be diffuse.

In involved lymph nodes in lymphoma the basic lymph node architecture is generally obliterated by the tumor. In lymphoma of small lymphocytes, however, complete obliteration of the architecture is exceptional. The lymph sinus system is usually partially maintained, especially the subcapsular and larger radiating sinuses. If the section is prepared in a way to show the hilar area, the proliferation is seen in a leukemia manner extending from the hilus into the intersinusoidal tissues. Larger vascular channels may be retained in their usual position, although the lymphoid proliferation encroaches on the vessel walls, and small lymphocytes may fill sinus and vascular channels. The process in lymph node thus may resemble a leukemic proliferation (Figure 35). This type of lymph node involvement supports the concept that the distinction between lymphoma and leukemia in this process may be artifactual with well differentiated lymphocytic lymphoma and well differentiated leukemia being terms interchangeable with the traditional term 'chronic lymphocytic leukemia.' It has been reported that a small number of cases may involve tissue independently without leukemic manifestations [286]. Yet when carefully evaluated, and when the absolute lymphocyte count is considered, most cases in which lymph node biopsy is interpreted as lymphoma of small B cells are associated with lymphocytosis (over 3500 lymphocytes mm^{-3}) in adults over the age of 60 years.

The lymphoma is composed of small lymphocytes with essentially no nuclear irregularity and scant cytoplasm (Figure 36). On imprints the cytoplasm is clear and granule free in contrast to lymphoma of small T lymphocytes in which azurophilic granules may be observed [288]. The cytoplasm appears to be of low density and PAS negative; surprisingly, occasionally the rim may be intensely pyroninophilic. The nuclei are characterized by dense chromatin and lack of discernible nucleoli. The scant cytoplasm allows for a tumbled appearance of the lymphocytes in tissue section with cell margins overlapping one another, in contrast to the discrete appearance of more cytoplasmic cells, i.e. plasmacytic-lymphocytic proliferations in tissue and normoblasts in bone marrow sections.

Mitoses and phagocytic histiocytes are very few in number in this slowly progressive lesion, and some observers have called this a tumor of accumulation. Plasma cells, if found at all, are in perivascular sites, but they generally are found with great difficulty in this process and reflect the lack of the modulation of the small lymphocyte to the immunoglobulin-producing cell. The scantiness of plasma cells is manifested by hypogammaglobulinemia frequently in association with this tumor [289]. Diagnosis in some instances may be confusing when niduses of larger cells with more abundant cytoplasm and fine nuclear chromatin lead to the erroneous interpretation of reactive follicles. Such niduses of cells are commonly present in lymph nodes in this lymphoma, and have been called *pseudofollicles* [286].

Plasmacytic-lymphocytic lymphoma: This lesion has been called well differentiated lymphocytic lymphoma with immunoglobulin inclusions. This diffuse process is also a lesion of low aggressiveness, and the alteration of the involved lymph nodes is similar to that of lymphomas of small B lymphocytes. Follicular centers are absent, and mitotic activity and phagocytosis are scant. Some sparing of the usual lymph node architecture may occur, especially preservation of the subcapsular sinus, and inspection of the hilus of the lymph node microscopically may reveal the leukemic type of involvement. The cellular detail in this lesion differs from the small cell proliferation of lymphomas of small B lymphocytes in cytoplasmic and nuclear detail (Figure 37). The cells in this tumor are a heterogeneous combination of plasma cells, small lymphocytes and mainly plasmacytoid lymphocytes, the latter with nuclei resembling those of lymphocytes, but eccentric and associated with abundant cytoplasm which is at least moderately pyroniphilic. Periodic acid Schiff positive inclusions may be observed in cytoplasm as Russell bodies [290] or in the nucleus as Dutcher bodies [291]. Immunological markers demonstrate a monoclonal pattern of the cellular proliferation. The prototype for this lesion is macroglobulinemia of Waldenström [292]; however, the lesion may occur as a monoclonal gammopathy expressed as heavy chain abnormalities other than mu (IgM). Serum immunoglobulin values are usually, but not invariably, increased, reflecting the monoclonicity of the tumor in tissue.

In Lukes' schema, the plasmacytic-lymphocytic lymphoma cell occurs as the end result of lymphocyte transformation in tissue [18] and thus functionally is far removed from the small unstimulated B lymphocytes which is presumed to be involved in the majority of cases of lymphoma of small lymphocytes. Certainly, the function of this cell as an active immunoglobulin producer is often associated with hypergammaglobulinemia, in contrast to tumors of small B lymphocytes in which the patient is often hypogammaglobulinemic.

Plasmacytic-lymphocytic lymphomas of the IgM type (Waldenström's) have been associated with amyloidosis in which the paraprotein in staining properties and distribution tends to resemble primary amyloidosis more than the secondary type [293–295].

Unlike lymphomas of small B lymphocytes in which peripheralization of the lesion is expressed as leukemia (chronic lymphocytic leukemia), the peripheral blood in plasmacytic-lymphocytic lymphoma may not be characterized by identifiable tumor cells. It has been shown, however, that idiotype-bearing lymphocytes in the peripheral blood can be demonstrated in cases of Waldenström's macroglobulinemia, as in multiple myeloma [296].

Immunoblastic sarcoma of B cells: As a large cell tumor, this has been included with the histiocytic group of Rappaport. Presumably, this process arises in the interfollicular tissue and is therefore diffuse [18] when the lymph node is completely involved. Partial or focal involvement is common, however, for the lesion may arise in an abnormal immune process [297, 298]. Focal involvement is characterized by monomorphous cellular aggregates which lie in a heterogeneous background of smaller lymphocytes and inflammatory cells, making diagnosis difficult. Cytologically the lesion is composed of large transformed B lymphocytes, with a moderate amount of dense cytoplasm which is intensely pyroninophylic. The cell is easiest to identify when it has the additional plasmacytoid features of eccentric nuclei with chromatin similar to that of the plasma cell. Clues to diagnosis and subclassification of this lesion lie in the recognition that the tumor is composed of (1) cells resembling plasma cells, or (2) a spectrum of cells from distinct plasma cells through large immunoblasts can be recognized (Figure 38). However, the lesion may lack distinctive plasma cell features or plasma cell association in the tissue, making diagnosis more difficult. The cell in any milieu, however, does have dense pyroninophilic cytoplasm and a nucleus which is generally pleomorphic with single and multiple nucleoli which vary in size and which may be huge. The cytoplasm contains immunoglobulin, which is demonstrated with the immunoperoxidase method, and which is often but not invariably monoclonal [82]. The immunoglobulin-producing character of the cell is occasionally emphasized in proliferations in which the transformed cells contain cytoplasmic and nuclear inclusions (Figure 39).

This lesion of large transformed lymphocytes may present a problem in differential diagnosis (1) from the large transformed cell of the follicular center (large noncleaved follicular center cell lymphoma), and (2) from T immunoblastic sarcoma. Also to be distinguished from this tumor are immunoblastic reactions. In distinguishing this process from lymphomas of large noncleaved follicular center cells, the appreciation of the background milieu is important, for immunoblastic sarcoma of B cells is associated with small lymphocytes and plasma cells, while the lymphoma of large non-cleaved follicular center cells has a background population of small and large cleaved and small noncleaved lymphocytes. Distinguishing immunoblasts of T and B cell type depends on appreciation of differences in cytoplasm and nuclear detail. The cytoplasm of T immunoblasts, in contrast to that of the B cell lesion, is pale in routine sections, suggesting low density, and the pyroninophilia of the transformed T cell is generally mild, in contrast to the dense markedly pyroninophilic cytoplasm of the B immunoblast. Nucleoli of B immunoblasts tend to be quite pleomorphic, while the nucleoli of T immunoblasts tend to be small, located close to the nuclear membrane, and resemble typical immunoblasts (Figure 40).

The differentiation of immunoblastic sarcoma of B cells from severe immunoblastic reactions may be difficult. In severe immunoblastic reactions, necrosis is always present in some degree, but necrosis may occur also in immunoblastic sarcoma. In severe immunoblastic reactions, the lymph node architecture is preserved, in areas other than those involved in necrosis, but this may be very difficult to determine in routine sections alone. In immunoblastic sarcoma the interfollicular focal proliferation of neoplastic immunoblasts may be impossible to distinguish from interfollicular reactive proliferations. In such instances, rebiopsy is often necessary, and demonstration of monoclonal cytoplasmic immunoglobulin with the immunoperoxidase method may be helpful in establishing a diagnosis of neoplasia.

Immunoblastic sarcomas of B cells have been found in individuals with abnormal immune systems [297–300] and is the usual lymphoma evolving in patients with immunoblastic lymphadenopathy [297]. Other processes associated with lymphoma, some of which appear to be immunoblastic sarcoma of B cell type (from their reported descriptions), include: immunodeficiency states [301], organ transplantation [302, 303], autoimmune disease including rheumatoid arthritis [304] and Sjögren's syndrome [305, 306].

3.1.2. Follicular Expressions. Lymphomas of follicular center cells may be follicular or diffuse [307]. It is apparent, however, that the more indolent lesions are likely to be follicular lymphomas, while the more actively proliferating cell populations, when first seen, are more often diffuse processes. Thus lymphomas of small cleaved follicular center cells show some degree of nodularity in 75% of the cases, and lymphomas of large cleaved follicular cells are first diagnosed in follicular form in 50% of the cases. Lymphomas of noncleaved follicular center cells representing Burkitt and Burkitt-like lesions and large noncleaved follicular center cell lymphomas appear in a follicular expression infrequently (about 10% show some degree of follicularity at diagnosis).

Lymphomas of small cleaved follicular center cells: These lesions have been included in the category poorly differentiated lymphocytic lymphoma. These lesions have been of low aggressiveness [21], but nevertheless are generally found in Stage IV disease. This phenomenon relates to the indolency of the tumor cells as can be appreciated by observance of the paucity of mitoses and phagocytic activity (Figure 41). The tumor even after years of growth in an individual may retain a discretely nodular form. The nodules are generally easily recognized as lymphomatous because of their cellular homogeneity and lack of distinctive lymphoid mantles. However, varying degrees of follicularity are noted, and the degree of follicularity has been reported to be of prognostic significance [254]. As the nodules become less discrete, there may be an increase in noncleaved cells which can be demonstrated with the methyl green pyronin stain. As the number of noncleaved follicular center cells increase in a tumor, the numbers of mitoses and phagocytes also increase.

The small cleaved follicular center cell varies in size from that of the small lymphocyte to the size of the nucleus of the phagocytic histiocyte. Smaller cells have more dense chromatin, but the cells generally are characterized by irregular nuclear contour, indistinct and usually non-discernible nucleoli and scant cytoplasm. The lack of cytoplasm allows a tumbling effect of the cells in tissue, which helps to distinguish this lesion from small cytoplasmic cell proliferations, namely plasmacytic-lymphocytic proliferations in which the abundant cytoplasm allows for a pattern in which the nuclei are distinct and separate. The tumbling and overlapping effect of cells in this proliferation also aid in the distinction from convoluted cell lymphomas; in convoluted cell lymphomas, the cells, although with irregular nuclear outline and scant cytoplasm, tend to lie definitely separate from one another.

Cytoplasm, when identified at all, is of low density, is not pyroninophilic, and is periodic acid Schiff negative. Cytoplasmic immunoglobulin is not demonstrated by immunoperoxidase methods, although surface markers of cell suspensions prepared from the lymphoma tissue and circulating lymphocytes illustrate the B cell character of the process which generally is reflected in IgG monoclonal immunofluorescent pattern [82, 307].

The architecture of the lymph node is usually completely obliterated by this tumor, whether the tumor is expressed in follicular or in diffuse form. Rarely is a lymph node involved in a leukemic pattern, and uncommonly the process may incompletely involve a reactive node. The distinction between reactive and lymphomatous follicles in the same lymph node section requires careful attention to cellular detail and an appreciation that lymphoma cells of small cleaved follicular center cell type may appear to have exaggerated nuclear clefts and greater nuclear irregularity than normal cells. Involved follicles are either homogeneous in their small irregular-nucleus cell content, or the proportion of small cleaved follicular center cells is distinvtly greater than in the reactive follicles. The distinction of reactive follicles from heterogeneous lymphomatous follicles (mixed nodular lymphoma) remains, for some of us, the most difficult differential problem in lymphoma diagnosis.

The importance of recognizing this proliferation relates to the separation from other lesions which have been called lymphosarcoma or poorly differentiated lymphocytic lymphoma, and which have included a variety of lesions of diverse proliferative activity. Rappaport's poorly differentiated lymphocytic lymphoma (PDLL) as initially reported was a heterogeneous group of lesions, mainly referring to an indolent process which might present in nodular or diffuse form, but which included aggressive lesions, namely the convoluted cell lymphoma [30] curently called lymphoblastic lymphoma by some observers [241]. Clinically the lesions grouped as PDLL represented tumors spanning all age groups from childhood through old age. It has become apparent that the typical poorly differentiated lymphocytic lymphoma or small cleaved follicular center cell lymphoma is extremely unusual in childhood [308] and that the lymphomas of childhood are essentially those of active cellular proliferations.

The nodules of follicular non-Hodgkin lymphoma are rarely discernible on gross examination of the surgical specimen, but the pathologist may suspect a nodular lymphoma, when on gross examination there appears to be extension of nodules into perinodal fat. The tissue on gross examination is moderately firm, but not hard, and the tissue is easily sliced with little resistance to the knife's cutting edge.

Mixed nodular lymphoma of Rappaport is usually included in follicular lymphomas of small cleaved follicular center cell type of Lukes, since Lukes includes no mixed group in his terminology and states that large cells may comprise up to 15–20% of the cellularity in the lymphomas of small cleaved follicular center cell type [18]. Arbitrary figures, which may cause some confusion especially in borderline cases, nevertheless serve as guidelines for correlation in interpretation between observers. Mixed lymphomas, when classified as small cleaved follicular center cell lymphomas by Lukes, are associated with more mitoses and phagocytes than are expected for the typical lymphoma of this cell type. An understanding by the pathologist of the spectrum of cellular patterns is important in his/her attempt to classify lesions in a consistent manner.

Large cleaved follicular center cell lymphoma: This lesion has been included with the histiocyte lymphomas of Rappaport. This lesion represents a lymphomatous proliferation of large, but incompletely transformed, cells of the follicular center (Figure 42). The lesion may present in follicular or diffuse form, but when follicular the lesion has a peculiar pattern that is a clue to the type of cell involved. The follicles, which usually are not discrete, are distributed uniformly throughout the lymph node, as is often apparent in lymphomas of small cleaved follicular center cell type. In the lesion of larger cells, at least some of the follicles merge into one another and characteristically at low magnification present a serpentine or serpiginous pattern (Figure 43). While not pathognomonic for the lesion, we have found the recognition of this pattern very helpful as a clue in subclassification and helpful in the distinction of this cellular proliferation from that of tumors of large lobated T cells [33], which may be confused cytologically with this large B cell lesion.

Cytologically, lymphomas of large cleaved follicular center cells are distinctive. The typical cell is larger than the nucleus of a phagocytic histiocyte in the same section, and the nuclear contour is irregular, but the outlines of the cell are generally softer and less angular than in the small cleaved follicular center cell. The chromatin is typically pale and fine, and nucleoli are indistinct, if even discernible. Cytoplasm varies in quantity, but when present it is of low density. Artifactual ballooning of cytoplasm in formalin-fixed tissue may cause confusion in diagnosis, especially with the large lobated T cell. In formalin-fixed tissues, the cell may appear to contain a wide rim of clear cytoplasm, and in such instances when there is a serpiginous pattern of involvement, the lesion may be confused with metastatic carcinoma in lymph node. The cytoplasm is non-pyrininophilic and is periodic acid Schiff negative. Immunoglobulin is occasionally demonstrated in immunoperoxidase studies of such proliferations [82]. The lesion is seldom homogeneous and is diagnosed when this particular cell type is the predominant poliferation. Other cellular elements of the follicular center are invariably present, and distinction from the lymphoma of large noncleaved follicular center cells may be difficult, especially in less than ideally prepared material. Recognition of the cellular details are the basis for the diagnosis. Mitoses and phagocytic activity are more pronounced in this lesion than in lymphomas of small follicular center cells, and the acitivity probably relates to active proliferation of some large transformed cells which are always present.

This lesion is often associated with sclerosis and the retroperitoneum is a common site of involvement [309]. In reviewing sclerosing lymphomas, we have found that most of the lesions are predominantly or partially composed of large cleaved follicular center cells. It has been suggested that of the 'histiocytic' lymphomas, the large cleaved follicular center cell type is associated with the best prognosis of the group [267, 278]. I wonder if certain features may relate to the better prognosis: (1) the common association of sclerosis, which in itself may be a favorable feature [309]; (2) the finding of large cleaved follicular center cell lymphomas with or without sclerosis as Stage I extranodal disease as a common presentation [309, 310]; (3) the large cleaved follicular center cell itself is probably not very active, as demonstrated by low mitotic activity in the more homogeneous examples of the process, in contrast to the other histiocytic lymphomas, which essentially are neoplasms of large transformed lymphocytes and are actively proliferating.

Small noncleaved follicular center cell lymphoma: This lesion has been called undifferentiated lymphoma. This lesion almost always is diagnosed as a diffuse process, probably because of the high cell turnover rate and the rapid expansion of the tumor with loss of capability to form follicles by the time of tissue diagnosis. A small number of tumors with 'nodular' pattern have been reported and serve to emphasize the B cell nature of this lesion [307, 311].

This lymphoma in its most orderly cytologic form is Burkitt lymphoma [18, 51], described first in a fascinating saga of recognition of the tumor in African children by Denis Burkitt [281]. The Burkitt lymphoma, however, is one of a heterogeneous group of lesions included in the undifferentiated lymphomas of Rappaport. Other lesions in that group included more heterogeneous proliferations of follicular center cells and T cell lymphomas now recognized as convoluted cell or 'lymphoblastic' lymphomas.

In the Lukes' classification, two lesions are included in the category of small noncleaved follicular center cell lymphoma: Burkitt type and non-Burkitt type. The Burkitt type lymphoma is a homogeneous, actually monotonous, proliferation of small transformed lymphocytes with nuclei and cell size and shape showing minimal variation. The nuclear membrane is dense and sharply defined with nucleoli in close proximity to the nuclear membrane or appearing to contact the nuclear membrane when observed with light microscopy. Nucleoli vary in number from cell to cell and are small but distinct. Nuclear chromatin is fine and appears 'open' or 'vesiculated' in formalin-fixed tissue. Cytoplasm is not abundant and is seen as a distinct pyroninophilic margin around the centrally placed round or oval nucleus. The lesion has a cohesive appearance, and cell margins appear adherent to form a mozaic or tile-like appearance of the tumor in tissue (Figure 44). The cytoplasm stains diffusely, but minimally, with the periodic acid Schiff stain, and with immunoperoxidase staining invariably demonstrates a monoclonal IgM cytoplasmic immunoglobulin pattern with no propensity for either light chain. Surface markers reflect the same monoclonicity; serum and urine immunoglobulin values are usually normal.

The non-Burkitt type of small noncleaved follicular center cell lymphoma definitely differs from the Burkitt type in several ways. In pattern involvement, this process involves the lymph node diffusely as does the Burkitt lymphoma. Large areas of necrosis may be observed, however, in contrast to the findings in the Burkitt lymphoma. The cellular proliferation, while composed mainly of small transformed lymphocytes, lacks the monotony of the Burkitt lesion. In this process, the cells, while similar in size, vary considerably in nuclear contour and size of nucleoli. The lesion does not have the cohesive appearance of the Burkitt lesion, and the cellular proliferation may appear much looser than the small noncleaved follicular center cell lymphoma of Burkitt type (Figure 45). This process, in contrast to the Burkitt lesion, spans all age groups, although together with the Burkitt type, the small noncleaved follicular center cell lymphomas may comprise a little less than half of the non-Hodgkin lymphomas of childhood [308]. The starry sky pattern, as in the Burkitt type, is a common but not pathognomonic feature of this tumor. Histochemical and immunochemical features of the tumor are similar to those of the Burkitt lesion. Indeed, the major cytological difference between the two processes is the more loose pattern of the non-Burkitt type and its heterogeneous cell mixture, which suggests a mixed proliferation of small noncleaved and large cleaved follicular center cells.

As described for the Burkitt lymphoma [51], thymus, peripheral lymph nodes, and spleen tend to be spared early in the disease. Bone marrow is spared early, and presentation as acute B cell lymphocytic leukemia is rare [312, 313]. The central nervous system is involved early in the course [51].

The term undifferentiated lymphocytic lymphoma in the Rappaport classification refers to the size of the cell in this process, as compared to the nuclei of phagocytic histiocytes. In this lesion of small noncleaved follicular center cells, the tumor cell size approximates that of the nucleus of the phagocytic histiocyte. Some confusion has occurred with the term noncleaved cell when the term is thought to mean small unstimulated B lymphocytes. The small noncleaved cell of the follicular center is definitely a transformed lymphocyte with marked proliferative capability and is a large cell compared to the small B lymphocyte, i.e. three to four times the size of the small B lymphocytes.

Large noncleaved follicular center cell lymphoma: This tumor, because of its origin in the follicular center, is the lesion we have recognized traditionally as nodular histiocytic lymphoma. The fact that the lesion is observed more in follicular or 'nodular' form than is the lymphoma of small noncleaved follicular center cells suggests that the mitotic or proliferative rate is less than that of the small noncleaved follicular center cell. This premise is supported by cellular kinetic studies [93], in which the proliferation of the cell is reported as less than that of the smaller transformed cell.

In the uncommon instances when this lesion is diagnosed in follicular form, we have found the follicles usually to be discrete. However, we have also observed the lesion with the peculiar serpiginous pattern often associated with lymphomas of large cleaved follicular center cells. Cytologically this large cell (four to five times the size of the small B lymphocyte) has a small rim of moderately pyroninophilic cytoplasm which may demonstrate monoclonal or anomalous staining by the immunoperoxidase method [82] (Figure 46). The tumor is more likely than other non-Hodgkin lymphomas, in our experience, to be associated with marked necrosis, a feature which makes it very difficult to obtain viable cells in suspension for study of surface markers and other functional parameters. The interfollicular tissue, as with the other follicular lymphomas, generally contains small cleaved follicular center cells which are assumed to be neoplastic. As with rapidly proliferating tumors, a starry sky effect may be observed.

The process is usually diffuse and obliterates normal lymph node architecture. Classification of the lesion as a large noncleaved follicular center cell lymphoma, as distinguished from other large cell lymphomas, is based on (1) recognition of the pale cytoplasm as contrasted with that of the small noncleaved follicular center cell and the B immunoblast; (2) the presence of other follicular center cell elements, especially small and large cleaved follicular center cells in the commonly encountered heterogeneous milieu of this lesion; (3) the recognition of some degree of follicularity in some of the lesions, which allows assumption of the follicular center origin of the lymphoma.

Interrelationship of the B cell lymphomas: In discussing the evolution of follicular center cell lymphomas, Lukes and Parker suggest that follicularity proceeds to diffuseness in parallel with expansion of the pool of the actively proliferating cells of the follicular center [307]. Thus, it is to be expected over a period of time that follicular lesions become diffuse, and small indolent cell populations (small cleaved follicular center cells) give way to noncleaved or transformed lymphocytes of the follicular centers [307]. It is apparent in reviewing lymphomas of follicular center type that purely follicular lesions are indeed rare, and in most cases, small cleaved follicular center cells infiltrate into the interfollicular tissue, as well as into the lymph node capsule in many instances. The above authors suggest that the less cohesive quality of the small cleaved cell outside of the follicular center, as contrasted to the same cell type within the follicle, allows for a seeding phenomenon reflected in the high incidence of marrow involvement in follicular center cell lymphomas. It is interesting that lymphomatous involvement of the bone marrow and circulating lymphoma cells in the peripheral blood appear to be mainly of the small cleaved follicular center cell type, despite the nodal expression of the tumor.

In evaluating follicular center cell lymphoma, the pathologist may observe small cleaved follicular center cell lesions initially, with recurrence or extension of the tumor at a later date as a larger cell expression. Likewise, as already indicated, initial presentation may be as a follicular lymphoma, which later is manifested as a diffuse lymphoma of the same cell type. The basically diffuse B cell lymphomas may evolve to more aggressive cell types, i.e. lymphoma of small B lymphocytes may evolve to immunoblastic sarcoma of B cells, and plasmacytic-lymphocytic lymphoma likewise may terminate as immunoblastic sarcoma of B cells. While the former may be explained as 'switch-on' or transformation of small indolent cells to active proliferating cells, the mechanism of the process is not clear. Since both small B lymphocytes and plasmacytic lymphocytes appear and may both terminate in immunoblastic sarcoma, it is suspected that the process represents modulation of cell types, in a sense dedifferentiation of end stage cells to the precursor immunoblasts. Such evidence of changing cell types in an individual suggests that lymphomas of small lympocytes which have already gone through the transformation process and the plasmacytoid cells, as end stage cells, are involved, rather than the unstimulated earliest recognized small B lymphocytes, as described in Lukes' schema of the follicular center cell concept of lymphomas [18].

3.2. T Cell Lymphomas

T cell lymphomas are always diffuse, although a pseudonodular expression has been suggested [314]. The lesions arise in the paracortical zones or interfollicular areas in lymph nodes and in other T cell selective areas, i.e.

skin. Just as the B cell proliferations have certain distinguishing cytological features, the T cell proliferations have a certain theme of similarity in all but the definitely transformed cells or immunoblasts. The common theme in the T cell lesions is nuclear irregularity.

3.2.1. Lymphoma of Small T Lymphocytes. Lymphoma of small T lymphocytes has been identified [307], and like the B cell counterpart of this lesion, the separation of lymphoma and leukemia may be artificial. Some investigators pèrefer to include the small lymphocyte proliferations as one process, with occasional distinctive separation (i.e. as small B cell or small T cell lymphomas without peripheralization). While a sufficient number of cases of lymphoma/leukemia of small T lymphocytes has not been reported to allow for the definite recognition of the cell type on a cytological basis, and to distinguish it readily from small B lymphocyte lymphoma/leukemia, nevertheless certain clues help the pathologist to predict the nature of the lesion. In lymph node sections, several features are very helpful: (1) Residual follicular centers may be observed (Figure 47); (2) Plasma cells may be observed, especially in perivascular location in T cell lymphomas; (3) On a cytological basis, small T lymphocytes do seem to display a slight nuclear irregularity, unlike the smooth nuclear contour observed in small B cells. In imprint preparations, the demonstration of focal acid phosphatase and non-specific esterase activity suggests a T cell proliferation [42–44]. In imprints also, as in circulating cells in peripheral blood smears, it has been suggested that the presence of azurophilic granules indicate a T cell proliferation [288].

The lymph node architecture is generally obliterated in this process, and in the absence of residual follicular centers, the distinction from the small B cell lymphoma may be impossible. It has been suggested that in small T cell proliferations, the lack of 'pseudonodules' is a feature distinguishing the T cell lesion from the B cell counterpart in which pseudonodules are a common feature [141]. Lack of absolute peripheral lymphocytes and the presence of marked splenomegaly are features which may help to distinguish some cases of small T cell lymphoma/leukemia [141].

The approach to the diagnosis of leukemia has not been resolved. Based on the observations of others [315–318], and our own limited experience with T cell proliferations, we believe that the lesions of small T lymphocyte type should be approached in this manner: as a single entity with some variation in manifestations, rather than as distinctive lymphoma implying mainly organ involvement or as leukemia with systemic distribution.

3.2.2. Convoluted Cell Lymphoma. This lesion has been called undifferentiated lymphoma or poorly differentiated lymphocytic lymphoma. Barcos and Lukes [30], (Figures 48–51] described this lymphoma based on the cytologic features of abnormal cells which have (1) nuclear delineations, (2) fine or 'stippled' chromatin, (3) small, if distinguishable, nucleoli, and (4) scant cytoplasm (Figure 48). Other authors subsequently challenged the indication that convolutions of the nuclei are present in all cases and reported the lesion as lymphoblastic lymphoma with and without nuclear convolutions [241]. Subsequently, the literature has included reports using both terminologies for this lesion. The lesion in tissue is distinctive not only on the basis of the features listed above, but also because of other features which become obvious to the pathologist as he/she reviews multiple cases. In addition to the cytologic features noted above, the process involves the lymph node in a peculiar manner. The process is essentially interfollicular, and a clue to the diagnosis, as for other T cell proliferations in lymph node, is the recognition of partial involvement with sparing of reactive follicles. The cells have scant cytoplasm, yet in well-prepared tissue, the proliferation appears somewhat loosely cellular with little overlapping of cellular or nuclear borders (in contrast to the tumbling effect observed in lymphomas of small B cells and lymphomas of small cleaved follicular center cells in tissue sections). The background of the convoluted cell lymphoma, therefore, has a clear appearance, a feature which can be recognized at low magnification. This rapidly proliferating lesion extends readily through the lymph node capsule, and in most biopsies the pericapsular tissue is involved. Additional cytological details include a peculiarity of populations, generally of two cell sizes, a distinctly small cell population (cells at least twice the size of small lymphocytes or 8 μm in tissue sections), and a larger cell population with cells approaching the size of small transformed lymphocytes of B or T cell systems. The proliferation usually is homogeneous other than for cell size, but on occasion, transformed T lymphocytes (or T immunoblasts may be observed in tissue sections). Most subtypes of lymphomas of B and T cell type occur primarily in older individuals. The convoluted cell lymphoma, while occurring in all age groups [319–321], is essentially a disease of young adult males with a male:female ratio of 3:1 when cases including mediastinal involvement are reviewed [30]. The reason for the distinctive male predominance is unclear, but it is a definite phenomenon; the median age in Barcos' paper being 16 years. The tumor is rapidly proliferating, and patients will note rapid growth of lymph nodes or rapidly increasing symptoms of respiratory distress. The lesion often presents first in the mediastinum and may cause death of respiratory failure before diagnosis is made [30]. The patient often presents initially with leukemia with or without mediastinal and/or massive lymph node involvement. However, in those individuals who do not have leukemia initially, leukemic manifestations occur during the course of the disease in a predominant number of cases [30].

The lesion was included in the Rappaport classification under the subgroups of undifferentiated lymphoma or poorly differentiated lymphocytic lymphoma [16, 241]. The process is very different from the usual 'poorly differentiated lymphocytic lymphoma' which appears to represent Lukes' small cleaved follicular center cell lymphoma, an indolent B cell proliferation. In the undifferentiated lymphocytic lymphoma group, this lesion is distinguished by surface markers (easily detected T cell markers with tight sheep red blood cell rosette formation and lack of surface immunoglobulin), lack of cytoplasmic immunoglobulin with the immunoperoxidase method, and characteristic ultrastructure, and focal cytoplasmic acid phosphatase activity in imprint preparations in some cases. Prominent periodic acid Schiff stained inclusions may be observed in some cases, as in some acute lymphocytic leukemias of childhood.

The distinction of convoluted cell lymphomas from T cell acute leukemias has become obscured, and as for small T and B cell proliferations, there has been a trend to report this process as convoluted cell lymphoma/leukemia or lymphoblastic lymphoma/leukemia [321].

This rapidly proliferating lesion, with abundant mitoses and phagocytic histiocytes, may result in a starry sky pattern similar to that of Burkitt's lymphoma. In optimally prepared tissue sections, the distinction between the two lesions is clear, but the methyl green pyronin stain is particularly useful for reviewing routine histological sections and notably for distinguishing the markedly pyroninophilic Burkitt cells and Burkitt-like cells from the non-pyroninophilic, minimally cytoplasmic, convoluted cell lymphoma cells.

3.2.3. Sézary's Syndrome and Mycosis Fungoides. Sézary's syndrome was the first reported T cell disorder [322, 323], and mycosis fungoides was soon afterwards placed in the same category [324]. Historically mycosis fungoides was described first in 1835 as a tumor of the skin [325]; the name of the lesion referred to the character of the lesion rather than to its etiology as an expression of fungal infection. The lesion itself was recognized by the same author thirty years before when the process was included with infections of the skin [326]. Sézary's syndrome was first described in 1938, by Sézary, as a chronic leukemia characterized by generalized erythroderma [327]. Sézary's cells have been reported in mycosis fungoides' lesions for years [328, 329], but the mycosis fungoides and Sézary's syndrome have been regarded as separate entities until recently. In the past decade, the distinction between the two processes has become blurred and both are now considered within the spectrum of cutaneous T cell lymphoma [324, 330–335].

These lesions have always been reported as having a predilection for the skin, with the presumption that the process arises in the skin and then spreads or metastasizes to other organs. Recent kinetic studies indicate that this presumption is not likely and that the abnormal cells originate in sites other than skin, probably in lymph node [335]. The skin has been identified as a homing tissue for T lymphocytes [336], which supports the premise that the abnormal cells migrate or 'home' to the skin and are then expressed as cutaneous lymphoma [337]. The skin has a similar reticular framework as thymic and other thymic-dependent areas, i.e. interdigitating cells with dendritic processes, a feature regarded as pertinent to the observation that T cells 'home' to the skin [336].

The lesions of Sézary's syndrome and mycosis fungoides are characterized by abnormal lymphocytes with bizarre serpentine or cerebriform nuclei and scant cytoplasm (Figures 52 and 53). The Sézary cell generally has the most extreme nuclear irregularity, but in both lesions the changes appear to be part of the spectrum of nuclear irregularity observed in the lymphocytes of T cell lymphomas other than in immunoblasts of T cells. Nuclear irregularity is noted in small T lymphocytes, convoluted T lymphocytes, large lobated T lymphocytes, and lymphocytes of the lymphoepithelioid lymphoma. The pathognomonic feature of mycosis fungoides is the presence of bizarre cells in the skin and other tissues while the pathognomonic feature of Sézary's syndrome is the bizarre cell in the peripheral blood.

Although the two lesions are part of one disease process, the pathologic description is better applied to the processes separately. The skin lesion of mycosis fungoides is most easily recognized in the tumor stage, but the disease involves several patterns of skin involvement which have been described as three distinct stages [338]. The *premycotic,* or erythematous stage, does not allow for a definite interpretation of lymphoma. In this stage, characterized by variable sized erythematous patches on the skin, the superficial dermis is infiltrated by lymphocytes and histiocytes, and characteristic cerebriform cells of mycosis fungoides are not usually recognized. In the *plaque* stage, the infiltration contains large bizarre cerebriform cells as part of a heterogeneous proliferation of lymphocytes, histiocytes, and eosinophils, and involves the epidermis as well as the dermis. In this stage, the epidermis is characterized by Pautrier abscesses which contain mycosis cells. The *tumor* stage presents as a fungating ulcerating skin lesion which extends from epithelial surface through the dermis and into the subcutaneous tissue. The cellular infiltrate, while heterogeneous, contains many bizarre cells, the mycosis cells.

The plaque stage usually develops at the site of a premycotic lesion, but distinct, presumably normal, skin areas may be involved. Tumor nodules usually do develop in sites of previous plaques [339].

Lymph node involvement is common in mycosis fungoides, but other extracutaneous sites are often involved as well [340, 341]. Extracutaneous sites reported to be involved in order of decreasing frequency are: lymph node, lung, spleen, liver, kidney, thyroid, and pancreas [340]. Bone marrow is generally thought to be involved rarely in the early part of the course after diagnosis, but while not obviously involved, microscopic involvement may be frequent [340, 342]. Lymph node enlargement is common in mycosis fungoides and is an ominous sign, although disease is not demonstrated in all biopsies in such cases. Many lymph node biopsies are non-diagnostic for tumor and represent reactive changes, particularly dermatopathic lymphadenitis, a well-recognized histologic entity which occurs in individuals with chronic skin afflictions [343, 344].

The identification of mycosis fungoides in lymph nodes is not difficult when the node is partially or completely involved by the tumor. The problem lies in identifying minimal tumor involvement in lymph nodes characterized generally by dermatopathic lymphadenitis [340, 345–347]. A recent report suggests that lymph nodes in this disease be classified according to involvement or non-involvement, with the extent of involvement considered in the evaluation, the conclusion being that patients with lymph nodes in which there is no detectable mycosis fungoides have a good response to therapy [348]. This approach necessarily means that multiple lymph nodes may have to be sampled in order to reach a conclusion and may be discouraging when the patient has generalized lymphadenopathy in which complete sampling cannot be achieved. The indication that cells with abnormal karyocytes may be identified in specimens from skin and lymph nodes identified as dermatopathic lymphadenitis in the same individual is another parameter for diagnosis [349]. That is, enlarged lymph node not diagnostic for mycosis fungoides may be demonstrated as involved by cytogenetic studies.

These lesions have been called cutaneous T cell lymphomas, but 75% have extracutaneous lesions [340, 342]. In the more recent literature, it has been suggested that in using staging procedures similar to those for Hodgkin's disease and other non-Hodgkin lymphomas, liver is the most frequent site of extracutaneous involvement after lymph node involvement [350, 351].

The abnormal cells of mycosis fungoides and Sézary's syndrome originally were described by electron microscopy [352], but these cells can be readily seen in optimally prepared sections using light microscopy. Sézary cells have been more precisely described with their thin rim of cytoplasm which is finely vacuolated and is PAS positive. The cells have been described as having positive acid phosphatase staining, and we have observed the characteristic focal acid phosphatase activity characteristic of T lymphocytes [42–44] in Sézary cells. Tartrate resistant acid phosphatase has also been reported in Sézary's cells [351].

The abnormal cells of Sézary's syndrome and mycosis fungoides have more recently been further subclassified as 'helper' T cells; that is, they apparently have the ability to promote immunoglobulin synthesis by normal B cells [334, 354–357].

Sézary's syndrome differs from mycosis fungoides in presentation, with the skin in Sézary's syndrome showing a generalized erythroderma, biopsy of which may reveal the abnormal cells. Variable numbers of Sézary cells may be present in the circulation, with some cases being essentially aleukemic. In some cases, white cell counts approximate those of 'chronic' lymphocytic leukemia.

The bizarre cerebriform cell was thought to be a distinctive abnormal cell characteristic for mycosis fungoides and Sézary's syndrome. Unfortunately, this is not the case, for similar cells may be observed in other skin lesions [356, 358, 359]. Special studies may be useful in equivocal cases to determine the neoplastic basis of the process. In lymphocyte transformation studies, which indicated that the abnormal appearing cells were indeed lymphocytes [360], the cytogenetic evaluation revealed cells with abnormal chromosomes. While some observers reported no specific clones of cells [361], others confirmed the clonal nature of Sézary cells [360, 362]. A variety of chromosome abnormalities using Giemsa-banding techniques have been demonstrated in buffy coat preparations and presumably uninvolved lymph nodes [335].

Other studies which may prove useful in the diagnosis of these lesions include cytophotometric measurement of nuclear DNA [363] and evaluation of the electrophoretic mobility of Sézary's cells (which is reported as higher than for other lymphocytes in clonal proliferation [364]).

Staging classification of cutaneous T cell lymphomas has been proposed by the Mycosis Fungoides Cooperative Group [335].

Large and small cells in Sézary's syndrome have been described [361], and the observations are supported by cytogenetic studies showing populations of cells which include diploid, triploid and tetraploid cells [360, 361].

3.2.4. Lymphoepithelioid Cell Lymphoma. Equivalent terms for this lesion were not included in the Rappaport classification, although some observers may have called this lesion mixed lymphocytic-histiocytic type. Other terms currently used for this process include malignant lymphoma with high content of epithelioid histiocytes and 'Lennert's lymphoma' [365–368]. The lesion apparently arises in lymph node, and afflicted individuals usually present with hepatosplenomegaly and often with bone marrow involvement [367, 369]. This process has emerged from a heterogeneous group of lymphoproliferative lesions associated with epithelioid histiocytes described by Lennert and Mestdagh [366], and the lymphoma was later called by Lennert 'lymphoepithelial cell lymphoma' [379]. This process has been included in the Lukes classification of lymphomas, since a small group of cases have been identified in which the lymphocyte components marked as T cells [34, 371].

In this lymphoma, the lymph node architecture is completely obliterated by a diffuse process in which lymphocytes intermingle with epithelioid histiocytes (Figure 54). The pattern of the epithelioid histiocyte proliferation is characteristic and can be recognized at low magnification by light microscopy, as the histiocytes appear to radiate into the center of the lymph node section from the periphery as if following the sinusoidal pattern of the node. The predominant lymphocyte population is expressed in one of two ways. In some cases, the major lymphocyte proliferation is that of a small cell with dense nuclear chromatin, mild but distinct nuclear irregularity, distinct nucleoli, and scant cytoplasm (Figure 55). In other cases, the predominant lymphocyte is a transformed cell or immunoblast with low density cytoplasm as observed in T immunoblasts (Figure 56). Mitoses may be abundant in cases of either cell type. Plasma cells usually are present, but in small numbers, and eosinophils are usually an obvious component. The process generally is similar in other organs and identified as a discrete lesion in bone marrow and in other extranodal sites. Transformation of 'Lennert's lymphoma' to immunoblastic sarcoma has been reported [368, 372].

The problem in interpretation of this process lies in its separation from Hodgkin's disease and from reactive lesions and abnormal immune processes. The process usually is associated with eosinophils and a small component of plasma cells, and differentiation from mixed Hodgkin's disease may present a problem. However, the presence of immunoblasts and the lack of diagnostic Reed-Sternberg cells generally allows exclusion of mixed Hodgkin's disease from the diagnosis. The distinction from lymphocyte predominant Hodgkin's disease may present more of a problem when immunoblasts, plasma cells and eosinophils are absent or in small numbers. In this instance, diagnosis depends on (1) the observer's awareness of the L & H cell as a diagnostic criterion for lymphocyte predominant Hodgkin's disease, and (2) that the L & H cell is absent in lymphoepithelioid cell lymphoma. The most difficult differential diagnosis is the distinction of this non-Hodgkin lymphoma from reactive processes and abnormal immune lesions, the latter causing more difficulties because of their place in the spectrum of neoplastic lymphoproliferative processes. Sarcoidosis and toxoplasmosis have been confused with this lymphoma because of their high epithelioid histiocyte content [373]. Sarcoidosis is unlike this lymphoma in its 'hard' granulomas and its heterogeneous lymphocyte populations. Toxoplasmosis may be confused with this lymphoma when the usual pattern of follicular hyperplasia, the peculiar clustering of epithelioid cells, and the peculiar monocytoid cell component (of toxoplasmosis) are not appreciated [373]. Reactive lesions generally do distort but do not obliterate lymph node architecture. Abnormal immune lesions, such as immunoblastic lymphoadenopathy [297], angioimmunoblastic lymphoadenopathy [374], and similar processes [34], however, do obliterate basic lymph node architecture. In the latter instances, differentiation from lymphoma may be particularly difficult when the pathologist cannot determine whether there is a monomorphous lymphocyte proliferation. The histiocytes are of secondary importance, and their role in T cell proliferations is poorly understood. In this lesion the histologic findings often are equivocal, and multiple biopsies may be necessary before a firm diagnosis can be stated.

3.2.5. Immunoblastic Sarcoma of T Cells. This lesion has been included with histiocytic lymphoma in Rappaport's classification. The large transformed T lymphocyte is recognizable in tissue section by its low density cytoplasm and characteristic immunoblast nucleus [53]. This lymphoma subgroup includes a spectrum of immunoblast forms, however [5, 307]. The usual immunoblastic sarcoma of T cells is composed of large cells with little nuclear pleomorphism. The cytoplasm is distinct in its abundance and pale hue in hematoxylin-eosin, periodic acid Schiff, and methyl green pyronin stained sections. The cell has distinct cell margins with apparent interlocking or adherent cell margins (Figure 57). Mitoses are abundant. Epithelioid histiocytes may also be abundant, and plasma cells and eosinophils are often present. In the background milieu, small T lymphocytes have slightly irregular nuclei similar to the small cell features in lymphocyte predominant Hodgkin's disease and in lymphoepithelioid cell lymphoma. Occasionally convoluted cells are observed in small number.

The lymph node may be involved completely in a diffuse pattern. More often the lymph node is involved partially in T cell areas, i.e. interfollicular, or as an expanding mass with focal involvement of interfollicular tissue in the less affected areas (Figure 58). When the interfollicular tissue is involved in a patchy focal manner, diagnosis of lymphoma may be difficult to establish with certainty, and rebiopsy may be necessary.

This tumor is easily recognized in tissue when the large cell variant is dominant. Its incidence in cases where the diagnosis is confirmed by surface marker studies equals that of B cell immunoblastic sarcoma [283], with fifteen cases of each type reported in a series of 425 cases of lymphoma and leukemia. Several other cases, classified cytologically and by surface marker studies, have been reported [375–377].

Evolution to immunoblastic sarcoma has been reported in mycosis fungoides [378, 379] and in lymphoepithelioid cell lymphoma [368, 372], and is known to occur in the course of lymphoma of small T lymphocytes [283].

3.2.6. Other Lymphomas of T Cell Origin
T-zone lymphoma is a process described by Lennert as a parallel to follicular center cell lymphoma [380]. The process destroys the lymph node architecture, although remnants of follicular centers may be observed. The cellular proliferation or sinusoidal areas are replaced by tumor. The cellular proliferation is heterogeneous with large T lymphocytes and immunoblasts, occasional giant cells, and plasma cells, and is associated with a marked increase in venules. The peculiar cell in this process is a large T cell with low

density cytoplasm and variably irregular nucleus (Figures 59 and 60). The process resembles other T cell lymphomas in description of cell types [381] and tumor distribution, and probably falls within the category of immunoblastic sarcoma as described by Lukes [283].

Large lobated T cell lymphoma has been included with the histiocytic lymphomas because of the large cell size. It has probably been included, based on cytology, in the large cleaved follicular center cell group of the Lukes terminology. This distinctive process involves lymph nodes completely, or partially, as an expanding mass with sparing of some peripheral architecture and follicular centers (Figures 61 and 62). The cellular proliferation is largely that of a large multilobated (nucleus) cell with fine chromatin and indistinct nucleoli. The lobation of the cell is much more extreme than the nuclear irregularity of the large cleaved follicular center cell, and it is associated with small irregular (nucleus) lymphocytes, convoluted lymphocytes, and T immunoblasts. The process involved lymph node as the primary site as in the first (4/4) cases reported with surface markers [33], but extranodal dissemination may be common. Despite the small number of cases initially reported, the lesion is so distinctive it can be separated cytologically from other large cell lymphomas.

3.3. Histiocytic Lymphoma

According to current immunological classifications [18, 19], histiocytic lymphoma refers to tumors of macrophages. This tumor is the rarest of all lymphomas, comprising less than 1% of the lymphoid neoplasms [283]. Lesions, which were studied with surface markers, cytochemical and immunochemical parameters, were characterized by diffuse obliteration of lymph node architecture by cells which cytologically differed markedly from the lymphocytic lymphomas [283]. The cells had round nuclei which lacked the distinctive nuclear membrane and prominant nucleoli of transformed lymphocytes, and the cytoplasm was abundant and pale staining on hematoxylin-eosin stained sections, resembling the cytoplasm of epithelioid and sinus histiocytes. The relationship of this lesion to malignant histiocytosis is not clear. Morphologically the two lesions differ in distribution with the latter presenting in a leukemia pattern in lymph node, spleen, liver and bone marrow (Figure 63), and histiocytic lymphoma presenting as discrete tumor masses (Figure 64). Cytologically the cases differ markedly, with malignant histiocytosis appearing to be a much more pleomorphic proliferation based on comparison with the few cases on histiocytic lymphoma so far identified.

3.4. Other Lymphomas

3.4.1. Sclerosing Lymphoma. Malignant lymphoma associated with sclerosis [309, 310] is usually of B cell type in our experience, and on a cytologic basis, follicular center cell lesions with large cleaved follicular center cells are represented in most cases (Figures 65 and 66). The process tends to be localized (Stage I or II disease), in contrast to non-Hodgkin lymphomas in general, in which less than half are associated with limited or localized disease [310].

We have found sclerosing lymphomas most commonly to be composed of large cleaved follicular center cells, predominantly, or as a mixed proliferation of large and small cleaved follicular center cells. A smaller number of cases were either predominantly of small cleaved follicular center cell type, or were of large noncleaved follicular center cell type. Rarely was a lesion cytologically classified as a T cell lymphoma associated with sclerosis.

3.6.2. Signet Ring Lymphoma. This lesion, as described recently [382, 383], includes a variety of B cell lesions associated with cytoplasmic immunoglobulin. The term 'signet-ring' is derived from the appearance of some cells in which large intracytoplasmic globular structures compress the nuclei against the cell membranes (Figures 67 and 68). The phenomenon was recognized many years ago as a probable expression of protein synthesis [384] and more recently has been described as a distinctive B cell neoplasm, probably of follicular center cell origin [382, 385]. The intracytoplasmic inclusions simulate intracytoplasmic immunoglobulin as 'Russell bodies' and intranuclear immunoglobulin as Dutcher bodies [384], structures described in reactive and neoplastic plasma cell proliferations. Inclusions have been reported in lymphoma/leukemia of small cells (well differentiated lymphocytic leukemia) [385] and in immunoblastic sarcoma [386]. In the more recent reports, the inclusions were observed in a variety of lymphomas including: immunoblastic sarcoma, small cleaved follicular center cell lymphoma, large cleaved follicular center cell lymphoma [382], in lymphomas reported as nodular and diffuse mixed cell type, and nodular and diffuse poorly differentiated lymphocytic type [383].

In instances of severe cellular distortion, the signet ring appearance may cause difficulty in diagnosis between lymphoma and adenocarcinoma, as the name 'signet-ring' implies.

3.4.3. Composite Lymphomas. The term composite lymphoma was proposed for lymphomas in situations in which more than one distinct type of cellular proliferation was present in a single biopsy, or in different biopsies, performed in one individual at the same time [387]. Using this criteria, the incidence of 'composite' lymphomas was frequent (16–35% in some series) [388, 389]. More recent discussion of this phenomenon emphasizes the relationships of the components of lymphocyte subtypes, i.e. T and B cells, and suggested a spectrum of cell forms at different maturation levels, particularly of B cells [390]. In two of ten reported cases in that series, a similarity in immunologic properties was observed to support the premise of a single basic lesion rather than distinctly separate processes in an individual who had Hodgkin's disease co-existing with non-Hodgkin lymphoma.

The indication that two or more expressions of a neoplasm may be observed in one individual seems to be a confirmation of the premise that all lymphomas, both Hodgkin's disease and non-Hodgkin lymphoma, are part of the spectrum of one neoplastic proliferation.

Figures 69 and 70 illustrate a composite lesion in the intestinal tract.

3.5. Extranodal Lymphomas

Non-Hodgkin's lymphoma, unlike Hodgkin's disease, occurs in all organ systems, and a significant number of non-Hodgkin lymphomas (10–25%) are believed to arise in extranodal sites [391–394]. Differential diagnosis from reactive lymphoid proliferations or pseudolymphoma may present a problem, but the key to lymphoma identification lies with an appreciation of a monomorphous cellular infiltrate. In circumscribed lesions composed of single cell types, the diagnosis of lymphoma is not difficult. Unfortunately, many sites of involvement are not distinct or separate from surrounding organ parenchyma and reactive elements. This is especially obvious in lymphomas of the gastrointestinal tract, when a distinctive lymphoma may be difficult to appreciate in the presence of reactive elements, including follicular centers and abundant plasma cells in the superficial mucosa.

The peculiarities of lymphoma at several extranodal sites justify special comment. Extranodal lymphoma must be evaluated from two aspects: (1) the distinction between peculiar reactive proliferations; and (2) the assessment of the extranodal lesion as a primary site of involvement or as an expression of extended disease.

In the gastrointestinal tract, primary lymphomas comprise 2–4% of all malignant neoplasms [395], and the great majority of lymphomas occur in the stomach, small intestine, and colon. The colon appears to be the least involved site of the three. Stomach as the site of most lymphoma is cited in North American series [396–398], while small intestine may have a small edge in reports from western Europe [399, 400]. Primary lymphoma of the lower duodenum and upper jejunum predominate in the Middle East and in poorer population groups [401–410]. The studies on 'Mediterranean lymphoma' and alpha heavy chain disease have been a fascinating episode in the investigation of lymphomas in the past two decades [411–415]. The varying pathology of these small intestinal lymphomas appears to depend largely on the patient's age and circumstances, suggesting that environmental conditions play an important role in the etiology of this group of lymphomas [417]. Gastrointestinal lesions are mainly of B cell type. Almost three-fourths are histiocytic lymphomas in the Rappaport classification [415]. We have found a predominance of large non-cleaved follicular center cell lymphomas and immunoblastic sarcoma of B cells in review of gastrointestinal lymphomas, although other cell types, including small cleaved follicular center cell type, large cleaved follicular center cell type, and plasmacyticlymphocytic type, are observed.

Lymphoma of the thyroid gland also is mainly 'histiocytic' or large non-cleaved follicular center cell type in one series [416]. These lesions emphasize the occurrence of neoplasia in previously immunologically altered tissue, i.e. Hashimoto's disease [416, 417].

Testicular lymphomas also appear to be mainly represented by 'histiocytic' lymphoma [418], as do lymphomas of the central nervous system [419].

Parotid lymphomas appear to be mainly on B cell type, as recorded in the literature [420] and in our review of a large series of parotid lesions [421].

Waldeyer's ring as a site of non-Hodgkin lymphoma merits special attention, mainly because it is rarely involved by Hodgkin's disease, as compared to its involvement in non-Hodgkin lymphoma [422]. The point might be argued that this is hardly extranodal tissue since the area is considered with lymph node sites for staging purposes and involvement of this area is usually an expression of extended disease rather than as a primary site of disease.

While most of the series of extranodal involvement appear to be at least presumptively characterized by B cell proliferation on the basis of histology alone, certain areas might be expected to be prime sites for T cell proliferations, especially the skin and mediastinum. Certainly Sézary's syndrome and mycosis fungoides are cutaneous T cell lymphomas arising in the skin. Cutaneous lymphoid proliferations of B cell type, however, do occur. Involvement of the skin in association with lymph node disease rather than as a primary disease is the more likely role for B cell neoplasms to the skin [423]. Surface marker studies and cytogenetic studies of skin lymphoma, as for lymphoma in other sites, may be useful in establishing a clonal origin for such lesions [424].

3.6. The Pathology of Staging

Staging procedures for non-Hodgkin lymphoma vary with different investigators. It has been suggested, however, that staging of non-Hodgkin lymphoma, in the mode of that for Hodgkin's disease with staging laparotomy, is of limited value [425]. Thorough search, short of laparotomy, is the general rule. Multiple biopsies of accessible lymph nodes and other masses and bone marrow examinations reveal surprising manifestations of the disease. Different cytologic patterns may be encountered at different sites, and the pathologist is asked to determine whether the patient has one or two tumors. As emphasized above, different cytology may mean different expressions of a single cellular proliferation. In this setting of varying cytology in the same patient, special studies to evaluate for clonal origin of the proliferation are of particular interest.

The lymphoma cell type in staging procedures in individual cases is generally predictable, and the tumor of the extended disease tends to mimic that of the initial biopsy, i.e. when small cleaved follicular center cell lymphoma nodular is diagnosed in the initial cervical biopsy, the same cytology is to be expected in a groin lymph node taken around the same time. Bearing in mind, however, that lymphocyte transformation is not a static phenomenon, it should not be surprising to encounter different cellular expressions at different sites. Nodular lymphomas become diffuse; small cleaved follicular center cell proliferations give way to lesions of large transformed cells.

Bone marrow involvement is a common phenomenon in non-Hodgkin lymphoma, an obvious reason for the avoidance of staging laparotomy in this disease [426]. Bone marrow involvement at the time of lymphoma diagnosis varies from 36 to 41% [427–429]; up to 76% of patients with 'poorly differentiated' lymphocytic lymphoma have bone marrow involvement at the time of diagnosis, in contrast to 30% of the patients with histiocyte lymphoma [430]. Support for the proposal that the small lymphocyte seeds to bone marrow and other sites in lymphoma comes with the observation of apparent poorly differentiated lymphocytic lymphoma involving the bone marrow in a patient whose lymph node diagnosis is 'histiocytic lymphoma.' Conversely, when lymphomas of small cleaved follicular center cell type (poorly differentiated lymphocytic lymphoma) 'switch-on,' the expression of the disease in the bone marrow may be that of a large transformed lymphocyte.

4. PRELYMPHOMATOUS LESIONS

Persistent reactive lymphadenopathy has been reported as leading to malignant lymphoma [431], and it has been suggested that abnormal immune lesions set the stage for lymphoma, especially immunoblastic sarcoma [297, 298]. Immunoblastic sarcoma has been observed to occur in individuals with a variety of lesions including: autoimmune disease [304, 305], other lymphomas, even nodular lymphoma [53], organ transplantation [302, 303], and alpha heavy chain disease [432]. Of particular interest has been the observations that immunoblastic sarcoma occurs in a number of individuals with the peculiar abnormal immune process *immunoblastic lymphadenopathy* (IBL) or the closely related process *angioimmunoblastic lymphadenopathy* (AILD), as well as in a spectrum of lesions which are similar to, but not identical to, immunoblastic lymphadenopathy [297, 298]. Lennert's 'lesion', which includes a definite T cell lymphoma (lymphoepithelioid lymphoma), and abnormal immune lesions which are not clearly defined, has been reported to progress to immunoblastic sarcoma [372]. We have observed this phenomenon of T cell immunoblastic sarcoma arising in peculiar lesions which resemble but are not identical to IBL, mainly differing in their abundant cellularity in contrast to the hypocellular process of IBL.

In our original series of immunoblastic lymphadenopathy (IBL), we noted immunoblastic sarcoma during the course of the IBL or at autopsy in 3/32 cases [297]. Since that publication we have noted a similar percentage of immunoblastic sarcoma arising in a larger series of IBL and IBL-like lesions [433]. Angioimmunoblastic (AILD), has been associated with approximately 30% incidence of immunoblastic sarcoma, according to one large series [298]. Since the original publications of IBL and AILD, other cases of each group have been reported as evolving to immunoblastic sarcoma.

4.1. Immunoblastic Lymphadenopathy

Immunoblastic lymphadenopathy is a clinicopathologic entity which reflects an abnormal immune system. The precise nature of the lesion is not clear, although abnormal immunoregulatory mechanisms seem to be implicated. There appears to be a decrease in circulating T cell populations [434, 435] and the question arises of a deficiency in suppressor T cells [436, 437]. The lesion was proposed first as a B cell proliferation because of the constant finding of hypergammaglobulinemia [297], but it has become apparent that the problem of pathogenesis is more complex than simple excessive proliferation or depression of cell types. The process is definitely associated with hypersensitivity states in some individuals, with drugs being incriminated as a triggering mechanism in about a third of the cases in the original series [297]. Chemical and environmental factors probably also may be inciting factors, the implication being gleaned from review of the histories of patients whose tissues have been reviewed in consultation.

Afflicted individuals present with sudden onset of lymphadenopathy, usually diffuse, with enlarged liver and spleen, often with bone marrow lesions [438], or with other manifestations as in skin [439] and lung [440]. Instances of involvement of peripheral nerve [441] and kidney [442] have been reported also. The lymphadenopathy is associated often with a maculopapular rash and with lymphoma symptoms, including chills, fever, night sweats, weight loss, and pruritis. Laboratory studies reveal protein abnormalities, mainly hypergammaglobulinemia. Anemia is usually present and often of the Coombs positive type. The leukocyte count varies but lymphopenia and/or eosinophilia may be profound. The course is generally progressive, leading to demise within two years in most cases [297]. Some success in obtaining remissions has been achieved with immunosuppressive therapy [297, 442].

The histopathology includes a diffuse involvement of lymph nodes with a triad of distinctive features including: (1) marked proliferation and arborization of small caliber vessels; (2) a mixed cellular proliferation which includes many immunoblasts and few small lymphocytes. Plasma cells and eosinophils, as well as reactive histiocytes, are present in variable numbers; (3) hypocellular, lymphopenic tissue with a background of amorphous interstitial material (Figures 71 and 72).

We have excluded, from the diagnosis, cases in which the lymph nodes are partially involved in singly or regionally affected lymph nodes, since the significance of partial involvement is unclear. Rebiopsy is suggested in such cases if the lymphadenopathy persists. We have observed immunoblastic sarcoma occurring in instances of partial lymph node involvement (Figure 73); but have, on the other hand, observed courses up to ten years with no recurrence in instances in which there was regional involvement characterized by partial lymph node involvement (Figure 74). In general, we have considered reactive follicles to be against the diagnosis of IBL in lymph node and to reflect a reactive state. Hypercellularity is considered to be definitely not characteristic of IBL, a lesion recognized by its lymphopenic tissue appearance. Nevertheless, cellular lesions with marked arborization of proliferating small vessels in a diffusely involved node are singled out as abnormal immune processes; some of these lesions have progressed to IBS in our experience.

The character of the interstitial amorphous material in IBL has been studied by electron microscopy, and is considered by some to represent cellular debris [444]. Amyloid has been documented in IBL [445].

4.2. Angioimmunoblastic Lymphadenopathy

This is a lesion within the spectrum of abnormal immune lesions, and some cases appear to be identical histologically and clinically to those identified as IBL. Anioimmunoblastic lymphadenopathy, while histologically similar to IBL, includes two other features: (1) abortive or abnormal follicles, and (2) very dense intensely positive periodic acid Schiff stained material, unlike the pale amorphous lightly PAS stained material described in IBL [374].

Since IBL and AILD were first described, a number of reports have appeared in the literature [435–453] and have added to the accumulating knowledge of the pathogenesis of these peculiar lesions, including confirmation of drugs as apparent triggering mechanisms [454–456] and demonstration of chromosome abnormalities [457].

Table 5. Hodgkin's disease in children – data from different case series 0 to 15 years.

Case Series (ref)	Lymphocyte Predominant		Mixed Cellularity		Lymphocyte Depletion		Nodular Sclerosis		Unclassified	
	M	F	M	F	M	F	M	F	M	F
Butler [474] 1969 M.D. Anderson Hosp.	6		20		7		23		—	—
Strum [470] 1970 Univ. Chicago	6	0	1	0	0	0	22	2	3	1
Burn [460] 1971 Manchester, England	9	7	21	5	3	2	4	2	—	—
East Africa	23	3	39	3	39	12	11	3	—	—
Schnitzer [472] 1973 Univ. Michigan	14	3	10	4	0	2	15	12	—	—
Lukes [475] 1974 Univ. S. California	13	0	2	2	0	0	11	10	1	1
Garwicz [476] 1974 Sweden	1	2	11	2	0	0	4	3	—	—
Norris [471] 1974 Mayo Clinic	17	5	19	5	1	2	43	24	0	0
Jenkin [477] 1975 Princess Margeret Hosp.	15		30		0		62		2	
Smith [480] Royal Marsten Hosp.	13		9		2		32		—	
Sobrinho-Simoes [478] Portugal 1978	4		18		3		10		—	
Armata [479] 1978 Poland	5		22		5		0		2	
Summary:	LP = 146 19%		MCT = 221 28%		LD = 78 10%		NSHD = 329 42%		Uncl = 10 1%	

5. LYMPHOMAS IN CHILDHOOD

5.1. Hodgkin's Disease

Hodgkin's disease in children is similar to the disease in adults as regards histopathology, course, and response to therapy, with some exceptions. This is in contrast to non-Hodgkin lymphoma in children, in which tumors are essentially diffuse lesions with a high degree of aggressiveness (while there is a heterogeneous group of non-Hodgkin lymphoma in adults). All the subtypes of Hodgkin's disease are encountered in children, but geography and particularly socioeconomic status are important factors [458]. In the 'western' countries, namely the United States and Europe, lymphocyte depletion Hodgkin's disease is seldom observed in the pediatric age group, while this subtype is common in children in Latin America and some eastern countries [459–461]. In Table II, data in Burn's study indicate the high incidence of lymphocyte depletion Hodgkin's disease in East African Children.

That two of the original seven cases described by Thomas Hodgkin's were in children bears little relationship to the incidence of the disease in children compared to that in adults, at this time. (In 1926 it was noted that one of the two children in Hodgkin's series had had tuberculosis rather than neoplasia [462]). While lymphomas account for about 8% of childhood cancer deaths [463], Hodgkin's disease accounts for less than 2% of the deaths, and non-Hodgkin lymphoma accounts for 6% [464]. In the United States the incidence of Hodgkin's disease in children is cited as 8.3% to 10.8% of the total number of cases of Hodgkin's disease in the general population [182, 196]. A higher percentage of children are reported in series of cases of Hodgkin's disease in 'non-western' countries. Some of the data for those countries include: in India 25% of the Hodgkin's disease cases are in children [459]; in Peru 40% of the Hodgkin's cases are in children [465]; children are afflicted in 36% of the cases in Uganda [466]; children comprise 23% of the cases in Lebanon [467]. It has been noted that the percentage of childhood Hodgkin's disease in the United States was greater several decades ago and was similar to that currently cited for non-western countries [459].

Early childhood Hodgkin's disease differs from the disease in the older age group in the major subtype observed (Tables 5 and 6) [460–484] and in a lower death rate in the younger group. The male:female ratio of afflicted individuals is greater in the early childhood group (Table 4) and decreases after the first decade. It has been suggested that the differences in the first decade, as compared to older children, reflect changing disease, actually an adult of the disease, occurring in the prepubescent period. The increase in number of girls afflicted after age 10 years and the increase in incidence of nodular sclerosing type in the 10–15 age group fit with the data of

Table 6. Hodgkin's disease in children – stage of disease at diagnosis – 0–15 years.

Case series	No. of cases	Stage I	Stage II	Stage III	Stage IV
Pitcock [473] 1959	44	17	12	15	0
Teillet [484] 1968	70	22	20	20	8
Strum [470] 1970	16	7	5	4	0
Santiago [483] 1970	32	3	8	13	7
Shah [481] 1979	57	20	21	6	10
Norris [482] 1972	113	30	50	24	9
Schnitzer [472] 1973	55	16	22	12	5
Norris [471] 1974	116	33	50	24	9
Jenkin [477] 1975	109	29	36	28	16
Smith [480] 1977	87	12	51	17	7*
Armata [479] 1978	34	7	14	10	3
Total	733 (100%)	196 (27%)	289 (39%)	173 (24%)	74 (10%)

* Stage IIIB and IV listed together.

Keller [182] which show a high incidence of nodular sclerosing Hodgkin's disease in young women. The sharp rise in mortality rate after age 11 years is similar in data from 1972 to 1974 [468] and in data from 1950 to 1959 [469]. The reason for the sharp rise in mortality rate after the first decade is not clear.

5.1.1. Histopathology. A review of several series of Hodgkin's disease in children is summarized in Tables 5 and 6. Data in individual series suggest predominance of particular subtypes of Hodgkin's disease in children, notably nodular sclerosing type in the report of Strum and Rappaport [470]. In composite data from several series, mixed cellularity type is the major subtype in the first decade and comprises 37% of the cases. Nodular sclerosing type comprised 29% in this group; lymphocyte predominant type occurred in 18%, lymphocyte depletion type in 12%, and unclassified lesions were reported in 4%.

In the pediatric age group generally, from zero to fifteen years, nodular sclerosis in the predominant type at 42%, mixed cellularity type comprises 28%, lymphocyte predominant type is reported in 19% of the cases, lymphocyte depletion is 10%, and unclassified Hodgkin's disease is reported in 1% (Table 5). In one series of 116 cases, 20 of 67 cases of nodular sclerosing Hodgkin's disease were reported as cellular phase [471]. This seems to be a large number of such cases as compared to this type in adults, and the significance of the large number of cases is not clear. There was no difference in age of patients, clinical findings, or survival in this group, as compared to the 47 individuals whose biopsies showed classical nodular sclerosis in section.

Strum and Rappaport [470] and Schnitzer [472] reported a high tissue lymphocyte content and low Reed-Sternberg cell component in their cases. Strum and Rappaport noted the worse courses in those individuals whose biopsy sections showed less than 80% lymphocyte content.

Lymphocyte depletion Hodgkin's disease is unusual in the western countries, and it appears to be a lesion which afflicted persons in less affluent societies. As indicated above, the incidence of Hodgkin's disease in children, in comparison to the afflicted population in general, has decreased in the recent decades. The reason for this decrease is not clear. Until the advent of modern therapeutic approaches, Hodgkin's disease is children was considered a progressive, and rapidly fatal lesion. Current modes of therapy are a major factor in decreasing the mortality rate of this neoplasm, but therapy does not explain the possible changing pattern of disease. In reviewing earlier literature, it is interesting that children with Hodgkin's disease had lesions classified as paragranuloma and granuloma mainly, with a paucity of cases of the lesion of Hodgkin's sarcoma. Pitcock *et al.* reported no sarcoma in a representative series of 46 cases [473]. The paucity of Hodgkin's sarcoma, as classified previously according to Jackson and Parker, may compare with the paucity of lymphocyte depletion Hodgkin's disease reported in certain populations at this time.

5.1.2. Stage of disease. Table 6 summarizes stage of Hodgkin's disease in children who have undergone laparatomy. Most of the children were found to have Stage II disease (39%), 27% were in Stage I, 24% were in Stage III, and 10% were in Stage IV.

5.1.3. Presentation. As for Hodgkin's disease generally, most lesions present in children as asymptomatic cervical lymph node enlargement.

Summary of Hodgkin's disease in the pediatric age group.
1. Mixed cellularity type is the major lesion in the first decade.
2. Nodular sclerosing type is the predominant form in the general group of afflicted children (0–15 years).
3. Lymphocyte depletion type is uncommon in children in the United States and in Europe and is more common in lower socioeconomic societies.
4. Childhood Hodgkin's comprises a small percentage of the total number of cases of Hodgkin's disease in the United States. In Latin American and eastern countries, the percentage of children with Hodgkin's disease is much higher.
5. The high male:female ratio in Hodgkin's disease in the first decade drops to compare with that of adult Hodgkin's disease after the tenth year.
6. There is a marked increase in the mortality rate after the 11th year, but overall remission and survival is good in terms of modern therapeutic approaches.

Table 7. Non-Hodgkin's lymphoma in children – histopathologic types – Rappaport.

Case series	Cases #	LB Conv	WDLL	PDLL	Undiffer.** B	Undiffer.** non-B	Histiocytic	Mixed	Unclass.***	N	D
Sullivan [490] 1973	51	–	0	0	13	30	8	0	9	0	51
Gladstein [491] 1974	32	–	0	11	0	4	14 (1N)	3	0	1	31
Garwicz [476] 1974	27	–	6	7	5		9 (1N)	0	0	1	26
Pinkel [492] 1975	64	–	0	2 (N)	2	41	19	0	0	2	62
Murphy [489] 1975	31	–	0	5	0	9	10	0	5	2	29
Landbag [493] 1975	27	–	0	13	0	5	8	0	0	1	26
Lemerle [494] 1975	190	0	0	126	10	0	63	0	0	1	189
Hausner [495] 1977	30	10	1	0	0	6	4	0	0	0	30
Jaffe [496] 1977	30	–	0	9	0	7	10	2	1	0	30
Brecher [497] 1978	31	–	0	19	0	3	7	1	0	0	31
Woolner [485] 1978	104	–	8 (3N)*	49 (8N)*	0	18 (1n)*	20	3 (2N)*	0	14*	90
Lukes [308] ----	114	56	0	0	13	33	12 (6B IBS) (4T IBS) (2 Hist)	0	0	±1	113
Total #	731	66	15	201	43	156	184	9	15	23* → 11	708 → 720

* On reclassification 12/14 were reclassified as diffuse. Some cases also reclassified as lymphoblastic.
** undifferentiated; *** unclassified; N = nodular; D = diffuse.
LB = lymphoblastic; Conv = convoluted;

5.2. Non-Hodgkin Lymphoma in Children

The terminology maze that has long surrounded the non-Hodgkin lymphomas has caused particular confusion in the understanding of lymphoproliferative lesions in children because of the use of terms which include heterogeneous groups of tumors. It has become apparent that certain lymphomas are observed in children, and that some types are essentially not observed in this age group. Unfortunately, the non-Hodgkin lymphomas in children are diffuse, aggressive lesions with high turnover rates and a propensity to disseminate early and widely. A growing awareness of the immunologic parameters of subtypes of lymphomas and leukemias has resulted in an appreciation of differences in course of disease immunologic subtype, especially in regards to the acute leukemias.

It has become obvious in the last decade that the tumors of lymphoid tissue in children are essentially diffuse (Table 7) and that lesions previously classified as nodular on re-inspection do not fit within the current of lesions having origin within follicular centers [485]. The variety of nodular lymphoma in childhood has been emphasized in a review of 318 cases of childhood lymphoma in which nodular lesions comprised 8/318 or 2.5% of the cases [486]. In the older literature, cases of poorly differentiated lymphocytic lymphoma are cited, but current reviews suggest that such terminology is not appropriate for childhood lymphoma because of the implication of indolent disease with low mitotic rate and a common 'nodular' pattern; Lukes and Collins, Bryne [487]. Aggressive B and T cell proliferations are represented in childhood lymphomas. The so-called undifferentiated lymphoma of Rappaport is now recognized as a B cell tumor (Burkitt or non-Burkitt type) or small transformed cell of the follicular center according to Lukes. T cell or null cell lesions, with the emphasis on T cell orientation, were also included formerly as undifferentiated or poorly differentiated lymphocytic lymphomas, and now are recognized as part of a clinicopathologic process called convoluted cell lymphoma by Barcos and Lukes [30] and lymphoblastic lymphoma by Nathwani and others [241]. Some uathors indicate a T cell lesion for all cases studied [488].

In the literature pertaining to lymphomas in children, lymphocytic lymphoma outnumbers histiocytic lymphomas 3:1 [489] to 9:1 [308]. The term 'histiocytic' is well recognized currently as including a variety of B and T cell lymphomas, and histiocytic proliferations as macrophage processes. In a retrospective study of 114 cases, 11 of 114 lesions would fall into the so-called histiocytic group and include immunoblastic sarcoma of B cells, immunoblastic sarcoma of T cells and two cases of 'true' histiocytic lymphoma, Lukes [308].

Table 7 [308, 489–497] summarizes various types of lymphomas recorded in several series, using the Rappaport classification. Note the paucity of lesions called well differentiated lymphocytic and the few cases called mixed lymphocytic-histiocytic type, 2% and 1% respectively. Of the 731 cases compiled from these several series, 481 or 66% were lymphocytic and 184 or 32% were histiocytic with a few unclassified lesions (2%), the mixed type is included with the lymphocytic lymphomas.

Few reports have been published so far that deal specifically with the immunologic classification specifically in children. In a series by Williams of 65 lymphomas/leukemias studied with surface markers, 49 were lymphoid in character, 36 being acute lymphocytic leukemia of childhood and 13 were non-Hodgkin lymphomas [498]. Kersey, in a series of 69 cases, reported 10 T-cell lesions and 7 B-cell lesions, all of which were lymphomas, and 52 cases which were essentially leukemias [488].

The Lukes' classification is primarily a morphologic one which has been supported by data from a large number of cases [283]. Thus in reviewing the 114 cases of lymphomas in children we believe there is merit in classifying the lesions as particular subtypes implying immunologic relationships. It seems obvious from these data and those compiled in Table 6 that certain lymphomas are usual in the pediatric age group and that others are rare.

If it is agreed that the term poorly differentiated lymphocytic lymphoma is a poor term for childhood lymphomas (and implies the small cleaved follicular center cell) and that essentially childhood lesions properly fall within the small non-cleaved follicular center cell group or are T or null cell lesions, we find that children are rarely afflicted with three of the four follicular center cell types. Children do not develop lymphomas of small B or T cell type, nor of plasmacytic-lymphocytic type, nor of Sézary's/mycosis fungoides types, nor of lymphocytic lymphoma associated with a high content of epithelioid histiocytes.

The bulk of childhood lymphomas, in summary, are of aggressive B or T cell types, often present as abdominal or mediastinal masses and have a propensity for dissemination to the central nervous system [308]. A small number of B and T immunoblastic proliferations are expected in series of childhood lymphoma cases, and histiocytic lymphomas of 'true histiocyte' or macrophage type are rare.

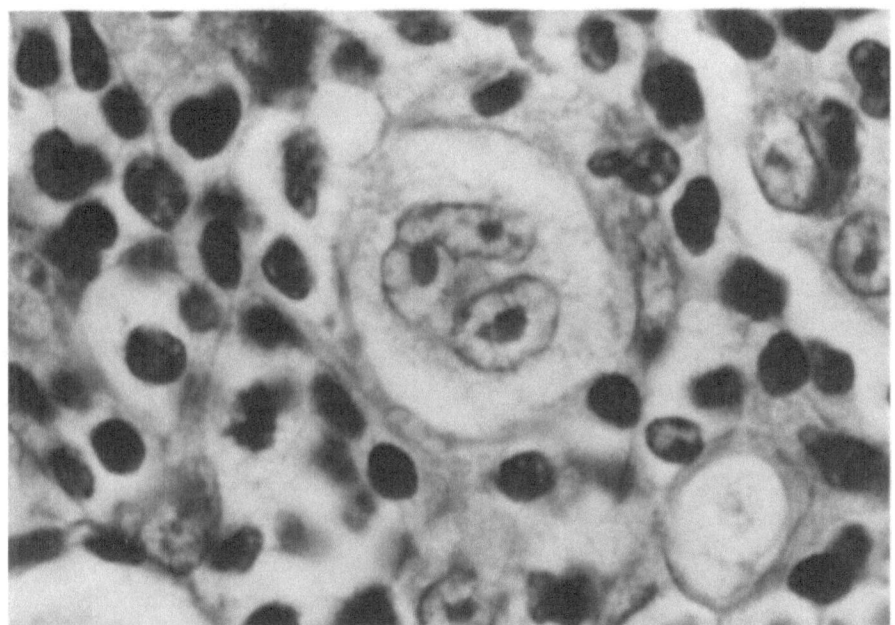

Figure 1. Diagnostic Reed-Sternberg cell with large inclusion-like nucleoli (H & ×1180).

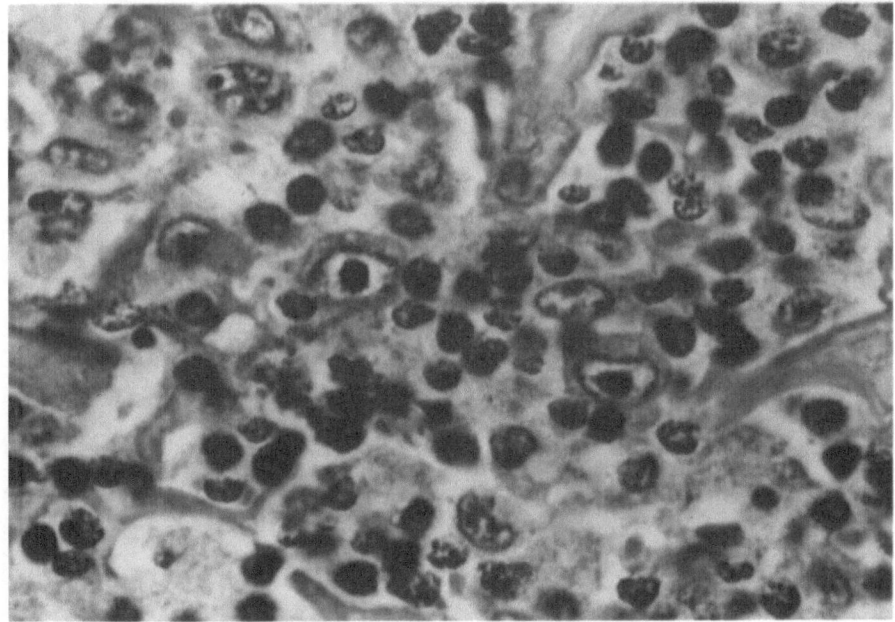

Figure 2. Reed-Sternberg cell variant, mononuclear type (H & E ×910).

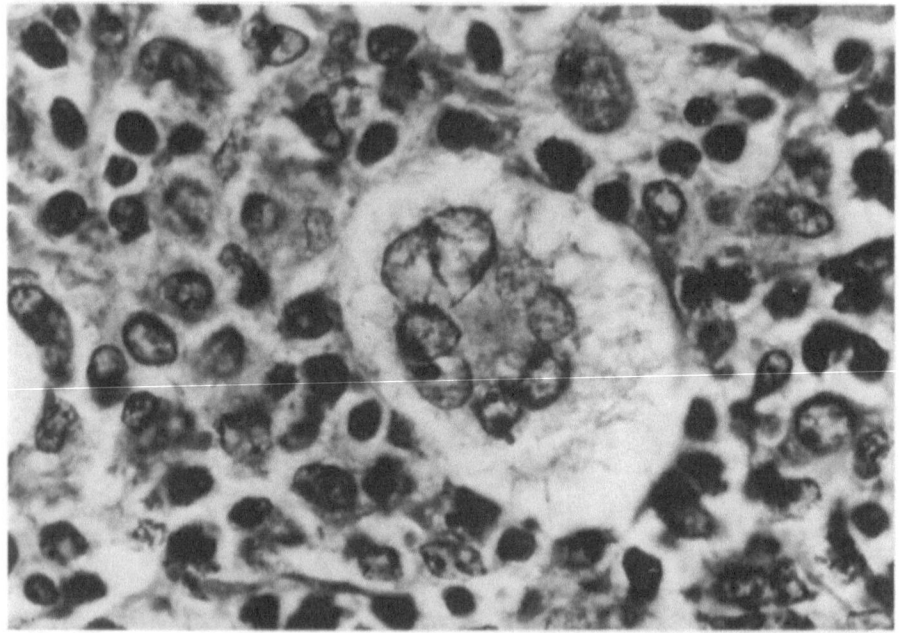

Figure 3. Reed-Sternberg cell variant, lacunar cell type (H & E ×2170).

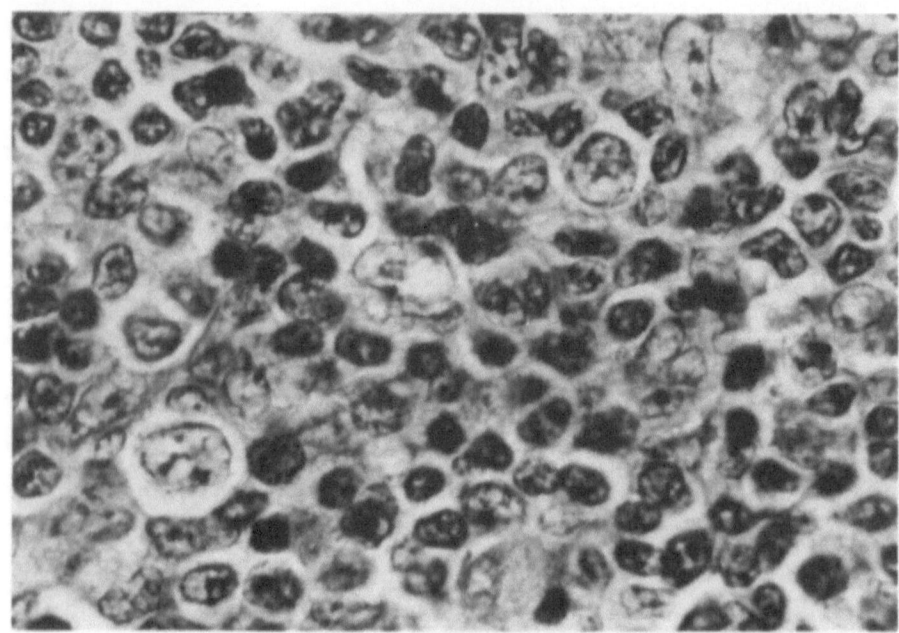

Figure 4. Reed-Sternberg cell variant, L & H cell (H & E ×910).

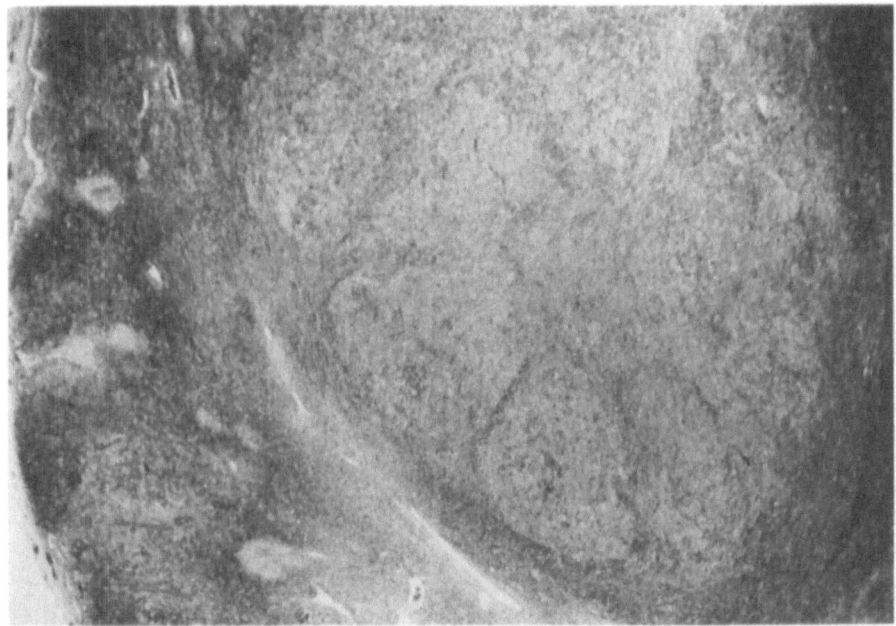

Figure 5. Lymphocyte predominant Hodgkin's disease with incomplete lymph node involvement (H & E ×22.72).

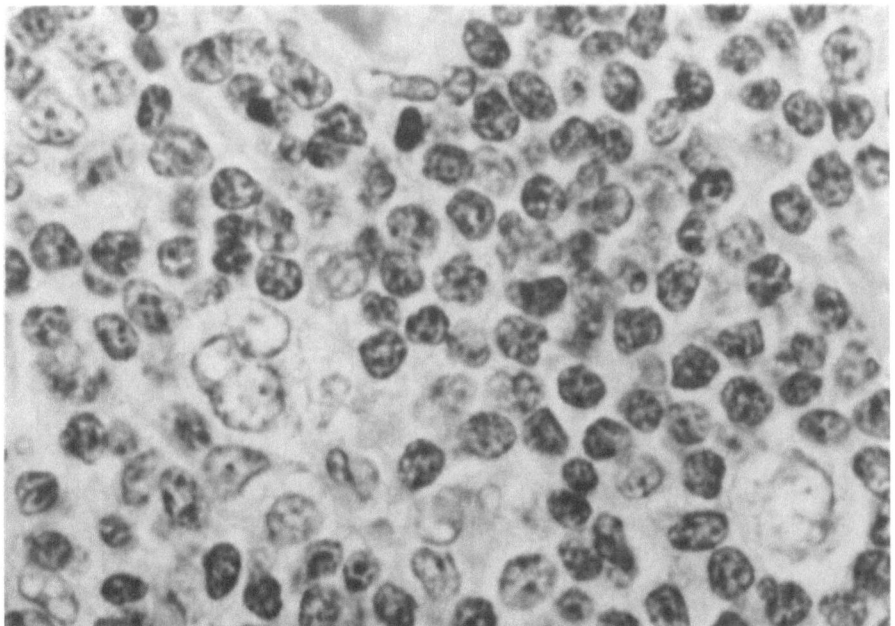

Figure 6. L & H cell in lymphocyte predominant Hodgkin's disease, nodular type (H & H cell in lymphocyte predominant Hodgkin's disease, nodular type (H & E ×910).

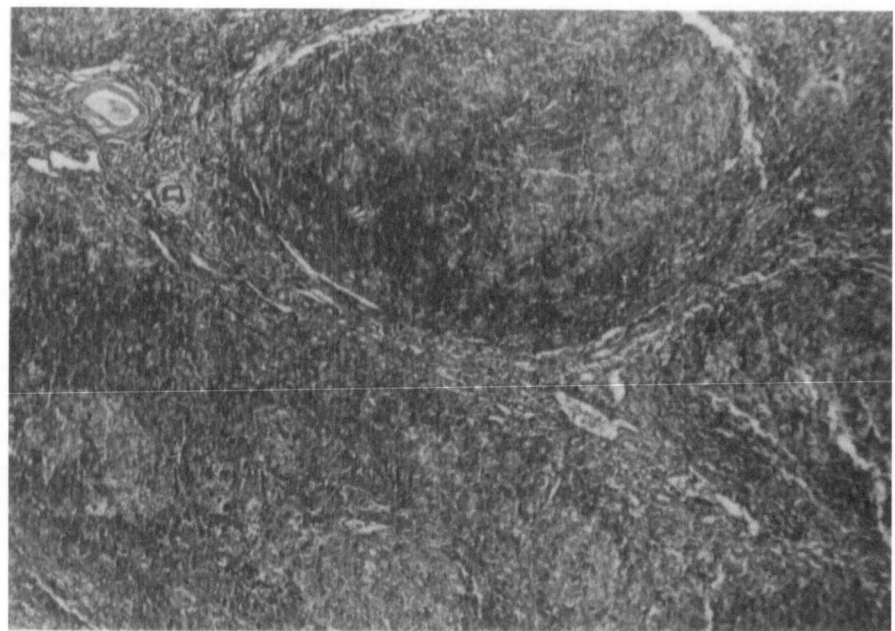

Figure 7. Lymphocyte predominant Hodgkin's disease with ill-defined nodules (H & E ×22.75).

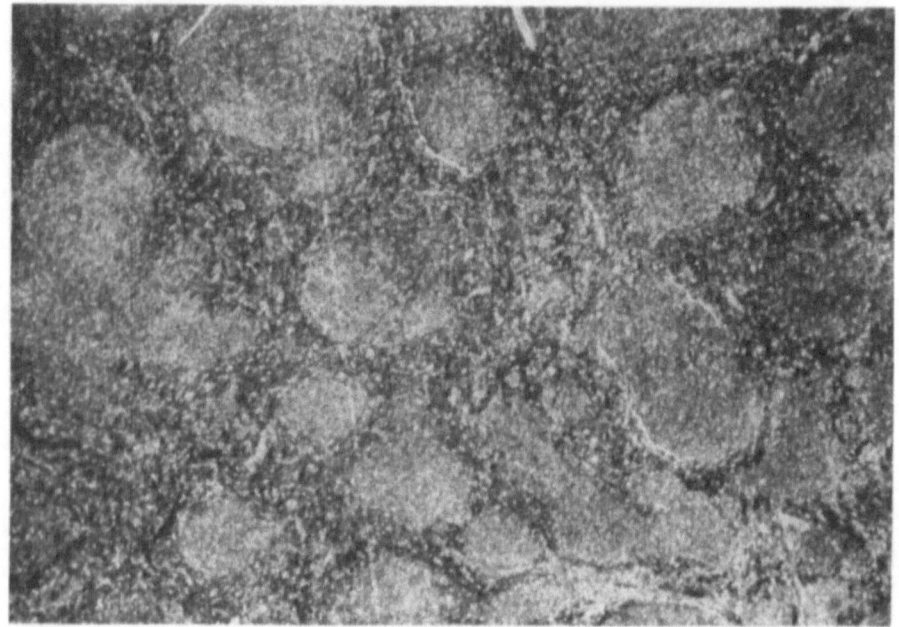

Figure 8. Non-Hodgkin's lymphoma, follicular type with discrete nodules representing neoplastic follicular centers (H & E ×22.75).

Figure 9. Lymphocyte predominant Hodgkin's disease, diffuse pattern (H & E ×22.95).

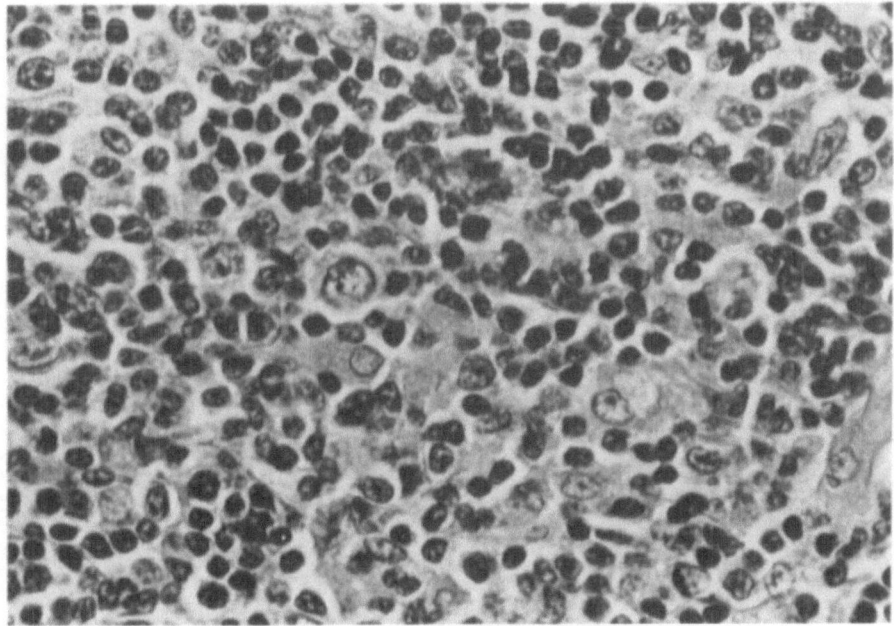

Figure 10. Lymphocyte predominant Hodgkin's disease, diffuse pattern. L & H cell (center) and reactive histiocyte (Lower left) in a background of small lymphocytes (H & E ×365).

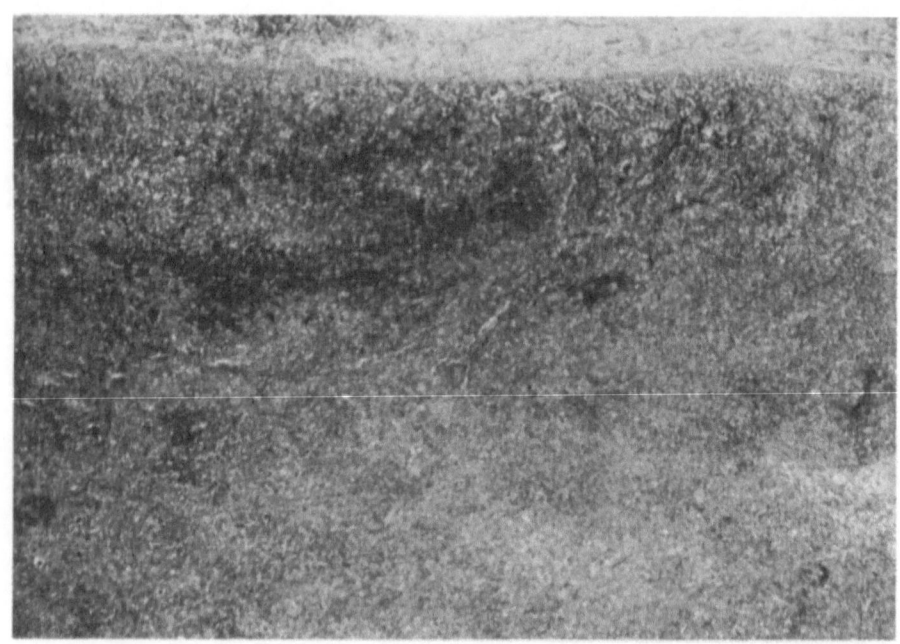

Figure 11. Hodgkin's disease, diffuse type (H & E ×22.75).

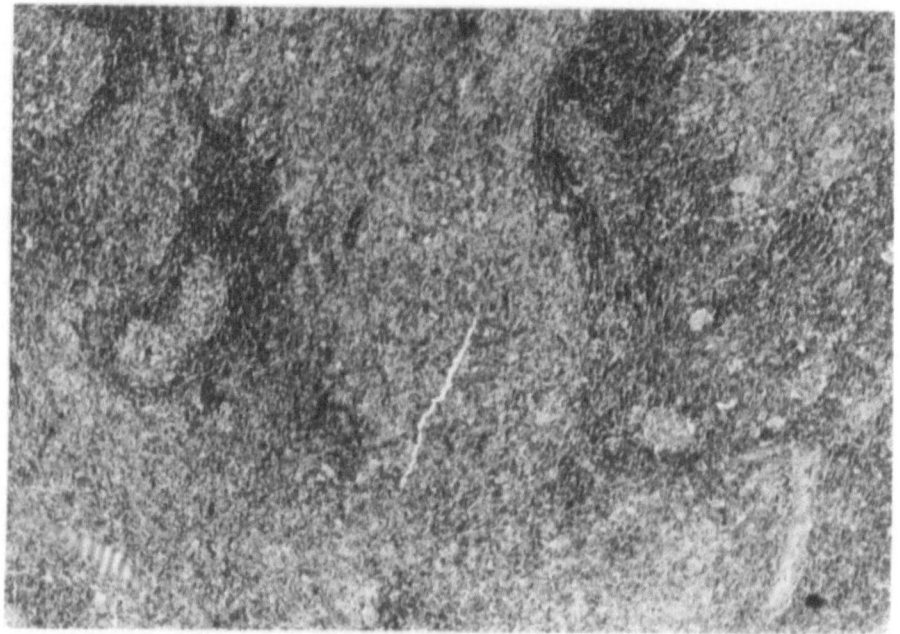

Figure 12. Mixed cellularity Hodgkin's disease, focal, with expansion of interfollicular tissue (H & E ×22.75).

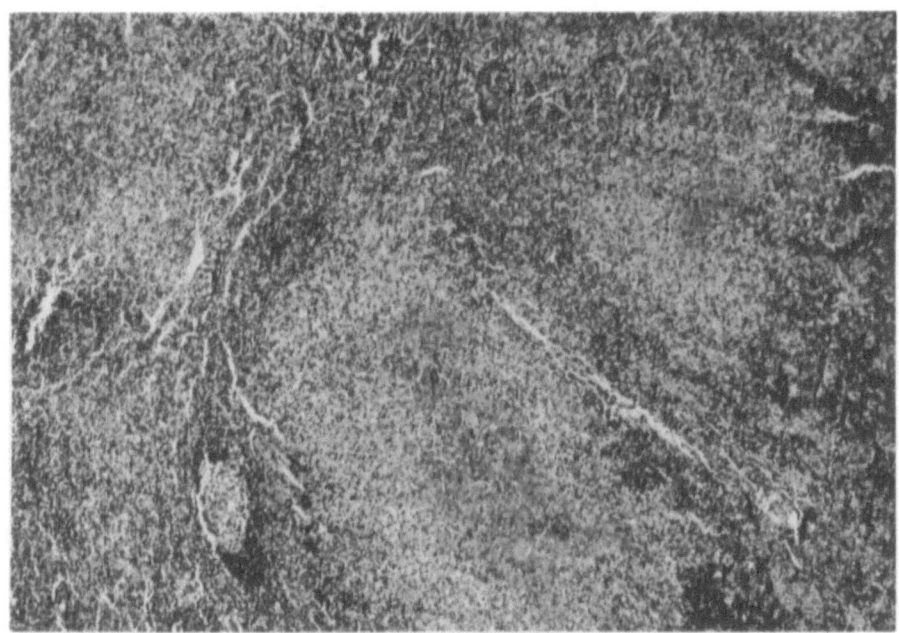

Figure 13. Eosinophilic necrosis in mixed cellularity Hodgkin's disease (H & E ×22.75).

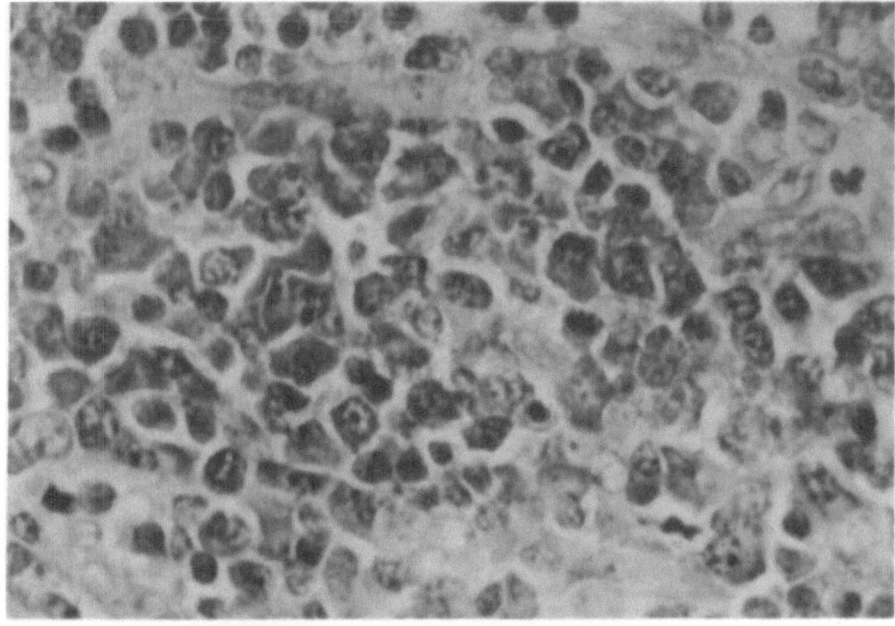

Figure 14. Plasma cell focus as part of a dramatic plasma cell proliferation in a case of mixed cellularity Hodgkin's disease (H & E ×910).

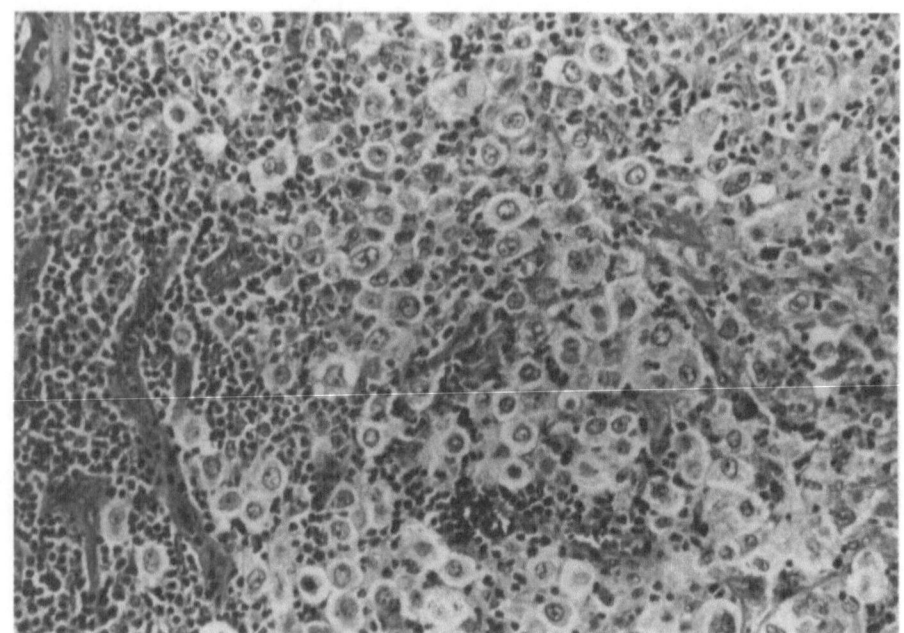

Figure 15. 'Cellular phase' of nodular sclerosing Hodgkin's disease not associated with collagen
bands (H & E ×145).

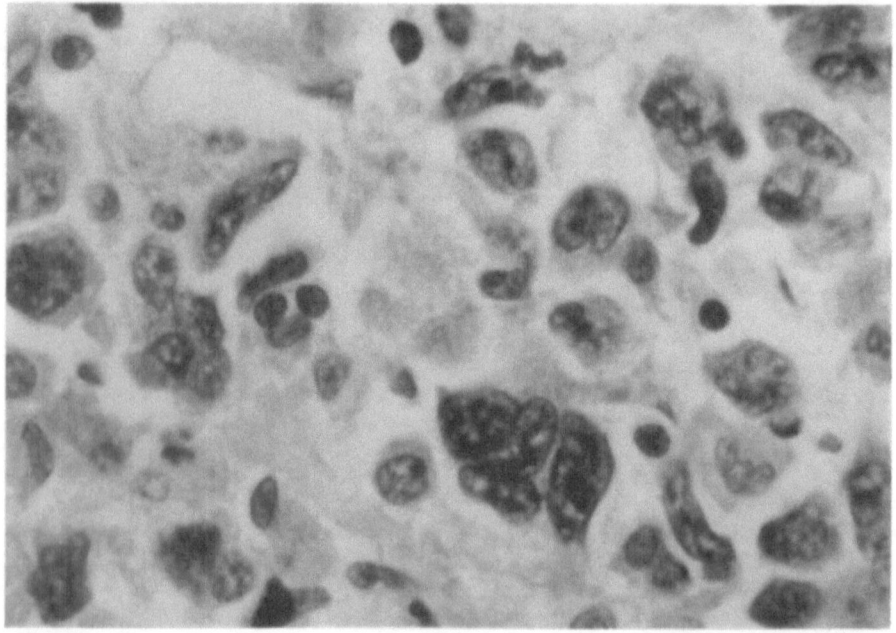

Figure 16. Pleomorphic Reed-Sternberg cell in lymphocyte depletion Hodgkin's disease (H & E
×580).

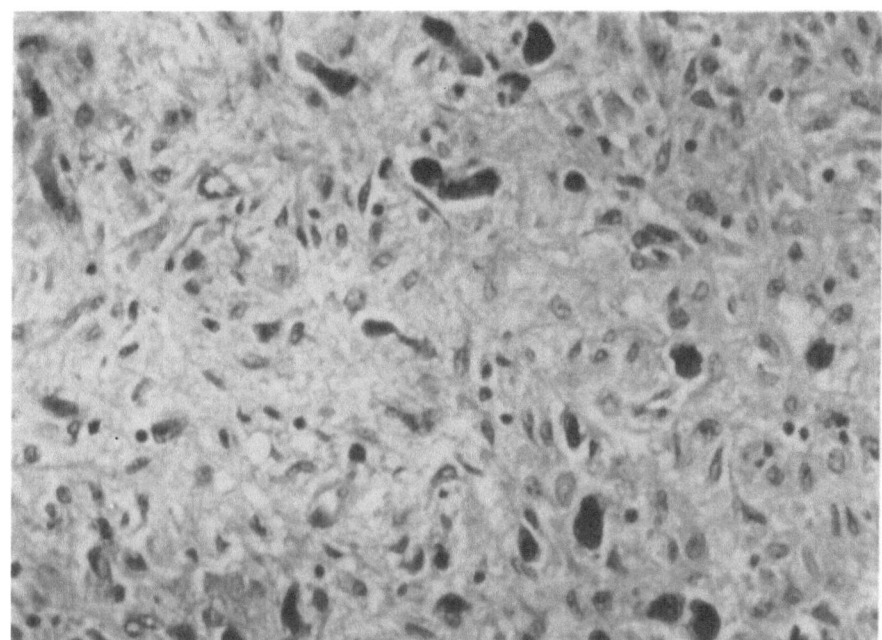

Figure 17. Hodgkin's disease, lymphocyte depletion diffuse fibrosis type (H & E ×365).

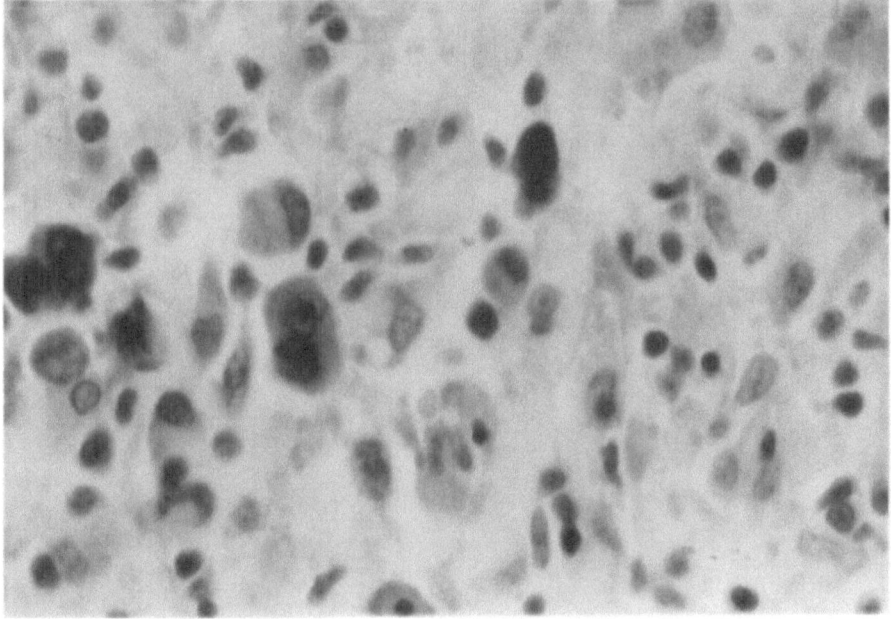

Figure 18. Reed-Sternberg cell in lymphocyte depletion Hodgkin's disease, diffuse fibrosis type (methyl green pyronin ×365).

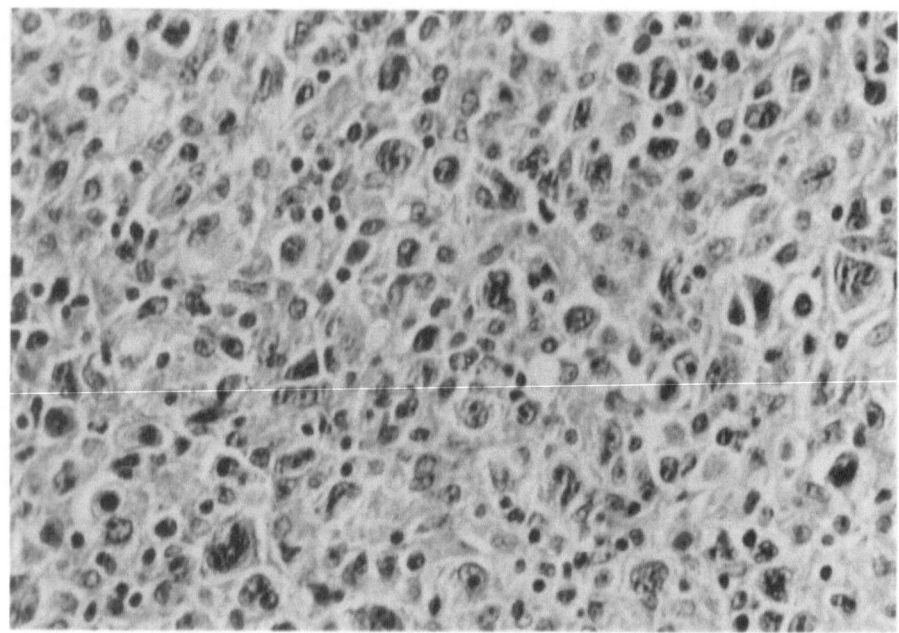

Figure 19. Hodgkin's disease, Lymphocyte depletion, reticular type (H & E ×145).

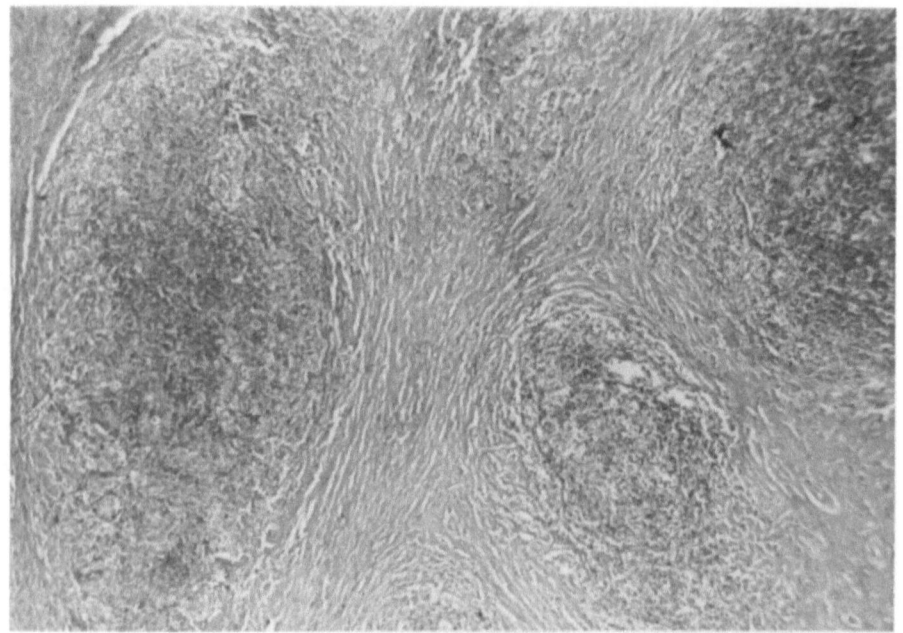

Figure 20. Nodular sclerosing Hodgkin's disease. Sclerosing collagen bands surround cellular nodules containing lacunar cells (H & E ×22.75).

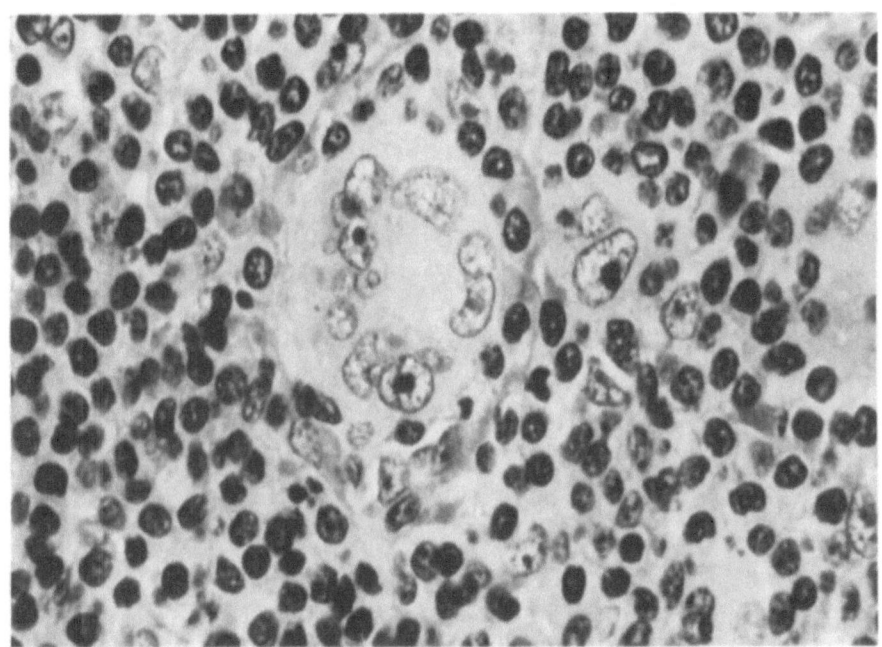

Figure 21. Lacunar cellin B-5 fixed tissue (H & E ×580).

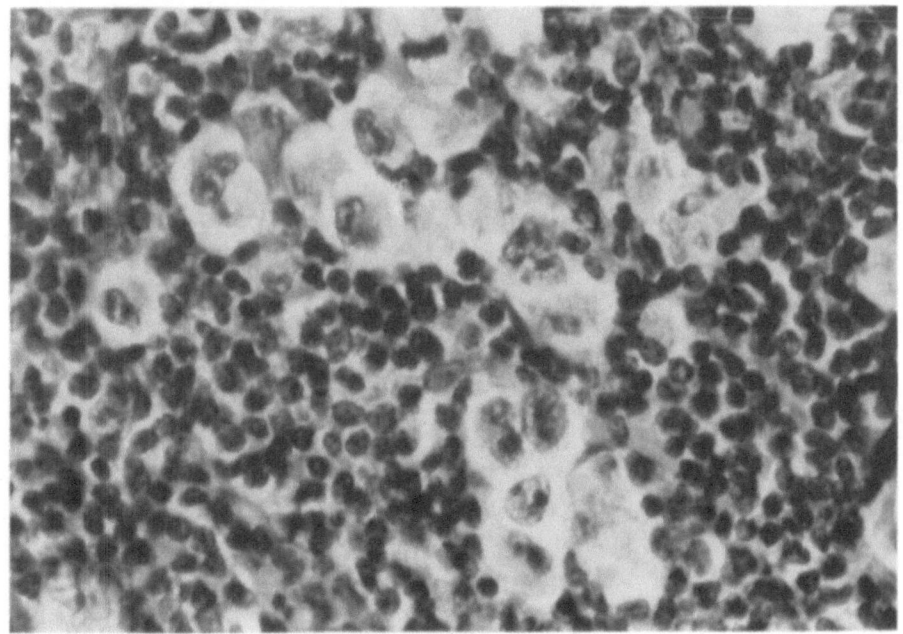

Figure 22. Lacunar cells in formalin fixed tissue (H & E ×365).

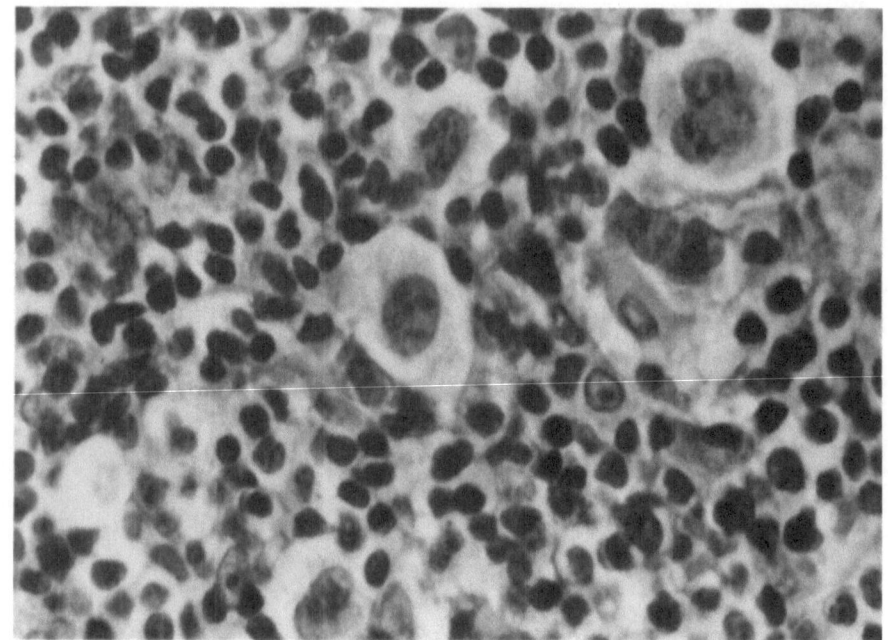

Figure 23. Lacunar cell, mononuclear type resembling a T immunoblast (H & E ×580).

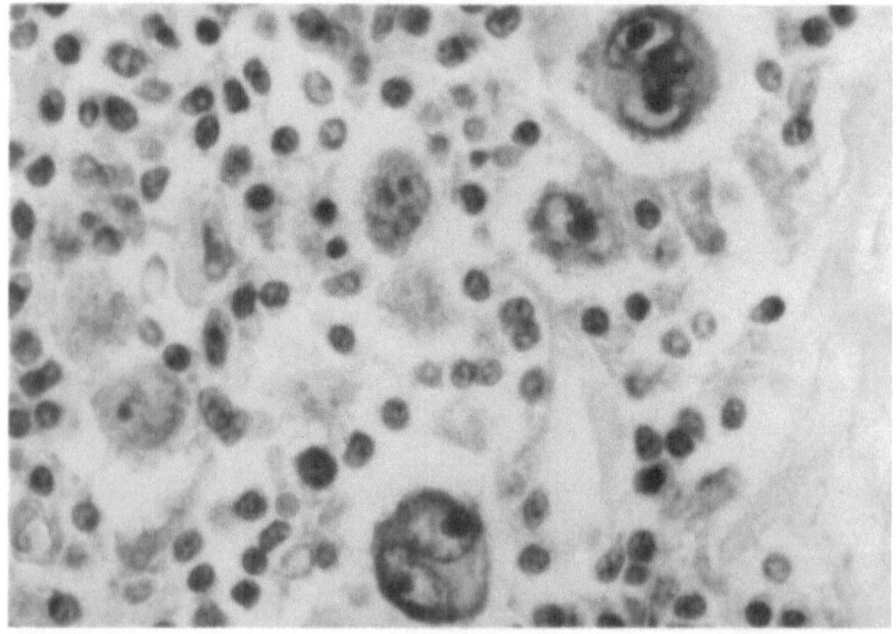

Figure 24. Lacunar cell as a diagnostic Reed-Sternberg cell (upper right) (H & E ×365).

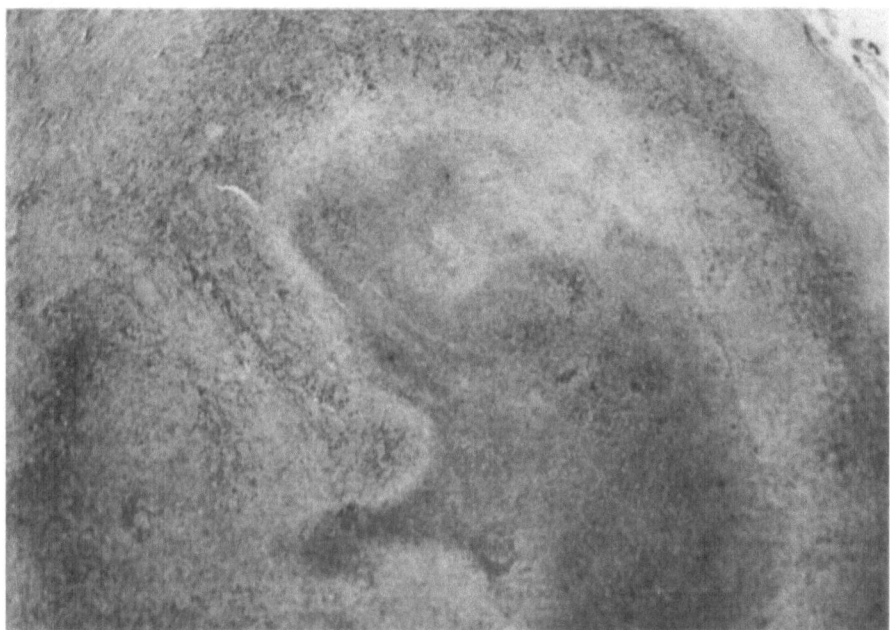

Figure 25. Extensive necrosis in nodular sclerosing Hodgkin's disease (H & E ×22.95).

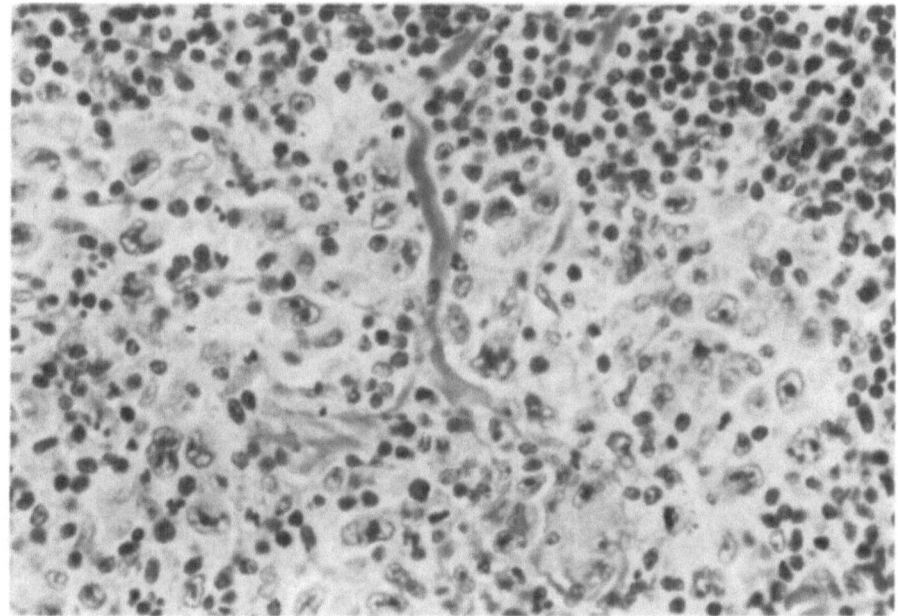

Figure 26. Hypocellular area with abnormal cells in nodular sclerosing Hodgkin's disease (H & E ×145).

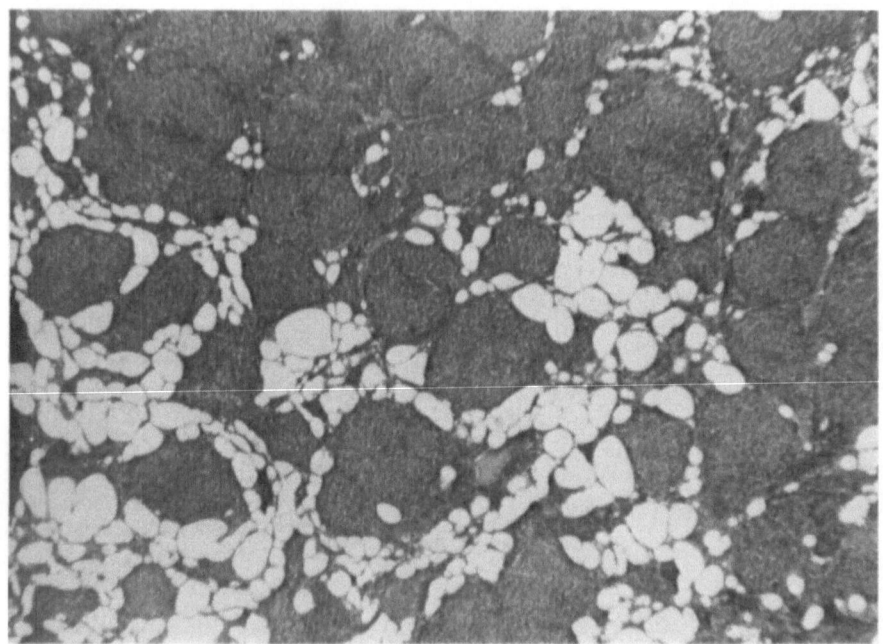

Figure 27. Post-lymphangiogram effect in abdominal lymph node (H & E ×22.75).

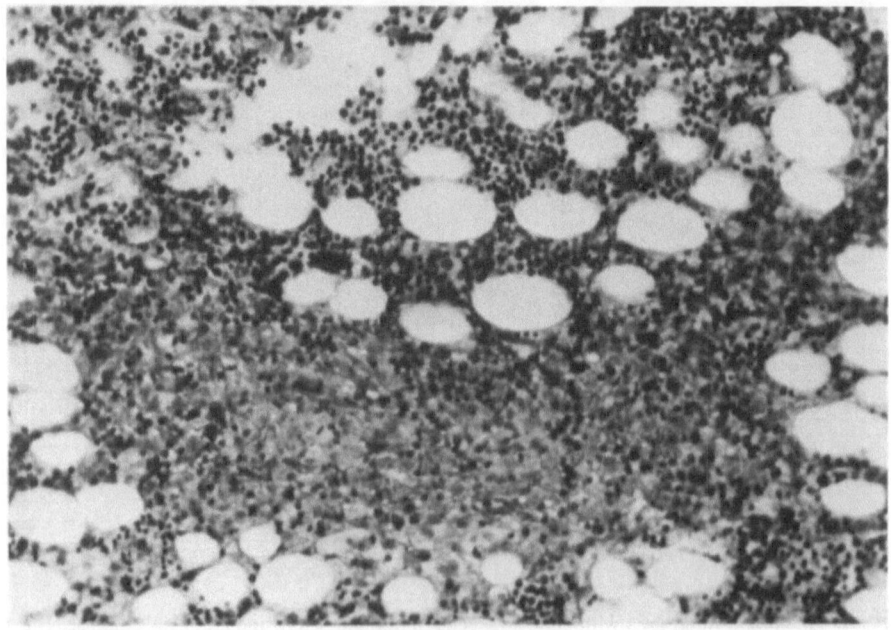

Figure 28. Bone marrow involvement with Hodgkin's disease (H & E ×90).

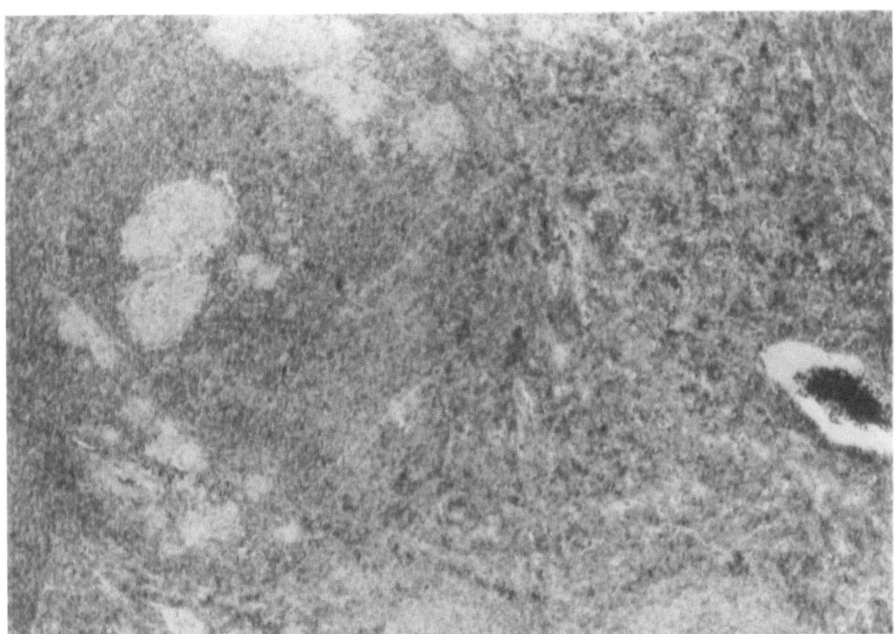

Figure 29. Spleen involvement in Hodgkin's disease (H & E ×22.75).

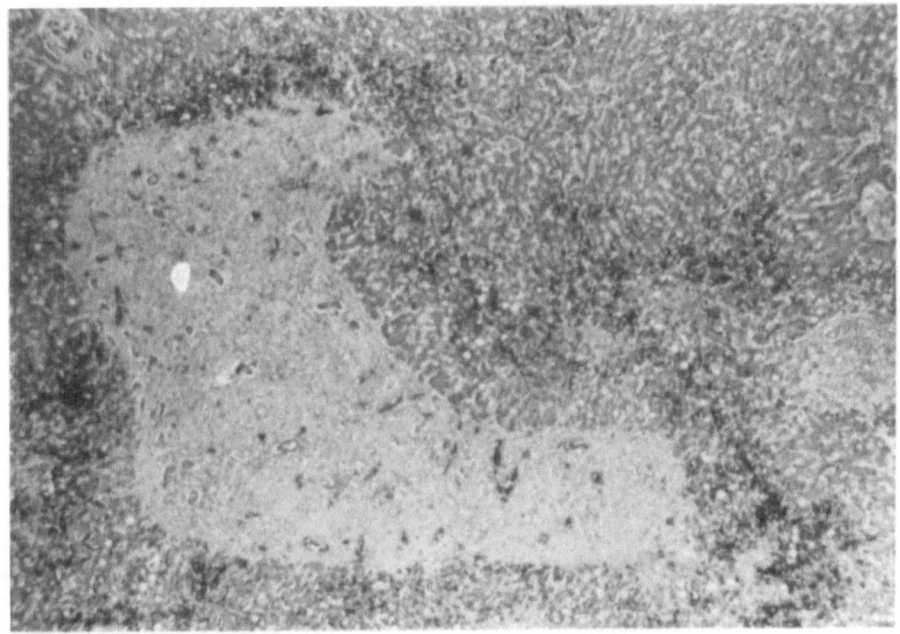

Figure 30. Liver involvement in Hodgkin's disease (H & E ×22.75).

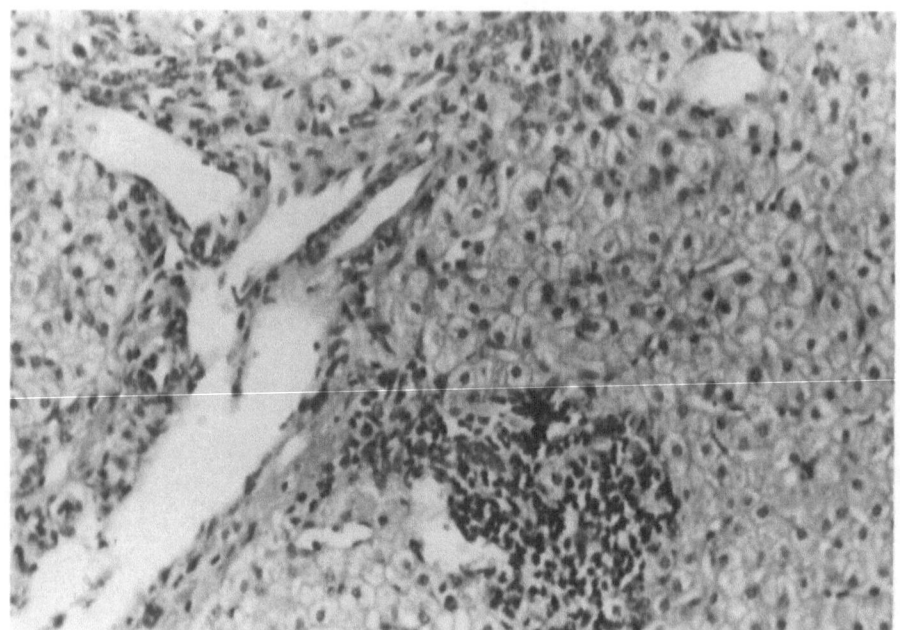

Figure 31. Portal area lymphocyte infiltration in liver section from a staging laparotomy for Hodgkin's disease (H & E ×90).

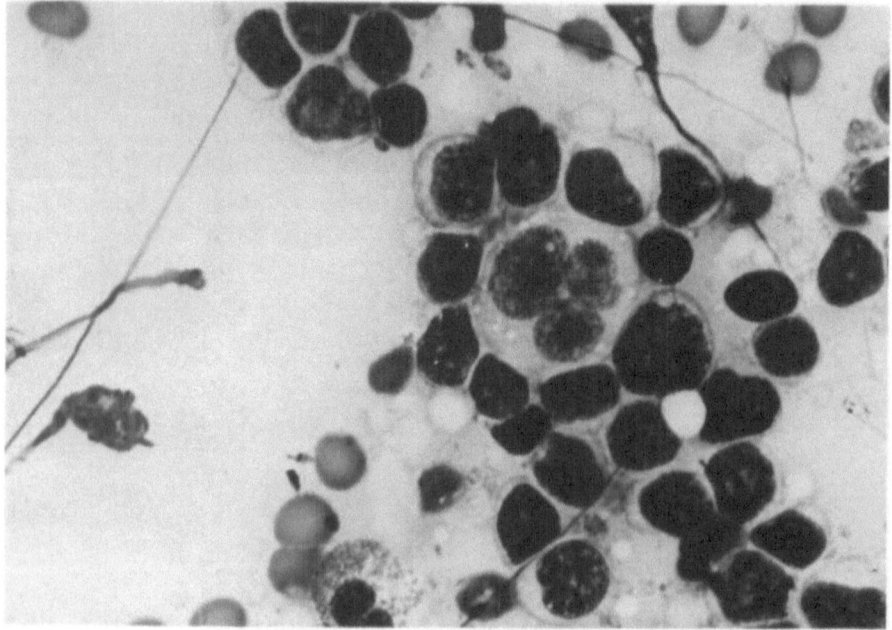

Figure 32. Reed-Sternberg cell in tissue imprint in Hodgkin's disease (H & E ×22.75).

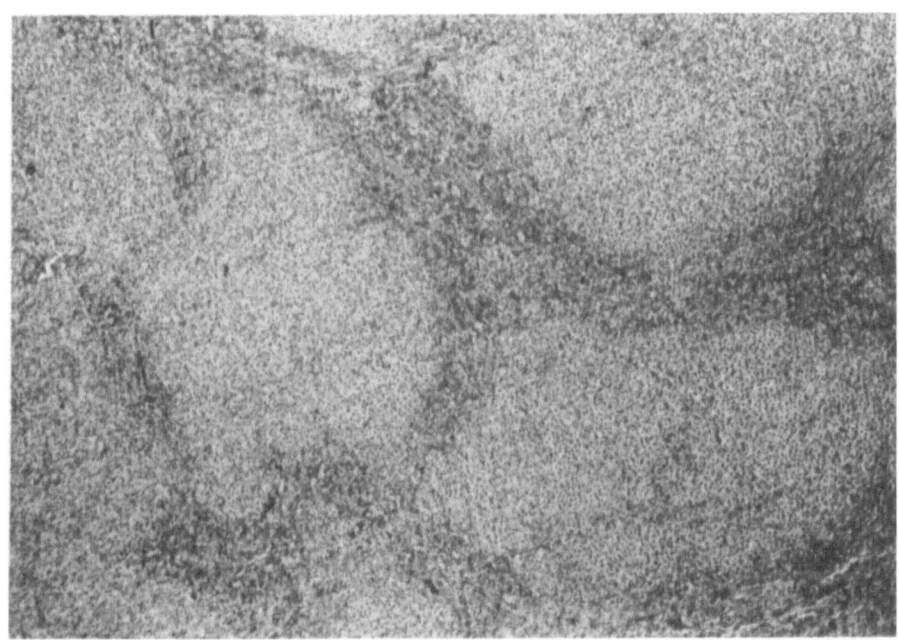

Figure 33. Non-Hodgkin's lymphoma, follicular pattern (H & E ×22.75).

Figure 34. Non-Hodgkin's lymphoma, diffuse pattern (H & E ×22.75).

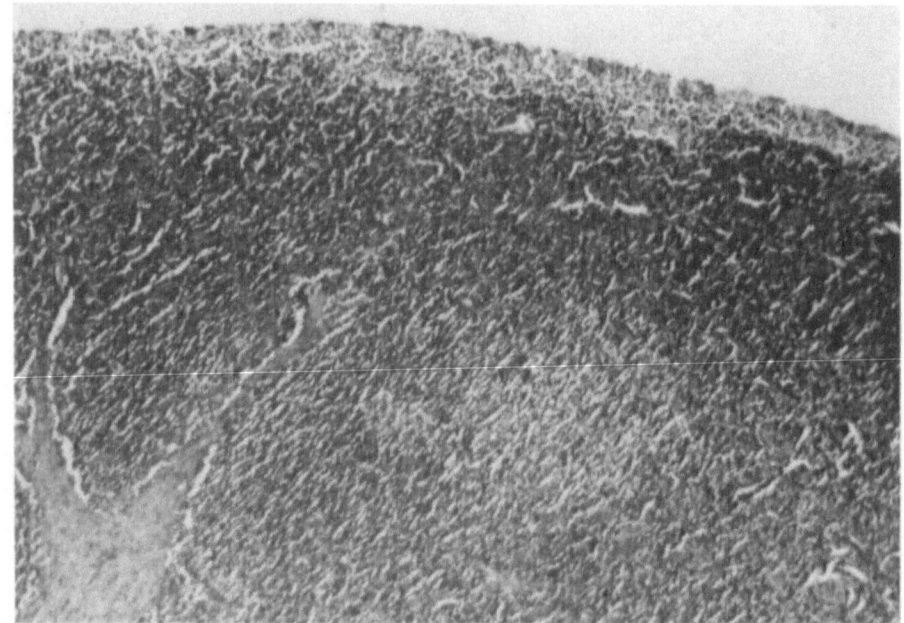

Figure 35. Lymphoma of small B cells. Diffuse pattern with some discernible sinuses (H & E ×22.75).

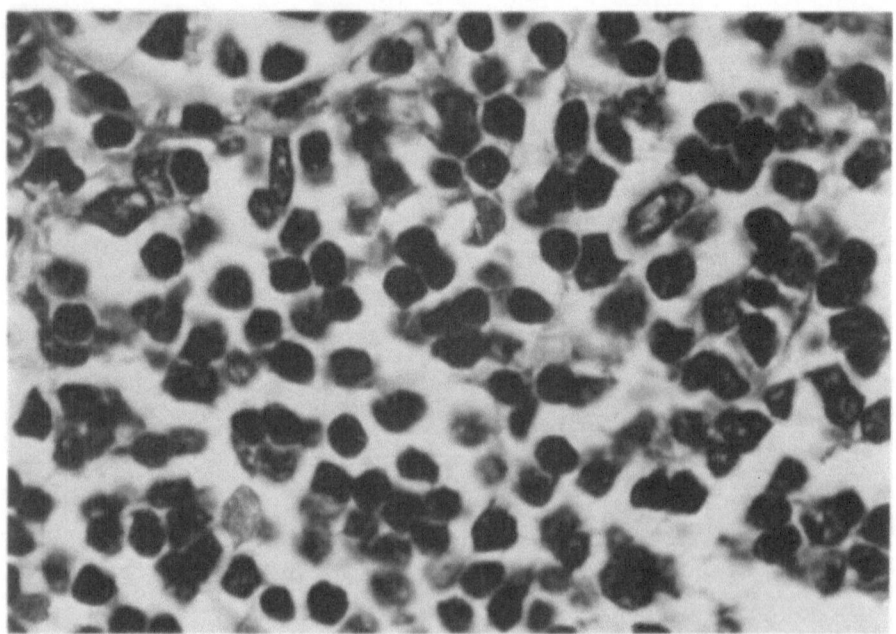

Figure 36. Lymphoma of small B lymphocytes (H & E ×910).

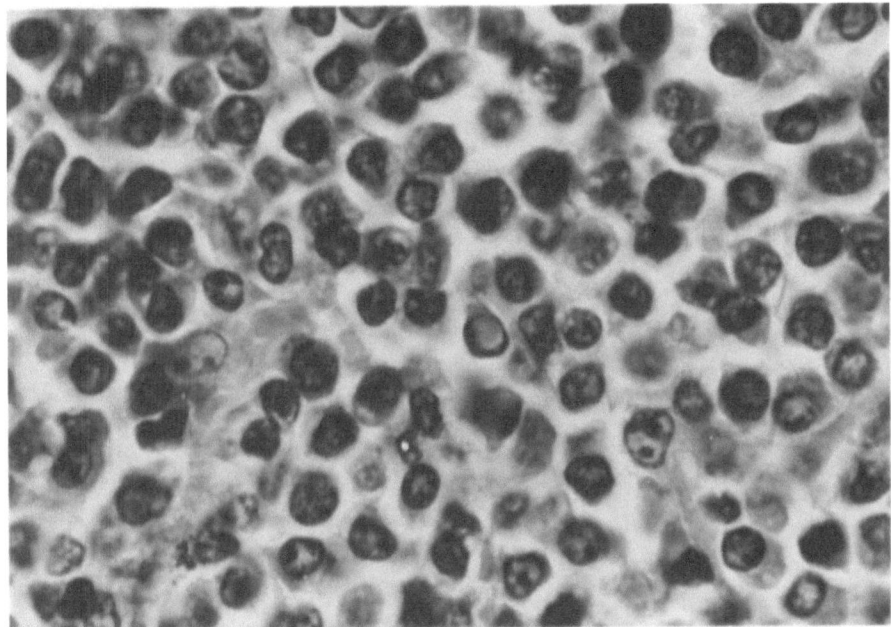

Figure 37. Lymphoma of plasmactyic-lymphocytic type. Ducther body in cell at center (H & E ×910).

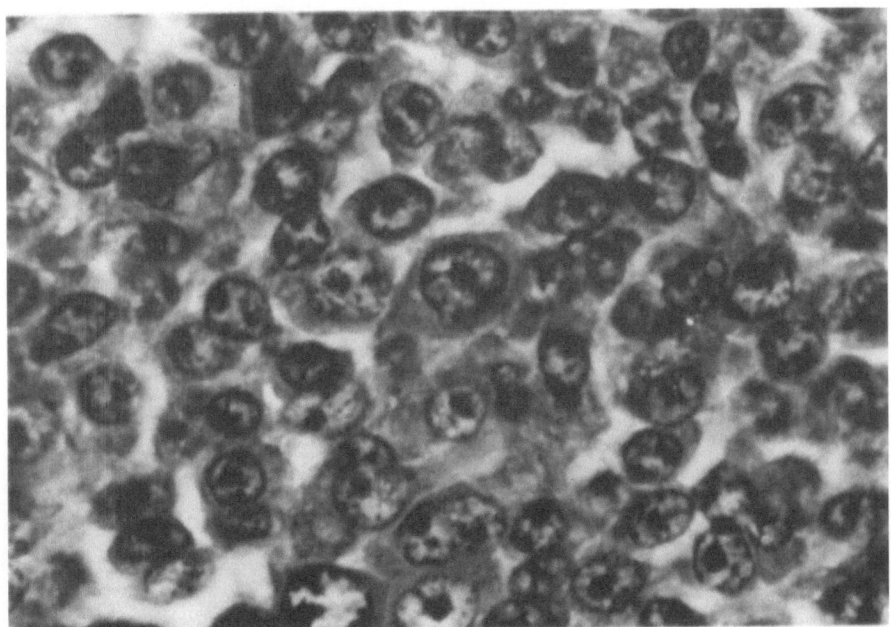

Figure 38. Immunoblastic sarcoma of B cell type (H & E ×910).

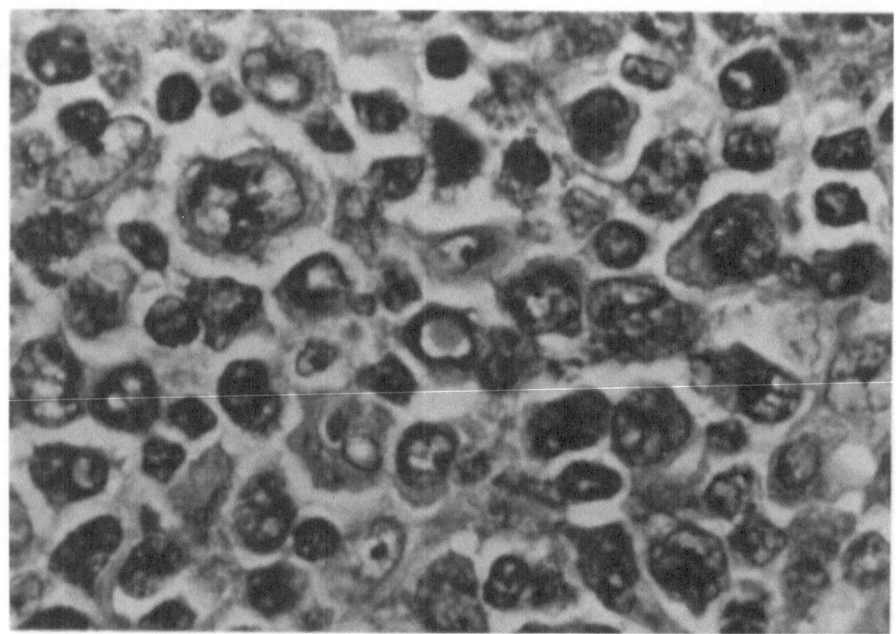

Figure 39. Immunoblastic sarcoma of B cell type. Nuclear inclusion (cell at center) and cytoplasmic inclusion (cell to lower left center) (H & E ×910).

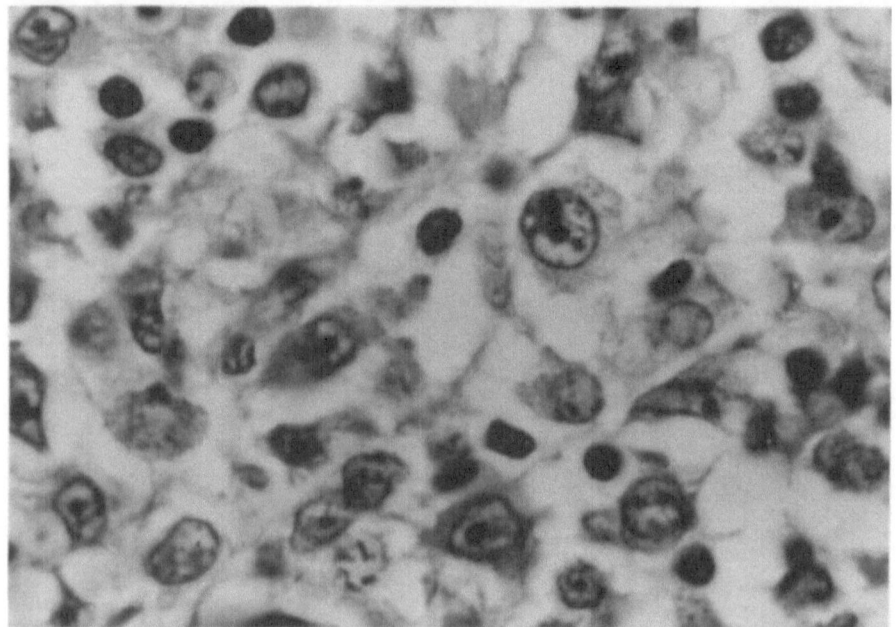

Figure 40. T immunoblasts (H & E ×910).

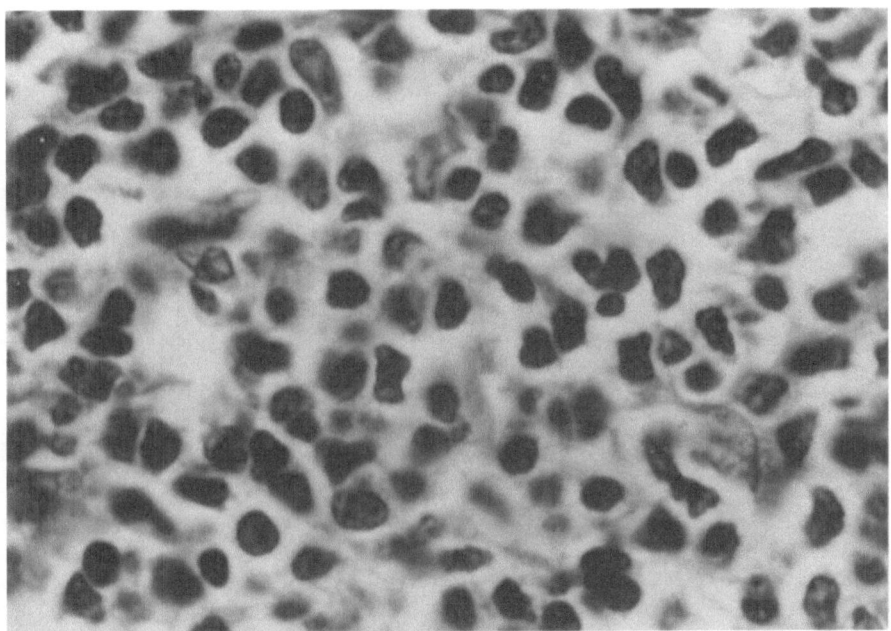

Figure 41. Follicular center cell lymphoma, small cleaved cell type (H & E ×910).

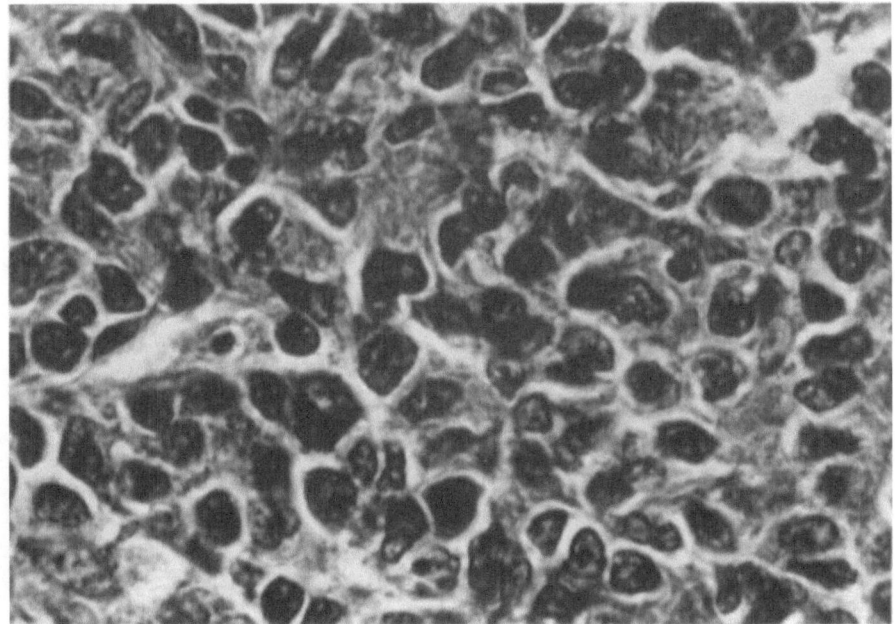

Figure 42. Follicular center cell lymphoma, large cleaved cell type (H & E ×910).

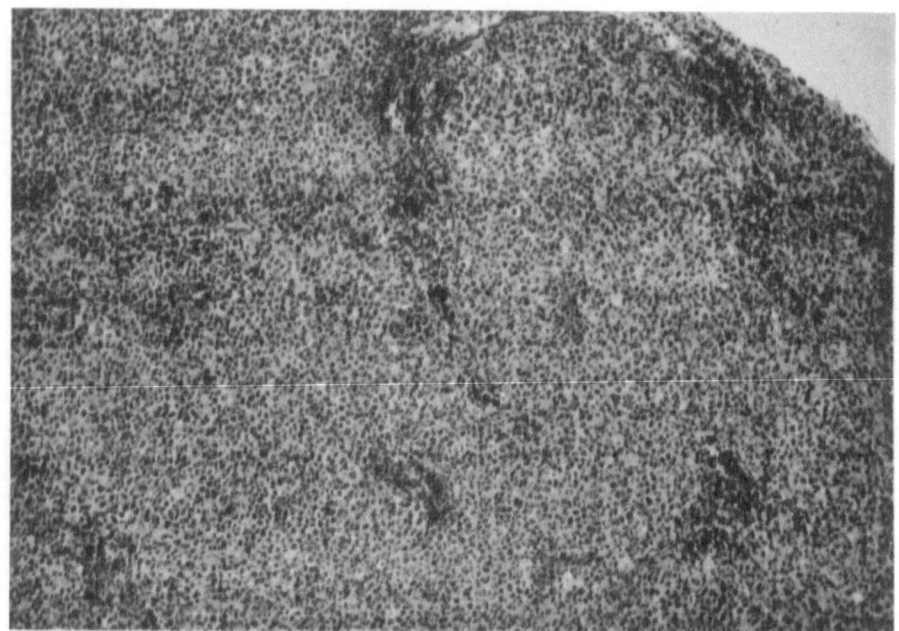

Figure 43. Large cleaved follicular center cell lymphoma with serpiginous pattern of lymph node involvement (H & E ×90).

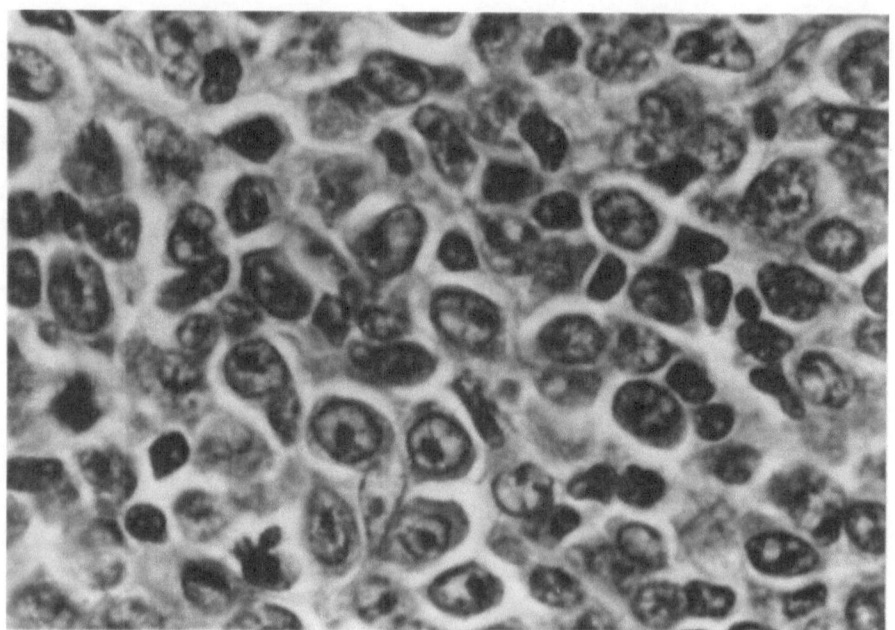

Figure 44. Follicular center cell lymphoma, small non-cleaved cell, Burkitt type (H & E ×910)

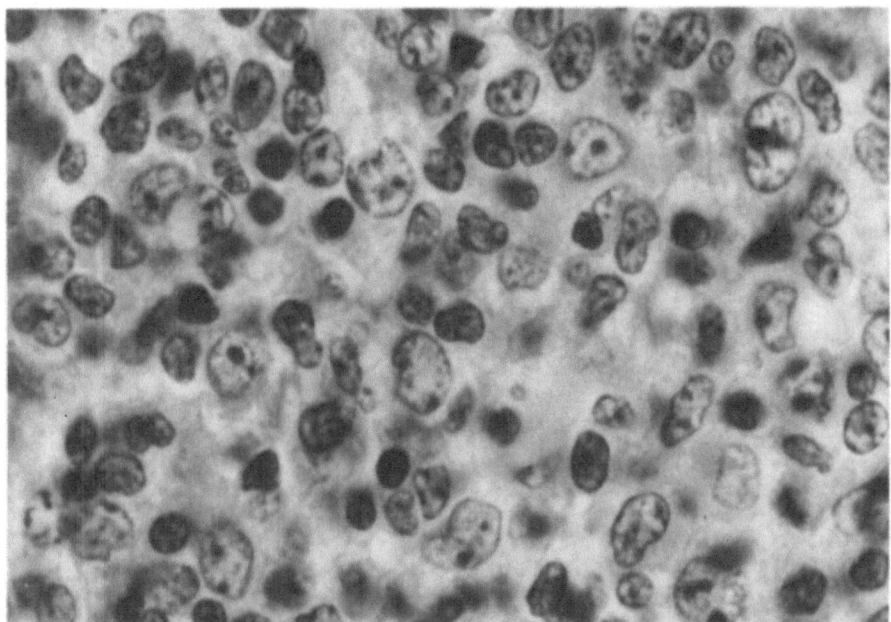

Figure 45. Follicular center cell lymphoma, small non-cleaved cell, non-Burkitt type (H & E ×910).

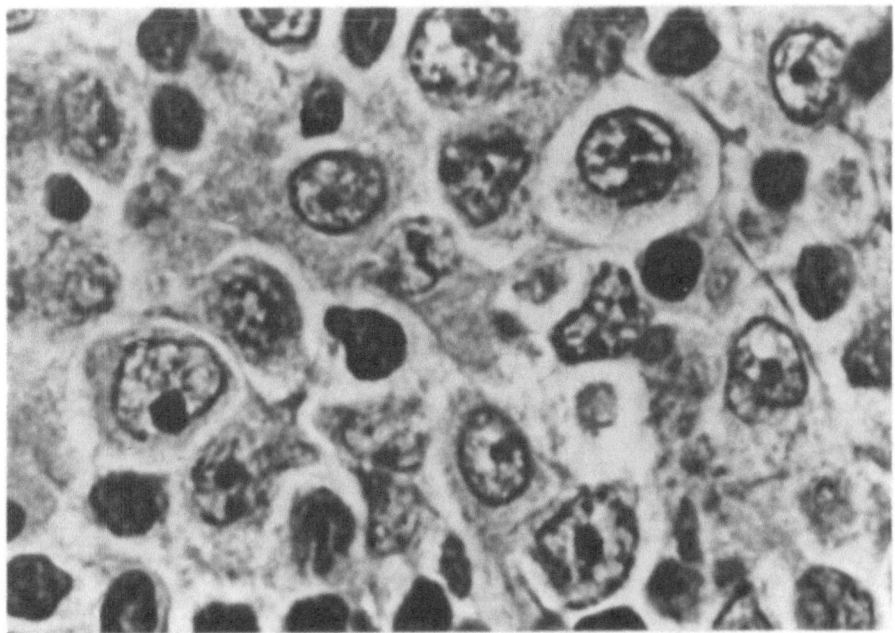

Figure 46. Follicular center cell lymphoma, large non-cleaved cell type (H & E ×1180).

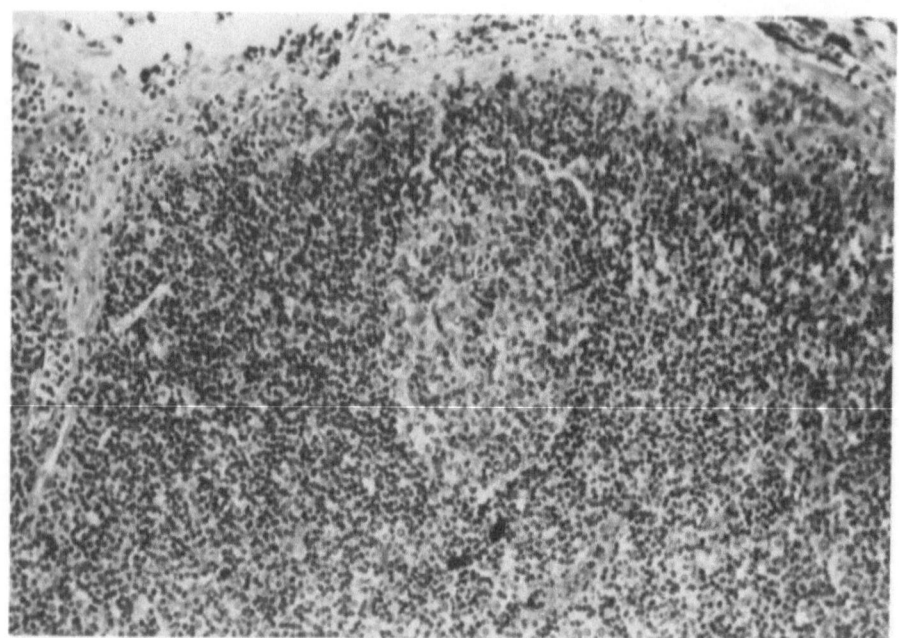

Figure 47. Lymphoma of small T lymphocytes. Residual follicular center in invloved lymph node (H & E ×90).

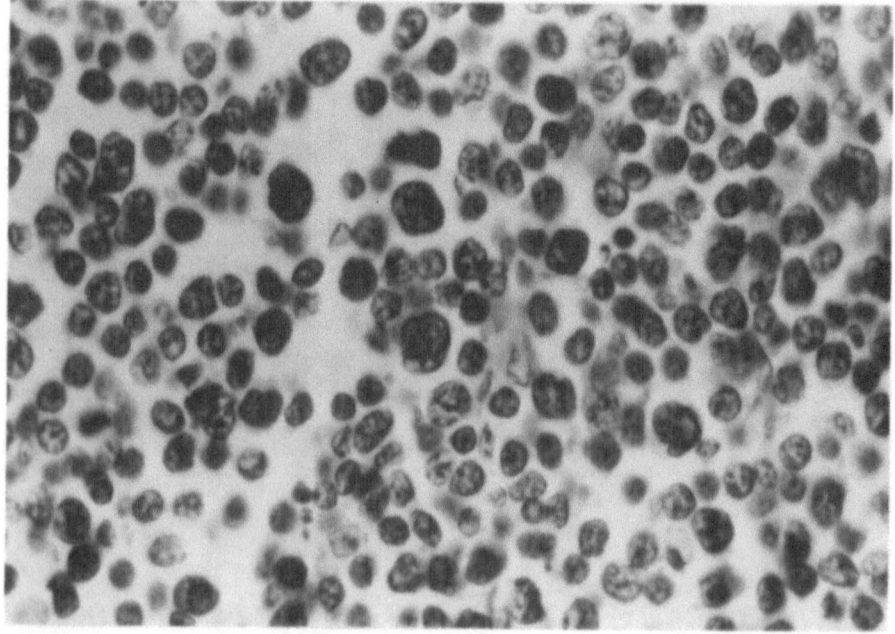

Figure 48. Convoluted cell lymphoma with two cell populations of small and large cells (H & E ×475).

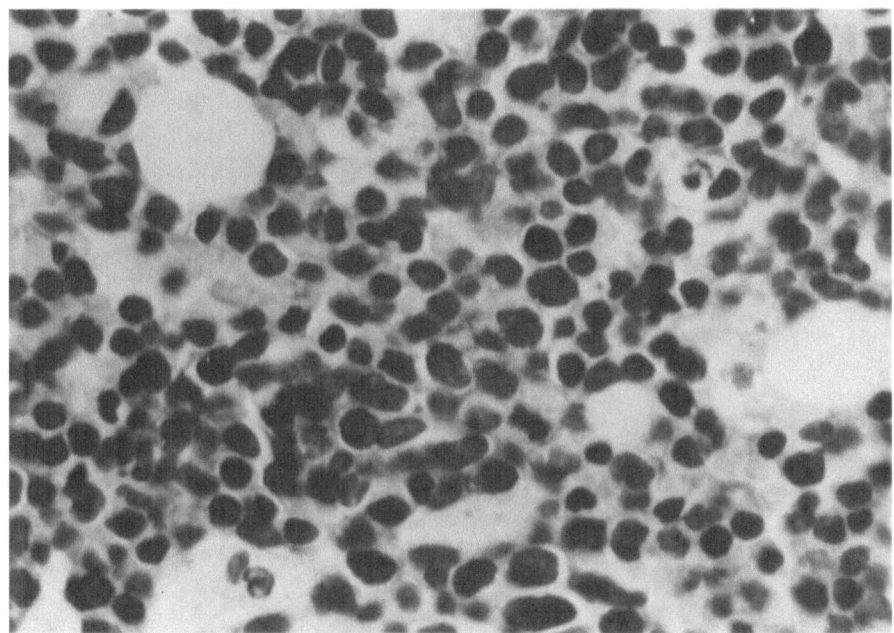

Figure 49. Convoluted cell lymphoma. Moderate degree of nuclear irregularity (H & E ×475).

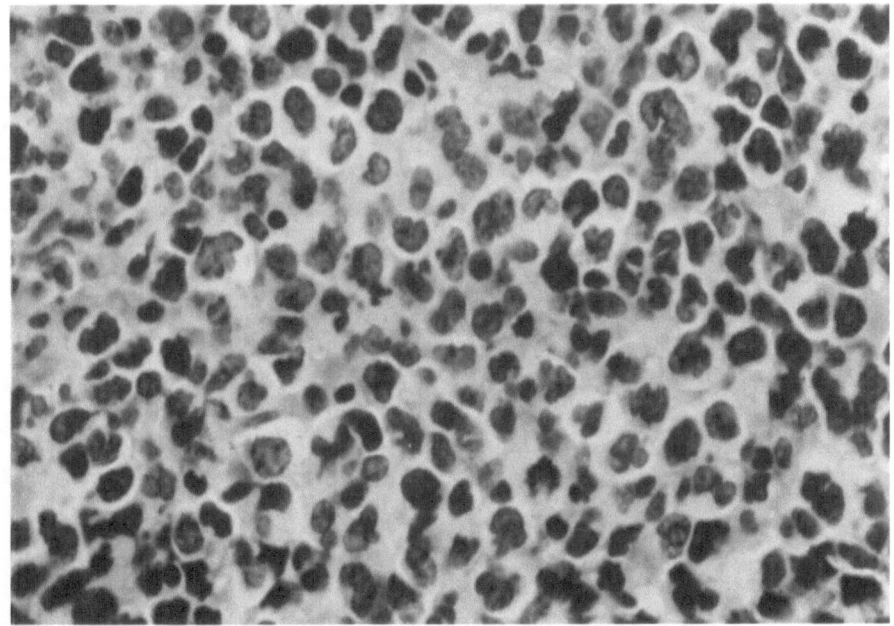

Figure 50. Convoluted cell lymphoma, Marked degree of nuclear irregularity (H & E ×365).

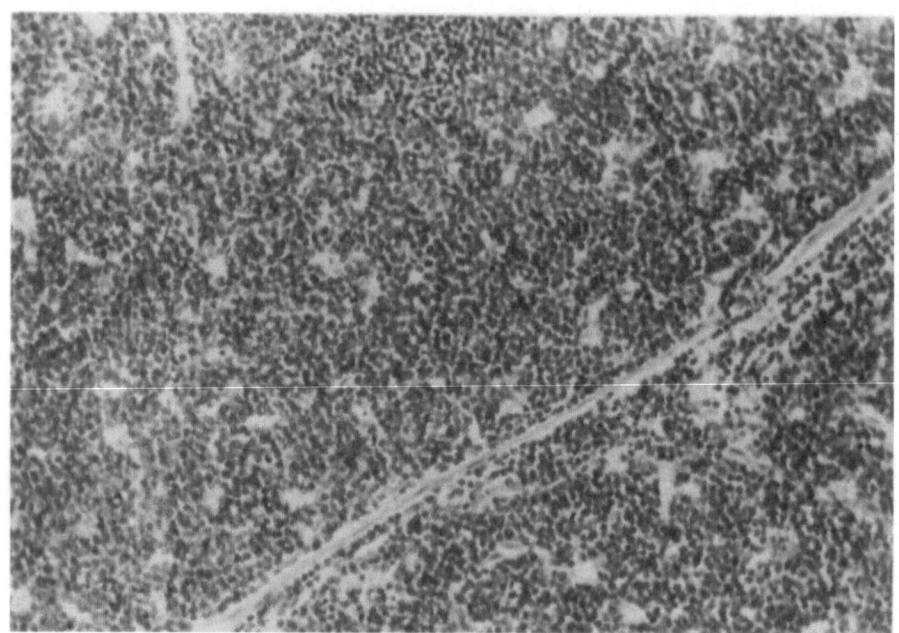

Figure 51. Convoluted cell lymphoma with starry sky phenomenon (H & E ×90).

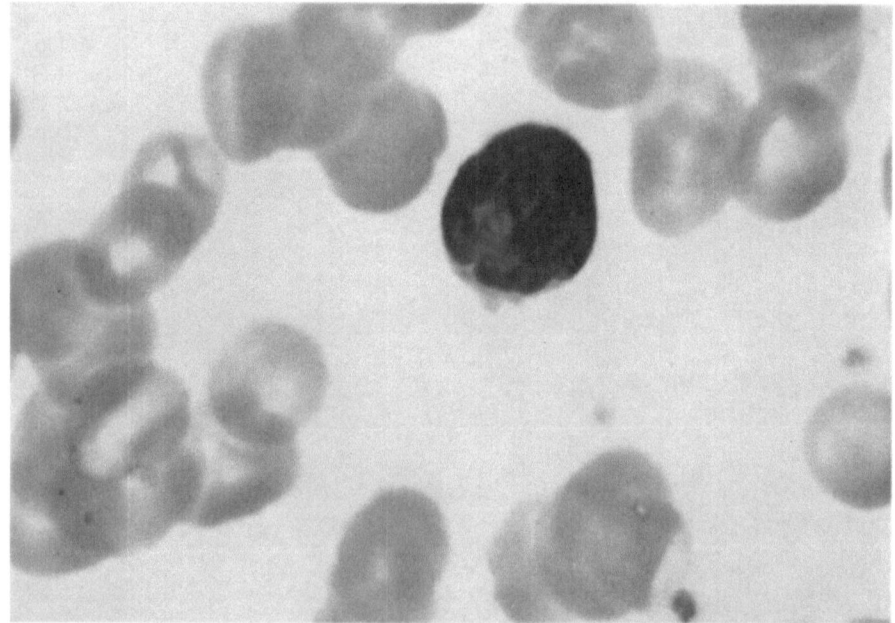

Figure 52. Sézary cell. Peripheral blood smear (H & E ×910).

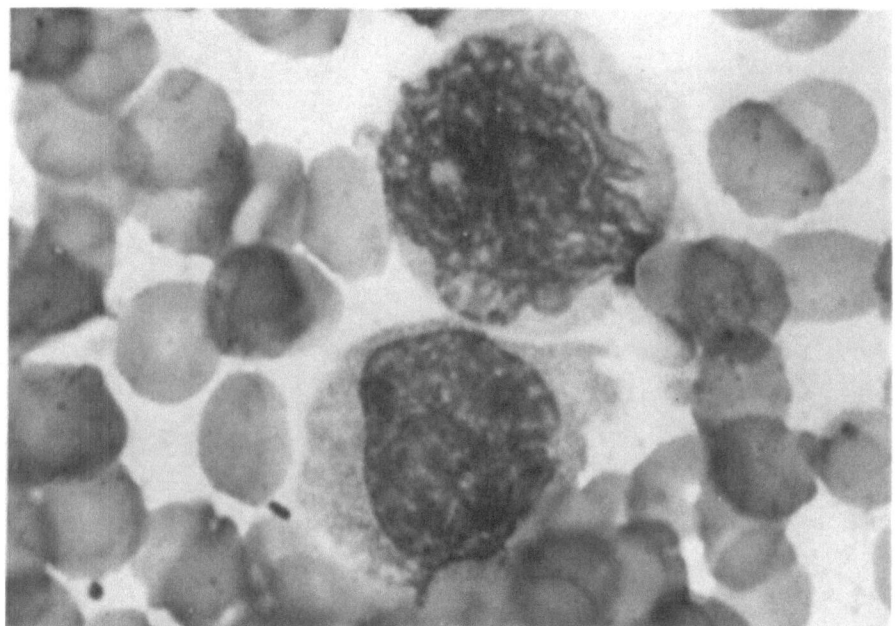

Figure 53. Mycosis fungoides cell. Buffy coat, peripheral blood smear (H & E ×910).

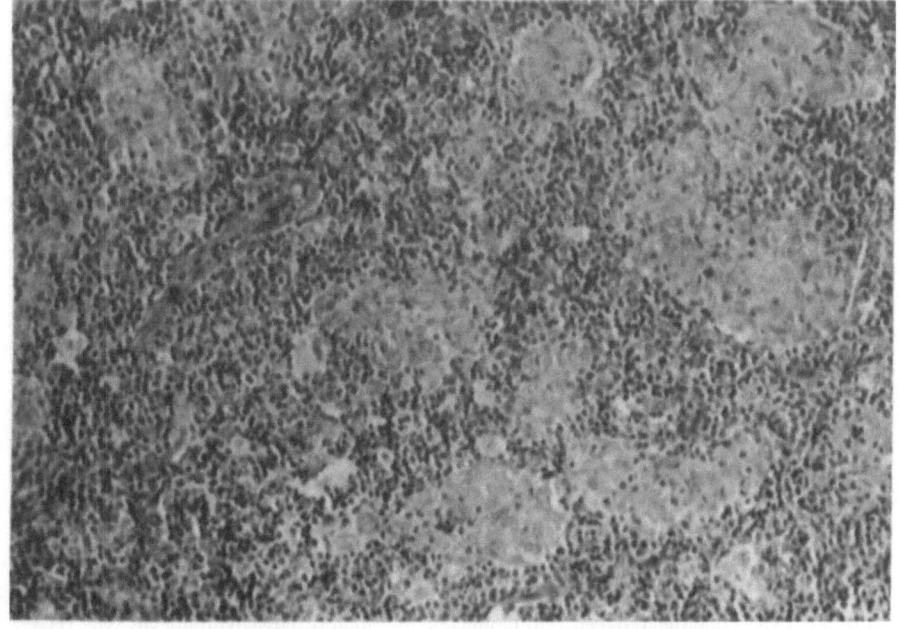

Figure 54. Lymphoepithelioid cell lymphoma (H & E ×90).

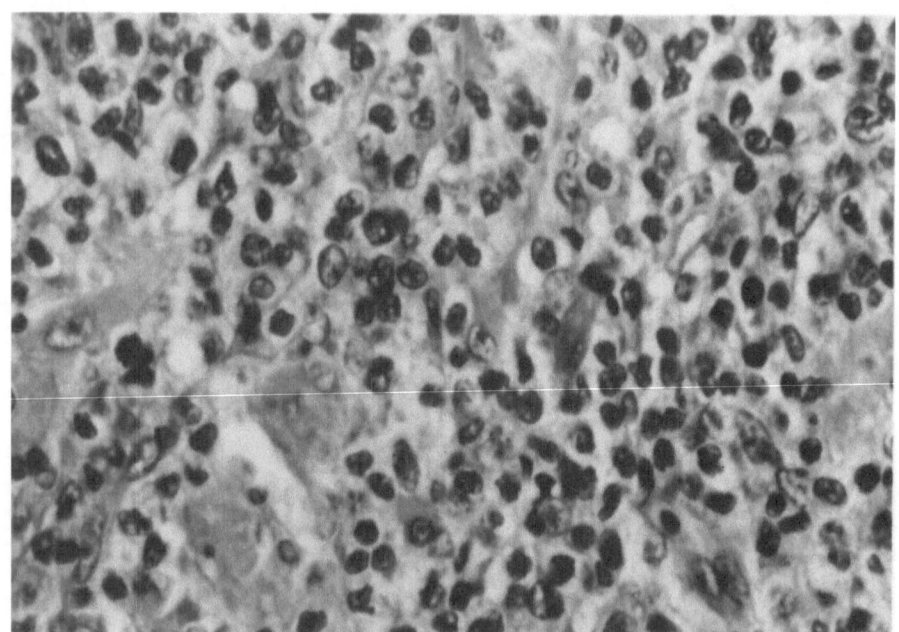

Figure 55. Lymphoepithelioid cell lymphoma, predominantly small lymphocyte type (H & E ×365).

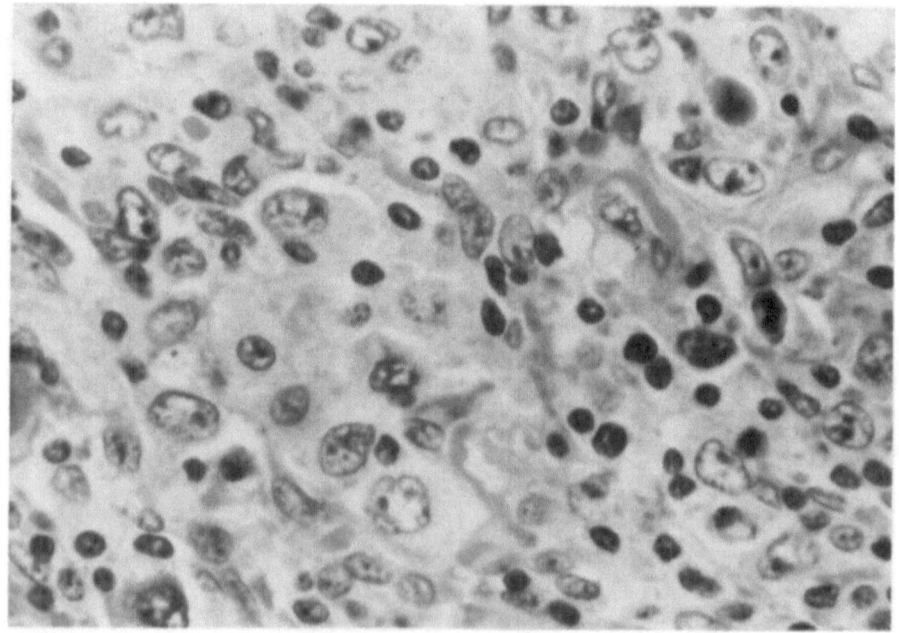

Figure 56. Lymphoepithelioid cell lymphoma, predominantly large lymphocyte type (H & E ×365).

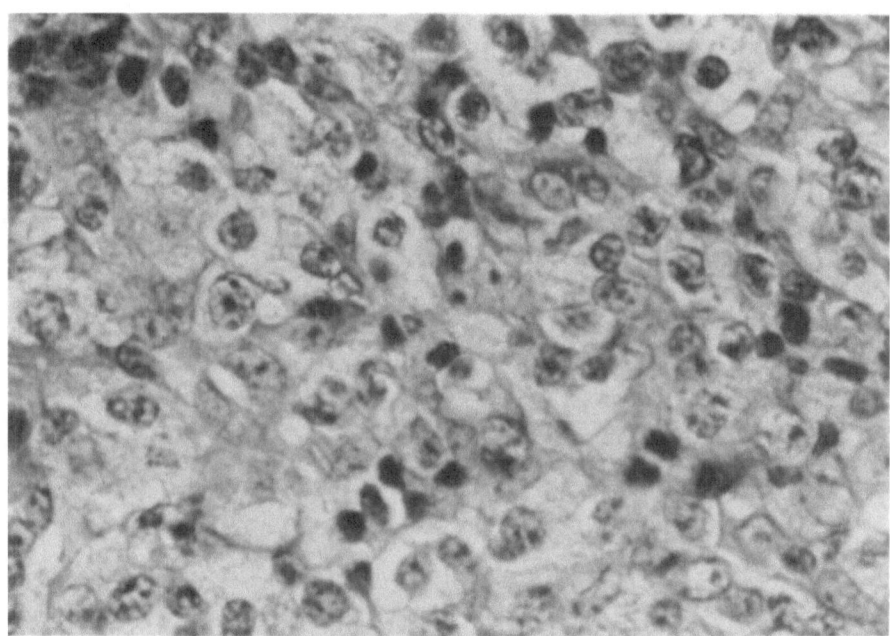

Figure 57. Immunoblastic sarcoma of T cell type (H & E ×365).

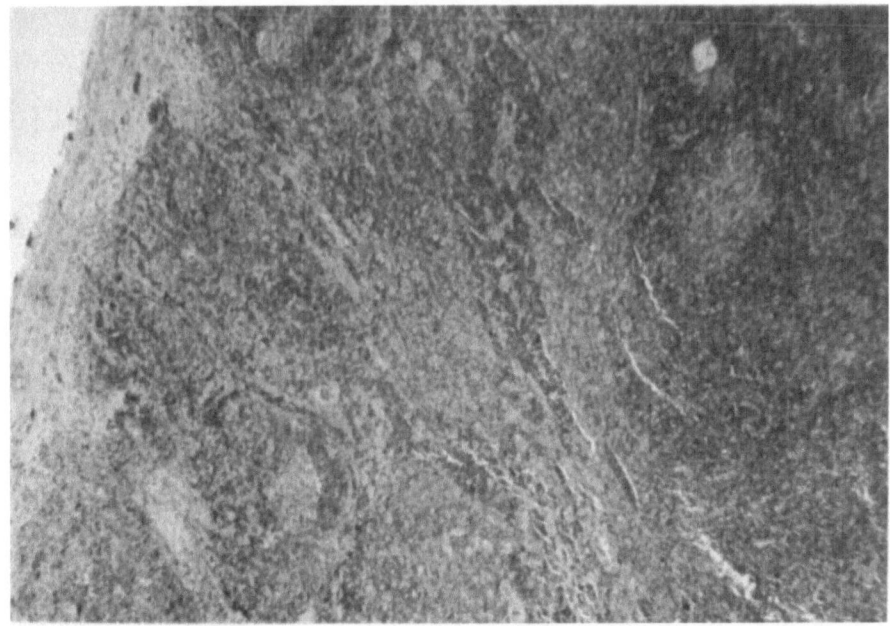

Figure 58. Immunoblastic sarcoma of T cell type. Partial lymph node involvement (H & E ×22.75).

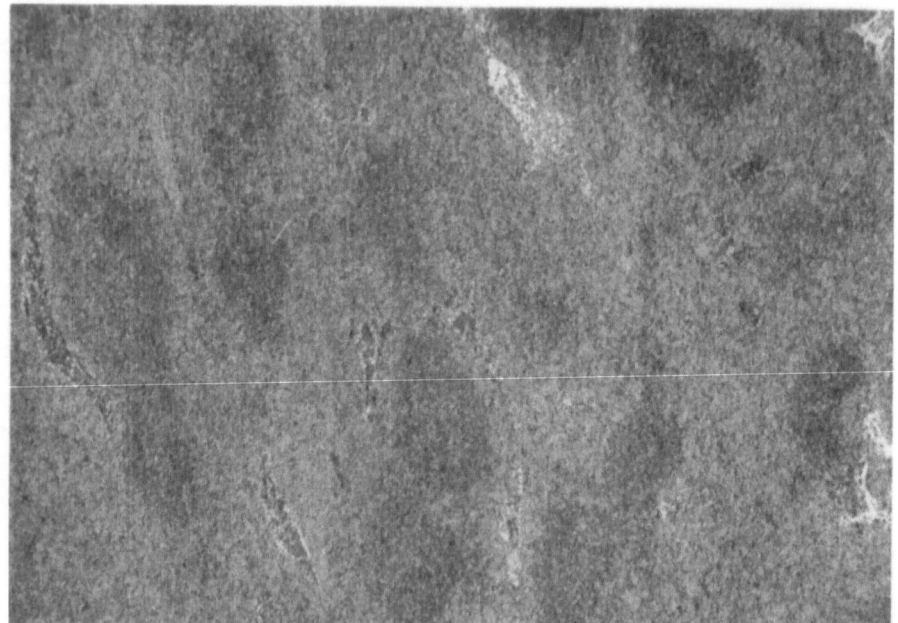

Figure 59. T zone lymphoma (H & E ×22.75).

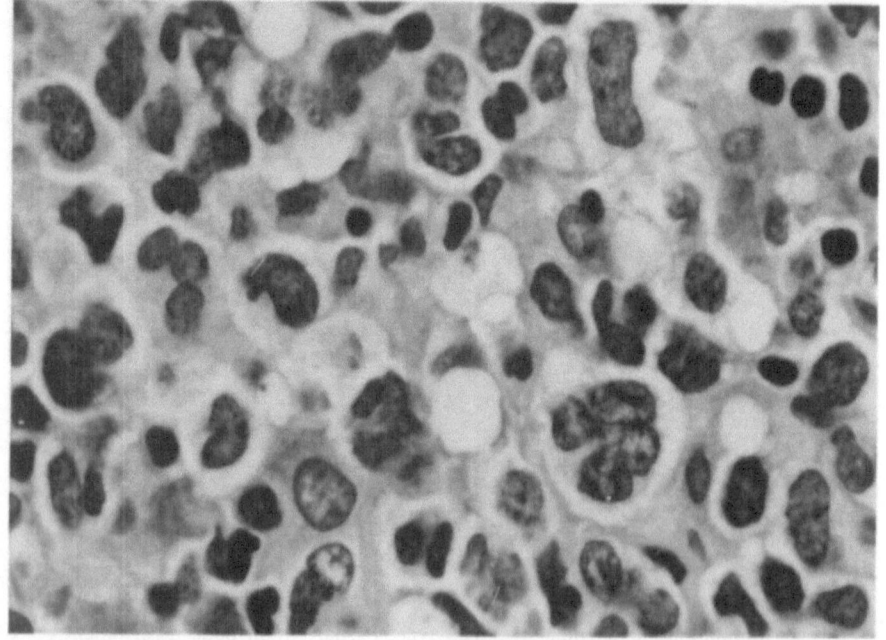

Figure 60. T zone lymphoma. Abnormal cells include bizarre large forms (H & E ×910).

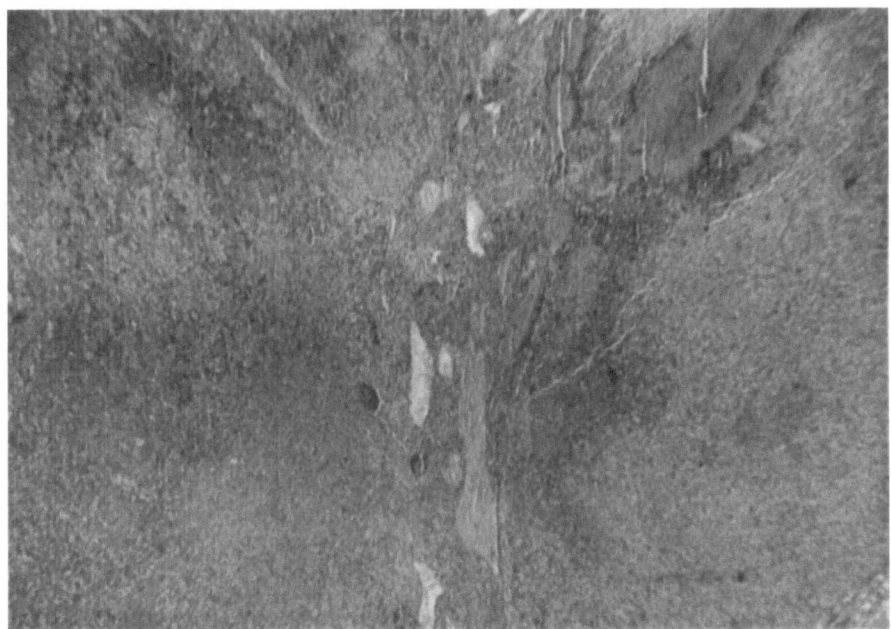

Figure 61. Malignant lymphoma. Large lobated T cell type (H & E ×22.75).

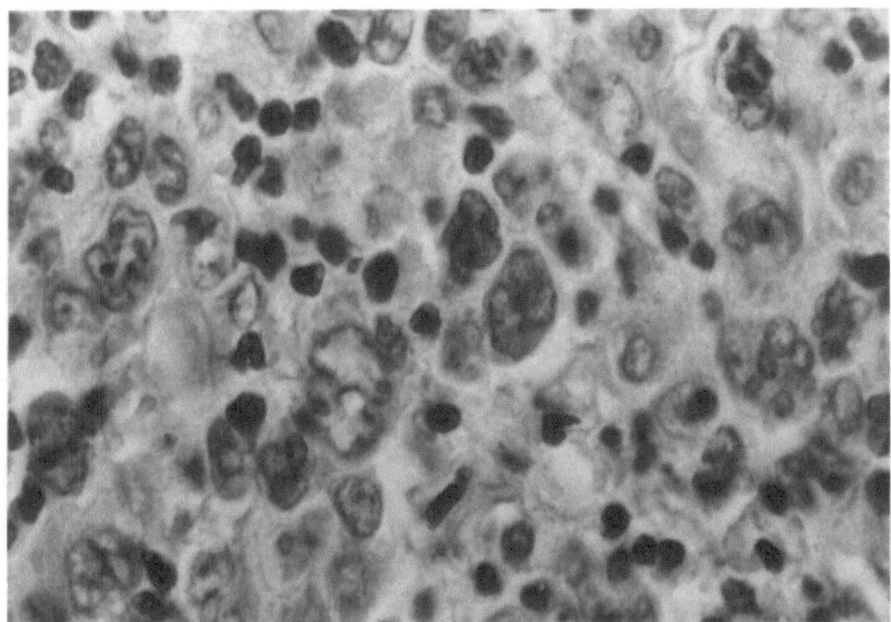

Figure 62. Malignant lymphoma. Large lobated T cell type (H & E ×580).

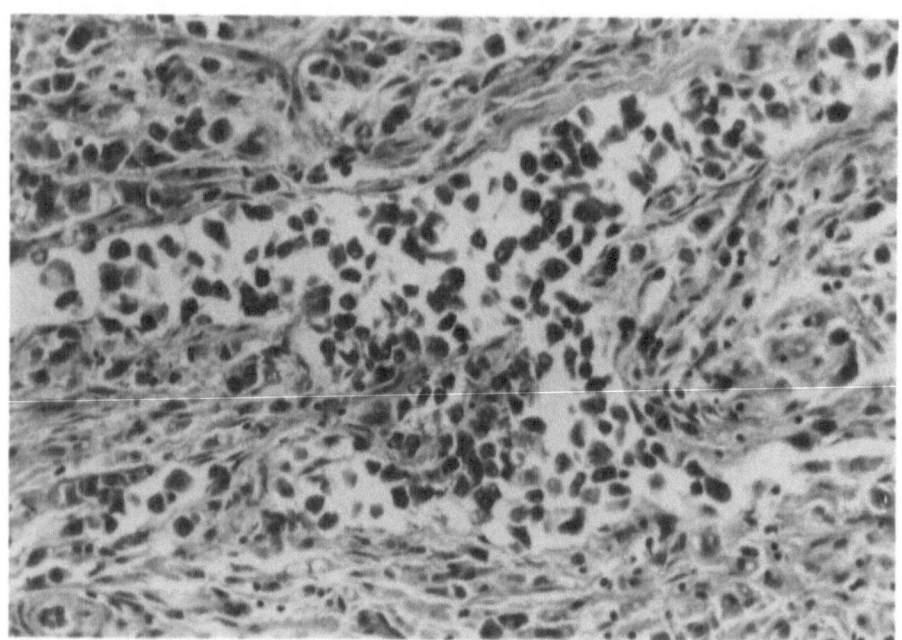

Figure 63. Malignant histiocytosis. Intrasinusoidal proliferation of neoplastic cells (H & E ×140).

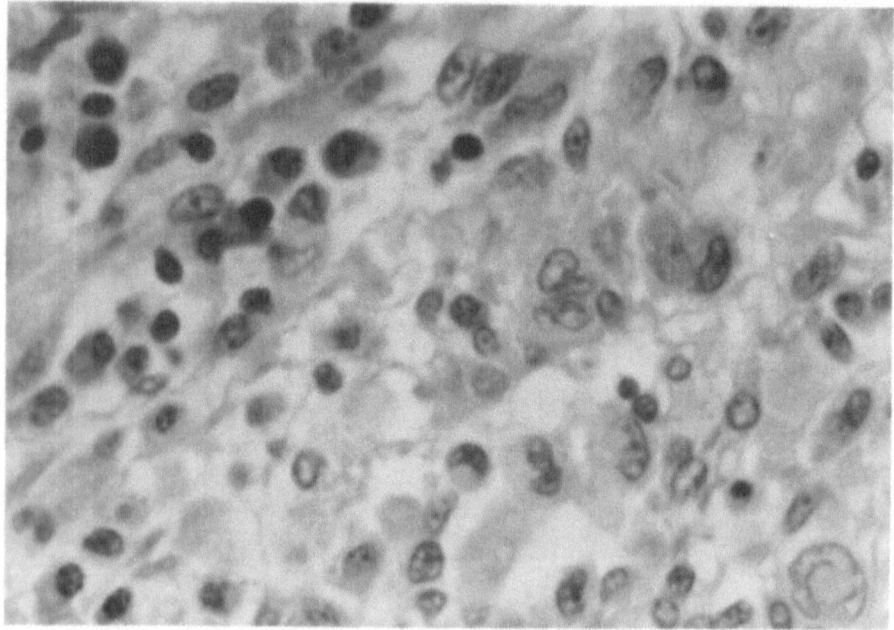

Figure 64. Histiocytic lymphoma. Large pale cells with indistinct cell margins (H & E ×365).

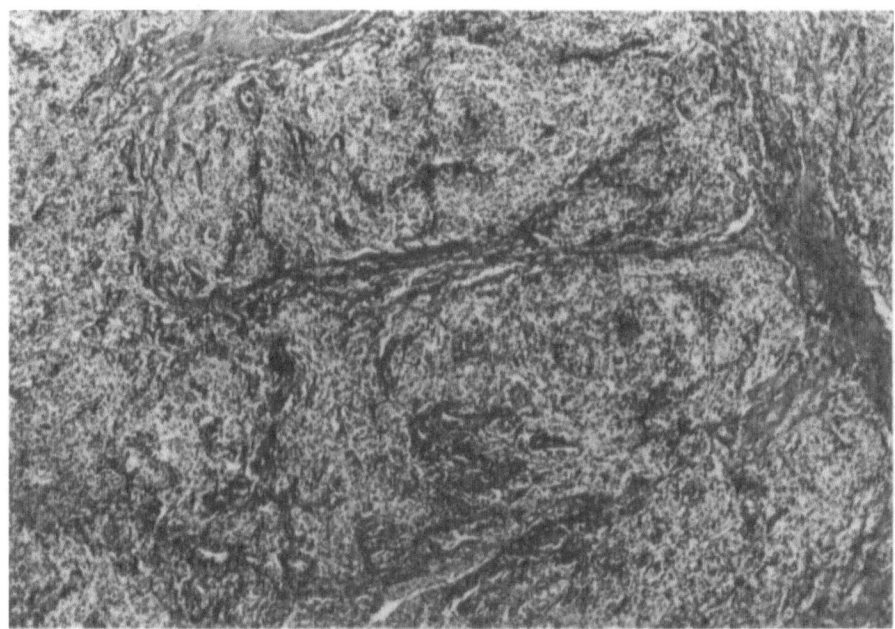

Figure 65. Sclerosing non-Hodgkin's lymphoma (H & E ×22.75).

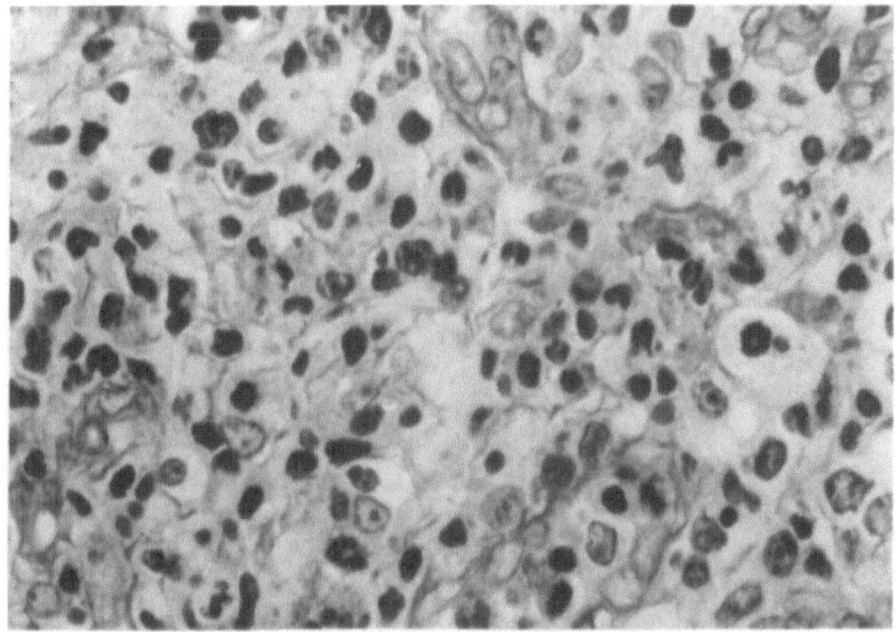

Figure 66. Sclerosing lymphoma, predominance of small cleaved follicular center cells (H & E ×365).

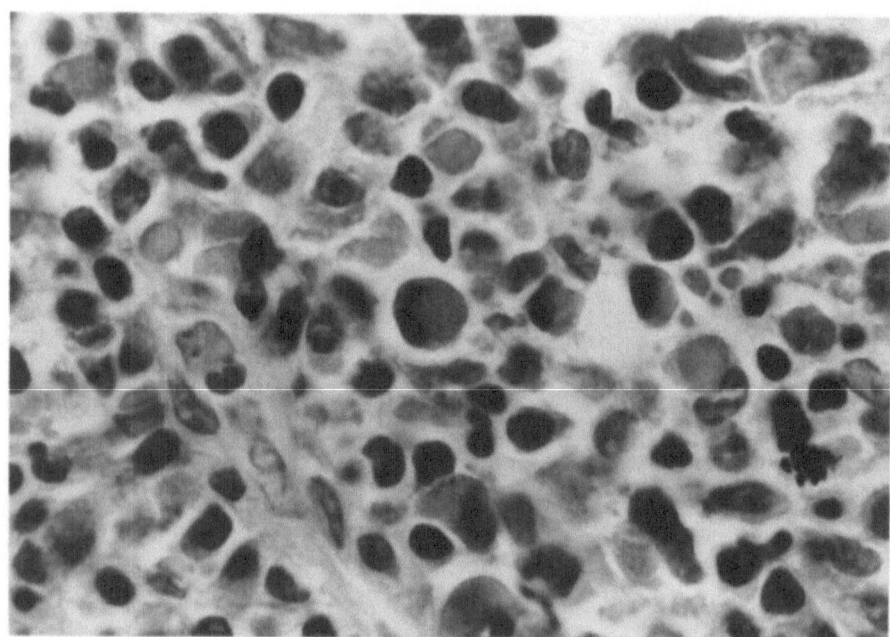

Figure 67. Signet ring lymphoma with cytoplasmic inclusions (center and center right) (immunoperoxidase-Ig kappa ×365).

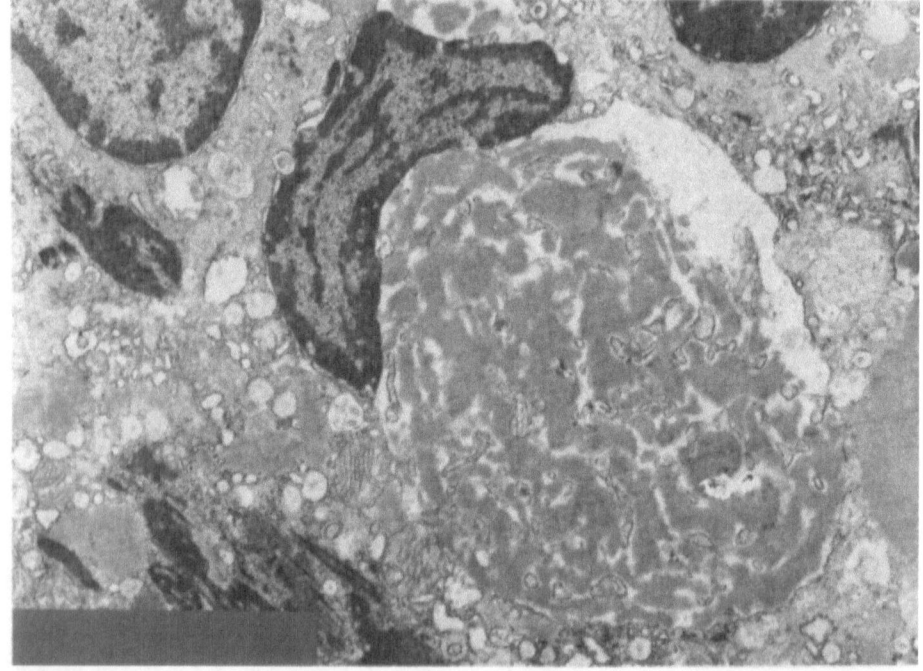

Figure 68. Signet ring lymphoma, ultrastructure on cell with cytoplasmic inclusion (×9800).

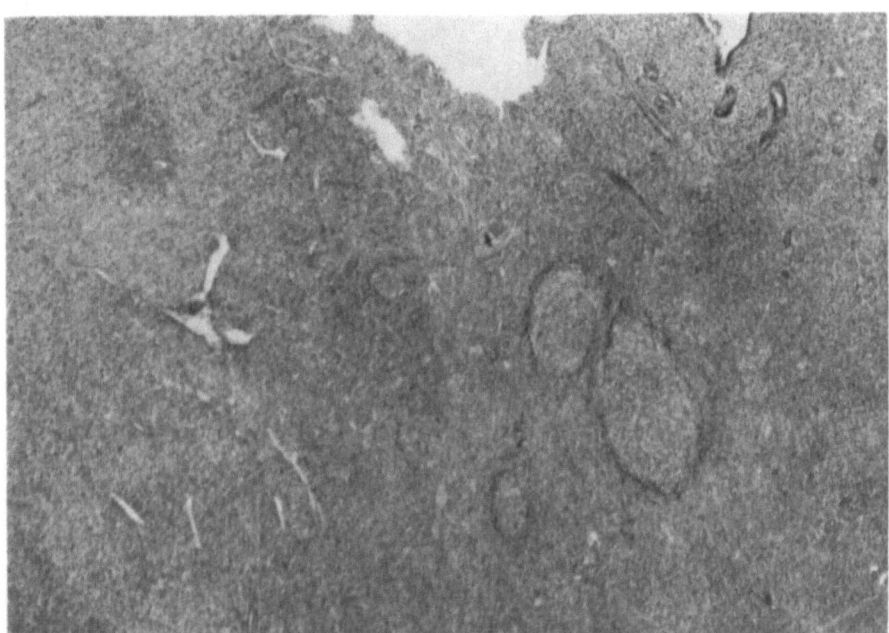

Figure 69. Composite lymphoma with diffuse and follicular components (H & E ×22.75).

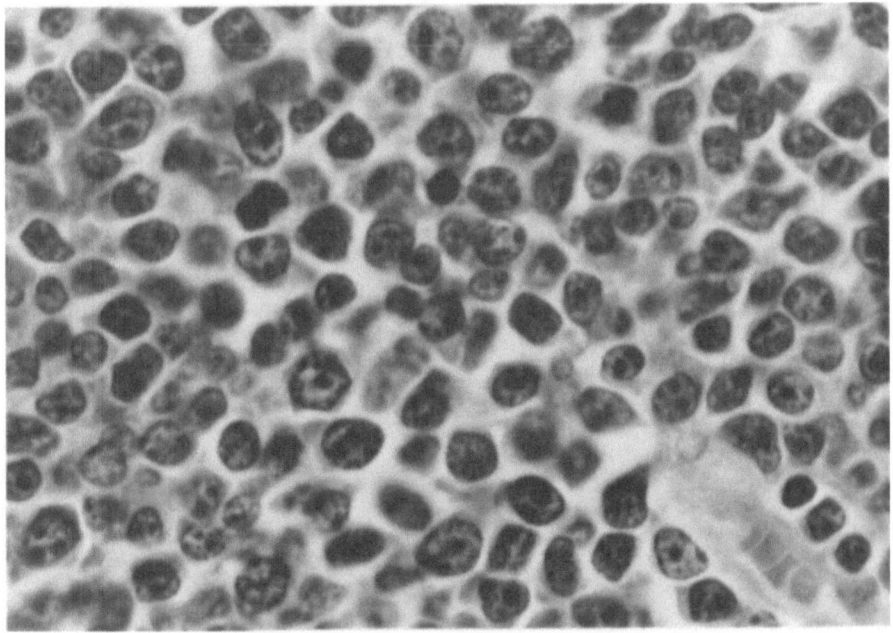

Figure 70. Composite lymphoma, diffuse area predominantly small non-cleaved follicular center cells; follicular areas predominantly small cleaved follicular

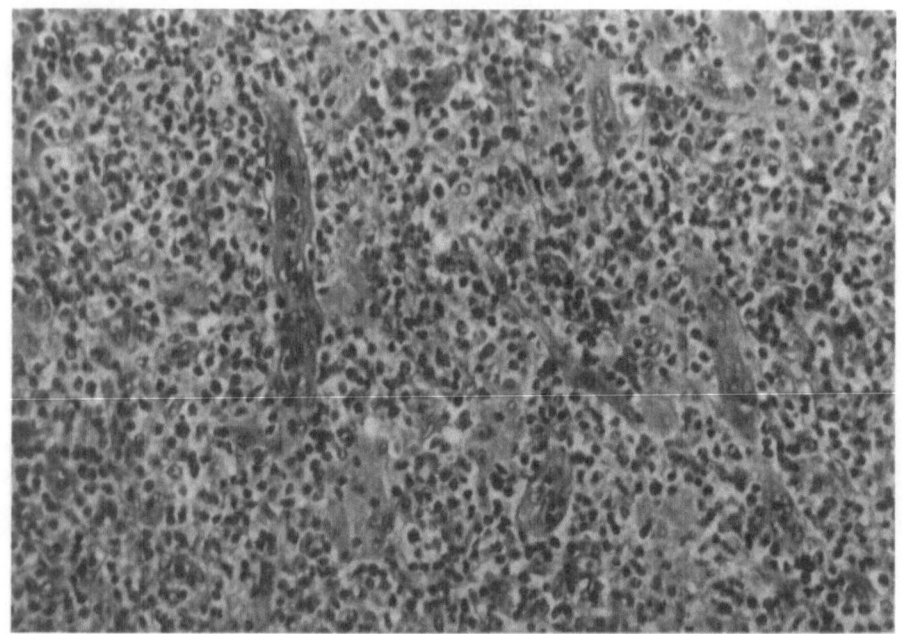

Figure 71. Abnormal immune lesion similar to, but more cellular than, typical immunoblastic lymphadenopathy (H & E ×145).

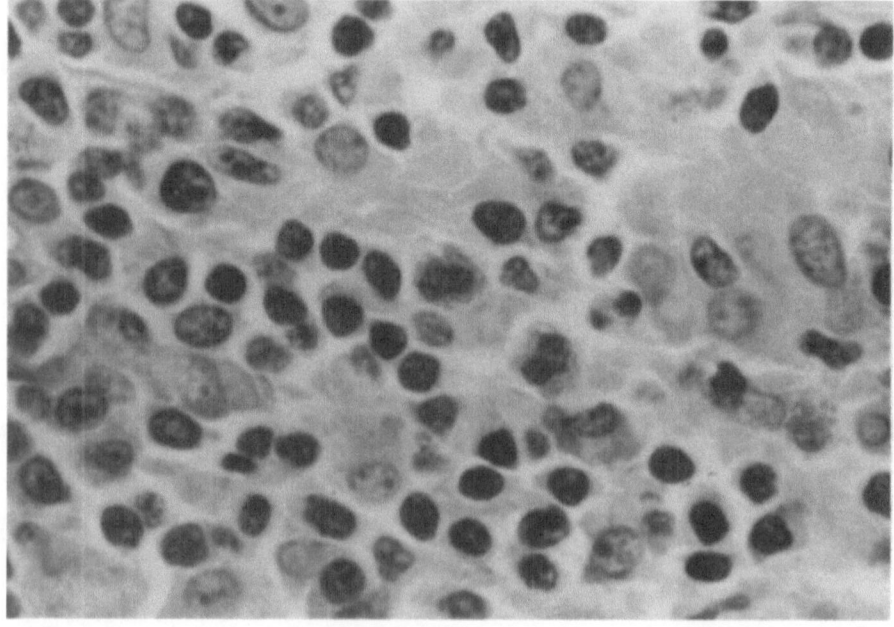

Figure 72. Immunoblastic lymphadenopathy. Mixed cellular proliferation and amorphous background material (H & E ×910).

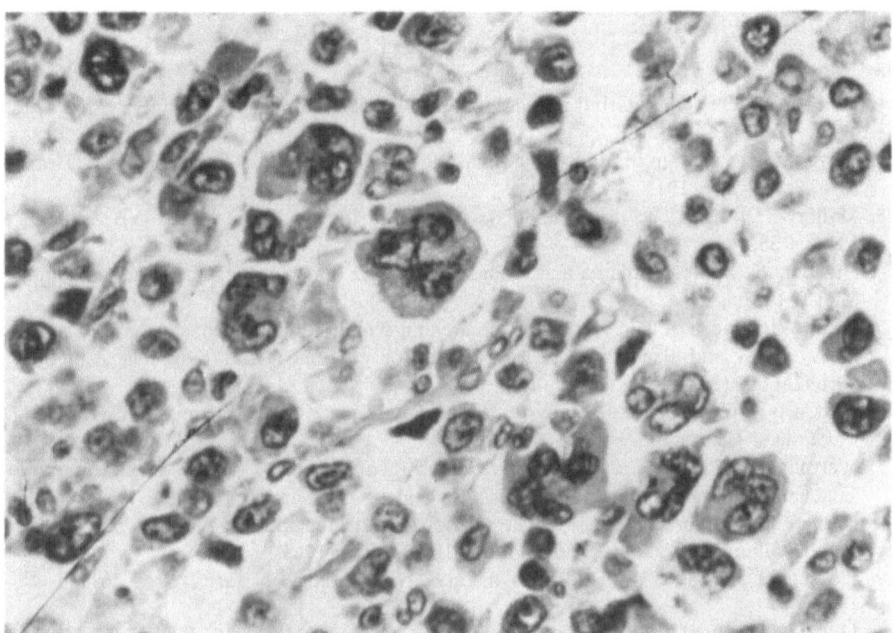

Figure 73. Immunoblastic sarcoma occurring after immunoblastic lymphadenopathy (H & E ×365).

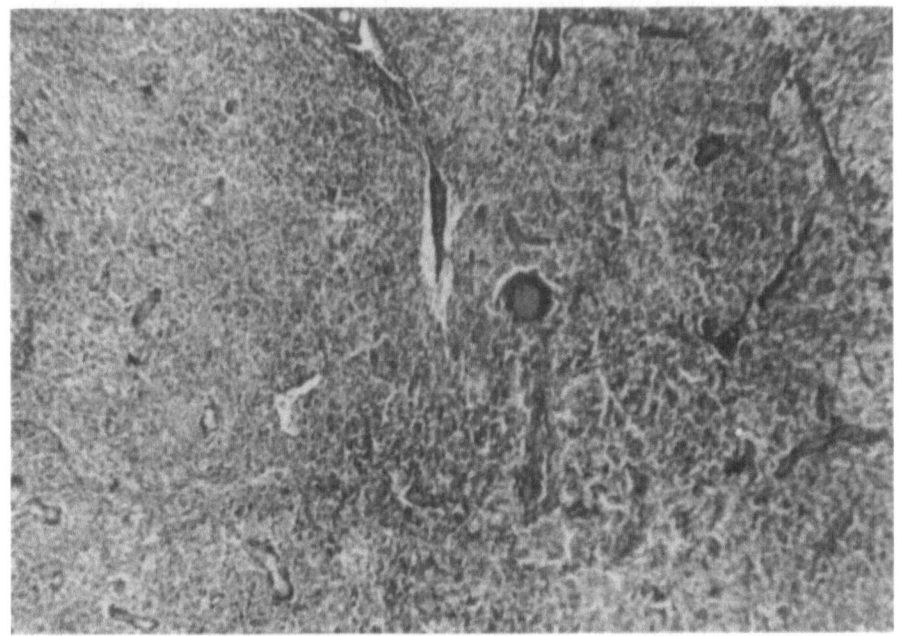

Figure 74. Immunoblastic lymphadenopathy in a partially involved lymph node (PAS ×22.75).

REFERENCES

1. Hodgkin T: On some morbid appearances of the absorbant glands and spleen. Med Chic Trans 17:68–114, 1832.
2. Oliver J: The relation of Hodgkin's disease to lymphosarcoma and endothelioma. J Med Res 29:191–207, 1913.
3. Mallory FBP: In: The principles of pathologic histology. Philadelphia: WB Saunders, 1914, p 333.
4. Ginsburg S: Lymphosarcoma and Hodgkin's disease: biologic characteristics. Ann Intern Med 8:14–36, 1934.
5. Coley WB: End results in Hodgkin's disease and lymphosarcoma treated by mixed toxins of erysipelas and Bacillus prodigiosus, alone or combined with radiation. Ann Surg 88:641–667, 1928.
6. MacCarty WC: A cytologic study of Hodgkin's disease, lymphosarcoma, and lymphatic leukemia. J Cancer Res 14:394–410, 1930.
7. Warthin AS: The genetic neoplastic relationship of Hodgkin's disease, aleukaemic and leukaemic lymphoblastoma and mycosis fungoides. Ann Surg 93:153–161, 1931.
8. Herbert PA, Miller FR, Erf LA: The relationship of Hodgkin's disease, lymphosarcoma and reticulum cell sarcoma. Am J Pathol 21:233–253, 1945.
9. Jackson H Jr, Parker F: Hodgkin's disease – II. Pathology. N Eng J Med 231:35–44, 1944.
10. Lukes RJ, Butler JJ: The pathology and nomenclature of Hodgkin's disease. Cancer Res 26:1063–1081, 1966.
11. Parker H, Jackson F: Hodgkin's disease and allied disorders. Oxford: Oxford University Press, 1947.
12. Custer RP, Bernhard WG: Interrelationship of Hodgkin's disease and other lymphatic tumors. Am J Med Sci 216:625–642, 1948.
13. Berman L: Malignant lymphomas, their classification and relation to leukemia. Blood 8:195–210, 1953.
14. Callender GR: Tumors and tumor-like conditions of the lymphocyte, the myelocyte, the erythrocyte and the reticulum cell. Am J Pathol 10:443–466, 1934.
15. Gall EA, Rappaport H: Seminar on diseases of lymph nodes and spleen. In: Proceedings of 23rd Seminar, American Society of Clinical Pathology, 1958, MacDonald JR, ed.
16. Rappaport H: Tumors of the hematopoietic system. Atlas of tumor pathology, section II, fascicle 8. Washington DC: Armed Forces Institute of pathology, 1966.
17. Jones SE, Fuks Z, Bull M, Kadin ME, Dorfman RF, Kaplan HS, Rosenberg SA, Kim H: Non-Hodgkin's lymphomas IV. Clinicopathologic correlation in 405 cases. Cancer 31:803–823, 1973.
18. Lukes RJ, Collins RD: Immunologic characterization of human malignant lymphomas. Cancer 34:1488–1503, 1974.
19. Lennert K, Mohri N, Stein H, Kaizerling E: Histopathology of malignant lymphomas. Br J Haematol 31:193–203, 1975.
20. Lukes RJ, Parker JW, Taylor CR, Tindle BH, Cramer AD, Lincoln TL: Immunologic approach to non-Hodgkin lymphomas and related leukemias. Analysis of the results of multiparameter studies of 425 cases. Semin Hematol 15:322–351, 1978.
21. Berard CW: Changing concepts and classification of the lymphomas a common language. Personal communication.
22. Tindle BH, Parker JW, Lukes RJ: 'Reed-Sternberg cells' in infectious mononucleosis? Am J Clin Pathol 58:607–617, 1972.
23. Slaughter DP, Economous SG, Southwick HW: Surgical management of Hodgkin's disease. Ann Surg 148:705–710, 1958.

24. Tao LC, Pearson FG, Delarue NC, Langer B, Sanders DE: Percutaneous llne-needle aspiration biopsy. I. Its value to clinical practice. Cancer 45:1480–1485, 1980.
25. Sinner WN: Pulmonary neoplasms diagnosed with transthoracic needle biopsy. Cancer 43:1533–1540, 1979.
26. Zajicek K: Aspiration cytology, part I. Cytology of supradiaphragmatic organs. Monographs in clinical cytology 4. New York: Karger, 1974, pp 97–107.
27. Betsill WL, Hajdu Si: Percutaneous aspiration biopsy of lymph node. Am J Clin Pathol 73:471–479, 1980.
28. Frable WJ, Frable MAS: Thin-needle aspiration biopsy. The diagnosis of head and neck tumors revisited. Cancer 43:1541–1548, 1979.
29. Bowling MC: Lymph node specimens: achieving technical excellence. Lab Med 10:467–467, 1979.
30. Barcos MP, Lukes RJ: Malignant lymphoma of convoluted lymphocytes. A new entity of possible T-cell type. In: Conflicts in childhood cancer, Sinks LF, Godden JE, eds. New York: Alan R Liss, 1975, pp 147–178.
31. Lutzner M, Edelson R, Schein P, Green I, Kirkpatrick C, Ahmed A: Cutaneous T-cell lymphomas: the Sézary syndrome, mycosis fungoides, and related disorders. Ann Intern Med 83:534–552, 1975.
32. Rosas-Urbide A, Variakajis D, Molnar Z, Rappaport H: Mycosis fungoides: an ultrastructural study. Cancer 34:634–645, 1974.
33. Pinkus GS, Said JW, Hargreaves H: Malignant lymphoma, T-cell type. A distinct morphologic variant with large multilobated nuclei, with a report of 4 cases. Am J Clin Pathol 72:540–550, 1979.
34. Tindle BH, Long J: Case records of the Massachusetts General Hospital. Case 30, 1977. N Eng J Med 297:206–211, 1977.
35. Said JW, Hargreaves Hk, Pinkus GS: Non-Hodgkin's lymphomas: an ultrastructural study correlating morphology and immunologic cell type. Cancer 44:504–528, 1979.
36. Levine GD, Dorfman RF: Nodular lymphoma: an ultrastructural study of its relationship to germinal centers and a correlation of light and electron microscopic findings. Cancer 35:148–164, 1975.
37. Sokol RJ, Durrant TE, Lambourne CA, Hudson G: Scanning electromicroscopy of exudative macrophages in malignant lymphomas. Scand J Haematol 22:129–140, 1979.
38. Skinnider LF: Scanning electron microscopic study follicular lymphoma. Arch Pathol Lab Med 103:276–278, 1979.
39. Pierce A, Everson G: Histochemistry, theoretical and applied, Vol I. Boston: Little-Brown, 1968, p 307.
40. d'Ablaing G, Rogers ER, Parker JW, Lukes RJ: A simplified and modified methyl green pyronin stain. Am J Clin Pathol 54:667–669, 1970.
41. Li CY, Yam LC, Lam KW: Studies of acid phosphatase isoenzyme in human leukocytes. Demonstration of isoenzyme cell specificity. J Histochem Cytochem 18:473–480, 1970.
42. Tamaoki M, Essner E: Distribution of acid phosphatase, beta-glucuronidase and M-acetyl-beta-glycosaminidase activities in lymphocytes of lymphatic tissue of man and rodents. J Histochem Cytochem 17:238–243, 1969.
43. Catovsky D: T-cell origin of acid phosphatase positive lymphoblasts. Lancet II:327–328, 1975.
44. Basso G, Cocito MG, Semenzato G, Pezzutto A, Zanesco: Cytochemical study of thymocytes and T lymphocytes. Br J Haematol 44:577–582, 1980.
45. Yam LT, Li CY, Lam KW: Tartrate-resistant acid phosphatase isoenzymes in the reticulum cells of leukemic reticuloendotheliosis. N Eng J Med 284:357–363, 1971.
46. Nanba K, Jaffe ES, Braylan RC, Soban EJ, Berard CW: Alkaline phosphatase-positive malignant lymphoma. A subtype of B-cell lymphomas. Am J Clin Pathol 68:535–542, 1977.

47. Li CY, Lam KW, Yam LT: Esterase in human leukocytes. J Histochem Cytochem 21:1–12, 1973.

48. Bennett JM, Reed CE: Acute leukemia cytochemical profite: diagnostic and clinical implications. In: Unclassifiable leukemias, Bessis M, Brecker G (eds). New York: Springer-Verlag, 1975, pp 101–113.

49. Hayhoe FGJ: Cytochemical aspects of leukemia and lymphoma. In: Leukemia and lymphoma, Holland JF, Miescher PA, Jaffe ERE (eds). New York: Grune & Stratton, 1969, pp 37–38.

50. Dacie JC, Lewis SM: Practical hematology, 5th edn. Edinburgh: Churchill Livingstone, 1975, p 120.

51. Berard CW, O'Connor GT, Thomas LB, Torloni H: Histopathological definition of Burkitt's tumor. Bull WHO 40:601–607, 1969.

52. Lukes RJ, Collins RD: New approaches to the classification of the lymphomata. Br J Cancer 31:Suppl II:1–28, 1975.

53. Lukes RJ: The immunologic approach to the pathology of malignant lymphomas. Am J Clin Pathol 72:657–669, 1979.

54. Ault KA, Karnovsky MJ, Unanue ER: Studies on the distribution of surface immunoglobulin on human B-lymphocytes. J Clin Invest 52:2507–1516, 1973.

55. Berken A, Benacerraf B: Properties of antibodies cytophilic for macrophages. J Exp Med 123:119–144, 1966.

56. Bianco C, Patrick R, Mussenzweig V: A population of lymphocytes bearing a membrane receptor for antigen-antibody-implement complexes: I. Separation and characterization. J Exp Med 132:702–720, 1970.

57. Beain P, Gordon J, Willetts WA: Rosette formation by peripheral lymphocytes. Clin Exp Immunol 6:681–688, 1970.

58. Dickles HB, Kunkel HG: Interaction of aggregated globulin with B lymphocytes. J Exp Med 136:191–196, 1972.

59. Raff MC: Two distinct populations of peripheral lymphocytes in mice distinguishable by immunofluorescence. Immunology 19:637–650, 1970.

60. Shevach EM, Herberman R, Frank MM, Green I: Receptors for complement and immunoglobulin on human leukemic cells and human lymphoblastoid cell lines. J Clin Invest 51:1933–1938, 1972.

61. Unanue ER, Grey HM, Rabellino E, Campell P, Schmidtke J: Immunoglobulins on the surface of lymphocytes: II. The bone marrow as the main source of lymphocytes with detectable surface-bound immunoglobulin. J Exp Med 133:1188–1198, 1971.

62. Weiner MS, Bianco C, Nussenzweig V: Enhanced binding of neuraminidase-treated sheep erythrocytes to human T lymphocytes. Blood 42:939–949, 1973.

63. Wybran J, Carr MC, Fudenberg HH: The human rosette-forming cell as a marker of a population of thymus-derived cells. J Clin Invest 51:2537–2543, 1972.

64. Jondal M, Holm G, Wigzell H: Surface markers on human T and B lymphocytes: I. A large population of lymphocytes forming non-immune rosettes with sheep red blood cells. J Exp Med 136:207–215, 1972.

65. Lay WH, Nussenzweig V: Receptors for complement on leukocytes. J Exp Med 128:991–1007, 1968.

66. Leech JH, Glick AD, Waldron JA, Flexner JM, Horn RD, Collins RD: Malignant lymphomas of follicular center cell origin in man. I. Immunologic studies. J Natl Cancer Inst 54:11–21, 1975.

67. Mason DY, Taylor CR: The distribution of muramidase (lyzosome) in human tissues. J Clin Pathol 28:124–132, 1975.

68. Halper JP, Knowles DM II, Wang CY: Ia antigen expression by human malignant lymphomas: correlation with conventional markers. Blood 55:373–382, 1980.

69. Pinkus GS, Said JW: Characterization of non-Hodgkin's lymphomas using multiple cell markers: immunologic morphologic and cytochemical studies of 72 cases. Am J Pathol 94:349-377, 1979.

70. Ross GD: Identification of human lymphocyte subpopulations by surface marker analysis. Blood 53:799-811, 1979.

71. Lukes RJ, Taylor CR, Parker JW, Lincoln TL, Pettengale Pk, Tindle BH: A morphologic and immunologic surface marker study of 299 non-Hodgkin lymphomas and related leukemias. Am J Pathol 90:461-486, 1978.

72. Stein H: The immunologic and immunochemical basis for the Kiel classification. In: Malignant lymphomas other than Hodgkin's disease, Lennert K, ed. New York: Springer-Verlag 1978, pp 529-657.

73. Whiteside T, Rowlands DT: T-cell and B-cell identification in the diagnosis of lympho-proliferative disease. A review. Am J Pathol 88:754-792, 1977.

74. Evans RL, Lazarus H, Penta AC, Schlossman SF: Two functionally distinct subpopulations of human T cells that collaborate in the generation of cytotoxic cells responsible for cell-mediated lympholysis. J Immunol 120:1423-1428, 1978.

75. Reinherz EL, Schlossman SF: Con A-inducible suppression of MLC: evidence for mediation by the TH2+ T cell subset in man. J Immunol 122:1423-1428, 1979.

76. Reinherz EL, Streikaukas AJ, O'Brien C, Schlossman SF: Phenotypic and functional distinctions between the TH2+ and JRA+ T cell subsets in man. J Immunol 123:83-86, 1979.

77. Reinherz EL, Kung PC, Goldstein G, Schlossman SF: Separation of subsets of human T cells by a monoclonal antibody. Proc Natl Acad Sci 76:4061-4065, 1979.

78. Reinherz EL, Kung PC, Goldstein G, Schlossman SF: Further characterization of the human inducer T cell subset defined by monoclonal antibody. J Immunol 123:2894-2896, 1979.

79. Reinherz EL, Kung PC, Goldstein G, Schlossman SF: A monoclonal antibody reactive with the human cytotoxic-suppressor T cell subset previously defined by a heteroantiserum termed TH. J Immunol 124:1301-1307, 1980.

80. Shevach EM, Jaffe ES, Green I: Receptors for complement and immunoglobulin on human and animal lymphoid cells. Transplant Rev 16:3-28, 1973.

81. Brown G, Greaves MFb: Enumeration of absolute numbers of T and B lymphocytes in human blood. Scand J Immunol 3:161, 1974.

82. Taylor, CR: Results of multiparameter studies of B-cell lymphomas. Am J Clin Pathol 72:687-698, 1979.

83. Grossi CE, Webb SR, Zicca A: Morphological and histochemical analyses of two human T-cell subpopulations bearing receptors for IgM and IgG. J Exp Med 147:1405-1417, 1978.

84. Taylor CR: Hodgkin's disease and the lymphomas, Vols 1, 2 and 3,. In: Annual research reviews, Horrobin DF, ed. Montreal: Eden Press, 1976, 1977, 1978; Edinburgh/London: Churchill, Longman, Livingstone, 1977, 1978, 1979.

85. Humphreys RE, McCune SM, Chess L: Isolation and immunologic characterization of a human B-lymphocyte specific, cell surface antigen. J Exp Med 144:98-112, 1976.

86. Arbect RD, Sacks DH, Amos DB, Dickler HD: Human lymphocyte alloantigen(s) similar to murine Ir region-associated (Ia) antigens. J Immunol 115:173-1175, 1975.

87. Billing R, Rafizadeh B, Drew I, Hartman G, Gale R, Terasau P: Human B lymphocyte antigens expressed by lymphocytic and myelocytic leukemia cells. I. Detection by rabbit antisera. J Exp Med 144:167-168, 1978.

88. Taylor CR: Immunocytochemical methods in the study of lymphoma and related conditions. J Histochem Cytochem 26:496-503, 1978.

89. Taylor CR: Immunohistological approach to tumor diagnosis. Oncology 35:189-197, 1978.

90. Nilsson K, Ponten J: Classification and biological nature of established human hemato-poietic cell lines. Int J cancer 15:321–327, 1975.

91. Cunningham-Rundles S, Hanier J, Dupont B: Lymphocyte transformation in vitro in response to mitogens and antigens. In: Clinical immunology, Vol 3, Back F, Good R, eds. New York: Academic Press 1976, p 151.

92. Shackney SE, Erickson B, Lukes RJ, Lincoln TL: Analysis of non-Hodgkin's lymphomas in dual parameter flow cytofluormetry (FCF). In: Proc 68th Ann Mtg Am Ass Cancer Res, Denver, Colorado 18:60, 1977.

93. Lukes RJ, Lincoln TL, Parker JW, Alavaikko MJ: An immunologic aproach to classification of malignant lymphomas: a cytokinetic model of lymphoid neoplasia. In: Differentiation of normal and neoplastic hematopoietic cells. Cold Spring Harbor Laboratory, 1978, pp 935–952.

94. Shackney SE, Skramstad K: A dynamic interpretation of multiparameter studies in the lymphomas. Am J Clin Pathol 72:756–764, 1979.

95. Rowley JD: Chromosomes in leukemia and lymphoma. Semin Hematol 15:301–319, 1978.

96. Fleischman EW, Prigognina El: Karyotype peculiarities of malignant lymphomas. Hum Genet 35:269–279, 1971.

97. Hossfeld DK, Schmidt CG: Chromosome findings in effusions from patients with Hodgkin's disease. Int J Cancer 21:1947–1956, 1978.

98. Fukuhara S, Rowley RD: Chromosome translocations in non-Burkitt's lymphomas. Int J Cancer 22:14–21, 1978.

99. Fukuhara S: Significance of 14g translocations in non-Hodgkin's lymphomas. Virchows Arch B Cell Pathol 29:99–106, 1978.

100. Douglass EC, Magraph IT, Lee EC, Whang-Ping J: Cytogenetic studies in non-African Burkitt lymphoma. Blood 55:148–155, 1980.

101. Chang LMS: Development of terminal deoxynucleotidyl transferase activity in embryonic calf thymus gland. Biochem Biophys Res Commun 44:124–131, 1971.

102. Coleman MS, Hulton JT, DeSimone P, Ballum FJ: Terminal deoxynucleotidyl transferase in human leukemia. Proc Natl Acad Sci USA 71:4404–4408, 1974.

103. Ballum FJ: Terminal deoxynucleotidyl transferase as a hematopoietic cell marker. Blood 54:1203–1215, 1979.

104. Staff SA, Veach S, Pasqual SM, Schumacker HR, Keneklas TP, Ballum FJ: Terminal deoxynucleotidyl transferase positive acute lymphoblastic leukemia with Auer rods. Lancet 1:1042–1043, 1978.

105. Marks SM, Baltimore D, McCaffrey R: Terminal transferase: a prediction of initial responsiveness to Vincristine and prednisone in blastic crisis in myelogenous leukemia. N Engl J Med 298:812–814, 1978.

106. Wilks Sir S: Cases of enlargement of the lymphatic glands and spleen (or, Hodgkin's disease) with remarks. Guy's Hosp Rep 11:56–78, 1865.

107. Reed DM: On the pathological changes in Hodgkin's disease with special reference to its relation to tuberculosis. Johns Hopkins Hosp Rep 10:133–140, 1902.

108. Robb-Smith AHT: Reticulosis and reticulosarcoma: a histologic classification. J Pathol Bact 47:457–480, 1938.

109. Kaplan HS, Smithers DW: Auto-immunity in man and homologous disease in mice in relation to the malignant lymphomas. Lancet 2:1–4, 1959.

110. Vianna MJ, Greenwald P, Brady J, Dwork A, Dolan A, Mauro T, Davies JNP: Hodgkin's disease: cases with features of a community outbreak. Ann Int Med 77:169–180, 1972.

111. Davies JNP: Epidemics of Hodgkin's disease. In: Current problems in the epidemiology of cancer and lymphomas. Res Results Cancer Res 39:227–233, 1972.

112. Grufferman S, Cole P, Smith PG, Lukes, RJ: Hodgkin's disease in siblings. N Engl J Med 296:248–250, 1977.

113. Torres A, Martinez F, Gomez P, Gomez C, Garcia JM, Nunez-Roldan A: Simultaneous Hodgkin's disease in three siblings with identical HLA-genotype. Cancer 46:838-843, 1980.

114. Peckham MJ, Cooper EH: Proliferation characteristics of the various classes of cells in Hodgkin's disease. Cancer 24:135-147, 1969.

115. Lukes RJ: Criteria for involvement of lymph node, bone marrow, spleen and liver in Hodgkin's disease. Cancer Res 31:1755-1767, 1971.

116. Seif GSF, Spriggs AI: Chromosome changes in Hodgkin's disease. J Natl Cancer Inst 39:557-570, 1967.

117. Boecker WF, Hossfeld DK, Gallneir WM, Schmidt CG: Clonal growth of Hodgkin cells. Nature 258:235-236, 1976.

118. Order SE, Hellman S: Pathogenesis of Hodgkin's disease. Lancet 1:571-573, 1970.

119. Johansson B, Klein G, Henle W, Henle G: Epstein-Barr virus (EBV) associated antibody pattern in malignant lymphomas and leukemias. I. Hodgkin's disease. Int J Cancer 6:450-462, 1970.

120. Goldman JM, Aisenberg AC: Incidence of antibody to EB virus, herpes simplex and cytomegalo virus in Hodgkin's disease. Cancer 26:327-331, 1970.

121. Mochanko K, Fejo M, Breazarsick P, Swarez A, Bachman AE: The relation between Epstein-Barr virus antibodies and clinical symptomatology and immunodeficiency in patients with Hodgkin's disease. Cancer 44:2065-2070, 1979.

122. Bichel J: Postvaccinial lymphadenitis developing into Hodgkin's disease. Acta Med Scand 199:523-525, 1976.

123. Kelly WD, Lamb DL, Galton DA, Varco RL: An investigation of Hodgkin's disease with respect to the problem of homotransplantation. Ann NY Acad Sci 87:187-202, 1960.

124. Aisenberg AC: Studies on delayed hypersensitivity in Hodgkin's disease. J Clin Invest 41:1964-1970, 1962.

125. Aisenberg AC: Hodgkin's disease - prognosis, treatment and etiological and immunologic considerations. N Engl J Med 270:508-514, 1964.

126. Aisenberg AC: Immunologic status of Hodgkin's disease. Cancer 19:385-391, 1966.

127. Casazza AR, Duvall CP, Carbone PP: Summary of infectious complications occurring in patients with Hodgkin's disease. Cancer Res 26:1290-1296, 1966.

128. Eltringham JR, Kaplan HS: Impaired delayed hypersensitivity responses in 154 patients with untreated Hodgkin's disease. Natl Cancer Inst Monogr 36:107-115, 1973.

129. Sugden PJ, Lilleyman JS: Impairment of lymphocyte transformation by plasma from patients with advanced Hodgkin's disease. Cancer 45:899-905, 1980.

130. Wegener OJ Th, Geestman E, Bosjonjen H: T and B lymphocytes in spleens in Hodgkin's disease. Lancet 1:1378-1379, 1975.

131. Holm G, Millstedt H, Bjorkholm M, Johansson B, Killander D, Sundblod R, Soderberg G: Lymphocyte abnormalities in untreated patients with Hodgkin's disease. Cancer 37:751-762, 1976.

132. Gajl-Peczalska KJ, Bloomfield CD, Soson H, Kersey JH: B and T lymphocytes in Hodgkin's disease; analysis at diagnosis and following therapy. Clin Exp Immunol 23:47-55, 1976.

133. Lang JM, Bigel P, Oberling F, Mayer SE: Decreased active rosette-forming cells during remission in Hodgkin's disease. Biomedicine 29:83-84, 1978.

134. Willson JKV, Zaremba JL, Pretlow TG II: Functional characterization of cells separated from suspensions of Hodgkin's disease tumor cells in an isokinetic gradient. Blood 50:783-798, 1977.

135. Pinkus GS, Barbrito D, Said JW, Churchill WH: Lymphocyte subpopulations of lymph nodes and spleens in Hodgkin's disease. Cancer 42:1270-1279, 1978.

136. Taylor CR: A history of the Reed-Sternberg cell. Biomedicine 28:198-203, 1978.

137. Lukes RJ: Relationship of histologic features to clinical stages in Hodgkin's disease. Am J Roent 90:944-955, 1963.

138. Lukes RJ, Butler BB, Hicks EB: Natural history of Hodgkin's disease as related to its pathologic picture. Cancer 19:317-344, 1966.

139. Rappaport H, Berard W, Butler JJ, Dorfman RF, Lukes RJ, Thomas LB: Report of the committee on histopathological criteria contributing to the staging of Hodgkin's disease. Cancer Res 31:1864-1865, 1971.

140. Rosenthal SA: Significance of tissue lymphocytes in prognosis of lymphogranulomatosis. Arch Pathol 21:628-643, 1936.

141. Berard CW, Thomas LB, Axtell LM, Kruse M, Nuvell G, Kagan R: The relationship of histopathologic subtype to clinical stage of Hodgkin's disease at diagnosis. Cancer Res 31:1776-1785, 1971.

142. Greenfield WS: Specimens illustrative of the pathology of lymphadenoma and leukocythaemia. Trans Path Soc London, 272, 1878.

143. Sternberg C: Über eine Eigenartige unter dem Bilde der preudoleukam Verlaufende. Tuberkulose des lymphatischen Apparates. Z Hulk 19:21, 1898.

144. Robb-Smith AHT: Reticuloses and reticulosarcoma: A histological classification. J Pathol Bact 47:457-480, 1938.

145. Strum SB, Park JK, Rappaport H: Observations of cells resembling Reed-Sternberg cells in conditions other than Hodgkin's disease. Cancer 26:176-190, 1970.

146. Tindle BH: The hematopoietic system. In: Surgical pathology, Coulson WC, ed. Philadelphia: JB Lippincott, 1978.

147. Taylor CR: An immunohistological study of follicular lymphoma, reticulum cell sarcoma and Hodgkin's disease. Europ J Cancer 12:61-75, 1976.

148. Reynes M, Paczynski V, Galtier M, Diebold J: Ultrastructural and Immunocytochemical localization of immunoglobulin synthesis in tumor cells in Hodgkin's disease. Int J Cancer 23:474-481, 1979.

149. Bouvet JJ, Buffe D, Oriol R, Liacopoulos P: Two myeloma globulins IgGi-lambda and IgGl-kappa from a single patient. II. Their common cellular origin as revealed by immunofluorescence studies. Immunology 2:1095-1101, 1974.

150. Preval C, de Fougereau M: Absence of preferential reassociation between heavy and light chains of two human immunoglobulins from common cellular origin. Biochem Biophys Res Comm 67:236-239, 1974.

151. Payne SV, Jones DB, Haegert DG, Smith JL, Wright DH: T and B lymphocytes and Reed-Sternberg cells in Hodgkin's disease lymph node and spleen. Clin Exp Immunol 24:280-286, 1976.

152. Landaas JO, Godal T, Halvorsen TB: Characterization of immunoglobulin in Hodgkin's cells. Int J Cancer 20:717-722, 1977.

153. Curran RC, Jones EL: Immunoglobulin in Reed-Sternberg and Hodgkin cells. J Path 126:35-37, 1978.

154. Poppema S, Elema JD, Halie MR: The significance of intracytoplasmic proteins in Reed-Sternberg cells. Cancer 42:1793-1893, 1978.

155. Staples WG, Visser AE: Hodgkin's disease – a 'B' neoplasm? S Afr Med J 54:186-188, 1978.

156. Biniaminou M, Ramoti B: Possible T Lymphocyte origin of Reed-Sternberg cells: Lancet 1:368, 1974.

157. Sinkovics JG, Schullenberger CC: Hodgkin's disease. Lancet 2:506-507, 1975.

158. Kaplan HS, Gartner S: Reed-Sternberg giant cells of Hodgkin's disease: cultivation in vitro heterotransplantation, and characterization as neoplastic macrophages. Int J Cancer 19:511-525, 1977.

159. Wilson JKV Jr, Zaremba JL, Pretlow TG: II. Functional characteristics of cells separated from suspensions of Hodgkin's disease tumor cells in an isokinetic gradient. Blood 50:783-797, 1977.

160. Kadin ME, Asbury AK: Long term culture of Hodgkin's tissue. A morphologic and radioautographic study. Lab Invest 28:181-192, 1973.

161. Kadin ME, Stiles DD, Levy R, Warnke R: Exogenous immunoglobulin and the macrophage origin of Reed-Sternberg cells in Hodgkin's disease. N Engl J Med 299:1208-1214, 1978.

162. Anagnostou DA, Parker JW, Taylor CR, Tindle BH, Lukes RJ: Lacunar cells of nodular sclerosing Hodgkin's disease. An ultrastructural and immunohistologic study. Cancer 39: 1032-1043, 1977.

163. Brooks JS: Leukoerythrophagocytosis by Reed-Sternberg cells in Hodgkin's disease. N Engl J Med 300:115-116, 1979.

164. Sherwin RP, Morgolick JB: Emperipolesis or phagocytosis in Reed-Sternberg cells? N Engl J Med 301:1348-1349, 1979.

165. Poppema S: Sternberg-Reed cells with intracytoplasmic lymphocytes: phagocytosis or emperipolesis? Virchows Arch Pathol Anat 380:355-359, 1979.

166. Archibald RB, Frenstee, JH: Quantitative ultrastructural analysis of *in vivo* lymphocyte-Reed-Sternberg cell interactions in Hodgkin's disease. Natl Cancer Inst Monogr 36:239-245, 1973.

167. Braylan RC, Jaffee ES, Berard CW: Surface characteristics of Hodgkin's lymphoma cells. Lancet 2:328-1329, 1974.

168. Kay MMB, Kadin M: Surface characteristics of Hodgkin's cells. Lancet 1:748-749, 1975.

169. Pretlow TG II: Isolation of lymphocyte populations. Natl Cancer Inst Monogr 49:79-84, 1978.

170. Belpomme D, Joseph R, Noruares L, Gearad-Marchant R, Huchet R, Botto I, Grandjon D, Mathe G: T cells and Reed-Sternberg cells in spleens of Hodgkin's disease. N Engl J Med 291:1417, 1974.

171. Bakowski RH, Noguchi S, Hewlett JS, Doadhar S: Lymphocyte transformation in Hodgkin's disease. Am J Clin Pathol 65:31-39, 1976.

172. Gajl-Peczalska KJ, Bloomfield CD, Sosin H, Kersey JH: B and T lymphocytes in Hodgkin's disease: Analysis at diagnosis and following therapy. Clin Exp Immunol 23:47-55, 1976.

173. Kaur J, Catowsky D, Spiers ASD, Galton DA: Increase of T lymphocytes in the spleen in Hodgkin's disease. Lancet 2:800-802, 1974.

174. Grifoni V, DelGiacco GS, Manconi PE, Tognella R, Mantonvani G: Lymphocytes in spleen in Hodgkin's disease. Lancet 1:332-333, 1975.

175. Payne SV, Jones DB, Haegert DG, Smith JL, Wright DH: T and B lymphocytes and Reed-Sternberg cells in Hodgkin's disease lymph nodes and spleen. Clin Exp Immunol 24:280-286, 1976.

176. Hunter CP, Pinkus GS, Woodward L, Maloney WC, Churchill WH: Increased T lymphocytes and Ig MEA receptor lymphocytes in Hodgkin's disease spleens. Cell Immunol 31:193-198, 1977.

177. Poppema S, Kaiserling E, Lennert K: Epidemiology of nodular paragranuloma (Hodgkin's disease with lymphocyte predominance, nodular). J Cancer Res Clin Oncol 95:57-63, 1979.

178. Neiman RS: Current problems in the histopathological diagnosis and classification of Hodgkin's disease. Pathology annual part 2, Sommers and Rosen, eds. New York: Appleton-Century-Crofts, 1978, pp 289-328.

179. Schnitzer B: Malignant lymphomas. Univ Mich Med Center J 36:23-28, 1970.

180. Lukes RJ: Prognosis and relationship of histologic features to clinical stage. In: Current cancer concepts. JAMA 190:914–915, 1964.
181. Franssela KO, Kalima TU, Voutelainen A: Histologic classification of Hodgkin's disease. Cancer 20:1954–1601, 1967.
182. Keller AR, Kaplan HS, Lukes RJ, Rappaport H: Correlation of histopathology with other prognostic indicators in Hodgkin's disease. Cancer 22:487–499, 1968.
183. Desforges JF, Rutherford EJ, Puo A: Hodgkin's disease. N Engl J Med 301:1212–1222, 1979.
184. Baroni CD, Malchiodi F: Histology, age, and sex distribution and pathologic correlations of Hodgkin's disease. A study of 184 cases observed in Rome, Italy. Cancer 45:1549–1555, 1980.
185. Churg J, Strauss L: Allergic granulomatosis, allergic angiitis and periarteritis nodosa. Am J Pathol 27:277–301, 1951.
186. Gorton G, Linill F: Malignant tumors and sarcoid reactions in regional lymph nodes. Acta Radiol 47:381–392, 1957.
187. Ohose NW: Delayed-type hypersensitivity and the immunology of Hodgkin's disease with a parallel examination of sarcoidosis. Cancer Res 26: Part I. 1097–2003, 1966.
188. Brincker H: Epithelioid-cell granulomas in Hodgkin's disease. Acta Path Microbiol Scand Sect A 78:19–32, 1970.
189. Kadin MF, Donaldson SS, Dorfman RF: Isolated granulomas in Hodgkin's disease. N Engl J Med 283:859–861, 1970.
190. Strum SB, Rappaport H: Significance of focal involvement of lymph nodes for the diagnosis and staging of Hodgkin's disease. Cancer 25:1314–1319, 1970.
191. Rappaport H, Berard CW, Butler JJ, Dorfman RF, Lukes RJ, Thomas LB: Report of the committee on histopathological criteria contributing to staging of Hodgkin's disease. Cancer Res 31:1864–1865, 1971.
192. Neiman RS, Rosen PJ, Lukes RJ: Lymphocyte-depletion Hodgkin's disease, a clinicopathologic entity. N Engl J Med 288:751–755, 1973.
193. Bearman RM, Pangalis GA, Rappaport H: Hodgkin's disease, lymphocyte depletion type. A clinicopathologic study of 39 patients. Cancer 41: 293–302, 1978.
194. Cross RM: A clinicopathological study of nodular sclerosing Hodgkin's disease. J Clin Pathol 21:303–330, 1968.
195. Keller AR, Kaplam HS, Lukes RJ, Rappaport H: Correlation of histopathology and other prognostic indicators in Hodgkin's disease. Cancer 22:487–499, 1968.
196. Patchesfsky AS, Brodousky H, Southard M, Menduke H, Gray S, Hock WS: Hodgkin's disease. A clinical and pathological study of 235 cases. Cancer 32:105–161, 1973.
197. Cionini L, Arganini L, Mugal V, Biti GP, Bondi R: Prognostic significance of histologic subdivision of Hodgkin's disease nodular sclerosis. Acta Radiol Oncol 17:65–73, 1978.
198. Musshoff K: Prognostic and therapeutic implications of staging in extranodal Hodgkin's disease. Cancer Res 31:1814–1827, 1971.
199. Rosenberg SA, Kaplan HS: Hodgkin's disease and other malignant lymphomas. Calif Med 113:23–38, 1970.
200. Bardhan KD, McArthur D, Righy C: Hodgkin's disease of the duodenum presenting with hemorrhage and perforation. Postgrad Med J 51:180–182, 1975.
201. Portmann VV, Dunne EF, Hazard JB: Manifestations of Hodgkin's disease of the gastrointestinal tract. Am J Roentgenol Radiother Nucl Med 72:772–787, 1954.
202. Elrich An, Slatder G, Galler W, Sherlock P: Gastrointestinal manifestations of malignant lymphoma. Gastroenterology 54:1115–1121, 1968.
203. Cuttner J, Meyer R, Huang YP: Intracerebral involvement in Hodgkin's disease. Cancer 43:1497–1506, 1979.
204. Reagan T, Derby B: Intracerebral Hodgkin's disease. Dis Nev Siples 32:843–847, 1971.

205. Parker JC Jr: Intramedullary spinal cord involvement in Hodgkin's disease with an atypical systemic distribution. Cancer 30:545-552, 1972.

206. Blubarb SM: Cutaneous manifestations of the malignant lymphomas. Sprinfield: Charles C. Thomas, 1960, pp 240-294.

207. Benninghoff DL, Medone A, Alexander L, Carmel MR: The mode of the spread of Hodgkin's disease to the skin. Cancer 26:1135-1140, 1970.

208. Smith JL, Butler JJ: Skin involvement in Hodgkin's disease. Cancer 45:354-361, 1980.

209. Szur L, Harrison CV, Levene GM, Sannmon DD: Primary cutaneous Hodgkin's disease. Lancet 1:1016-1020, 1970.

210. MacCaulay WL: Lymphomatoid papulosis. Int J Dermatol 17: 204-212, 1978.

211. Strum SB, Hutchinson GB, Park JK, Rappaport H: Further observations on the biologic significance of vascular invasion in Hodgkin's disease. Cancer 27:1-6, 1971.

212. Rappaport H, Strum SB: Vascular invasion in Hodgkin's disease: its incidence and relationship to the spread of the disease. Cancer 25:1304-1313, 1970.

213. Todd GB, Michaels L: Hodgkin's disease involving Waldeyer's lymphoid ring. Cancer 34:1769-1778, 1974.

214. Glatstein E, Guernsey JM, Rosenberg SA, Kaplan HS: The value of laparotomy and splenectomy in the staging of Hodgkin's disease. Cancer 24:709b-718, 1969.

215. Aisenberg A, Qazi R: Abdominal involvement at the onset of Hodgkin's disease. Am J Med 57:870-874, 1974.

216. Lee Y-TN, Lukes RJ, Fink EJ, Feinstein DT, Powers DR: Staging laparotomy and splenectomy for Hodgkin's disease. Am Surgeon 40:215-225, 1978.

217. Sweet DL, Kinnealey A, Ultmann JE: Hodgkin's disease: problems of staging. Cancer 42:957-970, 1978.

218. Tubiana M, Attie E, Flamant R, Gerard-Marchant R, Hayat M: Prognostic factors in 454 cases of Hodgkin's disease. Cancer Res 31:1801-1810, 1971.

219. Farrer-Brown G, Bennett MH, Harrizon CV, Millett Y, Jelliffe AM: The diagnosis of Hodgkin's disease in surgically excised spleens. J Clin Pathol 25:294-300, 1972.

220. Kim TH, Lui V, K.S, Woodruff RD, Ragab AH: The spleen in Hodgkin's disease. VM J Ped Hem/Oncol 2:53-60, 1980.

221. Kadin M, Glatstein E, Dorfman RF: Clinicopathologic study of 117 untreated patients subjected to laparotomy. cancer 24:1277-1294, 1971.

222. Michel J, Ardichrili D, Omerhouse M, Kenis Y, Heuson JC: Hodgkin's disease with massive liver involvement and uninvolved spleen. Europ J Cancer 9: 701-702, 1973.

223. Salks A, Benjamin RS, Luna MA: Liver replacement with Hodgkin's disease, lymphocyte-depleted type, with an uninvolved spleen. Europ J Cancer 15:373-377, 1979.

224. Connel MJ, Schimpt SF, Kirschner RH, Abt AB, Wernik PH: Epithelioid granulomas in Hodgkin's disease. A favorable prognostic sign? JAMA 233:886-889, 1975.

225. Sacks EL, Donaldson SS, Goedson J, Dorfman RF: Epithelioid granulomas associated with Hodgkin's disease. Cancer 41: 562-567, 1978.

226. Geogii AV, Konpil KF: Unspecific mesenchymal reaction in bone marrow in patients with Hodgkin's disease. In: Diagnosis and therapy of malignant lymphomas. Rec Res Cancer Res 46:39-44, 1974.

227. Oehlert W: The unspecific mesenchymal reaction of the liver in patients with Hodgkin's disease. In: Diagnosis and therapy of malignant lymphomas. Rec Res Cancer Res (46:31-38, 1974.

228. Champion M, Richards RL: Amyloidosis in Hodgkin's disease: a Scottish survey. Scot Med J 24:9-12, 1979.

229. Cardell BS: Role of cytologic agents in production of amyloidosis in Hodgkin's disease. Br Med J 1:1145-1148, 1961.

230. Falkson G, Falkson G, HC: Amyloidosis in Hodgkin's disease. S Afr Med J 47:62-64, 1973.

231. Hanson TAS: Histological classification and survival in Hodgkin's disease. A study of 251 cases with special reference to nodular sclerosing Hodgkin's disease. Cancer 17:1595-1603, 1964.

232. Lundberg T, Larson L: Hodgkin's disease. Retrospective clinicopathologic study of 149 cases. Acta Radiol 8:389-414, 1969.

233. Lehmann HJ: Prognostic significance of histopathology of Hodgkin's granuloma. Acta Pathol Microbiol Scand 64:16-30, 1965.

234. Colby TV, Warnke RA: The histology of the initial relapse of Hodgkin's disease. Cancer 45:289-292, 1980.

235. Friedman M, Kim U, Shimoka K, Panahon A, Han T, Stutman L: Appraisal of aspiration cytology in management of Hodgkin's disease. Cancer 45:1653-1663, 1980.

236. Lukes RJ: The pathologic picture of the malignant lymphomas. In: Proc Int Conf on Leukemia-Lymphoma. Philadelphia: Lea & Febiger, 1968, pp 333-356.

237. Lukes RJ: A review of the American concept of malignant lymphoma. In: Progress in lymphology, Ruttiman A, ed. Stuttgart: George Thieme, 1967, pp 109-120.

238. Gall EA: Enigmas in lymphoma, reticulum cell sarcoma and mycosis fungoides. Minn Med 38: 674-683, 1955.

239. Gall EA: The reticulum cell, the cytologic identity of mesenchymal cells of lymphoid tissue. N Y Acad Sci 73:120-130, 1958.

240. Warren S, Picena JP: Reticulum cell sarcoma of lymph nodes. Am J Pathol 17:385-394, 1941.

241. Nathwani BM, Kim H, Rappaport H: Malignant lymphoma, lymphoblastic. Cancer 38:964-983, 1976.

242. Richter MH: Generalized reticular cell sarcoma of lymph nodes associated with lymphatic leukemia. Am J Pathol 9:285-296, 1928.

243. Trump DL, Mann RB, Phelp R, Roberts H, Conley Cl: Richter's syndrome: diffuse histiocytic lymphoma in patients with chronic lymphatic leukemia. A report of 5 cases and review of the literature. Am J Med 68:539-548, 1980.

244. Gall EA, Mallory TB: Malignant lymphomas. A clinicopathologic survey of 618 cases. Am J Pathol 18:381-429, 1942.

245. Baehr G, Rosentahl N: Malignant lymph follicle hyperplasia of spleen and lymph nodes. Am J Pathol 3:550-551, 1927.

246. Symmers D: Giant follicular lymphadenopathy with or without splenomegaly. Its transformation into polymorphous cell sarcoma of the lymphofollicles and its association with Hodgkin's disease, lymphatic leukemia, and an apparently unique disease of the lymph node and spleen – a disease entity heretofore undescribed. Arch Pathol 26:603-647, 1938.

247. Gall EA, Morrison HR, Scott AT: The follicular type of malignant lymphoma; a survey of 63 cases. Ann Intern Med 14:2073-2085, 1941.

248. Brill NE, Baehr F, Rosenthal N: generalized giant lymph follicle hyperplasia of lymph nodes and spleen: a hitherto undescribed type. JAMA 84:668-671, 1925.

249. Symmers D: Follicular lymphadenopathy with splenomegaly: a newly recognized disease of the lymphatic system. Arch Pathol 3:816-820, 1927.

250. Rudders RA, Kaddis M, Dehellis RA, Casey H Jr: Nodular non-Hodgkin's lymphoma (NHL): Factors influencing prognosis and indications for aggressive treatment. Cancer 43:1643-1651, 1979.

251. Portlock CS, Rosenberg SA: Chemotherapy of the non-Hodgkin's lymphomas: the Stanford experience. Cancer Treatment Reports 61:1049-1055, 1977.

252. Ezdinli EZ, Costello WG, Icli F, Silverstein M, Berard CW, Bennett JM, Carbone PP: Nodular mixed lymphocytic-histiocytic lymphoma (N.M.) response and survival. Cancer 45:261-267, 1980.

253. Jones SE, Fuks Z, Bull M, Kadin ME, Dorfman RF, Kaplan HS, Rosenberg SA, Kim H: Non-Hodgkin's lymphomas IV. Clinicopathologic correlation. Cancer 31:806-823, 1973.

254. Patchefsky As, Brodovsky HS, Menduke A, Southard M, Brooks J, Nichlos D, Hock WS: Non-Hodgkin's lymphomas. A clinicopathologic study of 293 cases. Cancer 34:1173-1186, 1974.

255. Rosenberg SA, Kaplan HS: Clinical trials in the non-Hodgkin's lymphomata at Stanford University: experimental design and preliminary results. Br J Cancer 31:Suppl II. 456-464, 1975.

256. Rappaport H: Tumors of the hematopoietic system. Atlas of tumor pathology, sect III, fascicle 8. Washington, DC: Armed Forces Institute of Pathology, 1966, p 428.

257. Jaffee ES, Shevach EM, Frank MM, Berard CW, Green I: Nodular lymphoma: evidence for origin from follicular B lymphocytes. N Engl J Med 290:813-819, 1974.

258. Leech JH, Glick AD, Waldron JA, Flexner JM, Horn RG, Collins RD: Malignant lymphomas of follicular center cell origin in man I. Immunologic studies. J Natl Cancer Inst 54:11-21, 1975.

259. Warnke RA, Kim H, Fuks Z, Dorfman RF: Immunology of follicular lymphomas: a model of B-lymphocyte homing. N Engl J Med 298:481-486, 1978.

260. Peters MV: The contribution of radiation therapy in the control of early lymphomas. Am J Roentgen 90:956-967, 1963.

261. Taylor CR: Classification of lymphoma: 'new thinking' on old thoughts. Arch Pathol Lab Med 102:549-554, 1978.

262. Bennett MY, Farrer-Brown G, Henry K: Classification of non-Hodgkin's lymphomas. Lancet 2:405-406, 1974.

263. Dorfman RF: Classification of non-Hodgkin's lymphomas. Lancet 1:1295-1296, 1974.

264. Mathe G, Belpomme D, Dantcher D, Puoillart P: Progress in the classification of lymphoid and/or monocytoid leukaemias of lympho and reticulosarcomas (non-Hodgkin's lymphomas). Biomedicine 22:177-185, 1975.

265. Mathe G, Rappaport H, O'Conor GT, Totloni H: Histological and cytological typing of neoplastic diseases of hematopoietic and lymphoid tissues. In: WHO international histological classification of tumors, No. 14. Geneva: World Health Organization, 1976.

266. Mann RB, Jaffee ES, Berard CW: Malignant lymphomas – a conceptional understanding of morphologic diversity – a review. Am J Pathol 94:105-192, 1979.

267. Nathwani BN, Kim H, Rappaport H, Solomon J, Fox M: Non-Hodgkin's lymphomas, a clinicopathologic study comparing two classifications. Cancer 41:303-325, 1978.

268. Nathwani BN: A critical analysis of the classification of non-Hodgkin's lymphomas. Cancer 44:347-384, 1979.

269. Ezdinli EZ, Costello W, Wasse LP, Lenhard RE, Berard CW, Hartsock R, Bennett JM, Carbone PP: Eastern Cooperative Oncology Group experience with the Rappaport classification of non-Hodgkin's lymphomas. Cancer 43:544-550, 1979.

270. Lukes RJ, Collins RD: A functional approach to the classification of the lymphomas. Rec Res Cancer Res 46:18-30, 1974.

271. Lukes RJ, Collins RD: Immunologic characterization of human malignant tumors. Cancer 34:1488-1503, 1974.

272. Stein N, Lennert K, Parwareschi MR: Malignant lymphomas of B-cell type. Lancet 1:855-858, 1972.

273. Frizzera G, Gajl-Peczalska KJ, Bloomfield CD, Kersey JH: Predictability of immunologic phenotype of malignant lymphomas by conventional morphology – a study of 60 cases. Cancer 43:1216-1224, 1979.

275. Galton DAG, Catovsky D, Wiltshaw E: Clinical spectrum of lymphoproliferative diseases. Cancer 42:901-910, 1978.

276. Risdall R, Hoppe RT, Warnke R: Non-Hodgkin's lymphomas, a study of the evaluation of disease based on 92 autopsied cases. Cancer 44:529–542, 1979.
277. DeVita VT Jr, Canellos GP, Chabner B: Advanced diffuse histocytic lymphoma, a potentially curable disease: results with combination chemotherapy. Lancet 1:248–250, 1975.
278. Strauchen JA, Young RE, DeVita VT, Anderson T, Fantone JC, Berard CW: Clinical relevance of the histopathological subclassification of diffuse 'histiocytic' lymphoma. N Engl J Med 299:1382–1387, 1978.
279. Bitran JD, Kinzie J, Sweet DL, Variakojis D, Griem ML, Golomb HM, Miller JB, Oetzel N, Ultmann JE: Survival of patients with localized histiocytic lymphoma. Cancer 39:342–346, 1977.
280. Warnke R, Miller R, Grogan T, Pederson M, Dilley J, Levy R: Immunologic phenotype in 30 patients with diffuse large-cell lymphoma. N Engl J Med 303:293–300, 1980.
281. Burkitt D: A sarcoma involving the jaws in African children. Br J Surg 46:218–223, 1958.
282. Klein E, Klein G, Nadkarni JS, Nadkarni JJ, Wigzell H, Clifford P: Surface IgM-kappa specificity on a Burkitt lymphomas cell *in vivo* and in derived cell lines. Cancer Res 28:1300–1310, 1968.
283. Lukes RJ, Parker JW, Taylor CR, Tindle BH, Cramer AD, Lincoln TL: Immunologic approach to non-Hodgkin's lymphomas and related leukemias. Analysis of the results of multiparameter studies of 425 cases. Semin Hematol 5:322–351, 1978.
284. Bom-van Noorloos AAAB-v, Splinter TAW, van Heede P, van-Beek AAM, Melief CJM: Surface markers and functional properties of non-Hodgkin's lymphoma cells in relation to histology. Cancer 42:1804–1817, 1978.
285. Dorfman RF: The non-Hodgkin's lymphomas. In: The reticuloendothelial system. IAP Monograph No. 16, Rebuck JW, Berard CW, Abell MR, eds. Baltimore: Williams & Wilkins, 1975, pp 262–281.
286. Pangalis GA, Nathwani BM, Rappaport H: Malignant lymphoma, well differentiated lymphocytic; its relationship with chronic lymphocytic leukemia and macroglobulinemia of Waldenstrom. Cancer 39:999–1010, 1977.
287. Dorfman RF: Pathology of the non-Hodgkin's lymphomas: new classifications. Cancer Treat Rep 61:945–951, 1977.
288. McKenna RW, Parkin I, Kersey JH, Gajl-Peczalska KJ, Peterson L, Brunning RD: Chronic lymphoproliferative disorder with unusual clinical, morphologic, ultrastructural and membrane surface marker characteristics. Am J Med 62:588–596, 1977.
289. Cone L, Uhr JW: Immunological deficiency disorders associated with chronic lymphocytic leukemia and multiple myeloma. J Clin Invest 43:2241–2248, 1964.
290. Brunning RO, Parkin J: Intranuclear inclusions in plasma cells and lymphocytes from patients with monoclonal gammopathies. Am J Clin Pathol 66:10–21, 1976.
291. Dutcher TF, Fahey JL: The histopathology of the macroglobulinemia of Waldenstrom. J Natl Can Inst 22:887–917, 1959.
292. Waldenstrom J: Incipient myelomatosis or 'essential' hyperglobulinemia with fibrinogeno-penia – a new syndrome? Acta Med Scan 117:216–247, 1944.
293. Forget BG, Squires JW, Sheldon H: Waldenstrom's macroglobulinemia with generalized amyloidosis. Arch Int Med 118:363–378, 1966.
294. Bottomly JP, Bradley J, Whitehouse GH: Waldenstrom's macroglobulinemia and amyloidosis with subcutaneous calcification and lymphographic appearances. Br J Radiol 17:232–235, 1974.
295. Steven DW, Whitehouse GH: Waldenstrom's macroglobulinemia with amyloidosis – lymphographic findings. Lymphology 9:142–144, 1976.
296. Schedel I, Peest D, Stichkel K, Friche M, Eckert G, Deisher H: Idiotype-bearing peripheral blood lymphocytes in human multiple myeloma and Waldenstrom's macroglobulinemia. Scan J Immunol 11:437–444, 1980.

297. Lukes RJ, Tindle BH: Immunoblastic lymphadenopathy. A new hyperimmune entity resembling Hodgkin's disease. N Engl J Med 292:1-8, 1975.

298. Nathwani BN, Rappaport H, Moran EM, Pangalis GA, Kim H: Malignant lymphoma arising in angioimmunoblastic lymphadenopathy Cancer 41:578-606, 1978.

299. Fisher RI, Jaffee ES, Braylan RC, Anderson JC, Tan HK: Immunoblastic lymphadenopathy evolution into a malignant lymphoma with plasmacytoid features. Am J Med 61:553-559, 1976.

300. Fayemi AO, Ali M, Brown EV, DeCecio T: Angioimmunoblastic lymphadenopathy: termination as diffuse lymphosarcoma with plasmacytoid features. Mt Sinai J Med 46:39-43, 1979.

301. Jones SE, Griffith K, Dombronski P, Gaine JA: Immunodeficiency in patients with non-Hodgkin's lymphoma. Blood 49:335-344, 1977.

302. Penn I: Malignant tumors in organ transplant recipients. Berlin: Springer-Verlag, 1970.

303. Penn I: Tumors arising in transplant recipients. In: Advances in cancer research, Klein G, Weinhouse S, eds. New York: Academic Press 1978, vol 28, pp 31-61.

304. Isomaki HA, Hakulinen T, Joutsenlahti U: Excess risk of lymphomas, leukemias and myelomas in patients with rheumatoid arthritis. J Chron Dis 31:691-696, 1978.

305. Pierce DA, Stern R, Jaffee R, Zulman J, Talal M: Immunoblastic sarcoma with features of Sjogren's syndrome and systemic lupus erythematosus in a patient with immunoblastic lymphadenopathy. Arthritis and Rheumatism 22:911-916, 1979.

306. Aizawa Y, Zawadzki ZA, Micolonghi TS, McDowell JW, Neiman RS: Vasculitis and Sjogren's syndrome with IgA-IgG cryoglobulinemia terminating in immunoblastic sarcoma. Am J Med 67:160-166, 1979.

307. Lukes RJ, Parker JW: The pathology of lymphoreticular neophasms. In: The immunopathology of lymphoreticular neoplasms, Twomey JJ, Good RA, eds. New York: Plenum Medical, 1978, PP 239-279.

308. Lukes RJ: Lymphomas in childhood. A review of 114 cases. Personal communication.

309. Bennett MH, Millett YL: Modular sclerotic lymphosarcoma, a possible new clinicopathologicial entity. Clin Radiol 20:339-346, 1969.

310. Bennett MH: Sclerosis in non-Hodgkin's lymphomata. Br J Cancer 31:Suppe II, 44-52, 1975.

311. Mann RD, Jaffee ES, Braylan RC, Nanba K, Ziegler JL, Berard CW: Non-endemic Burkitt's lymphoma: a B cell tumor related to germinal centers. N Engl J Med 295:685-691, 1976.

312. Flandrin G, Brouet JC, Daniel MT, Preud'homme JL: Acute leukemia with Burkitt tumor cells. A study of six cases with special reference to lymphocyte surface markers. Blood 45:183-188, 1975.

313. Prokocimer M, Matzner Y, Ben-Bassat H, Polliack A: Burkitt's lymphomas presenting as acute leukemia. (Burkitt's lymphoma cell leukemia). Report of two cases in Israel. Cancer 45:2884-2889, 1980.

314. Ioachim HL, Finkbeimer JA: Pseudonodular pattern of T-cell lymphoma. Cancer 45:1370-1378, 1980.

315. Nair KG, Han TH, Minowada J: T-cell chronic lymphocytic leukemia. Report of a case and review of the literature. Cancer 44:1652-1655, 1979.

316. Lennert K: Chronic lymphocytic leukemia, T-cell type (T-CLL). In: Malignant lymphomas other than Hodgkin's disease. New York: Springer-Verlag 1978, pp 141-145.

317. Vchiyama T, Yodoi S, Sagawa, Takatsuki K, Uchino H: Adult T-cell leukemia: clinical and hematologic features of 16 cases. Blood 50:481-492, 1977.

318. Brouet JC, Flandrin G, Sasportes M, Preud'homme JL, Seligmann M: Chronic lymphocytic leukemia of T-cell origin. Immunological and clinical evaluation in eleven patients. Lancet 2:890-894, 1975.

319. Rosen PJ, Feinstein DJ, Pattengale PK, Tindle BH, Williams AH, Cain MJ, Bonnorris JB, Parker JW, Lukes RJ: Convoluted lymphocytic lymphoma in adults; a clinicopathologic entity. Ann Int Med 80:319-324, 1978.

320. Long JC, McCaffrey RP, Aisenberg AC, Marks SM, Kung PC: Terminal desoxynucleotidal transferase positive lymphoblastic lymphomas in a study of 15 cases. Cancer 440:2127-2139, 1979.

321. Boucheix CB, Brebold S, Bermadon A, Reynes M, Tulbrez M, Cadion M, Paczynski V, Capron F, Bilski-Pasquier G: Lymphoblastic lymphoma/leukemia with convoluted nuclei. The question of its relation to the T-cell lineage studied in 13 patients. Cancer 45:1569-1577, 1980.

322. Broome JP, Zucker-Franklin D, Weiner MS, Bianco S, Nunen-Zweig V: Leukemia cells with membrane properties of thymus derived (T) lymphocytes in a case of Sézary's syndrome: morphologic and immunological studies. Clin Immunol Immunopath 40:319-329, 1973.

323. Brouet VC, Flandrin G, Seligmann M: Indications for the thymus derived nature of the proliferating cells in six patients with Sézary's syndrome. N Engl J Med 289:341-344, 1973.

324. Edelson RL, Kirkpatrick CH, Shevach EM, Schein PS, Smith RW, Green I, Lutzner M: Preferential cutaneous infiltration by neoplastic thymus-derived lymphocytes. Morphological and functional studies. Ann Int Med 80:865, 1974.

325. Alibert JLM: Monographic des dermatoses, 2nd edn. Paris: G. Baillier, 1885, p 413.

326. Alibert JLM: Descriptions des malades se la peace observées à l'Hospital Saint Louis. Paris: Barrors, 1906, p 153.

327. Sezary A, Bouvrain Y: Erythrodermis avec presence de céllules monstrés dans derme et dans sang currulaialt. Bull Soc Fr Dermatol Syphiligr 45:254-260, 1938.

328. Clendenning WE, Brecher G, Van Scott EJ: Mycosis fungoides, relationship to malignant cutaneous reticulosis and the Sézary syndrome. Arch Dermatol 89:785-792, 1964.

329. Lutzner MA, Hobbs JW, Harvath P: Ultrastructure of abnormal cells in Sézary's syndrome, mycosis fungoides, and parapsoriasis en plaque. Arch Dermatol 103:275-386, 1971.

330. Lutzner MA, Edelson RL, Schem R, Kirkpatrick CH, Ahmed A: Cutaneous T-cell lymphoma: the Sézary syndrome, mycosis fungoides and related disorders. Ann Int Med 83:534-552, 1975.

331. Edelson RL: Cutaneous T-cell Lymphoma: clues of a skin-thymus interaction. J Invest Dermatol 67:419-424, 1976.

332. Claudy AG, Schmitt D, A-aico A, Brochier J, Purot H, Thevolet J: Immunological characterization of the mycosis fungoides tumor cell. Bull Cancer 64:241-248, 1977.

333. Brouet JC, Flandrin G: Clinical and hematological heterogeneity of T-cell derived lymphoproliferative disorders. Bull Cancer 64:267-274, 1977.

334. Berger CL, Warburton D, Raafat J, LaGerfo P, Edelson RL: Cutaneous T-cell lymphoma: neoplasm of T cells with helper activity. Blood 53:642-651, 1979.

335. Lamburg SI, Bunn PA: Cutaneous T-cell lymphomas: summary of the Mycosis Fungoides Cooperative Group - National Cancer Institute Workshop. Arch Dermatol 115:1103-1105, 1979.

336. deSousa M: Ecotaxis, ecotaxopathy, and lymphoid malignancy: facts and predictions. In: The immunopathology of lymphoreticular neoplasms.

337. Goos M, Kaizerling E, Lennert K: Mycosis fungoides: mode for T-cell homing to the skin? Br J Dermatol 94:221-233, 1976.

338. Cawley EP, Curtis AC, Leech JER: Is mycosis fungoides a reticulo-endothelial neoplastic entity? Arch Dermatol Syph 64:255-261, 1951.

339. Bosler RSW, Lynch PJ: Mycosis fungoides: clinical and therapeutic review. J Family Prac 8:281-286, 1979.

340. Rappaport H, Thomas LB: Mycosis fungoides: the pathology of extracutaneous involvement. Cancer 34:1198-1206, 1974.
341. Rappaport H: The pathology of the extracutaneous lesions of mycosis fungoides. Bull Cancer 64:275-278, 1977.
342. Epstein EH, Levin DZ, Croft JD Jr, Lutzner MA: Mycosis fungoides: survival, prognostic feature, response to therapy and autopsy findings. Medicine 51:61-82, 1972.
343. Pautrier LM, Woringer F: Contribution à l'étude de l'histophysiologie cutanie. A prapos d'un aspect histopathologique nouveau du ganglion lymphatique: la réticular lipmélanique accompagagnant certaines dermatoses généralisées. Les exchanges entre le peau et le ganglion. Ann Dermatol Syph, Paris 8:256-276, 1937.
344. Hurvitt E: Dermatopathie lymphadenitis. J Invest Dermatol 5:197-210, 1942.
345. Rosas-Uribe A, Variakojis D, Molna Z, Rappaport H: Mycosis fungoides: an ultrastructural study. Cancer 34:634-645, 1974.
346. Thomas LB, Rappaport H: Mycosis fungoides and its relationship to other malignant lymphomas. The reticuloendothelial system. International Academy of Pathology Monograph. Baltimore: Williams & Williams, 1975, Chap 12.
347. Variakojis D, Rosas-Uribe A, Rappaport H: Mycosis fungoides: Pathologic finfings in staging laparotomies. Cancer 33: 1589-1600, 1974.
348. Scheffer E, Meyer CJLM, Van Vloten WA: Dermatopathic lymphadenopathy and lymphnode involvement in mycosis fungoides. Cancer 45:137-148, 1980.
349. Erkman-Balis B, Rappaport H: Cytogenetic studies in mycosis fugoides. Cancer 34:626-633, 1974.
350. Levi, Wiernik PH: Management of mycosis fungoides. Current status and future prospects. Medicine 54:73-88, 1975.
351. Huberman MS, Bunn PA, Matthew MJ, Ihde DC, Gazdar AF, Cohen MH, Minna JD: Hepatic involvement in the cutaneous T-cell lymphomas. Results of percutaneous biopsy and peritoneoscopy. Cancer 45:1683-1688, 1980.
352. Lutzner MA, Hobbs JW, Harvath P: Ultrastructure of abnormal cells in Sézary's syndrome, mycosis fungoides, and parapsoriasis en plaque. AMA Arch Dermatol 103:375-384, 1971.
353. Narim I, Capostagno JS, Johnson CE Jr, Schreu R, Gatto RA: Sézary syndrome; tartrate-resistant acid phosphatase in the neoplastic cells. Am J Clin Pathol 71:528-533, 1979.
354. Broder S, Edelsen RL, Lutzner MA, Nelson DL, MacDermott RP: The Sézary syndrome: a malignant proliferation of helper T cells. J Clin Invest 58:1297-1304, 1976.
355. Lawrence EC, Broder S, Jaffee ES, Braylan RC, Dobbins WO, Young RC, Waldman TA: Evolution of a lymphoma with helper T cell characteristics in Sézary syndrome. Blood 52:481-492, 1978.
356. Berger CL, Waburton D, Raafat J, LoGerto P, Edelson RL: Cutaneous T-cell lymphoma: neoplasm of T cells with helper activity. Blood 53:642-651, 1979.
357. Siegal FP, Siegal M: Enhancement by irradiated T cells of human plasma cell production: dissection of helper and suppressor functions in vitro. J Immunol 118:642-653, 1977.
358. Schneiderman P, Edelson R, Lutzner M: Lymphomatoid papulosis: immunologic and ultrastructural studies (abstract). Clin Res 23:455, 1975.
359. Flaxman BA, Zelazny G, Van Scott EJ: Nonspecificity of characteristic cells in mycosis fungoides. Arch Dermatol 104:141-147, 1971.
360. Crossen PE, Mella JEL, Finley AG, Ravich RB, Vincent PC, Gunz FW: The Sézary syndrome, cytogenetic studies and identification of the Sézary cell as an abnormal lymphocyte. Am J Med 50:24-34, 1971.
361. Lutzner MA, Emerit I, Duprepaire R, Flandrin G, Grupper CL, Prunieras M: Cytogenetic, cytophotometric, and ultrastructural study of large cerebriform cells of the Sézary syndrome and description of a small cell variant. J Natl Cancer Inst 50:1145-1162, 1973.

362. Winklemann RK: The Sézary cell symposium. Mayo Clin Proc 49:513-519, 1974.
363. Van Vloten WA, Schaberg A, vander Plaeg M: Cytophotometric studies on mycosis fungoides and other cutaneous reticuloses. Bull Cancer 64:249-258, 1977.
364. Wioland M, Hajman A: Sézary cell: characterization of a biophysical parameter. Biomedicine 31:29-30, 1979.
365. Burke JS, Butler JJ: Malignant lymphoma with a high content of epithelioid histiocytes (Lennert's lymphoma). Am J Clin Pathol 66:1-9, 1976.
366. Lennert K, Mestagh J: Lymphogranulomatosem mit konstant Hohem epithelioid Zellgehalt. Virchows Arch Pathol Anat Physiol 2344:1-20, 1968.
367. Kim H, Nathwani BN, Rappaport H: So-called 'Lennert's lymphoma'. Is it a clinicopathologic entity? Cancer 45:1379-1399, 1980.
368. Hayers P, Robertson JH: Malignant lymphomas with a high content of epithelioid histiocytes. J Clin Pathol 32:675-680, 1979.
369. Kim H, Jacobs C, Warnke RA, Dorfman RF: Malignant lymphoma with a high content of epithelioid histiocytes. A distinct clinicopathologic entity and a form of so-called 'Lennert's lymphoma'. Cancer 41:620-635, 1978.
370. Lennert K, Mohri N, Stein H, Kaizerling E: The histopathology of malignant lymphomas. Br J Haematol 31:Suppl 2, 103-203, 1975.
371. Lukes RJ, Parker JW: The pathology of lymphoreticular neoplasms. In: The immunopathology of lymphoreticular neoplasms, Twomey JJ, Good RA, eds. New York: Plenum Medical, 1978, pp 239-279.
372. Klein MA, Jaffe R, Neiman RS: 'Lennert's lymphoma' with transformation to malignant lymphoma, histiocytic types (immunoblastic sarcoma). Am J Clin Pathol 68:601-605, 1977.
373. Dorfman RF, Remington JS: Value of lymph-node biopsy in the diagnosis of acute acquired toxoplasmosis. N Engl J Med 289:878-881, 1973.
374. Frizzera G, Moran EM, Rappaport H: Angio-immunoblastic lymphadenopathy with dysproteinemia. Lancet 1:1070-1073, 1974.
375. Braylan RC, Jaffee ES, Mann RB, Frank MM, Berard CW: Surface receptors of human neoplastic lymphoreticular cells. In: Immunological diagnosis of leukemias and lymphomas. Haematology and blood transfusion, Vol 20, Thierfelder S, Rardt H, Thiel E, eds. New York: Springer-Verlag, 1977, pp 47-52.
376. Brouet JC, Preud-homme JL, Flandrin G, Chellone N, Seligmann M: Membrane markers in 'histiocytic' lymphomas (reticulum cell sarcomas). J Natl Cancer Inst 56:631-633, 1976.
377. Frizzera G, Gajl-Peczaeska KJ, Bloomfield CD, Kersey JH: Predictability of immunologic phenotype of malignant lymphomas by conventional morphology. A study of 60 cases. Cancer 43:1216-1224, 1979.
378. Lennert K: Mycosis fungoides. In: Malignant lymphomas other than Hodgkin's disease. New York: Springer-Verlag, 1978, pp 182-184.
379. Schwartz E-W, Ude P: Immunoblastic sarcoma with leukemic blood picture in the terminal stage of mycosis fungoides. Virchows Arch A 369:165-172, 1975.
380. Lennert K: Malignant lymphoma, lymphocytic, T-zone type. In: Malignant lymphomas other than Hodgkin's disease. New York: Springer-Verlag, 1978, pp 196-209.
381. Waldron JA, Leech JH, Glick AD, Flexner JM, Collins RD: Malignant lymphomas of peripheral T-lymphocyte origin. Immunologic, pathologic and clinical features in six patients. Cancer 40:1604-1617, 1977.
382. van den Tweel JG, Taylor CR, Parker JW, Lukes RJ: Immunoglobulin inclusions in non-Hodgkin's lymphomas. Am J Clin Pathol 69:306-313, 1978.
383. Kim H, Dorfman RF, Rappaport H: Signet ring cell lymphoma. A rare morphologic and functional expression of nodular (follicular) lymphoma. Am J Surg Pathol 2:119-132, 1978.

384. Rappaport H, Johnson FB: Intracellular protein resembling Russell bodies in malignant lymphomas associated with acquired hemolytic anemia. Blood 10:132–144, 1955.

385. Cawley JC, Smith J, Goldstone AH: IgA and Igm cytoplasmic inclusions in a series of chronic lymphocytic leukemia. Clin Exp Immunol 23:78–82, 1976.

386. Brunning RD, Parlin J: Intranuclear inclusions in plasma cells and lymphocytes from patients with monoclonal gammopathies. Am J Clin Pathol 66:10–21, 1976.

387. Custer RP: Pitfalls in the diagnosis of lymphoma and leukemia from the pathologist's point of view. Proc 2nd Natl Cancer Conf, Vol I. American Cancer Society, 1954, pp 554–557.

388. Custer RP: The changing pattern of lymphocytic malignancies. In: The lymphocyte and lymphocytic tissue. International Academy of Pathology Monograph, Rebuck JW, ed. New York: Hoeber, 1960, PP 181–193.

389. Gall EA: The cytological identity and interrelation of mesenchymal cells of lymphoid tissue. Ann NY Acad Sci 216:120–130, 1958.

390. van den Tweel JG, Lukes RJ, Taylor CR: Pathophysiology of lymphocyte transformation. A study of so-called composite lymphomas. AM J Clin Pathol 71:509–520, 1979.

391. Rudders RA, Ross ME, DeLellis RA: Primary extranodal lymphoma; response to treatment and factors influencing prognosis. Cancer 42:406-416, 1978.

392. Freeman C, Berg JW, Cutler SJ: Occurrence and prognosis of extranodal lymphoma. Cancer 29:252–260, 1972.

393. Newall J, Fiedman M, de Narvaez F: Extra-lymph-node reticulum cell sarcoma. Radiology 91:708–712, 1968.

394. Salzstein SL: Extranodal malignant lymphomas and pseudolymphomas. Pathol Ann 4:159–184, 1969.

395. Loehr WJ, Mujahed Z, Zahan FD, Gray GF, Thorbjarnarson B: Primary lymphoma of the gastrointestinal tract: a review of 100 cases. Ann Surg 170:232–238, 1969.

396. Lewin KJ, Ranchard M, Dorfman RF: Lymphomas of the gastrointestinal tract. A study of 117 cases presenting with gastrointestinal disease. Cancer 42:693–707, 1978.

397. Rosenfeld F, Rosenberg SA: Diffuse histiocytic lymphomas presenting with gastrointestinal tract lesions. The Stanford experience. Cancer 45:2188–2193, 1980.

398. Novak S, Caraoneo J, Sirowbridge A, Peterson RE, White RR III: Primary lymphomas of the gastrointestinal tract. South Med J 72:1154–1158, 1979.

399. Blackledge G, Bush H, Dodge OG, Crowther D: A study of gastrointestinal lymphoma. Clin Oncol 5:209–219, 1979.

400. Issacson P, Wright DH, Judd MA, Mepham BL: Primary gastrointestinal lymphomas, a classification of 66 cases. Cancer 43: 1805–1819, 1979.

401. Dutz W, Asuadi S, Sadri S, Kohout E: Intestinal lymphoma and sprue: a systematic approach. Gut 12:804–812, 1971.

402. Kewin K, Kahn LB, Novis B: Primary intestinal lymphoma of 'Western' and 'Mediterranean' type, alpha chain disease and massive plasma cell infiltration. A comparative study of 37 cases. Cancer 38:2511–2525, 1976.

403. WHO memorandum. Alpha chain disease and related small intestinal lymphomas. Bull WHO 54:3558–3560, 1976.

404. Plasnicai S, Sumi-Kriznik T, Goulouh R: Abdominal lymphoma with alpha-heavy chain disease. Isr J Med Sci 11:832–840, 1975.

405. Chantar C, Escartin P, Plaza AG, Corugedo AF, Arenas JJ, Sanz E, Anaya A, Bootello A, Segouia JA: Diffuse plasma cell infiltration of the small intestine with malabsorption associated to IgA monoclonal gammopathy. Cancer 34:1620–1630, 1974.

406. Ezechieli S, Ranz T, Ale G: Linfoma maligno dell intestino tinue con sindrome di malassorbimento. Recent Prog Med (Roma) 54:444–452, 1973.

407. Manousos ON, Economidou JC, Georgiadou DE, Pratsika-Ougorloglou IG, Kadziannis SJ, Merikas GE, Henry K, Doe WF: Alpha chain disease with clinical, immunological,

histological recovery. Br Med J 2:409–415, 1974.

408. Kahn LB, Selzer G, Kashula R: Primary gastrointestinal lymphoma. A clinicopathological study of 57 cases. Am J Dig Dis 17:219–230, 1972.

409. Ibarra R, Bondi JL, Rosse JC, de Larecchia I: Alteraciones de la mucosa del intestino delgado en el linfoma intestinal. Medicina (B Aires) 30:234–244, 1970.

410. Harris OD, Cooke WT, Thompson H, Waterhouse JAH: Malignancy in adult celiac disease and idiopathic steatorrhea. Am J Med 42:889–912, 1967.

411. Ramot B, Shahnin N, Bubis JJ: Malabsorption syndrome in lymphoma of the small bowel. Isr J Med Sci 1:221–226, 1965.

412. Seligmann M, Danon G, Hurez D, Mihaesco E, Preud'homme JL: Alpha-chain disease: a new immunoglobulin abnormality. Science 162:1396–1397, 1968.

413. Rappaport H, Ramot B, Hulu N, Park JK: The pathology of the so-called Mediterranean abdominal lymphoma with malabsorption. Cancer 29:1502–1511, 1972.

414. Ramot N, Levanon M, Hahn Y, Lahat N, Moroz C: The mutual clonal origin of the lymphoplasmacytic and lymphoma cell in alpha heavy chain disease. Clin Exp Immunol 27:440–445, 1977.

415. Selzer G, Sherman G, Calihan TR, Schwartz Y: Primary small intestinal lymphoma and alpha-heavy-chain disease. A study of 45 cases from a pathology department in Israel. Isr J Med Sci 15:111–123, 1979.

416. Maurer R, Taylor CR, Terry R, Lukes RJ: Non-Hodgkin lymphoma of the thyroid. A clinico-pathological review of 29 cases applying the Lukes-Collins classification and an immunoperoxidase method. Virchows Arch A Path Histol 383:293–317, 1979.

417. Sirota DK, Segal RL: Primary lymphomas of the thyroid gland. JAMA 242:1743–1746, 1979.

418. Paladugu RR, Bearman RM, Rappaport H: Malignant lymphoma with primary manifestation in the gonad. A clinicopathologic study of 38 patients. Cancer 45:561–571, 1980.

419. Herman TS, Hammond N, Jones SE, Butler JJ, Byrne GE Jr, McKelvey EM: Involvement of the central nervous system by non-Hodgkin's lymphoma. The Southwest Oncology Group experience. Cancer 43:390–397, 1979.

420. Colby TV, Dorfman RF: Malignant lymphomas involving the salivary glands. Pathology Annual Part 2, Somers and Rosen, eds. New York: Appleton-Century-Crofts, 1979, pp 307–324.

421. Tindle BH, Pinkus GS, Terry R: Unpublished data concerning lymphomas presenting as salivary gland masses.

422. Hoppe RT, Burke JS, Glatstein E, Kaplan HS: Non-Hodgkin's lymphoma. Involvement of Waldeyer's ring. Cancer 42:1096–1104, 1978.

423. Goldberg J, Davey FR, Lowenstein F, Gottliev AJ: Lymphoma cutis of apparent B cell origin. Arch Pathol Lab Med 102:15–18, 1978.

424. Edelson RL, Berger CL, Raafat J, Warburton J: Karyotype studies of cutaneous T cell lymphoma: evidence for clonal origin. J Invest Dermatol 73:548–550, 1979.

425. Chabner BA, Johnson RE, Young RC, Canellos GP, Hubbard SP, Johnson SK, DeVita VT: Sequential nonsurgical and surgical staging of non-Hodgkin's lymphoma. Cancer 42:922–925, 1978.

426. Brunning RD, McKenna RN: Bone marrow manifestations of malignant lymphoma and lymphoma-like conditions. Pathology Annual Part 1. New York: Appleton-Century-Crofts, 1979, pp 1–59.

427. Stein RS, Ultmann JE, Bryne GE Jr, Moran EM, Golomb HM: Bone marrow involvement in non-Hodgkin's lymphoma. Implications for staging and therapy. Cancer 37:629–636, 1976.

428. Rosenberg SA: Bone marrow involvement in the non-Hodgkin's lymphomata. Br J Cancer 31 Suppl. 2:261–264, 1975.

429. Brunning RD: Bone marrow and peripheral blood involvement in non-Hodgkin's lymphomas. Geriatrics 29:52–59, 1974.

430. Ribas-Mundo M, Roseberg SA: The value of sequential bone marrow biopsy and laparotomy and splenectomy in a series of 200 consecutive untreated patients with non-Hodgkin's lymphoma. Europ J Cancer 15:941-952, 1979.
431. Dawson PJ, Rambo DN: Diagnosis of malignant lymphoma, a clinicopathological analysis of 158 difficult lymph node biopsies. Cancer 17:1405-1413, 1964.
432. Pangalis GA, Rappaport H: Common clonal origin of lymphoplasmacytic and immunoblastic lymphoma in intestinal alpha chain disease. Lancet ii:880, 1977.
433. Lukes RJ, Tindle BH: Immunoblastic lymphadenopathy: a prelymphomatous state of immunoblastic sarcoma. In: Lymphoid neoplasias I. Rec Res Cancer 64:241-246, 1978.
434. Kosmidas PA, Axelrod AR, Palacas C, Stahl M: Angioimmunoblastic lymphadenopathy. A T-cell deficiency. Cancer 42:447-452, 1978.
435. Paluke M, Khilanani P, Weise R: Immunologic and electron-microscopic characteristics of a case of immunoblastic lymphadenopathy. Am J Clin Pathol 65:929-941, 1976.
436. Cullen MH, Stansfeld AG, Oliver RTD, Lister TA, Malpas JS: Angio-immunoblastic lymphadenopathy: reports of 10 cases and review of the literature. Quart J Med 48:151-177, 1979.
437. Krakauer RS, Waldmann TA, Strober W: Loss of suppressor T cells in adult NZB/NZW mice. J Exp Med 144:662-673, 1976.
438. Pangalis GA, Moran EM, Rappaport H: Blood and bone marrow findings in immunoblastic lymphadenopathy. Blood 51:71-83,
439. van Voorst Vader PC, Folkers E, van Rhenen DJ: Craquele-like eruption in angioimmunoblastic lymphadenopathy. Arch Dermatol 115:370, 1979.
440. Myers TJ, Cole SR, Pastuszak WT: Angioimmunoblastic lymphadenopathy: pleural pulmonary disease. Cancer 40:266-271, 1978.
441. Tredici G, Minazzi M, Lampugnani E: Peripheral neuropathy in angioimmunoblastic lymphadenopathy with dysproteinemia. J Neurol Neurosurg Psych 42:519-523, 1979.
442. Wood WG, Harkins MM: Nephropathy in angioimmunoblastic lymphadenopathy. Am J Clin Pathol 71:58-63, 1979.
443. Newcom SR, Kadin ME: Prednisone in treatment of allergen-associated angioimmunoblastic lymphadenopathy. Lancet I:462-464, 1979.
444. Neiman RS, Dervan P, Haudenchild C, Jaffe R: Angioimmunoblastic lymphadenopathy. An ultrastructural and immunologic study with review of the literature. Cancer 41:507-518, 1978.
445. Madri JA, Fromowitz F: Amyloid deposition in immunoblastic lymphadenopathy. Human Pathol 9:157-162, 1978.
446. Bluming AC, Cohen HE, Sazon A: Angioimmunoblastic lymphadenopathy with dysproteinemia. A pathogenetic link between physiologic lymphoid proliferation and malignant lymphoma. Am J Med 67:421-427, 1979.
447. Shamoto M, Suchi T: Intracytoplasmic type A virus-like particles in angioimmunoblastic lymphadenopathy. Cancer 44:1641-1643, 1979.
448. Iseman M, Schwartz M, Stanford R: Interstitial pneumonia in angioimmunoblastic lymphadenopathy with dysproteinemia. A case report with special histopathologic studies. Ann Intern Med 85:752-755, 1976.
449. Narasimham P, Ahm BH, Levy RN, Glasberg SS: Immunoblastic lymphadenopathy. High serum toxoplasma titer. NY State J Med 79:241-244, 1979.
450. Shoback DM: Angioimmunoblastic lymphadenopathy with dysproteinemia. Johns Hopkins Med J 140:101-106, 1979.
451. McDougall BK, Weinerman BH: Immunoblastic lymphadenopathy. Patient with prolonged fever of unknown origin. JAMA 241:921-922, 1979.
452. Wechsler HL, Stavrides A: Immunoblastic lymphadenopathy with purpura and cyroglobulinemia. Arch Dermatol 113:363-371, 1977.
453. Tsung SH: Immunoblastic lymphadenopathy. J Indiana State Med Soc 71:1068-1069, 1978, nov.

454. Degg HJ, Singer JW, Huang TW: Angioimmunoblastic lymphadenopathy with retinitis and drug related exacerbations. A clinicopathological case study. Cancer 44:1745-1750, 1979.
455. Weisenberger DD: Immunoblastic lymphadenopathy associated with methyldopa therapy. A case report. Cancer 42:2322-2327, 1978.
456. Matz LR, Papadimitriou JM, Carroll JR, Barr AL, Dawkins RL, Jackson JM, Herrmann RP, Armstrong BK: Angioimmunoblastic lymphadenopathy with dysproteinemia. Cancer 40: 2152-2160, 1977.
457. Hossfeld DK, Hoffken K, Schmidt CG, Diedriche H: Chromosome abnormalities in angioimmunoblastic lymphadenopathy. Lancet i:198, 1976.
458. Correa P, O'Connor GT: Epidemiologic patterns of Hodgkin's disease. Int J Cancer 8:192-201, 1971.
459. Dawar R, Mangalik A: Hodgkin's disease: an analysis of 128 cases. Am J Hematol 4:209-215, 1978.
460. Burn C, Davies G, Dodge OG, Nias BC: Hodgkin's disease in English and African children. J Natl Cancer Inst 46:37-41, 1971.
461. Doll R, Payne P: Cancer incidence in five continents. A technical report. New York: Springer-Verlag, 1966.
462. Fox H: Presentation of microscopical preparations made from some of the original tissue described by Thomas Hodgkin, 1832. Ann Med Hist 8:370-374, 1926.
463. Silverberg E, Grant RN: Cancer statistics. New York: American Cancer Society, 1970.
464. Miller RW: Fifty-two forms of childhood cancer. United States mortality experience 1960-1966. J Pediatr 75:685-689, 1965.
465. Solidoro A, Guzman O, Chang A: Relative increased incidence of childhood Hodgkin's disease in Peru. Cancer Res 26:1204-1208, 1966.
466. Wright DH: Epidemiology and histology of Hodgkin's disease in Uganda. Nat Cancer Inst Monogr 36:25-30, 1973.
467. Azzam SA: High incidence of Hodgkin's disease in children in Lebanon. Cancer Res 26:1202-1203, 1966.
468. Silverberg E: Leukemia and lymphoma. Statistical and epidemiological information. The American Cancer Society Professional Education Publication, 1977, p 51.
469. Miller RW: Mortality in childhood Hodgkin's disease: an etiologic clue. JAMA 198:1216-1217, 1966.
470. Strum SB, Rappaport H: Hodgkin's disease in the first decade of life. Pediatrics 46:748-754, 1970.
471. Norris DG, Burgert EO, Cooper HA, Harrison EG: Hodgkin's disease in childhood. Cancer 36:2109-2120, 1975.
472. Schnitzer B, Nishiyama RH, Heidelberger KP, Weaver DK: Hodgkin's disease in children. Cancer 31:560-567, 1973.
473. Pitcock JA, Bauer WC, McGavron MH: Hodgkin's disease in children: a clinicopathological study of 46 cases. Cancer 12:1043-1051, 1959.
474. Butler JJ: Hodgkin's disease in children. In: Neoplasma in childhood. Chicago: The Year Book Publishers, 1969, p 267.
475. Lukes RJ: Personal communication.
476. Garwicz S, Landberg T, Akerman M: Malignant lymphomas in children: a clinicopathologic retrospective study. I. Hodgkin's disease. Acta Pediatr Scand 63:673-678, 1974.
477. Jenkin RDT, Brown TC, Peters MV, Sonley MJ: Hodgkin's disease in children: a retrospective analysis 1958-1973. Cancer 35:979-990, 1975.
478. Sobrinho-Simoes MA, Areias MA: Relative high frequency of childhood Hodgkin's disease in the north of Portugal. Cancer 42:1952-1956, 1978.
479. Armata J, Stopyrowa J, Depowski M, Strzeszynski J, Borkowski W, Kaczor Z, Depowska T: MVPP chemotherapy combined with radiotherapy in the treatment of Hodgkin's disease in children. Acta Pediatr Scand 67:269-273, 1978.

480. Smith TE, Peckham MJ, McElwain TS, Gazet JC, Austin DE: Hodgkin's disease in children. Br J Cancer 36:120–129, 1977.
481. Shah NK, Freeman AT: Hodgkin's disease in children. American Society of Hematology. Abstracts of the December 1972 meeting, Hollywood, Florida, p 138.
482. Norris DG, Burgert EQ Jr, Cooper HA, Harrison EG: Hodgkin's disease in children. Blood 40:974, 1972.
483. Santiago PJ, Velez G: Hodgkin's disease in children. Review of 31 patients. Abstracts of the 13th International Congress of Hematology, Munich, August 1970, p 225.
484. Teillet F, Schweisguth O: La maladie de Hodgkin chez l'enfant. Etude de 72 observations personelles. Arch Fr Ped 25:313–330, 1968,
485. Wollner N: Non-Hodgkin's lymphoma in children: historical review, pattern of disease, and future trends. In: The immunopathology of lymphoreticular neoplasms, Twomey JJ, Good RA, eds. New York: Plenum Medical 1978, pp 609–640.
486. Frizzera G, Murphy SB: Follicular (nodular) lymphoma in childhood: a rare clinical-pathological entity. Report of eight cases from four cancer centers. Cancer 44:2218–2235, 1979.
487. Bryne GE Jr: Rappaport classification of non-Hodgkin's lymphoma: histologic features and clinical significance. Cancer Treat Rep 61:935–944, 1977.
488. Kersey JM, Nesbit ME: Lymphoreticular malignancies in childhood. In: The immunopathology of lymphoreticular neoplasms, Twomey JJ, Good RA, New York: Plenum Medical 1978, pp 533–542.
489. Murphy SB, Frizzera G, Evans AE: A study of childhood non-Hodgkin's lymphoma. Cancer 36:2121–2131, 1975.
490. Sullivan MP: Non-Hodgkin's lymphoma of childhood. In: Clinical pediatric oncology, Sutow, Vietti, Ferbach, eds. St. Louis: C.V. Mosby, 1973.
491. Glatstein E, Kim H, Donaldson SS, Dorfman RF, Gribbe TS, Wilbur JR, Rosenberg SA, Kaplan HS: Non-Hodgkin's lymphoma. VI. Results of treatment in childhood. Cancer 43:202–211, 1974.
492. Pinkel D, Johnson W, Aur RJA: Non-Hodgkin's lymphoma in children. Br J Cancer 31 Suppl 2:298–323, 1975.
493. Landberg T, Garwicz S, Akerman M: A clinico-pathological study of non-Hodgkin's lymphomata in childhood. Br J Cancer 31 Suppl 2:332–336, 1975.
494. Lemerle M, Gerard-Marchant R, Sancho H, Schweisguth O: Natural history of non-Hodgkin's malignant lymphomata in children. Br J Cancer 31 Suppl 2:324–331, 1975.
495. Hausner RJ, Tosas-Uribe A, Wickstrum DA, Smith PC: Non-Hodgkin's lymphoma in the first two decades of life. A pathological study of 30 cases. Cancer 40:1533–1547, 1977.
496. Jaffe N, Buell D, Cassady JR, Traggis D, Weinstein H: Role of staging in childhood non-Hodgkin's lymphoma. Cancer Treat Rep 61:1001–1007, 1977.
497. Brecker ML, Sinks LF, Thomas RRM, Freeman AI: Non-Hodgkin's lymphoma in children. Cancer 41:1997–2001, 1978.
498. Williams AH, Taylor CR, Higgins GR, Quinn JJ, Schneider BK, Swanson V, Parker JW, Pattengale PK, Chandor SB, Powars D, Lincoln TL, Tindle BH, Lukes RJ: Childhood lymphoma-leukemia I. Correlation of morphology and immunological studies. Cancer 42:171–181, 1978.

2. Clinical Features and Clinical Evaluation of Hodgkin's Disease and the Non-Hodgkin's Lymphomas

RICHARD S. STEIN

1. OVERVIEW

While Hodgkin's disease and the non-Hodgkin's lymphomas constitute a diverse spectrum of lymphoproliferative malignancies, the disorders share a number of important similarities. Both Hodgkin's disease and the non-Hodgkin's lymphomas commonly present as solitary or generalized lymphadenopathy. For both Hodgkin's disease and the non-Hodgkin's lymphomas, accurate staging – determining the extent of disease - is the cornerstone for rationale therapeutic planning. Nevertheless, there are important major differences between Hodgkin's disease and the non-Hodgkin's lymphomas. In Hodgkin's disease, contiguous spread of tumor from node to node is the rule, and most patients present with disease limited to the lymph nodes or to the lymph nodes and the spleen. In contrast, the majority of patients with one of the non-Hodgkin's lymphomas present with advanced disease. For example, over 80% of patients with nodular poorly differentiated lymphocytic lymphoma (N-PDL) have lymphomatous involvement of the bone marrow at presentation. Also, while Hodgkin's disease is curable, regardless of stage, only certain histologic types of non-Hodgkin's lymphoma – primarily the lymphomas included in the category diffuse histiocytic lymphoma (DHL) – are curable when the disease is disseminated.

Because of this diversity with respect to major clinical features – as well as differences with respect to incidence, epidemiologic associations, and immunologic features – it seems most reasonable to consider Hodgkin's disease and the non-Hodgkin's lymphomas separately. In addition, as part of the discussion of the non-Hodgkin's lymphomas, important distinctions must be made between the different histologic types of non-Hodgkin's lymphoma which vary significantly in their clinical behavior.

J.M. Bennett (ed.), Lymphomas 1, 129–175. All rights reserved.
Copyright © 1981 Martinus Nijhoff Publishers, The Hague/Boston/London.

2.   HODGKIN'S DISEASE

2.1. Incidence and Epidemiology

Hodgkin's disease accounts for approximately 1 % of newly diagnosed malignancies in the United States, i.e. approximately 10,000 cases per year. However, the economic impact of Hodgkin's disease is disproportionate to this low incidence since Hodgkin's disease is the most common malignancy of young adults; the average age of cases in the United States is 32 years.

The age-related incidence of Hodgkin's disease differs substantially among nations. In the United States and other developed nations there is a bimodal incidence of Hodgkin's disease with one peak occurring near age 25 and another peak occurring after age 55, (Figure 1) [1]. However, in underdeveloped countries, Hodgkin's disease is more commonly seen in children under the age of ten rather than in early adulthood [2]. In underdeveloped countries mixed-cellularity and lymphocyte .depleted Hodgkin's disease are more frequently seen, as are more advanced stages of Hodgkin's disease. The occurrence of Hodgkin's disease in older adults seems to be relatively independent of economic development.

Numerous studies have found positive correlations between the incidence of Hodgkin's disease and social class [3, 4]. Both the cross-cultural and social

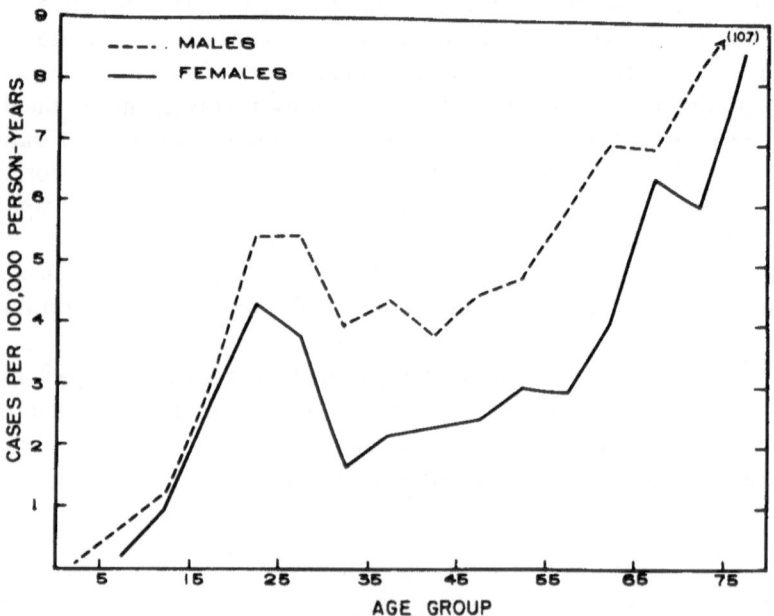

Figure 1. Age-specific incidence rates of Hodgkin's disease for 1969–1971, by sex [1].

class findings are compatible with the hypothesis that Hodgkin's disease is a rare consequence of a common viral infection – the probability of Hodgkin's disease occurring following exposure to the virus being higher when the initial exposure occurs in adolescence or young adulthood rather than in childhood [5, 6]. This model is the same epidemiologic model which was used to explain the incidence of paralytic polio in the pre-vaccine era. This model predicts that hygienic conditions in childhood homes as well as family size should be associated with the risk of Hodgkin's disease in adulthood. While recent evidence has supported these predictions [7, 8], the viral model of Hodgkin's disease remains a hypothesis as no specific viral etiology has been established. Specifically, efforts to link the Epstein-Barr virus to Hodgkin's disease have been unsuccessful [9, 10].

Efforts to show that Hodgkin's disease is contagious have also failed. A number of studies have demonstrated apparent 'links' between cases of Hodgkin's disease [11], However other investigators have suggested that the clusters of Hodgkin's disease are chance occurrences. Furthermore, despite extensive efforts, there has not been a consistent demonstration of a relationship between tonsillectomy and Hodgkin's disease [12]. In contrast, in recent years, a relationship has been demonstrated between Hodgkin's disease and occupational exposure to wood dust [13–15]. While the basis of this relationship has not been established, chronic antigenic exposure has been postulated.

In summary, Hodgkin's disease has a number of epidemiologic and clinical characteristics which suggest that in many cases Hodgkin's disease may be a complication of an infectious illness. However, efforts to identify a causative viral agent, or to demonstrate transmission between cases, have not been successful.

2.2. Immunologic Abnormalities

Hodgkin's disease has been associated with a wide array of immunologic abnormalities including autoimmune diseases – i.e. autoimmune hemolytic anemia and autoimmune thrombocytopenic purpura – deficiencies of immune function, and opportunistic infection.

Approximately 25% of patients with stage I Hodgkin's disease are lymphopenic, and the incidence of lymphopenia is higher among patients with advanced disease [16, 17]. Both peripheral blood T cells and B cells are decreased [18]. Cutaneous anergy has long been associated with Hodgkin's disease. However, when extensive batteries of skin tests have been used, only relative unresponsiveness rather than anergy has been detected. In one large series, no patients with stage I Hodgkin's disease were found to be anergic as compared to 26.6% of patients with stage IV disease [19].

Patients with Hodgkin's disease are at increased risk of developing infections. Part of this risk is attributable to the immunosuppressive effects of therapy and of splenectomy. However, patients with Hodgkin's disease seem to be unusually susceptible to infections by agents of low pathogenicity which do not usually affect normal hosts. These agents include parasites such as pneumocystis, fungi such as cryptococcus, mucor, and aspergillus, as well as bacteria such as nocardia and listeria. The incidence of these infections decreases markedly when patients are in remission. However, even in remission, the incidence of herpes zoster, shingles, is substantially increased in patients with Hodgkin's disease [20]. In one series which followed 78 patients for a 2-year period, 22% developed herpes zoster. An increased incidence was noted in higher stages of disease [20]. In addition, when herpes zoster occurs in a patient with Hodgkin's disease there is a greater risk of dissemination than when the infection occurs in a normal host [21].

Most of the observations of immunologic abnormalities in Hodgkin's disease have assumed that Hodgkin's disease causes the immunologic deficiency. Recently, however, immunologic function was assessed in a large number of patients who had been cured of advanced Hodgkin's disease by use of combination chemotherapy [22]. Although the patients had been cured, defects of T cell function could be detected. Decreased sheep red blood cell rosettes and decreased mitogen induced proliferation of lympho-cytes were observed. These defects were not noted in a group of patients with histiocytic lymphoma who had been cured by similar chemotherapy. While Hodgkin's disease may have caused an abnormality which persisted even when the disease was cured, this observation raises the possibility that an immunologic defect in T cell function is present prior to the development of Hodgkin's disease and may act as a predisposition to the disease.

2.3. Clinical Presentation

Hodgkin's disease presents as nodal disease in nearly all cases. In contrast to the non-Hodgkin's lymphomas, extranodal presentations occur in less than 2% of Hodgkin's disease patients. The cervical and supraclavicular nodes are most frequently involved – more than 70% of patients present with involvement of these areas. Axillary node involvement is the presentation in approximately 15% of patients. Subdiaphragmatic presentations are infre-quent in Hodgkin's disease as less than 10% of cases present as inguinal adenopathy. While some cases of Hodgkin's disease may present as medias-tinal involvement, physical examination often reveals enlarged right supra-clavicular nodes in these patients.

The lymph nodes in Hodgkin's disease are generally painless and have a rubbery consistency. However, these features are not pathognomonic for Hodgkin's disease. The differential diagnosis of Hodgkin's disease includes infectious disorders such as mononucleosis and toxoplasmosis, and – in the case of mediastinal presentations – tuberculosis and sarcoidosis. In older patients, the differential diagnosis includes other primary (mediastinal) and metastatic carcinomas. Although clinical features such as mediastinal and unilateral hilar disease may suggest the diagnosis of Hodgkin's disease, the diagnosis can be established only by biopsy and review of the pathologic material by a hematopathologist.

While Hodgkin's disease can present as a superior vena cava syndrome or as a spinal cord compression, these presentations are extremely rare. In such cases, or when Hodgkin's disease is diagnosed on a biopsy of Waldeyer's ring, an epitrochlear node, a primary gastrointestinal tumor, or a lesion of skin, bone, pancreas, or thyroid, one should be very certain that one has not mis-diagnosed a case of non-Hodgkin's lymphoma.

The majority of patients with Hodgkin's disease are asymptomatic except for their lymphadenopathy. However, approximately 25% of patients with Hodgkin's disease present with fever, night sweats, and/or weight loss, so-called 'B' symptoms. Less frequently, patients with Hodgkin's disease may present with Pel-Ebstein fever, a cyclical fever in which several days or weeks of fever alternates with an afebrile period. Patients who present with these symptoms have a worse prognosis than asymptomatic patients with Hodgkin's disease. While pruritis has been associated with Hodgkin's disease, and while its recurrence may herald clinical relapse patients in whom pruritis is the only symptom of Hodgkin's disease do not have a worse prognosis than asymptomatic patients. A rare symptom of Hodgkin's disease is the occurrence of pain in association with the ingestion of alcohol. Often, the pain occurs at a site of involvement of Hodgkin's disease. The mechanism of this alcohol induced pain is not understood, and there is some evidence that the incidence of this symptom has decreased during the past thirty years [23].

Table 1. Ann Arbor staging system for Hodgkin's disease.

Stage I	Involvement of a single lymph node region
Stage II	Involvement of two or more lymph node regions on the same side of the diaphragm
Stage III	Involvement of lymph node regions on both sides of the diaphragm, with or without splenic involvement
Stage IV	Diffuse or disseminated involvement of one or more extra-lymphatic organs or tissues, with or without associated lymph node involvement

The presence (B) or absence (A) of fever, night sweats, or weight loss of greater than 10% of body weight are denoted by the corresponding suffix letters B and A.

The subscript E (e.g. I_E or II_E) is used to denote involvement of an extralymphatic site by direct extension rather than by hematogenous spread, as in the case of a large mediastinal mass extending to involve the lung.

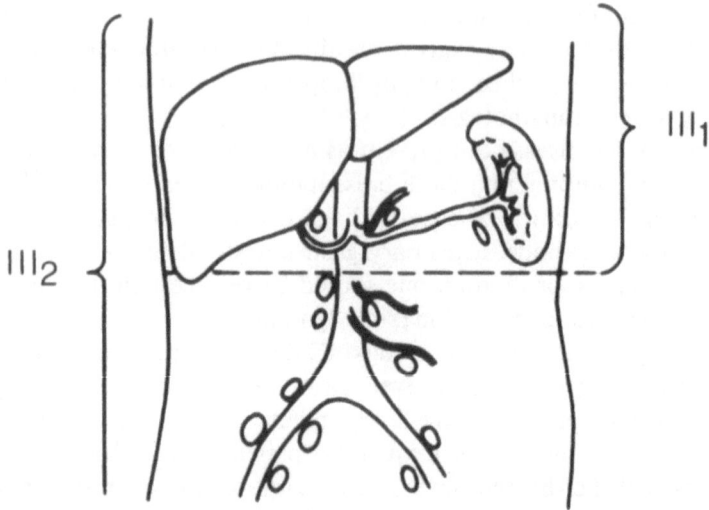

Figure 2. Representation of anatomic substages of Hodgkin's disease.

2.4. Staging

2.4.1. Rationale and Patterns of Spread. Staging (determination of the extent of disease) plays a critical role in the evaluation of the patient with Hodgkin's disease. The Ann Arbor staging system, which is most commonly used in Hodgkin's disease, is presented in Table 1. However, staging is not merely an academic exercise. Staging is first and foremost the basis for therapeutic planning. In this regard, several authors have recently suggested that with respect to the therapeutic options most commonly considered for patients with stage III Hodgkin's disease, division of this stage into anatomic substages (Figure 2) is necessary as a basis for planning therapy. This issue will be discussed elsewhere in this chapter.

Once enough information has been obtained to allow a decision to be made regarding therapy, additional staging procedures may still be necessary. Staging procedures may be needed to provide a baseline for restaging. For patients receiving chemotherapy, it is critically important to demonstrate that a complete remission has been obtained prior to the discontinuation of treatment. The completeness of remission can be assessed only when an adequate baseline has been obtained. Staging may also be used to provide more accurate information regarding prognosis. From an academic point of view, accurate staging may allow the results of therapy to be more meaningfully compared among institutions.

While the performance of staging procedures is guided by the principles stated above, it should be remembered that the approach to staging should

Table 2. Incidence of involvement of nodal sites, and occurrence of contiguous and non-contiguous nodal involvement.

Site	% cases involved	% sole site involved	% non-contiguous sites involved	% contiguous sites involved
Right axillary nodes	23	6.4	10.2	83.3
Left axillary nodes	26	3.3	3.3	93.3
Right cervical/supraclavicular nodes	59	6.0	0.5	93.4
Left cervical/supraclavicular nodes	71	9.5	2.5	88.0
Mediastinal nodes	62	2.4	0.5	97.1
Hilar nodes	11	0	0.0	100.0
Para-aortic nodes	34	0.9	0.9	98.2
Iliac, inguinal, femoral nodes	16	9.3	1.8	88.8

consider the fact that Hodgkin's disease tends to spread in a contiguous fashion (Table 2). With recognition of the anatomic connections between the left supraclavicular area and the upper abdomen, contiguous patterns of spread have been demonstrated in almost 95% of patients with Hodgkin's disease. It should be noted that for patients with only right supraclavicular presentations, abdominal disease is found in 8% of cases; for patients with left supraclavicular node presentations the incidence of abdominal disease is 40%; for patients with bilateral supraclavicular node involvement, further evaluation reveals disease below the diaphragm in 46% of cases.

Even within the abdomen, the pattern of disease involvement is generally consistent with the idea that disease spreads to the spleen by a hematogenous route and then spreads from the spleen in a contiguous fashion (Table 3). In

Table 3. Pattern of abdominal node involvement in stage III Hodgkin's disease.

Number of patients	Spleen	Nodes					
		Splenic	Celiac	Portal	Paraaortic	Iliac	Mesenteric
14	+	+ or −	−	−	−	−	−
2	+	+	+	−	−	−	−
3	+	+	+	+	−	−	−
3	+	+	−	−	+	−	−
5	+	+	+	+	+	−	−
6	+	+	+	+	+	+	−
4	+	+	+	+	+	+	+
8	+	Various nodes +					
7	−	Various nodes +					

one series of patients in whom staging laparotomies were performed, with rigorous attention to biopsy of all abdominal notal groups, the spleen and contiguous lymph nodes were involved in 71% of cases, the spleen and non-contiguous lymph nodes were involved in 16% of cases, and various lymph nodes were involved by Hodgkin's disease in the absence of splenic involvement in 13% of cases [24].

While discontinuous spread does occur, these results mean that when clinical evaluation suggests that a discontinuous pattern of disease is present, further confirmation of the abnormal findings may be indicated. For example, assume that an asymptomatic patient with Hodgkin's disease presents with right supraclavicular adenopathy and has a staging evaluation which is normal except for a lymphangiogram which shows only an abnormal *iliac* node; the remainder of the lymphangiogram is normal and there is no evidence of splenic enlargement on physical examination or by isotopic scan of the spleen. While clinical assessment can be a basis for therapeutic decisions in many cases, in this setting – i.e. apparent discontinuous spread – a staging laparoromy to assess the accuracy of the lymphangiogram would be a reasonable consideration.

2.4.2. Sites of Disease, Clinical Evaluation. As stated above, the staging of Hodgkin's disease is an analytical procedure designed to assist the planning of therapy, establish a baseline for re-evaluation following completion of therapy, and provide an accurate determination of prognosis. For this reason, the tests performed as part of a staging evaluation must be tailored to individual cases rather than performed as a check list. Nevertheless, the tests which are most commonly performed in the staging of Hodgkin's disease are presented in Table 4.

Table 4. Diagnostic evaluation of Hodgkin's disease.

History: Careful evaluation of fever, night sweats, and weight loss
Complete physical examination: Careful evaluation of all peripheral nodes, liver, spleen, and Waldeyer's ring
Laboratory tests: Complete blood count, platelet count, liver and renal function tests, alkaline phosphatase, erythrocyte sedimentation rate (optional)
Chest X-ray: Chest tomograms if findings on chest X-ray are equivocal
Lymphangiogram
Liver and spleen isotope scan
Bone marrow biopsy: May be omitted in patients with clinical stage I-A or II-A disease
Staging laparotomy with splenectomy: In selected patients
Other optional procedures: Abdominal CT scan, gallium scan, isotopic bone scan, immunologic evaluation – skin tests and/or peripheral blood lymphocyte typing, cytologic evaluation of effusions, biopsy of potential visceral sites of disease as suggested by clinical evaluation

Table 5. Incidence of Hodgkin's disease by stage, therapeutic options by stage, and potential for cure.

Stage	Estimated incidence	Therapeutic options	Estimated % of patients who are cured
I–A	10%	Involved field or extended field radiation therapy	95
II–A	30%	As for stage I–A	85
I–B, II–B	10%	Extended field radiation ± combination chemotherapy; total nodal radiation	70
III$_1$–A	15%	Total nodal radiation or extended field radiation	85
III$_2$–A	10%	Combination chemotherapy ± total nodal radiation	65
III–B	15%	As for stage III$_2$–A	60
IV–A, IV–B	10%	Combination chemotherapy	50

In addition, while a detailed discussion of therapy is beyond the scope of this chapter, staging occurs in a clinical context. Accordingly, Table 5, which presents the relative incidence of each stage of Hodgkin's disease, and the percentage of patients with that stage who are cured by either initial treatment or salvage therapy, also presents some of the therapeutic options which are commonly considered for patients with each stage of Hodgkin's disease.

History and physical examination: In taking the medical history, special attention must be given to those factors which determine prognosis, i.e. 'B' symptoms such as unexplained fever, night sweats, or weight loss. In order for a patient to be categorized as 'B', the weight loss must be equal to or greater than 10% of body weight. While this can usually be accurately documented, patients often give questionable histories regarding fever or night sweats. Fever may be undocumented, or may be attributed to a concurrent infectious illness. While drenching night sweats may be easily documented, patients may give a history of awakening to find only neck and chest dampness. In reality, there is a continuum ranging from the truly asymptomatic patient to the patient who has substantial fever, night sweats, and weight loss; the Ann Arbor system, however, arbitrarily classifies patients as either 'A' or 'B'. This is an oversimplification, but in the absence of any other suggested scale of symptoms, general practice is to consider patients with an equivocal history of symptoms as 'A.'

Therapy of the patients with Hodgkin's disease creates the potential of damage to a large number of organ systems, e.g. radiation therapy induced hypothyroidism, combination chemotherapy induced sterility, adriamycin induced cardiomyopathy, or bleomycin induced pulmonary fibrosis. Therefore, a complete history and physical examination, and review of systems, should be part of the baseline assessment of every patient with Hodgkin's

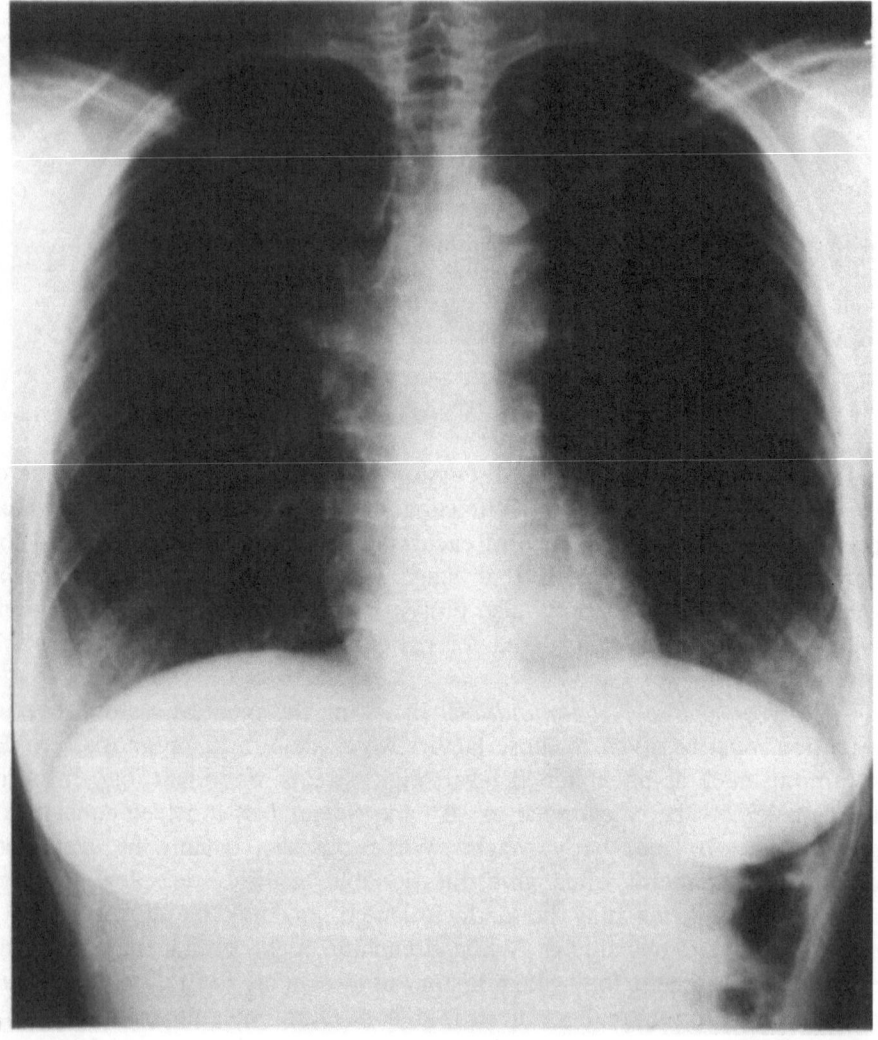

Figure 3. A: Chest X-ray in a 32-year-old woman with nodular sclerosis Hodgkin's disease showing widening of the mediastinum. The patient was also found to have liver involvement and received six months of combination chemotherapy. B: Upon completion of chemotherapy, the mediastinum had not returned to normal. Conceivably, this could be due to fibrosis rather than active Hodgkin's disease. However, the patient received radiation therapy – 4000 rads in four weeks – to a small mediastinal port and has remained in remission for two years.

disease. In addition, this evaluation will occasionally reveal unsuspected sites of disease, and establish the need for special diagnostic tests. For example, while bone involvement is infrequently observed, the sclerotic ivory vertebra has been well described as a manifestation of Hodgkin's disease. A history of bone pain is an indication for the performance of bone scans and X-rays which might ordinarily be omitted.

In addition to a careful examination of those nodal areas in which involvement by Hodgkin's disease is frequent, i.e. cervical, supraclavicular, axillary, and inguinal nodes, the physical examination should also include an evaluation of other less frequently involved lymph node regions such as epitrochlear, femoral, and submental nodes as well as Waldeyer's ring. While examination of the abdomen is part of the routine physical examination, it

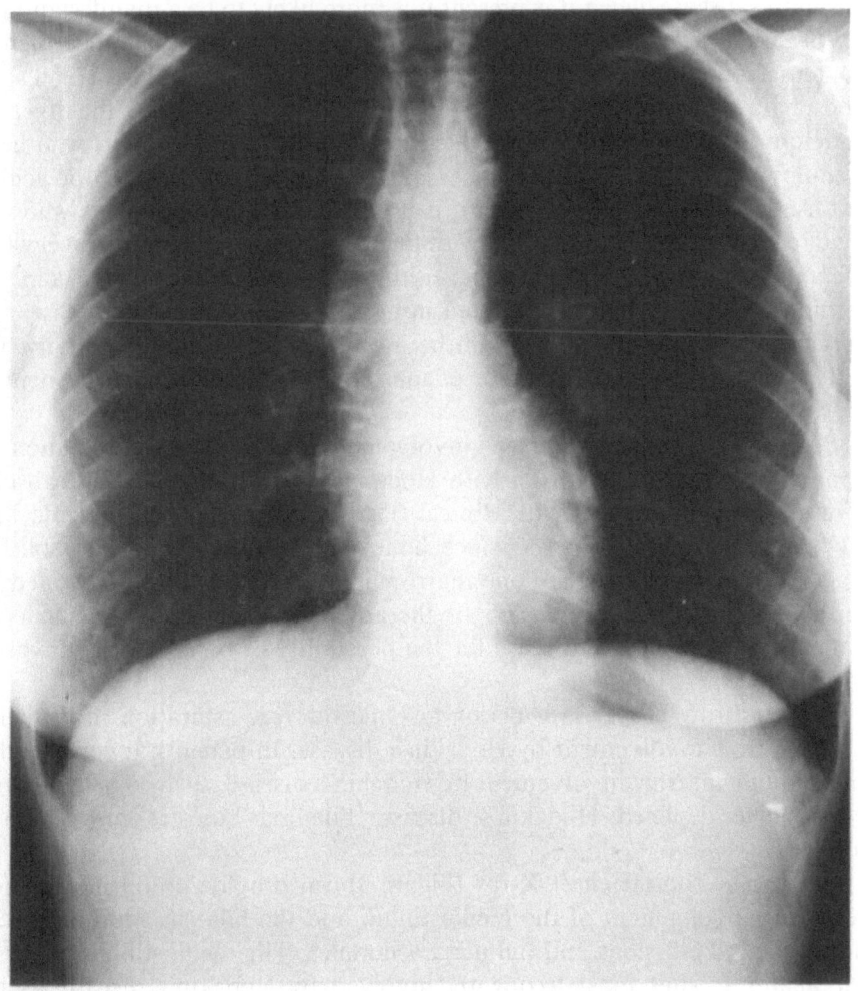

b

must be recognized that enlargement of the liver and spleen, in a patient with Hodgkin's disease, may merely be signs of non-specific hypertrophy of the monocyte-phagocyte system, rather than signs of involvement of these organs.

Laboratory tests: While a complete blood count, platelet count, liver and renal function tests, and serum uric acid level are part of the baseline evaluation of the patient with Hodgkin's disease, they are generally of limited value. Anemia in a patient with Hodgkin's disease is more likely to be the chronic anemia of malignancy, or the anemia of hypersplenism, than to be a sign of marrow involvement by Hodgkin's disease. However, since autoimmune hemolytic anemia has been associated with Hodgkin's disease, and may require specific therapy, evaluation of anemia is indicated. Similarly, while thrombocytopenia is infrequently seen at presentation in patients with Hodgkin's disease, when it is present it is more likely to be a manifestation of autoimmune thrombocytopenia or of hypersplenism than it is to be a sign of bone marrow involvement by Hodgkin's disease. While an elevated alkaline phosphatase may be a sign of Hodgkin's disease involving the liver or skeleton, the enzyme may be elevated non-specifically in patients who have granulomas, but not Hodgkin's disease, in their livers. While the uric acid is not useful as a staging procedure, it is useful in identifying patients who will require allopurinol therapy to prevent further elevation of the uric level when therapy is initiated. Although the erythrocyte sedimentation rate and the serum copper level may be elevated in patients with Hodgkin's disease, and are considered by some authors to be useful indices of disease activity, the tests are not specific enough to be of substantial value in the management of Hodgkin's disease.

Bone marrow: Bone marrow involvement is found at presentation in approximately 5% of patients with Hodgkin's disease and is almost exclusively limited to patients with clinical stage III disease and to patients with 'B' symptoms [28]. However, since bone marrow involvement establishes stage IV disease, and since bone marrow involvement can be reassessed by repeat biopsy at the conclusion of therapy, many authorities evaluate all patients with Hodgkin's disease for the possibility of bone marrow involvement.

Bone marrow biopsy is superior to bone marrow aspiration in detecting bone marrow involvement by Hodgkin's disease. In patients at considerable risk of bone marrow involvement by Hodgkin's disease, such as patients with lymphocyte depleted Hodgkin's disease, bilateral biopsies may be performed.

Chest: The routine chest X-ray (Figure 3) can provide useful information regarding involvement of the mediastinum and the hila; in addition, it can detect pleural effusions and pulmonary nodules. The mediastinum is one of the anatomic sites most frequently involved by Hodgkin's disease, as the incidence of mediastinal involvement is 60% in most series. In contrast, hilar disease is seen at presentation in less than 20% of cases of Hodgkin's disease. Hilar disease in the absence of mediastinal disease is rare. In fact, in a young patient with hilar adenopathy, in the absence of mediastinal enlargement, the working diagnosis should be sarcoidosis.

Pleural effusions in the patient with Hodgkin's disease do not necessarily indicate malignant involvement of the pleura. In addition to infectious complications such as tuberculosis, pleural effusions – often chylous – can result from compression of lymphatic structures by large mediastinal masses. The presence of a pleural effusion is an indication for thoracentesis with cytologic evaluation and routine bacterial cultures as well as cultures for tuberculosis and fungi. If no diagnosis is established by these procedures a pleural biopsy is indicated.

Pulmonary parenchymal lesions in a patient with Hodgkin's disease create a differential diagnosis which includes Hodgkin's disease, tuberculosis, and opportunistic infections, as well as coincidental benign and malignant nodules. Unless other clinical features dictate a therapeutic course, pathologic evaluation with bronchoscopy, transthoracic biopsy, and, eventually, open lung biopsy may be indicated.

Chest tomography is of marginal clinical value in the patient with Hodgkin's disease. Some authors feel that tomograms are indicated whenever the chest X-ray is equivocal, when the configuration of the chest obscures accurate interpretation of the plain film, when hilar adenopathy is present, or when a large mediastinal mass prevents evaluation of the lung parenchyma [29]. In one large series, tomography was able to provide additional information in approximately 20% of patients with Hodgkin's disease; however, this information changed the stage of the patient and the approach to therapy in only 1.2% of cases [30]. Furthermore, some studies have suggested that a large mediastinal mass – i.e. greater than 6 cm in diameter, or greater than one-third the diameter of the chest – may, by itself, be an indication for chemotherapy [31, 32]. While this approach necessitates a careful evaluation of thoracic disease, it may mean that the routine chest X-ray establishes the therapeutic plan in these patients, and that tomography adds little to their management.

Abdominal nodal disease: Evaluation of abdominal involvement by Hodgkin's disease is not only critical for therapeutic planning, it is also the most difficult aspect of staging. Since staging decisions can be guided to some degree by the likelihood of discovering involvement, the incidence of involvement of various abdominal sites is presented in Table 6.

Lymphangiography is the standard means of assessing retroperitoneal node involvement in Hodgkin's disease. While the accuracy of the lymphangiogram depends on the skill of the radiologist who interprets the procedure, the overall accuracy of lymphangiography is 80–90%. However, lymphangiogra-

Table 6. Incidence of involvement of abdominal sites in Hodgkin's disease.

Site	% of all cases with involvement
Spleen	35–40%
Liver	10%
Lymph nodes	
Splenic hilar	30–40%
Para-aortic	30–40%
Mesenteric	<5%
Portal	<5%

phy does not visualize lymph nodes above the second lumbar vertebra. Thus, when the lymphangiogram is read as normal, involvement of the splenic hilar, celiac nodes, and porta hepatis nodes – as well as splenic involvement – may occur in up to 30% of patients. When the lymphangiogram is abnormal, findings at staging laparotomy have generally confirmed the radiologic interpretation. Lymphangiography has the additional value that the lymphangiogram dye may remain in the lymph nodes for from 4 to 24 months following the procedure, thus enabling a flat plate of the abdomen to provide useful information regarding the response to therapy during this period (Figure 4).

Abdominal CT scanning has recently been suggested as a non-invasive means of assessing the retroperitoneum. Most studies have shown substantial correlations between the results of lymphangiography and the results of abdominal CT scanning [34, 35]. However, in one recent study, 'positive' CT scans, while confirmed by 'positive' findings at staging laparotomy, disagreed as to the level of nodal involvement [36]. Since the specific level of abdominal node involvement may be of critical clinical importance, the value of CT scanning as a staging procedure is apparently limited. Furthermore, in view of its cost, and intrinsic inability to detect normal sized nodes in which the internal architecture has been replaced – nodes which can be detected by lymphangiography – it seems unlikely that CT scanning will replace lymphangiography as the procedure of choice in the assessment of retroperitoneal Hodgkin's disease.

Spleen: The spleen is the most common site of abdominal involvement by Hodgkin's disease and is involved in 80% of patients with stage III Hodgkin's disease [27]. However, while clinical assessment of splenic involvement by physical examination and nuclear imaging is accurate in two-thirds of patients, these procedures are highly insensitive [37]. Since splenic involvement may consist of only a few microscopic nodules, it is easy to appreciate how a spleen which is clinically normal may actually be

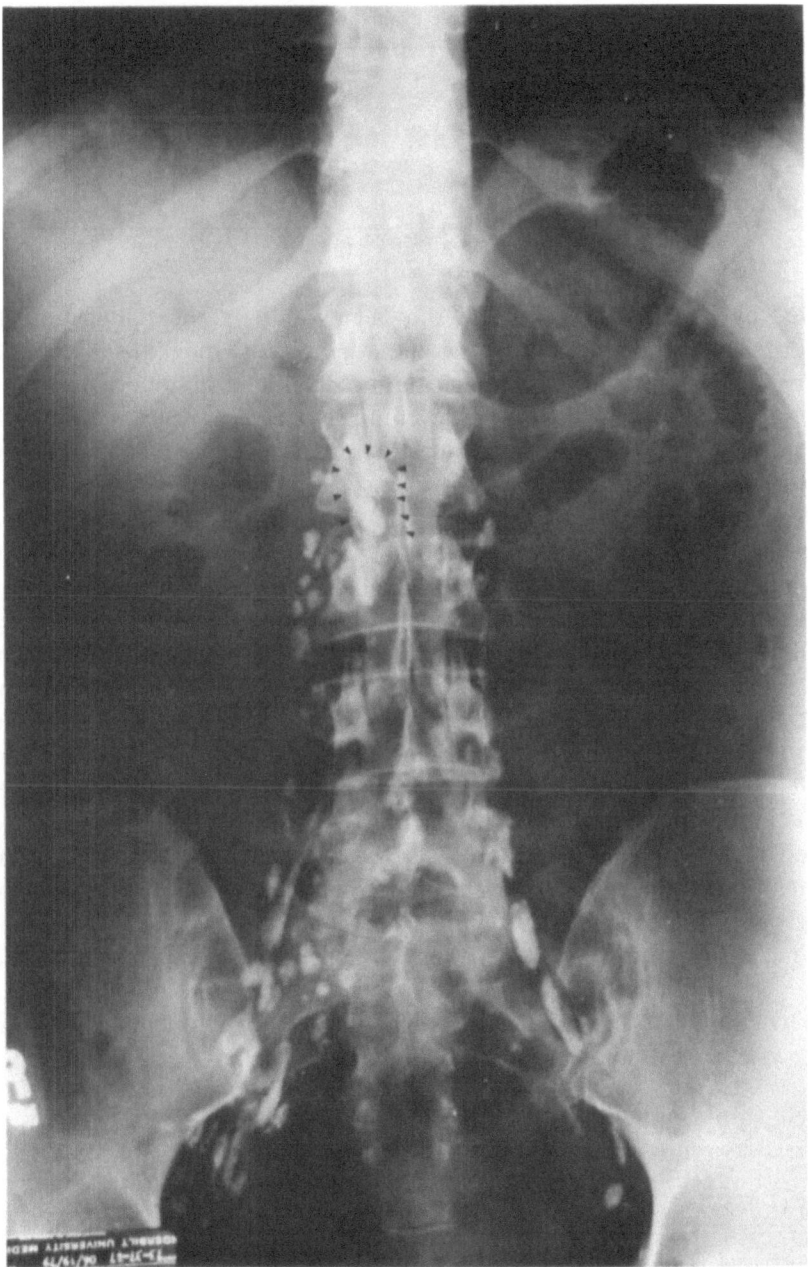

Figure 4. Lymphangiogram from a 48-year-old man with mixed cellularity Hodgkin's disease. The abnormal node, which is marked, is enlarged and its internal architecture is abnormal. As stated in the text, and illustrated by this figure, the lymphangiogram does not visualize lymph nodes above the second lumbar vertebra.

Table 7. Correlation of clinical and pathologic evaluation of splenic involvement.

Clinical evaluation	Pathologic evaluation	
	Positive	Negative
Positive	18%	10%
Negative	23%	49%

involved by Hodgkin's disease. As shown in Table 7, since clinical assessment of the spleen is usually negative in patients with Hodgkin's disease, the majority of patients in whom splenic involvement is found at staging laparotomy are actually felt to have clinically negative spleens. Similarly, since splenic enlargement may be due to granulomas, or other non-specific changes, splenomegaly is not diagnostic of splenic involvement by Hodgkin's disease.

Splenic involvement is considered a necessary condition for hepatic involvement by Hodgkin's disease to occur. Following a decade of staging laparotomies, hepatic involvement in the absence of splenic involvement remains a reportable phenomenon [38]. While it is recognized that splenic involvement predicts hepatic involvement, it is often not appreciated that splenic weight also pays a predictive role. Table 8 presents data compiled from some of the early series of staging laparotomies [39–45]. While liver involvement was noted in 18% of cases in which the spleen was involved, hepatic involvement was more frequently seen when the involved spleen weighed more than 400 g. It should also be noted, on the basis of the data presented in Table 8, that while *splenic* involvement was found in approximately one-third of spleens weighing less than 400 g, splenic involvement was detected in almost 90% of patients whose spleens weighed more than 400 g.

In recognition of the predictive value of splenic involvement, the Ann Arbor system treats the spleen as a special site, i.e. III-S is used to denote

Table 8. Liver involvement as related to splenic involvement and splenic weight.

	Liver involved/No. of cases
Spleen involved	
Weight >400 g	10/27 (37%)
Weight <400 g	6/61 (10%)
Spleen not involved	
Weight >400 g	0/4
Weight <400 g	4/112

splenic involvement. The assumption inherent in this approach is that stage III patients with splenic involvement will have a clinical course which is different from the course of stage III patients lacking splenic involvement.

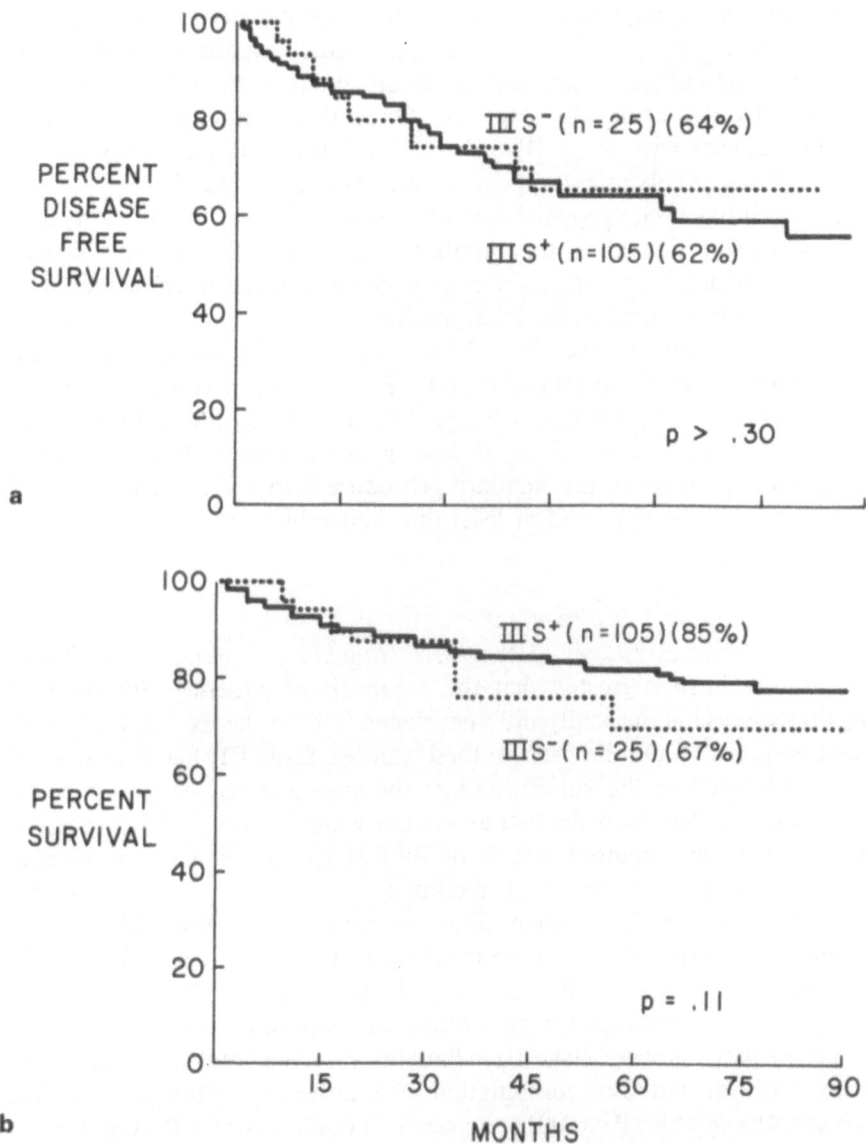

Figure 5. A: Actuarial disease free survival in Stage III Hodgkin's disease patients with splenic involvement (S+) and without splenic involvement (S−). B: Actuarial survival for the same patient groups. There is no statistically significant difference between S+ and S− patients with respect to either disease free survival or survival. Data are from collaborative study of 130 patients [27].

No evidence to support this hypothesis has ever been presented, and recent data suggest that this may not be the case. In a large series of stage III-A patients who were staged by laparotomy, both survival and disease free survival were statistically equivalent in stage III patients with splenic involvement as in stage III patients without splenic involvement (Figure 5) [27]. Although splenic involvement does predict hepatic involvement at laparotomy, patients in whom hepatic involvement is discovered at laparotomy are – by definition – in stage IV. Once these patients are excluded from the patients with stage III-S disease, the stage III patients with and without splenic involvement appear to have similar prognoses.

Recently, it has been suggested that while splenic involvement, *per se,* does not have prognostic value, the number of nodules of Hodgkin's disease which are detected in the spleen may predict the clinical outcome [46]. This finding awaits confirmation by other studies.

Liver: The liver is involved in 5–10% of patients with Hodgkin's disease, most of whom have 'B' symptoms. Liver involvement in Hodgkin's disease is usually so focal in nature that it can be detected only by the performance of open liver biopsies at the time of staging laparotomies. When a staging laparotomy is performed, the standard procedure is to obtain needle biopsies of both lobes of the liver and at least one wedge biopsy.

2.5. Special Staging Considerations

2.5.1. Anatomic Substages of Stage III Hodgkin's Disease. A number of recent studies have suggested that the prognosis of patients with stage III Hodgkin's disease is markedly different depending on the extent of abdominal disease [23–27]. On the basis of these studies, Stage III_1 has been defined as disease limited to the spleen, and/or the splenic hilar, celiac, or portal nodes. Stage III_2 has been defined as disease which involves the para-aortic nodes, iliac nodes, inguinal nodes, or mesenteric nodes, with or without involvement of sites in the upper abdomen.

A collaborative study involving four institutions, and designed to assess the clinical importance of anatomic substage, has been reported [27]. The study included 130 patients with pathologically staged III-A Hodgkin's disease. Median follow-up was 58 months. Seventy-four patients were stage III_1 and 56 patients were stage III_2. Patients received total nodal radiation therapy with or without combination chemotherapy. Both disease free survival (74% vs 46%, $P<0.001$) and survival (94% vs 65%, $P<0.001$) were better in stage III_1-A patients as compared to stage III_2-A patients (figure 6). These differences in favor of substage III_1 were also observed when the patients who received only radiotherapy were analyzed separately. The study also reported a slight but statistically insignificant tendency for stage III_2 patients to relapse in visceral rather than nodal sites.

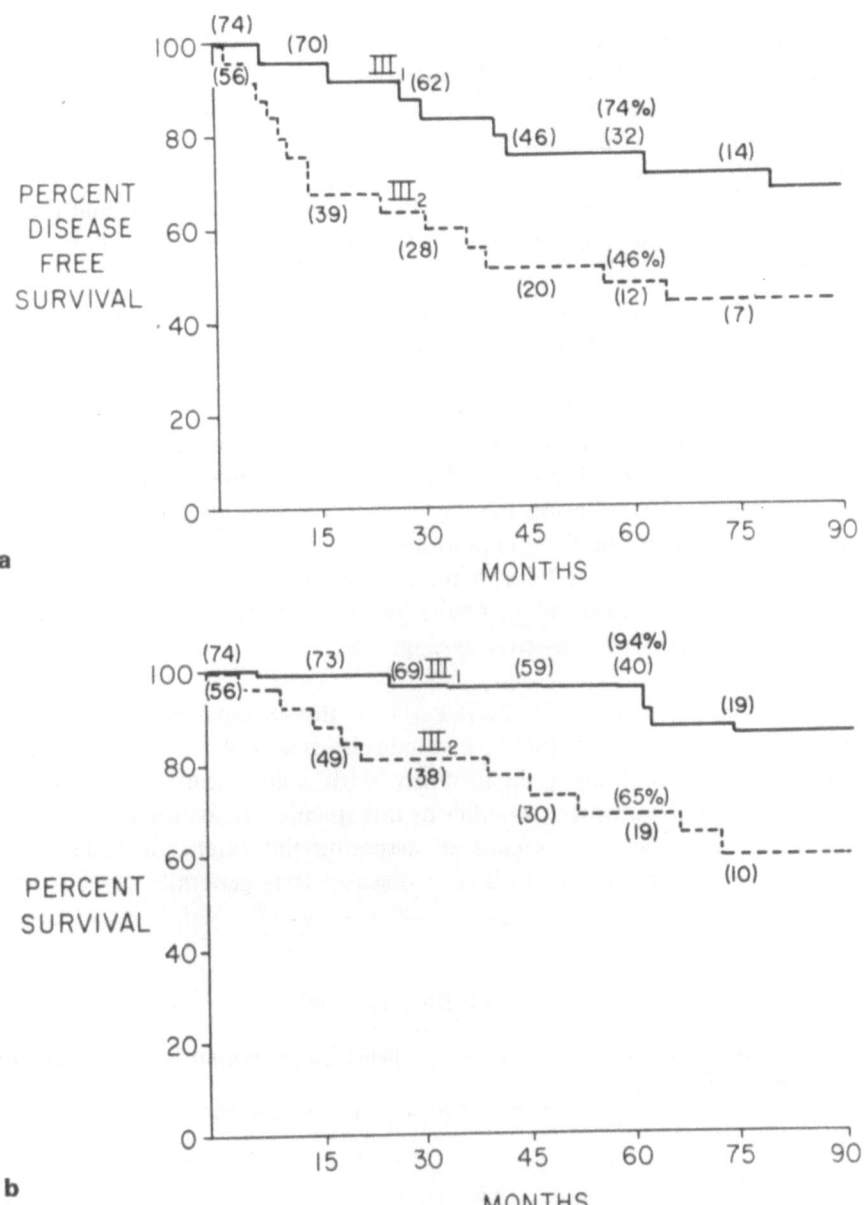

Figure 6. A: Actuarial disease free survival, Substage III₁ and Substage III₂, P<0.001. B: Actuarial survival, Substage III₁ and Substage III₂, P<0.001 [27].

The reason why stage III_2 patients should have a worse prognosis than stage III_1 patients is not established. Stage I and II patients who present with sub-diaphragmatic disease in the iliac or inguinal regions do no worse than other stage I or II patients [47]. It is therefore unlikely that there is something detrimental about having disease in these sites, *per se.* More likely, if abdominal Hodgkin's disease initially involves the spleen, and then spreads in a retrograde manner, involvement of the lower abdominal nodes reflects the fact that the host is doing a poor job controlling the tumor, or that the tumor is highly aggressive. Alternatively, stage III$_2$ disease may indicate that abdominal disease has been present for a longer period of time and that there has been, therefore, a greater risk that dissemination to occult sites may have occurred.

The distinction between stage III$_1$ and stage III$_2$ may be important with respect to therapeutic decisions. The survival of stage III$_1$ patients who receive radiation therapy is similar to the survival of stage II Patients treated by the same modality. By contrast, the survival of stage III$_2$ patients who have received standard total nodal irradiation is no better than the survival of stage IV patients who have received combination chemotherapy. Accordingly, extended field irradiation has been advocated for patients with stage III$_1$ disease, and combination chemotherapy – with or without radiation therapy – has been advocated for patients in stage III$_2$. If such a clinical approach is adopted, it becomes critically important to accurately distinguish patients in stage III$_1$ from patients in stage III$_2$.

2.5.2. Staging laparotomy. In the late 1960s, staging laparotomy (Table 9) was introduced as a research tool to evaluate the extent of Hodgkin's disease within the abdomen. Staging laparotomy with splenectomy is the most accurate means of determining whether or not splenic involvement is present and it is the most accurate means of assessing the extent of abdominal lymph node involvement by Hodgkin's disease. It is generally agreed that

Table 9. Procedures performed as part of a staging laparotomy.

1. Review of tests performed prior to laparotomy, including lymphangiography, to help guide the surgeon in planning biopsies
2. Complete consideration of the therapeutic options to determine if laparotomy is indicated in the individual patient

Surgery

3. Inspection of the abdomen
4. Liver biopsies of both lobes, wedge and needle biopsies
5. Splenectomy
6. Lymph node biopsies: splenic hilar, celiac, portal, para-aortic, iliac, mesenteric node biopsies
7. Placement of clips on splenic pedicle, sites of node biopsies, and margins of tumor masses if present
8. Oophoropexy in selected patients

staging laparotomy adds information regarding the extent of disease and changes the therapeutic plan in 30–40% of patients who undergo laparotomy. Nevertheless, routine use of staging laparotomy has never been proven to produce a clinical benefit. Staging laparotomy is of clinical benefit only if the changes in therapy produce better results (increased survival and/or decreased morbidity) and only if this improvement exceeds the morbidity of laparotomy [48]. Unfortunately, since the best treatment for each stage of Hodgkin's disease has not been established, it is difficult to assess the magnitude of the benefit which occurs when decisions are made on the basis of pathologic staging rather than clinical staging. The situation is complicated by the fact that salvage therapy at the time of relapse can compensate for some of the treatment errors which can result from initial errors in staging.

As an example of this problem we may consider a patient with clinical stage I-A or II-A nodular sclerosis Hodgkin's disease and a negative lymphangiogram. On the basis of previously published studies, we can estimate that if the patient underwent a staging laparotomy, there would be a 30% chance that disease would be found in the abdomen, changing the patient's stage to stage III-A [37]. However, to assess the benefit of laparotomy we must consider the fact that extended field irradiation has produced 5-year survivals of greater than 95% in clinical stage I-A and II-A patients with nodular sclerosis Hodgkin's disease who were not subjected to laparotomy [49, 50]. The reason for this apparent paradox is that the abdominal disease which is discovered in clinical stage I-A and II-A patients is usually limited to the upper abdomen [37], i.e. these patients are found to be in substage III_1. As we have stated previously, extended field radiation therapy may be adequate treatment for these patients. As a result, while laparotomy has increased the accuracy of staging, it may not have benefited the specific patients who were found to be in stage III. Furthermore, if the patient who is found to be in stage III_1 is given total nodal radiation therapy and chemotherapy on the grounds that this therapy is optimal for all stage III patients, this overtreatment may unnecessarily place him at risk for complications of therapy, such as acute leukemia.

Thus, the value of staging laparotomy cannot be considered apart from the therapeutic decision tree which is employed. Furthermore, the risks of staging laparotomy must also be considered. Splenectomy places patients at a small – approximately 1% – risk of fatal infections with encapsulated organisms, primarily pneumococcus and hemophilus [51–53]. In addition, laparotomy in major medical centers has a mortality rate of less than 1% with a 12% incidence of morbidity (pneumonia, pulmonary embolism, fecal fistulae, bowel obstruction, wound dehiscence, or ureteral transection) [54]. However, in institutions where staging laparotomies are performed infrequently, mortality rates greater than 6% and complication rates greater than

25 % have been observed. In summary, staging laparotomy can increase the
accuracy of staging in patients with Hodgkin's disease. However, the risk to
benefit ratio for laparotomy varies from case to case and from institution to
institution in conjunction with the skills of the surgical team and the clinical
decision tree which is employed.

2.6. Hodgkin's Disease in Children

Hodgkin's disease is relatively uncommon in children under five years of
age, especially in economically developed nations. When Hodgkin's disease
does occur in the first decade of life, 90 % of cases occur in males. While
non-Hodgkin's lymphoma in children differs substantially from its adult
counterpart, childhood Hodgkin's disease and adult Hodgkin's disease are
relatively similar with respect to histology [55], clinical presentations, and
stage [56]. However, two important clinical considerations must be made
with respect to childhood Hodgkin's disease. First, the risk of sepsis
following splenectomy is higher in children than in adults. Accordingly,
greater reliance may be placed on clinical staging than on pathologic staging
in children with Hodgkin's disease. Secondly, in children with Hodgkin's
disease, radiation therapy may produce growth retardation. As a result, stage
for stage, therapeutic decisions in childhood Hodgkin's disease may tend
towards the inclusion of chemotherapy to a greater extent than is the case in
adult Hodgkin's disease. When chemotherapy is part of the therapeutic plan,
the need to find occult visceral sites of disease is relatively limited.

3. NON-HODGKIN'S LYMPHOMA

3.1. Introduction

The non-Hodgkin's lymphomas are a group of malignancies which involve
lymphocytes. Although discussions of non-Hodgkin's lymphoma often consider the disorder as a single entity, critical differences among the disorders
exist. For example, some types of lymphoma are almost always disseminated
at presentation with a high rate of bone marrow and/or hepatic involvement;
other histologic types of lymphoma may frequently present with disease
limited to a single lymph node or to two adjacent sites. In some types of
non-Hodgkin's lymphoma, advanced disease is associated with a median
survival of 6 months unless combination chemotherapy produces a complete
remission. By contrast, in other lymphomas, advanced disease may be
associated with a survival of years with minimal therapy or – in the case of
asymptomatic patients – no therapy at all. In some types of non-Hodgkin's
lymphoma, a complete remission which is well documented by re-staging is
equivalent to cure; in other types of non-Hodgkin's lymphoma complete
remissions are never permanent and are eventually followed by relapses.

Table 10. Incidence of histologic types of lymphoma (Rappaport classification).

	Nodular	Diffuse
Well differentiated lymphocytic lymphoma (WDL)	---	2–5%
Poorly differentiated lymphocytic lymphoma (PDL)	20–30%	10–15%
Mixed cell (lymphocytic-histiocytic) lymphoma (MC)	5–15%	5–10%
Histiocytic lymphoma (HL)	3–7%	30–40%
Undifferentiated lymphoma	---	3–5%

Ironically, the lymphomas which appear to progress most rapidly in the absence of therapy, i.e. histiocytic lymphomas, may be associated with the highest cure rates when combination chemotherapy is used, while remissions in patients with slowly progressing lymphomas, such as nodular poorly differentiated lymphocytic lymphoma, are generally followed by relapses. These latter lymphomas may actually be incurable by present therapeutic approaches.

Because of these extensive differences, it is necessary to define biologically homogeneous categories of non-Hodgkin's lymphoma in order that the

Table 11. Incidence of common histologic types of lymphoma (Lukes-Collins classification)

		Incidence
B-cell disorders		
Small B cell lymphoma		
(including chronic lymphocytic leukemia)		10%
Plasmacytoid lymphoma		5%
Follicular center cell lymphomas		50%
Small cleaved cell lymphoma	20%	
Large cleaved cell lymphoma	15%	
Small transformed cell lymphoma	5%	
Large transformed cell lymphoma	10%	
Immunoblastic sarcoma of B-cells		5%
T-cell disorders		
Small T Cell lymphoma (T-cell CLL)		Rare
Convoluted lymphocytic lymphoma		10%
(lymphoblastic lymphoma)		
Cutaneous T-Cell lymphoma		3%
Immunoblastic sarcoma of T-cells		5%
(and other non-named lymphomas of node based T-cells)		
Undefined cell disorders (including acute lymphoblastic leukemia)		12%

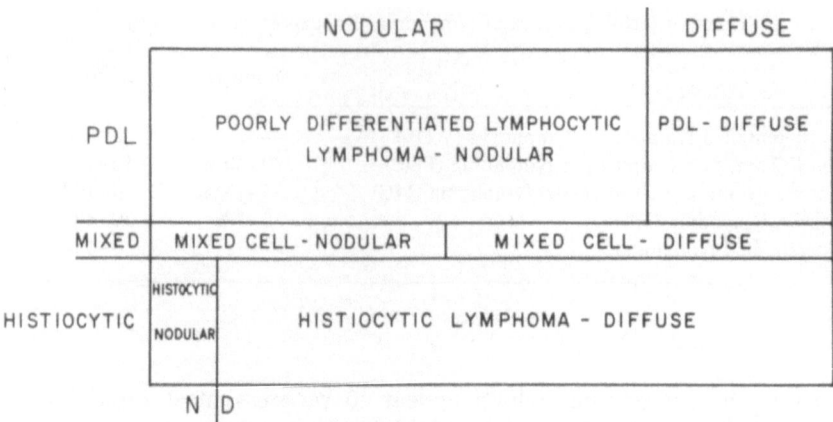

Figure 7. Rappaport classification of lymphoma. The area within each block is roughly proportional to the incidence of the lymphoma [71].

statements which are made regarding subtypes of non-Hodgkin's lymphoma have substantial scientific meaning. While the Rappaport classification system for lymphomas is widely used, certain categories of lymphoma defined by the Rappaport system, specifically diffuse poorly differentiated lymphocytic lymphoma [58–60], and diffuse histiocytic lymphoma [58–64], are heterogeneous categories. Furthermore, immunologically homogeneous entities [65–67], associated with more uniform clinical behavior [68, 69], can be identified within these heterogeneous groups by the use of immunologic

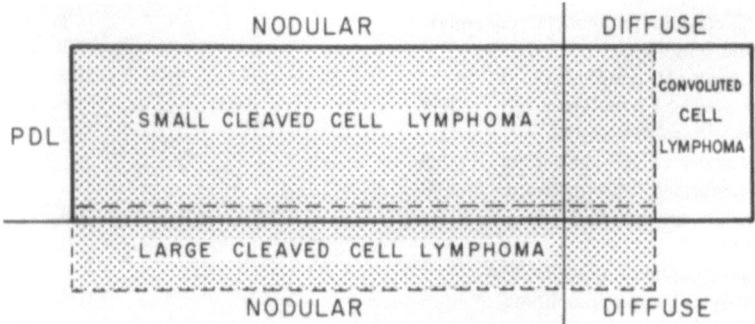

Figure 8. Subclassification of Rappaport category 'Poorly differentiated lymphocytic lymphoma', represented by heavy lines. Large cleaved cell lymphoma extends outside the heavy lines as this lymphoma is also included in the 'mixed- cell' and 'histiocytic' categories. B-cell lymphomas are shaded, T-cell lymphomas are not [71].

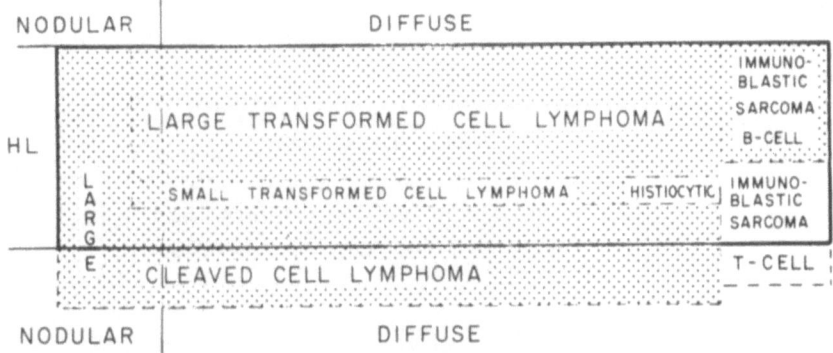

Figure 9. Subclassification of Rappaport category 'histiocytic' lymphoma, represented by heavy lines. Large cleaved cell lymphoma and immunoblastic sarcoma of T-cells extend outside the lines as these disorders are included in other categories. B-cell lymphomas are shaded, T-cell lymphomas are not [71].

markers or by the use of morphologic criteria derived from studies which have employed immunologic markers [70]. Since most studies performed during the past decade have presented their data in terms of the Rappaport system, it is used in the following discussion. Whenever it is appropriate, however, data will be presented regarding the immunologically homogeneous entities which can be delineated within the categories defined by the Rappaport system.

3.2. Incidence and Epidemiology

Approximately 15,000 new cases of non-Hodgkin's lymphoma occur in the United States each year. The breakdown by histologic subtype is shown in Tables 10 and 11 and in Figures 7–10 [71].

Most of the non-Hodgkin's lymphomas are diseases of older age groups as the median age of patients is in the fifth or sixth decade for most of the histologic subtypes. By contrast, lymphoblastic lymphoma, a T-cell lymphoma classified by the Rappaport system as part of diffuse poorly differentiated lymphocytic lymphoma, is most commonly seen in adolescents and young adults [65, 66]. Diffuse undifferentiated lymphoma also tends to occur in a somewhat younger age group than other types of non-Hodgkin's lymphoma.

An increased incidence of non-Hodgkin's lymphoma has been noted in patients with chronic immune deficiencies such as patients with ataxia telangectasia, as well as patients who have received renal transplants [72].

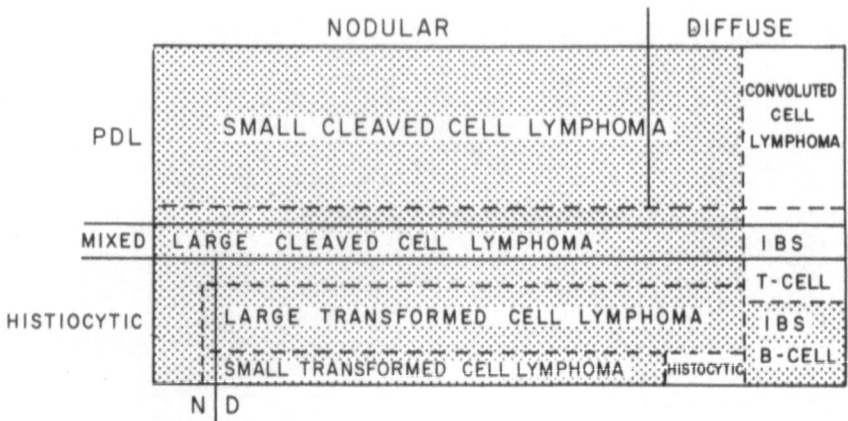

Figure 10. Lukes-Collins classification of lymphomas superimposed on Rappaport classification.

For unexplained reasons, these latter patients tend to develop diffuse histiocytic lymphomas in the central nervous system [72]. There is also an increased incidence of non-Hodgkin's lymphomas in patients with collagen vascular disease. Among patients with Sjogren's syndrome, the incidence of non-Hodgkin's lymphoma may approach 10%. Most of these lymphomas have been immunoblastic sarcomas [73]. An increased incidence of non-Hodgkin's lymphoma has also been reported in patients with Hodgkin's disease who received both radiotherapy and chemotherapy.

While epidemiologic associations do not exist for most of the common types of non-Hodgkin's lymphoma, the African form of Burkitt's lymphoma (a lymphoma of small transformed follicular center cells) has been associated with the Epstein-Barr virus. In Africa, the endemic area for Burkitt's lymphoma also corresponds to the area in which malaria is prevalent, suggesting that chronic stimulation of the immune system may be a predisposing factor for the occurrence of this lymphoma.

3.3. Presentations

Patients with non-Hodgkin's lymphoma may present with lymphadenopathy – which is more often generalized than solitary. As with Hodgkin's disease, cervical, supraclavicular ,and axillary nodes are frequently involved. In addition, inguinal, femoral, and epitrochlear nodes, as well as Waldeyer's ring – sites which are rarely involved in Hodgkin's disease – may be involved in non-Hodgkin's lymphoma. Predilections for specific types of non-Hodgkin's lymphoma to involve specific nodal sites has not been well documented except for the tendency of lymphoblastic lymphoma to involve the mediastinum. In contrast to Hodgkin's disease, the mediastinum is

Table 12. Stage at completion of staging evaluation as related to histology: non-Hodgkin's lymphomas.

	Stage			
	I	II	III	IV
	(% of patients)			
Histology				
Nodular				
Poorly differentiated lymphocytic	4	0	27	69
Mixed cell (lymphocytic-histiocytic)	0	8	24	68
Diffuse				
Poorly differentiated lymphocytic *	7	14	0	79
Histiocytic	8	23	25	45

* For lymphoblastic lymphoma (convoluted cell lymphoma), the T-cell subset of diffuse poorly differentiated lymphocytic lymphoma, essentially all cases are stage IV.

infrequently involved in other types of non-Hodgkin's lymphoma. While most patients with non-Hodgkin's lymphoma present with symptoms due to a slowly enlarging mass of nodes, non-Hodgkin's lymphoma may also present as an oncologic emergency such as a superior vena cava syndrome or a spinal cord compression.

The percentage of patients in each stage – at the time of presentation and following complete clinical and pathologic evaluation – is presented in Table 12 [74]. As can be seen from that table, at the time of presentation, the patient with a non-Hodgkin's lymphoma is more likely to have disseminated disease than is the patient with Hodgkin's disease. When assessing a patient with non-Hodgkin's lymphoma, therefore, it is reasonable to assume that disseminated disease is present until proven otherwise. Furthermore, while the Ann Arbor classification system for Hodgkin's disease is frequently used in the staging of non-Hodgkin's lymphoma, from the point of therapy most clinicians divide non-Hodgkin's lymphoma into two stages: limited and disseminated. While it has not been established where the line between limited and disseminated disease should be drawn, the low cure rates which have been reported using radiotherapy in some series suggest that it might be reasonable to consider even patients in stage II as having disseminated non-Hodgkin's lymphoma. Since non-Hodgkin's lymphoma is, of course, a group of diseases it may well be that the clinical distinction between limited and advanced disease may eventually be drawn at different points for the different types of non-Hodgkin's lymphoma.

Extranodal presentations have been frequently reported in patients with non-Hodgkin's lymphoma. In the Rappaport system these cases have usually been classified as diffuse, but this may be of limited meaning since a nodular pattern can generally be observed only when lymphoma is present in a lymph node. Extranodal non-Hodgkin's lymphoma may involve the gastrointestinal tract, the lung, bone, skin, thyroid, ovary or testis. Lymphomas of the stomach or of bone are most frequently diffuse histiocytic lymphomas, while lymphomas of the thyroid gland are most often immunoblastic sarcomas – a type of lymphoma which is also included within the category diffuse histiocytic lymphoma by the Rappaport system.

As a rough estimate, 10–20% of diffuse poorly differentiated lymphocytic lymphomas and 20–30% of diffuse histiocytic lymphomas arise at extranodal sites. These figures may, however, be overestimates of the incidence of extranodal disease. A study of patients with apparent extranodal non-Hodgkin's lymphoma involving cortical bone revealed that most of these patients had disseminated disease when complete staging was performed [75]. Thus, extranodal involvement, which is designated by the subscript 'E', may actually reflect visceral disease which should more correctly be regarded as stage IV. Since many of the studies in the literature which allegedly report patients with extranodal non-Hodgkin's lymphoma did not employ staging which was complete by present standards, all such studies should be interpreted cautiously.

3.4. Staging

3.4.1. Rationale. As in Hodgkin's disease, staging is the basis for therapeutic planning in non-Hodgkin's lymphoma, and staging also provides the physician with the ability to restage the patient upon the completion of therapy. However, there are several additional considerations regarding staging in non-Hodgkin's lymphoma.

First, patients with non-Hodgkin's lymphoma are often older than patients with Hodgkin's disease. This may not only limit therapeutic options,but it may also increase the morbidity associated with certain procedures, such as lymphangiography. For example, when diffuse histiocytic lymphoma (DHL) is disseminated, the usual survival is less than 6 months unless combination chemotherapy produces a complete remission [76–78]. For this reason, patients with DHL are usually staged in a manner similar to that used in Hodgkin's disease in order to be certain whether or not disseminated disease is present. However, patients more than 75 years of age, and in some cases patients greater than 70 years of age, cannot tolerate the combination chemotherapy regimens which are needed to produce cures in DHL. These patients not only have a limited marrow reserve, they are also more prone to complications such as vincristine induced paralytic ileus, and they are more susceptible to the infections which may be associated with neutropenia. Thus, if an 80 year old woman presents with DHL involving a cervical lymph node, only palliative therapy can be given if advanced disease is discovered. In this context, only minimal baseline evaluation should be obtained, and radiation therapy to the involved node should be considered. While complete staging could provide prognostic information, if the disease is disseminated there is no benefit to this patient in its detection.

Secondly, the idea that staging provides a basis for eventual restaging assumes that therapy will be given with the intent of inducing a complete remission. In diffuse histiocytic lymphoma, as in Hodgkin's disease, this is the case. In many of the indolent lymphomas, minimal therapy, or no therapy, may be given [79, 80]. If this therapeutic approach is going to be taken, there is little justification for an extensive and potentially expensive baseline evaluation. Once enough information is obtained to establish a therapeutic plan, other procedures can be deferred until the time that a more aggressive therapeutic approach is required.

Third, specific histologic subtypes of lymphoma are associated with different incidences of organ involvement, and therefore one may decide to search more diligently for involvement of a specific site based on the histology of the lymphoma. For example, both nodular and diffuse forms of poorly differentiated lymphocytic lymphoma (small cleaved cell lymphoma) have been associated with a high risk of bone marrow involvement [81, 82]. If the results of the procedure will influence therapy, a repeat bone marrow biopsy can easily be justified in a patient with one of these types of lymphoma when the inital biopsy is negative. Similarly, lymphoblastic

Table 13. Baseline evaluation in non-Hodgkin's lymphoma.

History: Careful evaluation of fever, night sweats, or weight loss; general medical history
Physical examination: Careful examination of all lymph node chains including epitrochlear, femoral, infraclavicular, and submental nodes; examination of Waldeyer's ring; examination of abdomen for abdominal masses, mesenteric nodes, or enlarged liver or spleen
Laboratory tests: Complete blood count, platelet count, liver and renal function tests, blood urea nitrogen, calcium, uric acid
Bone marrow biopsy, bone marrow aspiration
Chest X-ray
Assessment of the retroperitoneum: extent of evaluation depends on the therapeutic plan
    a) Procedures of low sensitivity – (useful to exclude massive disease if non-aggressive therapy is planned): intravenous pyelography, ultrasound
    b) Sensitive procedures – (useful to detect minimal disease, helpful as a baseline for restaging when aggressive therapy is planned): lymphangiography, CT scan
Optional procedures: Liver-spleen scan, gastrointestinal X-rays (if symptoms are present), skeletal X-rays, bone scan (if symptoms are present), cytologic evaluation of effusions (if present), quantitation of immunoglobulins, skin tests to evaluate immune competence, lumbar puncture (in Burkitt's lymphoma, small transformed cell lymphoma, and lymphoblastic lymphoma)
Staging laparotomy is rarely indicated in non-Hodgkin's lymphoma

lymphoma, Burkitt's lymphoma, and small transformed cell lymphoma (undifferentiated lymphoma) tend to behave like leukemias. In addition to baseline bone marrow evaluation, evaluation of the cerebrospinal fluid is an essential part of the evaluation of these patients.

While staging must be individualized on the basis of clinical circumstances, general guidelines for staging are presented in Table 13.

3.4.2. Sites of disease, clinical evaluation

History and physical examination: Once the diagnosis of non-Hodgkin's lymphoma has been established by review of the pathologic material by a hematopathologist, the evaluation of the patient with non-Hodgkin's lymphoma begins with a complete history and physical examination. The history should place special emphasis on the presence or absence of fever, night sweats, or weight loss. Although these events appear to have less prognostic meaning in non-Hodgkin's lymphoma as compared to Hodgkin's disease, in patients with indolent lymphomas, the presence of symptoms may be the only indication that therapy should be initiated. As non-Hodgkin's lymphomas often occur in older patients, the medical history should determine if a contraindication to a specific form of therapy exists, e.g. congestive heart failure as a relative contraindication to adriamycin, or chronic lung disease as a contraindication to bleomycin.

Since extranodal sites of disease are often present in non-Hodgkin's lymphoma, the history may also be the first clue of a specific site of lymphomatous involvement and may indicate that a specific evaluation is indicated. For example, the upper gastrointestinal X-ray series is not usually obtained as part of staging in patients with non-Hodgkin's lymphoma. However, symptoms of anorexia, or abdominal discomfort may be the first indication of lymphomatous involvement of the gastrointestinal tract, and in the presence of these symptoms radiographic evaluation of the gastrointestinal tract should be obtained. Similarly, skeletal pain may be the first indication of bone involvement in a patient with non-Hodgkin's lymphoma.

As stated previously, non-Hodgkin's lymphoma can involve any nodal site and special attention should be given to the examination of peripheral nodes and Waldeyer's ring. While physical examination is likely to detect large abdominal masses or substantial splenomegaly, as in Hodgkin's disease, the physical examination is not highly sensitive in the assessment of abdominal sites of disease in non-Hodgkin's lymphoma.

Following the history and physical examination, the direction of the staging evaluation depends on the specific clinical options which are being considered. The following discussion of the tests which are performed in staging provides a format for discussing various sites of organ involvement in non-Hodgkin's lymphoma.

Laboratory tests: Routine blood tests are part of the medical evaluation of the patient with non-Hodgkin's lymphoma, but are rarely specific enough to provide important staging information. Despite the high incidence of bone marrow involvement in certain types of non-Hodgkin's lymphoma, the peripheral blood counts are usually normal in these patients [81]. In fact, in one series of patients with non-Hodgkin's lymphoma who were evaluated at presentation, anemia and thrombocytopenia were observed as frequently in patients who did not have bone marrow involvement as in the patients whose bone marrows were found to contain lymphoma. Only in the terminal phases of nodular poorly differentiated lymphocytic lymphoma is marrow involvement likely to be extensive enough to produce anemia or other cytopenias.

Generally, anemia in non-Hodgkin's lymphoma is the chronic simple anemia of malignancy, or may represent a hemolytic anemia due to hypersplenism or an autoimmune process. Autoimmune hemolytic anemia is infrequent, however, and occurs in less than 5% of patients with non-Hodgkin's lymphoma. Due to the age of patients with non-Hodgkin's lymphoma, anemia may be the hint of a coincidental process, such as a malignancy of the gastrointestinal tract. Thrombocytopenia, which is not frequently seen in non-Hodgkin's lymphoma, may also be a manifestation of hypersplenism or of an auto-immune process.

Involvement of the peripheral blood may occur in non-Hodgkin's lymphoma, and may create some semantic problems, especially if the Rappaport system is used. Diffuse well differentiated lymphocytic lymphoma (D-WDL) and chronic lymphocytic leukemia (CLL) are, for practical purposes, diseases of the same cell, the small B lymphocyte. When peripheral blood involvement – arbitrarily defined as greater than 5000 cells/mm^3 or greater than 10,000 cells/mm^3 – is present, the disease process is considered CLL. However, clinical distinctions between CLL and D-WDL have not been firmly established. Furthermore, it is likely that sensitive tests, able to detect small monoclonal populations of lymphocytes, will be able to detect peripheral blood involvement in the 'non-leukemic' cases of D-WDL.

For cases of poorly differentiated lymphocytic lymphoma, involvement of the peripheral blood may be designated 'lymphosarcoma cell leukemia.' However, these cases are generally regarded as lymphoma, and are not treated as a separate entity. It is estimated that from 33% to 47% of patients with poorly differentiated lymphocytic lymphoma (small cleaved cell lymphoma) may have peripheral blood involvement at presentation [83–85]. These estimates are based on reviews of peripheral blood smears for cleaved lymphocytes, as the incidence of florid leukemia (greater than 5000 cells/mm^3) is probably between 5 and 10%. However, in view of the tendency for these lymphomas to be disseminated at presentation, sensitive procedures – such as the use of monoclonal antibodies – may reveal that the actual incidence of peripheral blood involvement is even higher.

In contrast to poorly differentiated lymphocytic lymphoma, with the exception of small transformed cell lymphoma, and lymphoblastic lymphoma, peripheral blood involvement in other types of lymphoma appears to be infrequent. Interestingly enough, in a series of patients whom we evaluated for the presence of surface immunoglobulins, we found the incidence of bone marrow involvement to be much higher in follicular center cell lymphomas in which IgM was the surface immunoglobulin than in cases in which IgG was the surface immunoglobulin [83]. This observation held true for all the major types of follicular center cell lymphomas.

While liver and renal function tests are not sensitive indicators of visceral involvement by non-Hodgkin's lymphomas, patients with non-Hodgkin's lymphoma should be screened for hypercalcemia and hyperuricemia. Hypercalcemia is an infrequent complication of non-Hodgkin's lymphoma, but minimal degrees of hyperuricemia are frequently seen. I have personally observed a patient who presented with lymphoma, acute renal failure, and a serum uric acid of 51 mg/dl prior to the initiation of therapy. With the initiation of therapy, hyperuricemia would be a frequent problem in non-Hodgkin's lymphoma were it not for the routine use of allopurinol. While other electrolyte abnormalities are infrequently seen in non-Hodgkin's lymphoma, patients with Burkitt's lymphoma can experience massive tumor lysis following the institution of chemotherapy. These patients may develop hyperphosphatemia, hypocalcemia, hyperuricemia, azotemia, and finally, fatal hyperkalemia [86, 87].

Table 14. Bone marrow involvement in non-Hodgkin's lymphoma.

Histology	Incidence of bone marrow involvement
Rappaport classification	
Nodular lymphomas	
Poorly differentiated lymphocytic lymphoma	55–85%
Mixed cell lymphoma	15–25%
Diffuse lymphomas	
Poorly differentiated lymphocytic lymphoma	30–60%
Histiocytic lymphoma	5–15%
Lukes-Collins classification	
Small cleaved cell lymphoma	55–75%
Large cleaved cell lymphoma	35–45%
Small transformed cell lymphoma	20–85%
Large transformed cell lymphoma	30–35%
Lymphoblastic lymphoma	50–70%

Evaluation of the bone marrow: The incidence of bone marrow involvement at the time of presentation in non-Hodgkin's lymphoma, as related to the histologic type of lymphoma, is presented in Table 14 [81, 82, 88–90]. It is well established that bone marrow biopsy is better than bone marrow aspiration in detecting non-Hodgkin's lymphoma. However, a bone marrow aspirate or touch preparation should be performed along with a bone marrow biopsy as these procedures can provide material for cytologic, immunologic, or histochemical studies.

While marrow involvement is often seen at presentation in certain forms of non-Hodgkin's lymphoma, suggesting hematogenous dissemination, it is rarely the only manifestation of disseminated disease. In one study in which patients with poorly differentiated lymphocytic lymphoma underwent extensive clinical staging, bone marrow involvement was detected in none of 11 patients who were in stage I or II, but marrow involvement was detected in 40 of 56 patients who were in stage III or IV on the basis of clinical evaluation, exclusive of marrow biopsy. While marrow involvement was noted in patients who were in stage I and II by clinical appearance, these patients were found to have evidence of stage III disease – usually retroperitoneal adenopathy – when complete staging was performed.

Bone marrow involvement in non-Hodgkin's lymphoma is generally focal. Therefore, one would expect that the probability of obtaining a positive marrow biopsy in non-Hodgkin's lymphoma would depend on the amount

Table 15. Mediastinal involvement in non-Hodgkin's lymphoma.

Histology	% with abnormal mediastinum on chest X-ray	% with primary mediastinal lymphoma
Nodular lymphomas		
Poorly differentiated lymphocytic lymphoma	12	0
Mixed cell lymphoma	20	0
Histiocytic lymphoma	14	0
Diffuse lymphomas		
Well differentiated lymphocytic lymphoma	0	0
Poorly differentiated lymphocytic lymphoma	35	22 *
Mixed-cell lymphoma	12	0
Histiocytic lymphoma	13	11 **
Undifferentiated lymphoma	11	0

* Of eleven cases, nine were convoluted cell lymphoma, two were small cleaved cell lymphoma.

** Of six cases, four were immunoblastic sarcoma, two were large transformed cell lymphoma.

of marrow which was sampled. It has been reported that in nodular poorly differentiated lymphocytic lymphoma, 14 of 32 patients had bilateral bone marrow involvement while six had only unilateral marrow involvement. This suggests that bilateral marrow biopsies should be routinely obtained in the staging of non-Hodgkin's lymphoma. However, since the amount of marrow which is sampled can be increased by increasing the diameter of the biopsy needle, or by increasing the depth of the specimen which is obtained, it is impossible to make definitive recommendations about the number of marrow biopsies which should be obtained in a patient with non-Hodgkin's lymphoma.

Although bone marrow involvement is infrequent in diffuse histiocytic lymphoma, the finding of bone marrow involvement in this disorder has special clinical importance as it identifies patients at high risk of developing leptomeningeal disease. In two series of patients with diffuse lymphomas – primarily histiocytic lymphomas and undifferentiated lymphomas – the incidence of central nervous system disease was 13 of 20 (65%) and 7 of 19 (35%) in patients with bone marrow involvement [91].

Chest: Mediastinal disease is less frequent in non-Hodgkin's lymphoma than in Hodgkin's disease (Table 15). Routine chest X-ray is generally adequate for assessment of disease and tomography is rarely indicated in non-Hodgkin's lymphoma. While lymphoblastic lymphoma (convoluted cell lymphoma) represents only 5% of all cases of non-Hodgkin's lymphoma, in one series this histology was observed in 9 of 17 cases of lymphoma presenting as a mediastinal mass [92].

Diffuse histiocytic lymphoma can also present as mediastinal disease. Attention has recently been drawn to the clinical pathologic syndrome of

Table 16. Incidence of involvement of abdominal sites of disease in non-Hodgkin's lymphoma.

| Histology | Abdominal lymph nodes | | | | |
	Para-aortic	Mesen-teric	Splenic Hilar	Spleen	Liver
All nodular lymphomas	60–80%	70%	60%	60%	40%
Poorly differentiated lymphocytic lymphoma	70–80%	80%		60%	50%
Mixed-cell lymphoma	50–80%	65%		50%	40%
All diffuse lymphomas	25–50%	30%	40%	15–20%	40%
Poorly differentiated lymphocytic lymphoma	30–40%	35%		15–20%	70%
Histiocyticlymphoma	20–60%	25%		15–20%	20%

diffuse histiocytic lymphoma with fibrosis presenting in association with a superior vena cava syndrome [93]. These patients tend to be refractory to chemotherapy. Review of these cases with respect to the Lukes-Collins system has shown these cases to be both large cleaved cell and large transformed cell lymphoma.

Abdominal nodal disease: Abdominal lymph nodes are frequently involved in non-Hodgkin's lymphoma, although the incidence of involvement varies among the types of lymphoma (Table 16). In contrast to Hodgkin's disease, lymph node involvement in non-Hodgkin's lymphoma is often extensive with massive enlargement of the abdominal nodes (Figure 11). Furthermore, while mesenteric nodes are involved in less than 5% of patients with Hodgkin's disease, these nodes are involved in 70% of patients with nodular lymphomas [94]. While lymphangiography usually detects other nodal disease in patients with mesenteric node involvement, this is not always the case. In one series of 55 patients with mesenteric node involvement, 46 had positive lymphangiograms while nine had negative lymphangiograms [94].

Since lymphangiography may miss common sites of nodal disease in the abdomen, and since the size of involved nodes is such that detection by CT scanning is feasible, many centers prefer abdominal CT scanning to lymphangiography in the staging of patients with non-Hodgkin's lymphomas (Figure 12). Definitive comparisons of lymphangiography and abdominal CT scanning are needed to establish the role of these procedures.

Spleen: Splenic involvement is a frequent occurrence in non-Hodgkin's lymphoma. Involvement may be either focal or generalized. While splenic involvement may be associated with only minimal splenic enlargement, splenic involvement in non-Hodgkin's lymphoma can occasionally produce massive splenomegaly of the type generally associated with myeloid metaplasia. Rare cases of non-Hodgkin's lymphoma apparently limited to the spleen have been described, and in a recent report a 'new' lymphoma composed of perifollicular cells in the spleen was described [95].

Hepatic involvement is more frequent in patients with non-Hodgkin's lymphoma having splenic involvement than in patients whose spleens are not involved. In one series, 50% of non-Hodgkin's lymphoma patients with splenic involvement were found to have liver involvement, while only 11% of patients without splenic disease were found to have involvement of the liver [96].

Liver: Hepatic involvement is frequently discovered in non-Hodgkin's lymphoma when an extensive staging evaluation is performed (Table 16). However, hepatic involvement by non-Hodgkin's lymphoma is generally not extensive enough to affect liver function tests or the appearance of the liver on liver scan. In one series, 24 of 38 patients with liver biopsies positive for lymphoma had normal liver scans, and 33 of 41 had normal liver function tests; however, when liver function tests or liver scans were abnormal, the

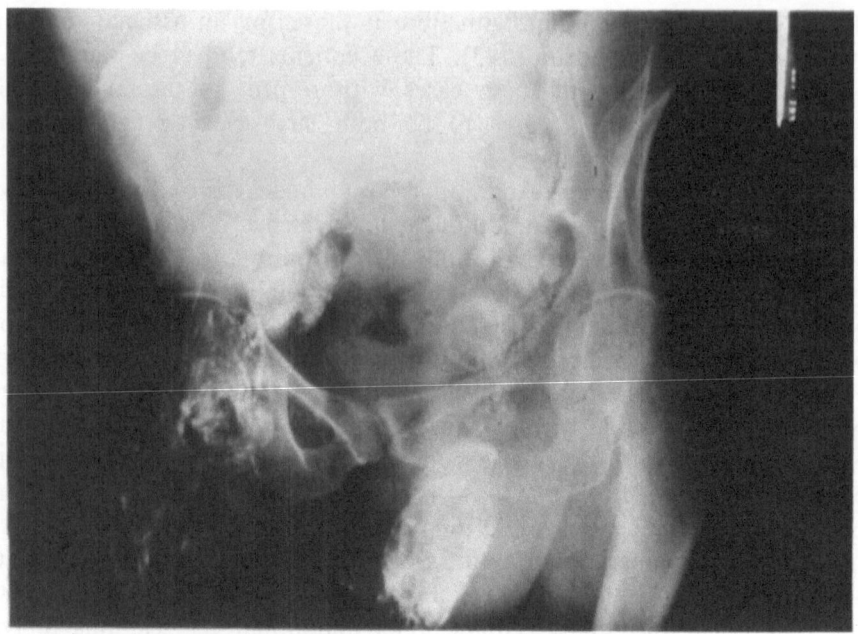

Figure 11. A: Lymphangiogram in a 59-year-old woman with histiocytic (large transformed cell) lymphoma. B: Following six months of chemotherapy the lymphangiogram was normal. The patient has remained in remission for five years.

liver was almost always involved [96].

The focal nature of hepatic involvement by lymphoma is further supported by the following observation. In a series of 77 patients studied at the National Cancer Institute, percutaneous liver biopsy was positive for lymphoma in only 16 patients. However, further evaluation – including sequential peritoneoscopy and open liver biopsy at laparotomy – revealed 17 additional cases of hepatic involvement by lymphoma which had been missed by closed needle biopsy.

Staging laparotomy in non-Hodgkin's lymphoma: In contrast to Hodgkin's disease, staging laparotomy is rarely, if ever, indicated in patients with non-Hodgkin's lymphoma. First, the pattern of disease spread is different in non-Hodgkin's lymphoma. The high incidence of bone marrow involvement in poorly differentiated lymphocytic lymphoma, for example, makes staging laparotomy unnecessary for most patients with that histologic type of lymphoma.

Second, clinical decisions in patients with non-Hodgkin's lymphoma are less likely to hinge on the findings at laparotomy than in patients with Hodgkin's disease. Clinical assessment of abdominal nodes is often less

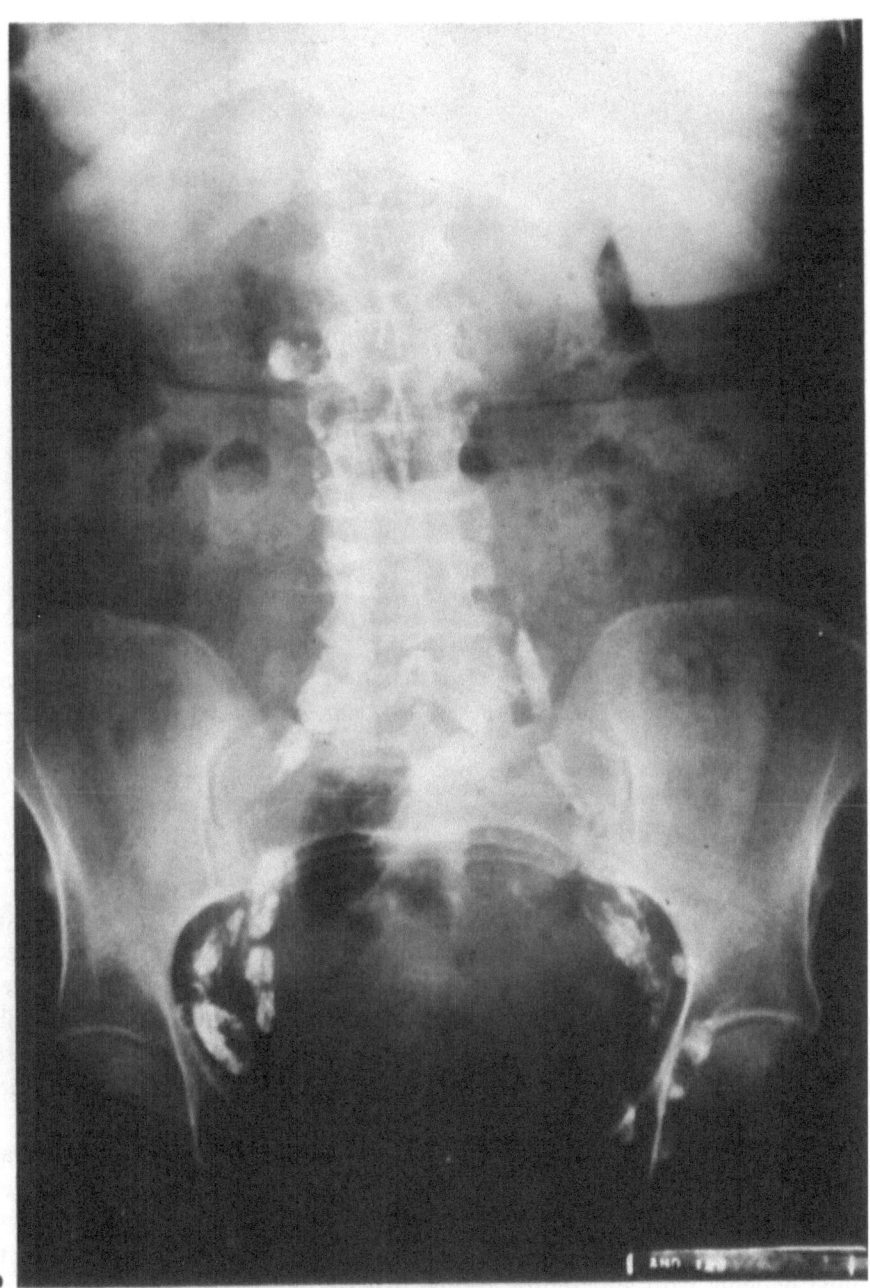

b

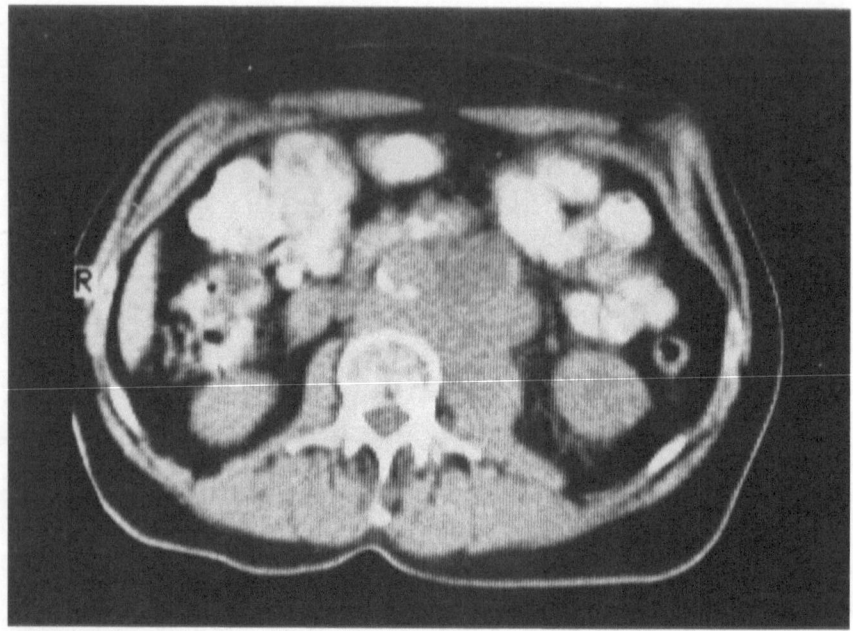

Figure 12. Abdominal CT scan in a 58-year-old man with histiocytic (large transformed cell) lymphoma. The patient presented with inguinal node disease and received radiation therapy. Evaluation including a CT scan was normal at that time, but one year later the patient developed severe leg pain. This CT scan shows massive retroperitoneal disease compatible with involvement of the lumbar plexus.

equivocal in non-Hodgkin's lymphoma than in Hodgkin's disease as the nodes are massively enlarged. With the use of CT scanning to detect mesenteric nodes, the limits of lymphangiography can often be corrected without staging laparotomy. Since stage III and stage IV disease are generally treated in a similar manner, once clinical staging establishes that stage III disease is present, further assessment regarding hepatic involvement is not necessary.

Third, patients with non-Hodgkin's lymphoma are generally older than patients with Hodgkin's disease, which means that the risks of staging laparotomy are higher in these patients.

Staging laparotomy in non-Hodgkin's lymphoma should be limited to young patients with apparently limited disease in whom aggressive therapy with curative intent will be given if advanced disease is discovered. For practical purposes, this limits laparotomy to the disorders included in the category histiocytic lymphoma. Even then, however, there is no evidence that laparotomy is of benefit. Only 10 % of patients with histiocytic lymphoma whose clinical staging suggests that disease is limited are found to have

Table 17. Incidence of histologic types of non-Hodgkin's lymphoma in children.

Histology	Incidence
Poorly differentiated lymphocytic lymphoma	47%
Mixed lymphocytic-histiocytic lymphoma	2%
Histiocytic lymphoma	33%
Lymphoblastic lymphoma	14%
Burkitt's lymphoma	3%
Unclassified lymphoma	2%

occult sites of disease at laparotomy. If, instead of laparotomy, these patients were to receive local radiotherapy and were then to receive chemotherapy only if they relpsed, their ultimate survival might be equivalent to that achieved by the early detection of advanced disease. Furthermore, the recent suggestion that chemotherapy should be the treatment of choice even for stage I histiocytic lymphoma [97] may make this entire consideration of staging laparotomy academic as in that context the value of staging would be limited to establishing a baseline for re-staging and the risks of laparotomy could not be justified.

3.5. Non-Hodgkin's Lymphoma in Children

Non-Hodgkin's lymphoma in children differs from non-Hodgkin's lymphoma in adults in several respects. First, the incidence of the histologic types of non-Hodgkin's lymphoma is markedly different. The incidence of pathologic types of non-Hodgkin's lymphomas seen in children – as based on a compilation of several series – is presented in Table 17 [96–104]. Nodular lymphomas are rarely observed in children.

Secondly, childhood non-Hodgkin's lymphoma has an even greater tendency than adult non-Hodgkin's lymphoma to be disseminated shortly after diagnosis [105]. A leukemic picture occurs in up to 35% of children with non-Hodgkin's lymphoma, and is often seen in patients who have disease which appears to be limited following staging [106, 107]. For this reason, most clinicians favor systemic therapy for children with non-Hodgkin's lymphoma, even if disease appears to be limited in extent [105]. The high incidence of leukemic transformation of childhood non-Hodgkin's lymphoma raises the point that the distinction between non-Hodgkin's lymphoma with marrow involvement and childhood lymphocytic leukemia with bulky extra-nodal disease may be arbitrary. In general, the cutoff of 25% leukemic cells in the bone marrow has been suggested as an upper limit for the diagnosis of non-Hodgkin's lymphoma; above this limit, leukemia is said to be present. In addition to the high incidence of bone marrow involvement in

Table 18. Staging system for childhood non-Hodgkin's lymphoma.

Stage I:	A single extranodal tumor, or single nodal area, with the exclusion of mediastinum or abdomen.
Stage II:	A single extranodal tumor with regional node involvement; two or more nodal areas on the same side of the diaphragm; two single extranodal tumors with or without regional lymph node involvement on the same side of the diaphragm; a primary gastrointestinal tumor, usually ileocecal, with or without involvement of mesenteric nodes.
Stage III:	Two single extranodal tumors on opposite sides of the diaphragm; two or more nodal areas above and below the diaphragm; all primary intrathoracic tumors – mediastinal, pleural, thymic; all extensive primary intra-abdominal disease.
Stage IV:	Any of the above with initial CNS and/or bone marrow involvement.

children with non-Hodgkin's lymphoma, there is also a high incidence of central nervous system involvement [109].

While the Ann Arbor staging system for Hodgkin's disease may be inadequate for adults with non-Hodgkin's lymphoma, it is certainly inadequate for children with non-Hodgkin's lymphoma. A modified staging system which has been proposed for use in children is presented in Table 18 [105]. The definition of stage I disease recognizes the fact that mediastinal disease has an extremely poor prognosis, as does gastrointestinal lymphoma – except for those cases in which a complete surgical excision is performed.

3.6. Mycosis Fungoides and the Sézary Syndrome (Cutaneous T-Cell Lymphoma)

Mycosis fungoides and Sézary's syndrome are malignant lymphomas of T-cell origin in which the malignant lymphocyte tends to involve the skin. Most patients with mycosis fungoides are in the fifth or sixth decade and the most common presentations are eczema, dermatitis, macular rashes, nodules, tumors, and exfoliative dermatitis. The disease generally progresses from flat plaque-like lesions to raised tumors. While limited and even generalized plaques may be associated with a 5-year survival in more than 50% of patients, the presence of tumors is associated with a markedly limited prognosis – generally less than 2 years [110]. Sézary syndrome – erythroderma with peripheral blood involvement – has been accepted as a leukemic variant of mycosis fungoides since the demonstration that both the Sézary syndrome and mycosis fungoides are diseases of T-cells having identical morphologic features [111].

Since mycosis fungoides involves multiple skin sites, it is always a stage IV disease with respect to the Ann Arbor staging system. However, since prognostic subgroups of mycosis fungoides can be identified, a staging system

Table 19. Staging system for cutaneous T-cell lymphomas.

Stage 0:	Premalignant lesions
Stage I:	Erythematous plaque or generalized erythema
Stage II:	Indurated plaque or exfoliative erythroderma, or both
Stage III:	Tumors with or without papules, plaques, or generalized erythroderma
Stage IV:	Histologically confirmed lymph node involvement
Stage V:	Visceral involvement
A:	Without a leukemic phase
B:	With a leukemic phase

specifically designed for mycosis fungoides and the Sézary syndrome has been proposed (Table 19). An alternative system based on TNM (tumor, node, metastases) considerations has also been suggested [112]. While lymph node enlargement is commonly present in mycosis fungoides, this finding is not equivalent to nodal involvement, as many enlarged nodes reveal only non-specific (dermatopathic) changes when biopsies are performed.

Extensive staging procedures have generally not been performed in patients with mycosis fungoides. In one study which used lymphangiography as a diagnostic procedure, however, abnormal nodes were detected in 64% of patients [113]. Not surprisingly, a higher incidence of abnormal lymphangiograms has been noted in patients with lymphadenopathy than in patients without enlarged nodes [113]. However, lymphangiography is unable to distinguish between dermatopathic adenopathy and involvement of lymph nodes by mycosis fungoides.

Staging laparotomies have rarely been performed in mycosis fungoides. In one study involving only 13 patients, four were found to have splenic involvement, three had involvement of abdominal nodes, and one had hepatic involvement [114]. The significance of these observations is tempered by the fact that all four patients with abdominal disease had involvement of the peripheral blood by Sézary cells. In one case this involvement was of leukemic proportions, and in the other cases the number of abnormal cells was not specified.

Visceral involvement in mycosis fungoides frequently occurs with progressive disease. In autopsy series, involvement of the lungs, liver, and spleen has been noted in more than one-half of patients while involvement of the kidney, heart, and pancreas has been noted in more than 20% of patients [115, 116]. While Sézary syndrome is a leukemic condition, these patients generally do not have bone marrow involvement until the terminal stages of the disease. This paradoxical situation of leukemia in the absence of bone marrow involvement has been exploited clinically by the use of leukapheresis to successfully debulk the skin lesions in patients with Sézary's syndrome [117].

Although mycosis fungoides is generally considered a cutaneous based disease, a recent study has suggested that the incidence of visceral involvement is much higher than generally appreciated. The use of immunologic tests for circulating T-cells, along with electron microscopy, and cytogenetic studies revealed the presence of extracutaneous disease in 43 of 49 patients with mycosis fungoides/Sézary syndrome, including 27 of 29 studied at presentation.

REFERENCES

1. Gutensohn N, Cole P: Epidemiology of Hodgkin's disease. Semin Oncol 7:92–102, 1980.
2. Correa P, O'Conor GT: Epidemiologic patterns of Hodgkin's disease. Int J Cancer 8:192–201, 1971.
3. MacMahon B: Epidemiology of Hodgkin's disease. Cancer Res 26:1189–1200, 1966.
4. Hoover R, Mason TJ, McKay FW, et al.: Geographic patterns of cancer mortality in the United States. In: Persons at high risk of cancer: an approach to cancer etiology and control, Fraumeni JH Jr, ed. New York: Academic, 1975.
5. Newell G: Etiology of multiple sclerosis and Hodgkin's disease. Am J Epidemiol 91:119–122, 1970.
6. Abramson JH: Childhood experience and Hodgkin's disease in adults. An interpretation of incidence data. Isr J Med Sci 10:1376–1370, 1974.
7. Abramson JH, Pridan H, Sacks MI, et al.: A case-control study of Hodgkin's disease in Israel. J Natl Cancer Inst 61:307–314, 1978.
8. Vianna NJ, Polan AK: Immunity in Hodgkin's disease: importance of age at exposure. Ann Intern Med 89:550–556, 1978.
9. Hesse J, Levine PH, Ebbesen P, et al.: A case-control study on immunity to two Epstein-Barr virus-associated antigens and to herpes simplex virus and adenovirus in a population-based group of patients with Hodgkin's disease in Denmark, 1971-1973. Int J Cancer 19:49–58, 1977.
10. Miller RW, Beebe GW: Infectious mononucleosis and the empirical risk of cancer. J Natl Cancer Inst 50:315–321, 1973.
11. Vianna NJ, Greenwald P, Davies JNP: Extended epidemic of Hodgkin's disease in high school students. Lancet 1:1209–1211, 1971.
12. Paffenbarger R Jr, Wing AL, Hyde RT: Characteristics in youth indicative of adult onset Hodgkin's disease. J Natl Cancer Inst 58:1489–1491, 1977.
13. Milham S Jr, Hesser JE: Hodgkin's disease in woodworkers. Lancet 2:136–137, 1967.
14. Petersen GR, Milham S: Hodgkin's disease mortality and occupational exposure to wood. J Natl Cancer Inst 53:957–958, 1974.
15. Greene MH, Brinton LA, Fraumeni JF, et al.: Familial and sporadic Hodgkin's disease associated with occupational wood exposure. Lancet 2:626–627, 1978.
16. Brown RS, Hayes HA, Foley HT, et al.: Hodgkin's disease: immunologic clinical and histologic features of 50 untreated patients. Ann Intern Med 67:291–301, 1967.
17. Swan HT, Knowlton J: Prognosis in Hodgkin's disease related to lymphocyte count. Br J Haematol 21:343–349, 1971.
18. Bukowski RM, Noguchi S, Hewlett JS, et al.: Lymphocyte subpopulations in Hodgkin's disease. Am J Clin Pathol 65:31–39, 1976.

19. Young RC, Corder MP, Hayes HA, *et al.*: Delayed hypersensitivity in Hodgkin's disease. Am J Med 52:63–73, 1972.
20. Schimpff S, Serpick A, Stoler B, *et al.*: Varicella-Zoster infection in patients with cancer. Ann Intern Med, 76:241–254, 1972.
21. Sokal JE, Firat D: Varicella-Zoster infection in Hodgkin's disease. Am J Med 39:452–463, 1965.
22. Fisher RI, DeVita VT Jr, Bostick F, *et al.*: Persistent immunologic abnormalities in long-term survivors of advanced Hodgkin's disease. Ann Intern Med 92:595–599, 1980.
23. Kaplan HS: Hodgkin's disease. Cambridge, Mass.: 1980.
24. Desser RK, Golomb HM, Ultman JE, *et al.*: Prognostic classification of Hodgkin's disease in pathologic stage III based on anatomic considerations. Blood 49:883–893, 1977.
25. Levi JA, Wiernik PH: The therapeutic implications of splenic involvement in stage IIIA Hodgkin's disease. Cancer 39:2158–2165, 1977.
26. Stein RS, Hilborn RM, Flexner JM, *et al.*: Anatomical substages of stage III Hodgkin's disease. Cancer 42:429–436, 1978.
27. Stein RS, Golomb HM, Diggs CH, *et al.*: Anatomical substages of stages III-A Hodgkin's disease: a collaborative study. Ann Intern Med 92:159–165, 1980.
28. Rosenberg SA: Hodgkin's disease of the bone marrow, Cancer Res 31:1733–1736, 1971.
29. Jones SE: Importance of staging in Hodgkin's disease. Semin Oncol 7:126–135, 1980.
30. Castellino RA, Filly R, Blank N: Routine full-lung tomography in the initial staging and treatment planning of patients with Hodgkin's disease and non-Hodgkin's lymphoma. Cancer 38:1130–1136, 1976.
31. Levi JA, Wiernik PH: Limited extranodal Hodgkin's disease: unfavorable prognosis and therapeutic implications. Am J Med 63:365–372, 1977.
32. Thar TL, Million RR, Hausner RJ, *et al.*: Hodgkin's disease, stages I and II: relationship of recurrence to size of disease, radiation dose, and number of sites involved. Cancer 43:1101–1105, 1979.
33. Mauch P, Goodman R, Hellman S: The significance of mediastinal involvement in early stage Hodgkin's disease. Cancer 42:1039–1045, 1978.
34. Redman HC, Glatstein E, Castellino RA, Federal WA: Computed tomography as an adjunct in the staging of Hodgkin's disease and non-Hodgkin's lymphomas. Radiology 124:381–385, 1977.
35. Jones SE, Tobias DA, Waldman RS: Computed tomographic scanning in patients with lymphoma. Cancer 41:480–486, 1978.
36. Best JK, Blackledge G, Forbes WStC, *et al.*: Computed tomography of abdomen in staging and clinical management of lymphoma. Br Med J 2:1675–1677, 1978.
37. Desser RK, Moran EM, Ultmann JE: Staging of Hodgkin's disease and lymphoma: diagnostic procedures including staging laparotomy and splenoctomy. Med Clin N Am 57:479–498, 1973.
38. Fialk MA, Jarowski CI, Coleman M, Mouradian J: Hepatic Hodgkin's disease without involvement of the spleen. Cancer 43:1146–1147, 1979.
39. Aisenberg AC, Goldman JM, Baker JW, *et al.*: Spleen involvement at the onset of Hodgkin's disease. Ann Intern Med 74:544, 1971.
40. Farrer-Brown G, Bennett MH, Harrison CV, *et al.*: Pathological findings following laparotomy in Hodgkin's disease. Br J Cancer 25:449, 1971.
41. Glatstein E, Guernsey JM, Rosenberg SA, *et al.*: The value of laparotomy and splenectomy in the staging of Hodgkin's disease. Cancer 24:709, 1969.
42. Glatstein E, Trueblood HW, Enright LP, *et al.*: Surgical staging of abdominal involvement in unselected patients with Hodgkin's disease. Radiology 97:425, 1970.
43. Hanks GE, Newsome JF, Lewis NT: The value of laparotomy in staging lymphomas. South Med J 64:585, 1971.

44. Lowenbraum S, Ramsey H, Sutherland J, *et al.*: Diagnostic laparotomy and splenectomy for staging Hodgkin's disease. Ann Intern Med 72:655, 1970.
45. Prosnitz LR, Nuland SB, Kiligerman MM: Role of laparotomy and splenectomy in the management of Hodgkin's disease. Cancer 29:44, 1972.
46. Hoppe RT, Cox RS, Rosenberg SA, Kaplan HS: Prognostic factors in pathologic stage IIIA Hodgkin's disease. Proc Am Soc Clin Oncol 19:429, 1979.
47. Krikorian JG, Portlock CS, Rosenbert SA, Kaplan HS: Hodgkin's disease, Stages I and II occurring below the diaphragm. Cancer 43:1866-1871, 1979.
48. Stein RS: Staging laparotomy in Hodgkin's disease: a critical appraisal of its value. South Med J 71:1553-1558, 1978.
49. Johnson RE, Zimbler H, Berard CW, *et al.*: Radiotherapy results for nodular sclerosing Hodgkin's disease after clinical staging. Cancer 39:1439-1444, 1977.
50. Griffin T, Gerdes A, Parker R, *et al.*: Are pelvic irradiation and routine staging laparotomy necessary in clinically staged IA and IIA Hodgkin's disease? Cancer 40:2914-2916, 1977.
51. Desser RK, Ultmann JE: Risk of severe infection in patients with Hodgkin's disease or lymphoma after diagnostic laparotomy and splenectomy. Ann Intern Med 77:143-146, 1972.
52. Schimpff SC, O'Connell MJ, Greene WH, *et al.*: Infections in 92 splenectomized patients with Hodgkin's disease. Am J Med 59:695-701, 1975.
53. Weitzman S, Aisenberg AC: Fulminant sepsis after the successful treatment of Hodgkin's disease. Am J Med 62:47-50, 1977.
54. Slavin R, Nelson TS: Complications from staging laparotomy for Hodgkin's disease. Natl Cancer Inst Monogr 36:457-459, 1973.
55. O'Connor GT, Correa P, Christine B, *et al.*: Hodgkin's disease in Connecticut: histology and age distribution. Natl Cancer Inst Monogr 36:3-8, 1973.
56. Smith KL, Johnson D, Hustu O, *et al.*: Concurrent chemotherapy and radiation therapy in the treatment of childhood and adolescent Hodgkin's disease. Cancer 38-46, 1974.
57. Bloomfield DC, Kersey JH, Brunning RD, Gajl-Peczalska KJ: Prognostic significance of lymphocytic surface markers and histology in adult non-Hodgkin's lymphoma. Cancer Treat Rep 61:963-970, 1977.
58. Nathwani BN, Kim H, Rappaport H, Solomon J, Fox M: Non-Hodgkin's lymphomas: a clinicopathologic study comparing two classifications. Cancer 41:303-325, 1978.
59. Berard CW, Jaffe ES, Braylan RC, Mann RB, Nanba K: Immunologic aspects and pathology of the malignant lymphomas. Cancer 42:911-921, 1978.
60. Mann RB, Jaffe ES, Berard CW: Malignant lymphomas – a conceptual understanding of morphologic diversity. Am J Pathol 94:105-192, 1979.
61. Brouet JC, LaBaume S, Seligmann M: Evaluation of T and B lymphocyte membrane markers in human non-Hodgkin's malignant lymphomata. Br J Cancer 31:Suppl II, 121-127, 1975.
62. Davey FR, Goldberg J, Stockman J, Gottlieb AJ: Immunologic and cytochemical cell markers in non-Hodgkin's lymphomas. Lab Invest 35:430-438, 1976.
63. Filippa DA, Lieberman PH, Erlandson RA, *et al.*: A study of malignant lymphomas using light and ultramicroscopic, cytochemical and immunologic technics. Am J Med 64:259-268, 1978.
64. Li CY, Harrison EG: Histochemical and immunohistochemical study of diffuse large.cell lymphomas. Am J Clin Pathol 70:721-732, 1978.
65. Nathwani BN, Kim H, Rappaport H: Malignant lymphoma, lymphoblastic. Cancer 38:964-983, 1976.
66. Rosen PJ, Feinstein DI, Pattengale PK, *et al.*: Convoluted lymphocytic lymphoma in adults: a clinicopathologic entity. Ann Intern Med 89:319-324, 1978.

67. Waldron JA, Leech JH, Glick Ad, Flexner JM, Collins RD: Malignant lymphoma of peripheral T-lymphocyte origin. Cancer 40:1604–1617, 1977.
68. Strauchen JA, Young RC, DeVita VT, Anderson T, et al.: Clinical relevance of the histopathologic subclassification of diffuse 'histiocytic' lymphoma. N Engl J Med 299:1382–1387, 1978.
69. Stein RS, Collins RD, Ultman JE: Diffuse histiocytic lymphoma: B-cell origin by Lukes-Collins criteria predicts favorable response to COMLA (cyclophosphamide, oncovin, methotrexate, leucovorin, cytosine arabinoside) chemotherapy. Proc Am Soc Clin Oncol 21:469, 1980.
70. Lukes RJ, Collins RD: Immunologic characterization of human malignant lymphomas. Cancer 34:1488–1503, 1974.
71. Stein RS, Cousar J, Flexner JM, Collins RD: Correlations between immunologic markers and histopathologic classifications: clinical implications. Semin Oncol 7:244–254, 1980.
72. Penn II: Tumor incidence in human allograft recipients. Transplant Proc 11:1047–1051, 1979.
73. Zulman J, Jaffe R, Talal N: Evidence that the malignant lymphoma of Sjogren's syndrome is a monoclonal B-cell neoplasm. N Engl J Med 299:1215–1220, 1978.
74. Chabner BA, Johnson RE, DeVita VT, et al.: Sequential staging in non-Hodgkin's lymphoma. Cancer Treat Rep 61:993–997, 1977.
75. Reimer RR, Chabner BA, Young RC, et al.: Lymphoma presenting in bone. Ann Intern Med 87:50–55, 1977.
76. Jones SE, Rosenberg SA, Kaplan HS, et al.: Non-Hodgkin's lymphomas II. Single agent chemotherapy. Cancer 30:31–38, 1972.
77. Schein PS, DeVita VT, Hubbard S, Chabner BA, Canellos GP, et al.: Bleomycin, adriamycin, cyclophosphamide, vincristine, and prednisone (BACOP) combination chemotherapy in the treatment of advanced diffuse histiocytic lymphoma. Ann Intern Med 85:417–422, 1976.
78. Sweet DL, Golomb HM, Ultmann JE, Miller JB, Stein RS, et al.: Cyclophosphamide, vincristine, methotrexate with leucovorin rescue, and cytarabine (COMLA) combination sequential chemotherapy for advanced diffuse histiocytic lymphoma. Ann Intern Med 1980, 92:785–790.
79. Portlock CS, Rosenberg SA, Glatstein E, Kaplan HS: Treatment of advanced non-Hodgkin's lymphomas with favorable histologies: preliminary results of a prospective trial. Blood 47:747–756, 1976.
80. Portlock CS, Rosenberg SA: No initial therapy for stage III and IV non-Hodgkin's lymphomas of favorable histologic types. Ann Intern Med 90:10–13, 1979.
81. Stein RS, Ultmann JE, Byrne GE, et al.: Bone marrow involvement in non-Hodgkin's lymphoma: implications for staging and therapy. Cancer 37:629–636, 1976.
82. Coller BS, Chabner NA, Gralnick HR: Frequencies and patterns of bone marrow involvement in non-Hodgkin lymphomas: observations on the value of bilateral biopsies. Am J Hematol 3:105–119, 1977.
83. Cousar JB, Stein RS, Flexner JM, Glick AD, Collins RD: Pathologic and immunologic features of bone marrow and peripheral blood involvement in follicular center cell lymphomas (abstract). Lab Invest 40:14, 1979.
84. Foucar K, McKenna RW, Frizzera G, Brunning RD: Incidence and patterns of bone marrow and blood involvement by lymphoma in relationship to the Lukes-Collins Classification. Blood 54:1417–1422, 1979.
85. McKenna RW, Bloomfield CD, Brunning RD: Nodular lymphoma: bone marrow and blood manifestations. Cancer 36:428–440, 1975.
86. Arseneau JC, Bagley CM, Anderson T, Canellos GP: Hyperkalemia. A sequel to chemotherapy of Burkitt's lymphoma. Lancer 1:10, 1973.

87. Cohen LF, Balow JE, MaGrath IT, Poplack DG, Ziegler JL: Acute tumor lysis syndrome: a review of 37 patients with Burkitt's lymphoma. Am J Med 68:486–491, 1980.
88. Dick F, Bloomfield CD, Brunning RD: Incidence, cytology, and histopathology of non-Hodgkin's lymphomas in the bone marrow. Cancer 33:1382–1398, 1974.
89. Rosenberg SA: Bone marrow involvement in the non-Hodgkin's lymphomata. Br J Cancer (Suppl II), 261–264, 1975.
90. Brunning RD, Bloomfield DC, McKenna RW, Peterson L: Bilateral trephine bone marrow biopsies in lymphoma and other neoplastic diseases. Ann Intern Med 82:365–366, 1975.
91. Bunn PA, Schein PS, Banks PM, DeVita VT Jr: Central nervous system complications in patients with diffuse histiocytic and undifferentiated lymphoma: leukemia revisited. Blood 47:3–10, 1976.
92. Lichtenstein AK, Levine A, Taylor CR, et al.: Primary mediastinal lymphoma in adults. Am J Med 68:509–514, 1980.
93. Miller JB, Variakojis D, Bitran JD, Sweet DL Jr, Golomb HM, Ultmann JE: Diffuse histiocytic lymphoma with sclerosis: a clinicopathologic entity with frequent occurrence of superior venacaval obstruction. Blood 52, Suppl 1:263, 1978.
94. Goffinet DR, Warnke R, Dunnick NR, Castellino R, et al.: Clinical and surgical (laparotomy) evaluation of patients with non-Hodgkin's lymphomas. Cancer Treat Rep 61: 981–992, 1977.
95. Cousar JB, McKee LC, Greco FA, Glick AD, Collins RD: Report of an unusual B-cell lymphoma, probably arising from the perifollicular cells (marginal zone) of the spleen (abstract). Lab Invest 42(1):109, 1980.
96. Chabner BA, Johnson RE, Chretien PB, Schein PS, et al.: Percutaneous liver biopsy, peritoneoscopy and laparotomy: an assessment of relative merits in the lymphomata. Br J Cancer 31, Suppl II, 242, 1975.
97. Miller TP, Jones SE: Chemotherapy of localized histiocytic lymphoma. Lancet, 1:358–360, 1979.
98. Landberg T, Garwicz S, Akerman M: Clinicopathological study of non-Hodgkin's lymphomata in childhood. Br J Cancer 31 (Suppl 2):332–336, 1975.
99. Lemerle M, Gerard-Marchant R, Sancho H, et al.: Natural history of non-Hodgkin's malignant lymphoma in children: retrospective study of 190 cases. Br J Cancer 31 (Suppl 2):324–331, 1975.
100. Pinkel D, Johnson W, Aur RJA: Non-Hodgkin's lymphoma in children. Br J Cancer 31 (Suppl 2):298–323, 1975.
101. Murphy SB, Frizzera G, Evans AE: Study of childhood non-Hodgkin's lymphoma. Cancer 36:2121–2131, 1975.
102. Hutter JJ Jr, Favara BE, Nelson M, et al.: Non-Hodgkin's lymphoma in children. Correlation of CNS disease with initial presentation. Cancer 36:2132–2137, 1975.
103. Glatstein E, Kim H, Donaldson SS, et al.: Non-Hodgkin's lymphoma. VI. Results of treatment in childhood. Cancer 34:204–211, 1974.
104. Dehner LP: Non-Hodgkin's lymphomas and malignant histiocytosis in children. Semin Oncol 4:273–286, 1977.
105. Murphy SB: Prognostic features and obstacles to cure of childhood non-Hodgkin's lymphoma. Semin Oncol 4:265–271, 1977.
106. Sullivan MP: Leukemic transformation in lymphosarcoma of childhood. Pediatrics 29:589–599, 1962.
107. Watanabe A, Sullivan MP, Sutow W, et al.: Undifferentiated lymphoma, Non-Burkitt's type meningeal and bone marrow involvement in children. Am J Dis Child 125:57–61, 1973.
108. Wollner N, Burchenal JH, Lieberman PH, et al.: Non-Hodgkin's lymphoma in children. Med Pediatr Oncol 1:235–263, 1975.

109. Hutter JJ, Favara BE, Nelson M, *et al.*: Non-Hodgkin's lymphoma in children. Correlation of CNS disease with initial presentation. Cancer 36:2132–2137, 1975.
110. Fuks ZY, Bagshaw MA, Farber EM: Prognostic signs and the management of mycosis fungoides. Cancer 32:1385–1395, 1973.
111. Lutzner M, Edelson R, Schein P, *et al.*: Cutaneous T-cell lymphomas: the Sézary syndrome, mycosis fungoides, and related disorders. Ann Intern Med 83:534–552, 1975.
112. Lamberg SI, Green SB Byar DP, *et al.*: Status report of 376 mycosis fungoides patients at 4 years: mycosis fungoides cooperative group. Cancer Treat Rep 63:701–707, 1979.
113. Castellino RA, Hoppe RT, Blank N, *et al.*: Experience with lymphography in patients with mycosis fungoides. Cancer Treat Rep 63:581–586, 1979.
114. Variakojis D, Rosas-Uribe A, Rappaport H: Mycosis fungoides: pathologic findings in staging laparotomies. Cancer 33:1589–1600, 1974.
115. Long JC, Mihm MC: Mycosis fungoides with extracutaneous dissemination: a distinct clinicopathologic entity. Cancer 34:1745–1755, 1974.
116. Epstein EH, Levin DL, Croft JD, Lutzner MA: Mycosis fungoides: survival, prognostic features, response to therapy, and autopsy findings. Medicine 15:61–72, 1972.
117. Edelson R, Facktor M, Andrews A, *et al.*: Successful management of the Sézary syndrome. N Engl J Med 291:293–294, 1974.
118. Bunn PA, Huberman MS, Whang-Peng J: Prospective staging evaluation of patients with cutaneous T-cell lymphomas. Ann Intern Med 1980:93:223–230, 1980.

3. Radiographic Approach to the Staging of Lymphoma, Including Hodgkin's Disease

DEREK J. HAMLIN

1. INTRODUCTION

The significant improvement in the prognosis of both Hodgkin's disease and non-Hodgkin's lymphoma, as reported over the preceding two decades, has resulted from greater accuracy in the demonstration of sites of involvement using improved diagnostic and staging techniques coupled with new forms of therapy, including intensive megavoltage radiotherapy, combination chemotherapy, and combined modality therapy. The staging and management of the malignant lymphomas is discussed here, with specific attention to the role of modern non-invasive radiological procedures, including computed tomography, in the delineation of extent of the disease, assessment of response to treatment, and evaluation of relapse.

Initial sites of presentation of the disease, and subsequent patterns of spread of Hodgkin's disease and the non-Hogkin's lymphomas are significantly different and the diagnostic workup should ideally be modified to reflect these differences.

2. LYMPHANGIOGRAPHY IN HODGKIN'S DISEASE AND NON-HODGKIN'S LYMPHOMA

Modern lymphangiography was developed following the introduction of techniques of visualization of the lymphomas of the lower extremities by water-soluble contrast media [1 and that of direct intranodal injection of iodinized oils [2.

Initially, the diagnostic accuracy of lower extremity lymphangiography was difficult to evaluate except by comparison with intravenous urography and inferior vena cavography [3, 4] (Figure 1). The resolution and diagnostic accuracy of lymphangiography was found to be far superior to these other two radiographic procedures.

J.M. Bennett (ed.), Lymphomas 1, 177–233. All rights reserved.
Copyright © 1981 Martinus Nijhoff Publishers, The Hague/Boston/London.

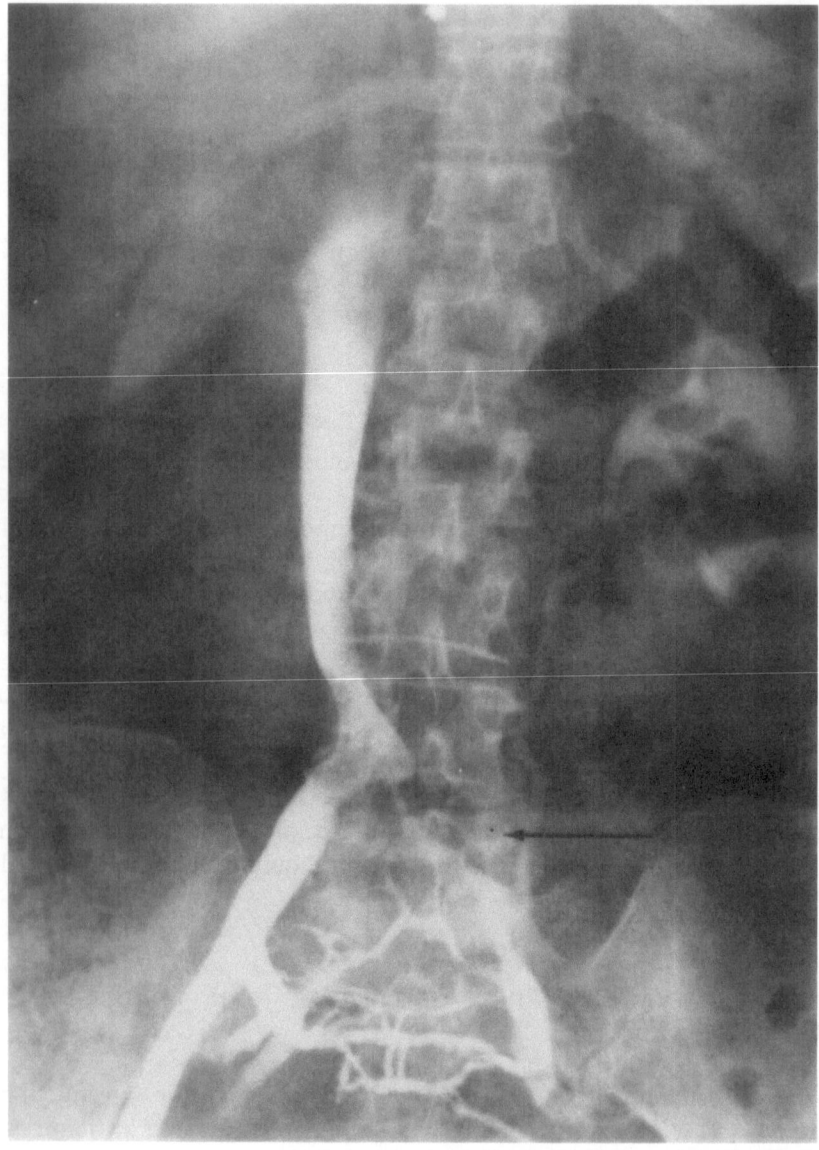

Figure 1. An inferior vena cavogram performed on a 59-year-old patient with diffuse non-Hodgkin lymphoma reveals compromised flow through left common iliac vein (arrow) with collateral flow across the pelvis to the right side. Also seen is extensive compression at the bifurcation of the inferior vena cava due to nodal masses.

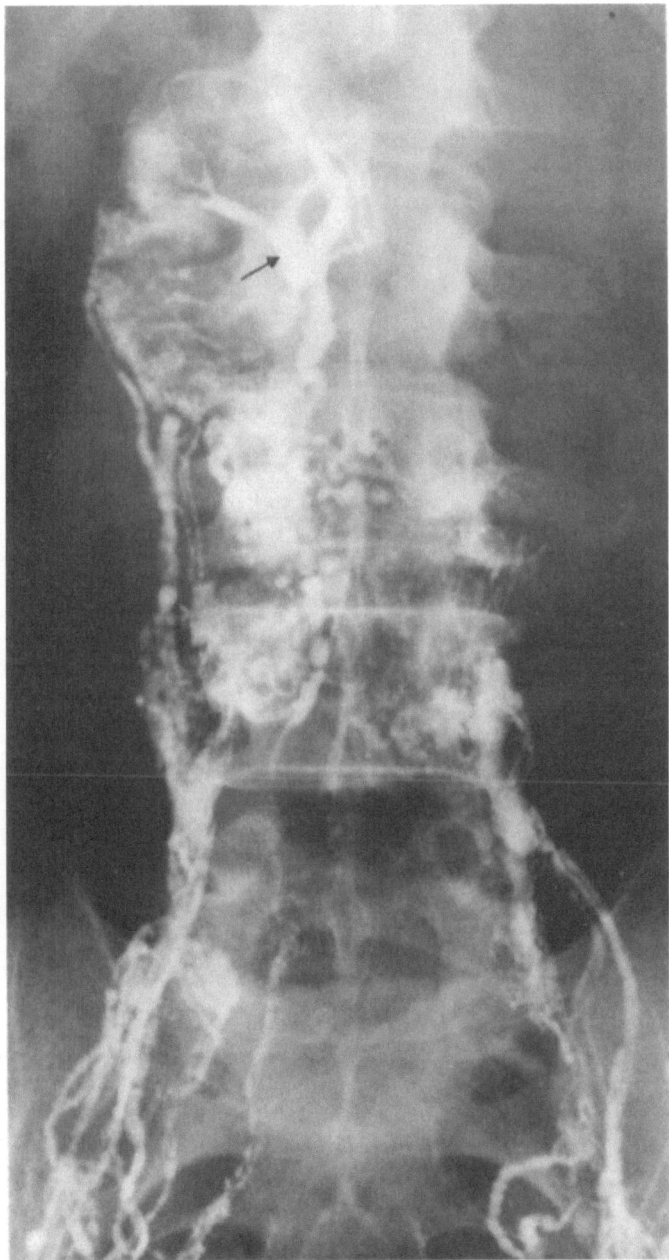

Figure 2. Tortuous, dilated cisterna chyli (arrowed) and other lymphatic vessels plus early filling of huge right para-aortic lymph node masses in this patient with diffuse histiocytic lymphoma. Lymphatic channel displacement around enlarged nodes is seen.

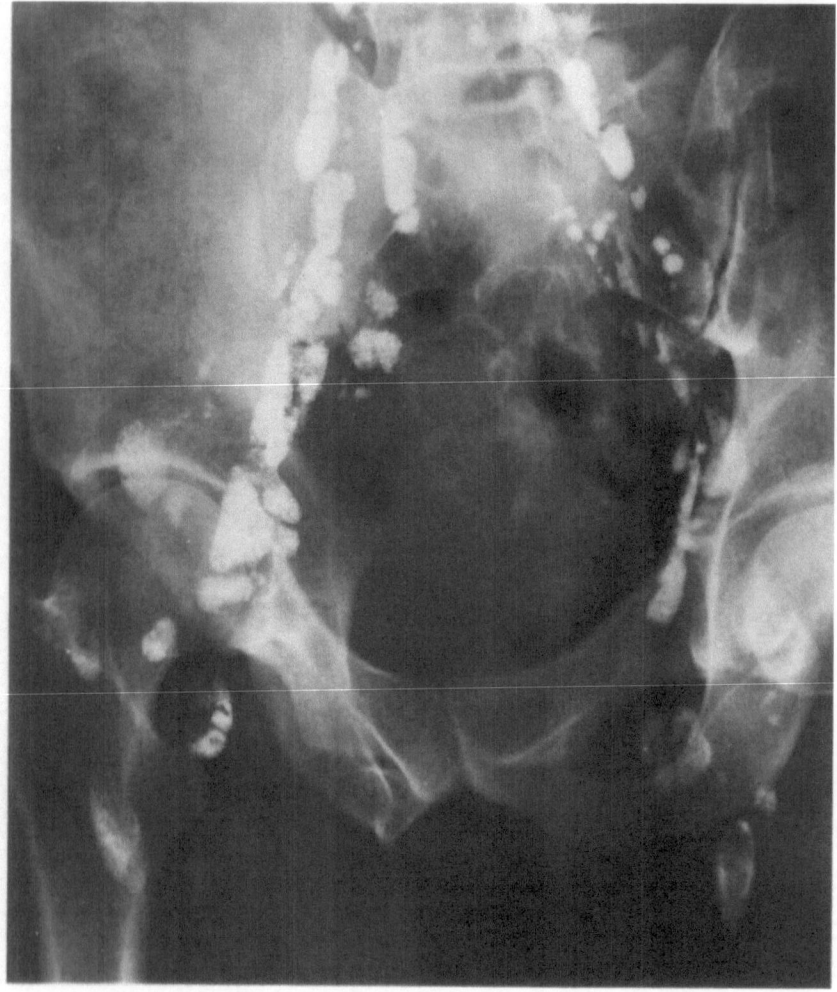

a

Figure 3. (a) Early lymphomatous replacement of normal nodal tissue results in coarsening of the granular texture of several lymph nodes, particularly right para-aortic and external iliac groups. (b) Same patient at the time of a CT scan showing slightly englarged contrast-filled external iliac nodes. Note that the CT scan does not reveal the architectural changes demonstrated by the lymphangiogram.

The lymphangiographic technique essentially involves the slow injection, using a carefully regulated pump pressure, of an oily iodinated radiographic contrast agent into the lymphatics of the dorsum of each foot via fine gauge needles or cannulas. Initially, the lymphatics are rendered visible by the

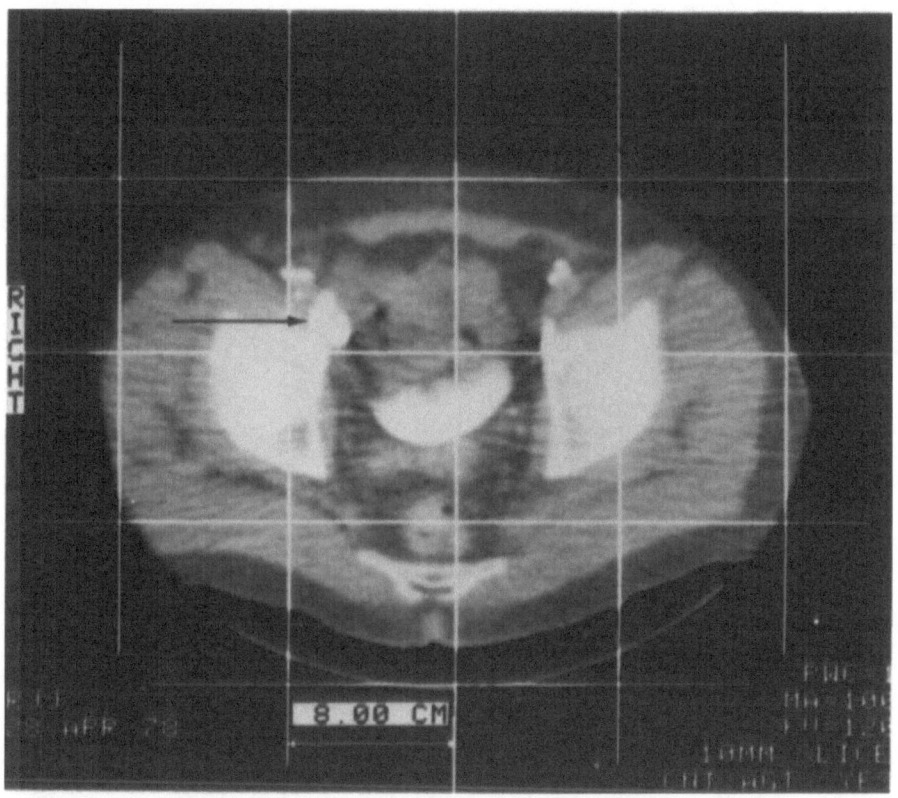

subcutaneous injection of a particulate dye. Important considerations include an awareness of the potential danger of this radiographic technique in patients with extensive bilateral chronic inflammatory or fibrotic disease of the lungs: embolization of oil to the lungs occurs at the time of the LAG which is therefore contraindicated in these patients. Other dangers include those associated with allergy to iodinated compounds. It is also important to ensure that the contrast agent is correctly administered into an appropriate lymphatic by fluoroscopic monitoring, during initial filling of the lymphatics, of the lower extremity and pelvis. Radiographs of the abdomen and pelvis are taken at the time of the injection and these are used to evaluate the size, course and general configuration of the para-aortic and pelvic lymphatic vessels. Twenty-four hours after injection further radiographs are obtained to enable the opacified abdominal and pelvic lymph nodes to be evaluated, particularly as regards size and internal architecture. Diagnostic criteria are essentially divided into those relating to the lymphatic channels and those

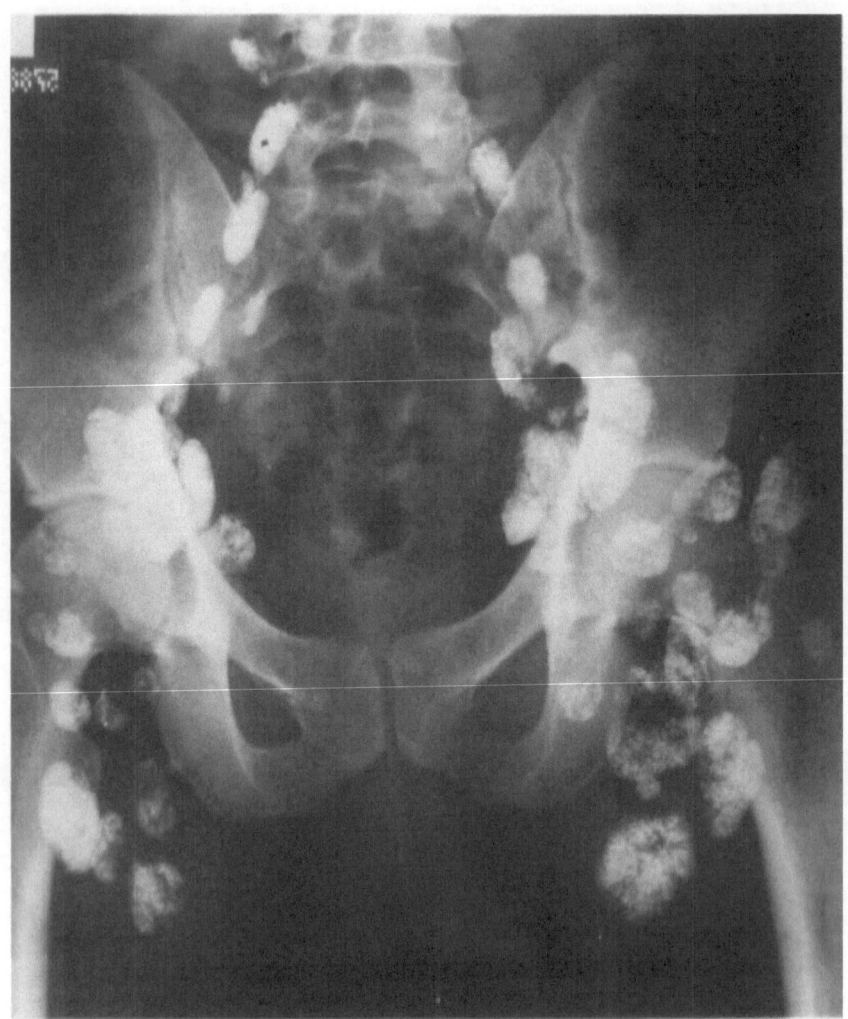

Figure 4. Twenty-four-year-old patient with non-Hodgkin lymphoma. All visualized nodes are enlarged but still relatively well maintained. Typical 'foamy' appearance with marginal sinus still identified on most nodes.

concerned with the lymph nodes themselves. *Lymphatic channels* may be displaced (Figure 2) and there may be relfux of contrast material into collateral channels. In addition, persistence of channel filling as evidenced by the presence of lymphatic channels on the 24 or 48 hours radiographs indicates lymphatic obstruction. Enlargement, displacement and altered

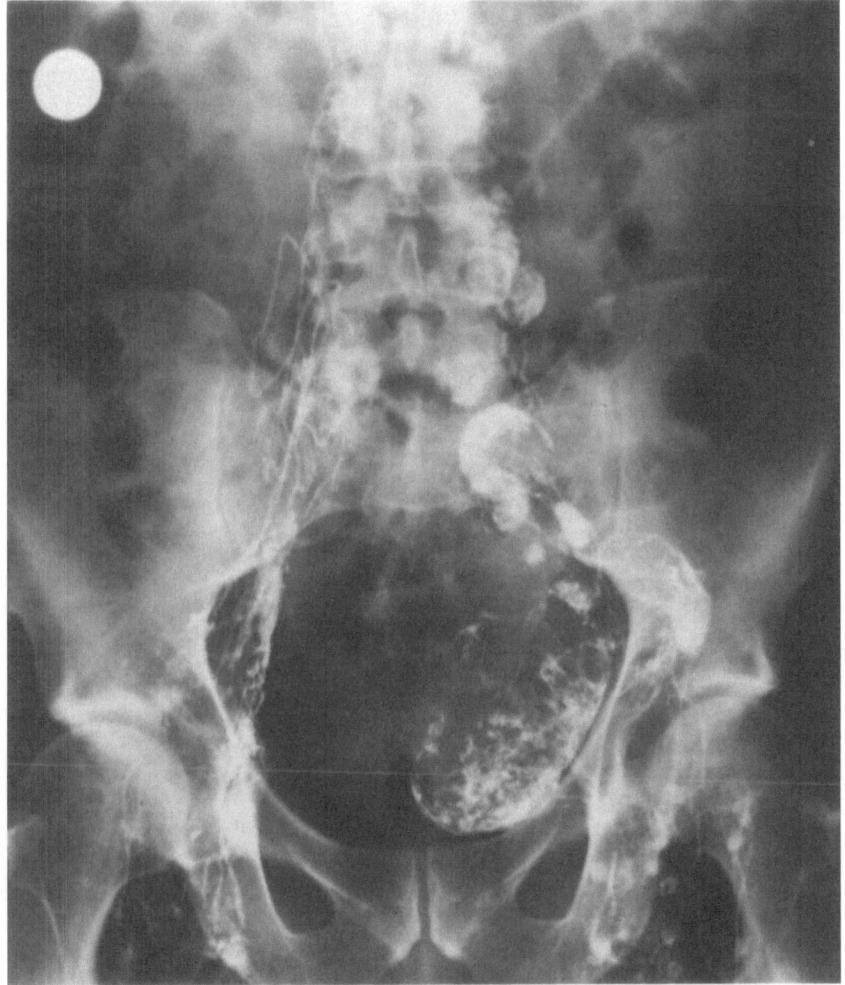

Figure 5. In this 44-year-old patient with Hodgkin's disease, extensive replacement of nodal tissue by tumor results in poor filling of pelvic nodes with contrast displaced out towards the periphery to form a thin rim.

architecture of the *lymph nodes* is optimally demonstrated on the 24 hour radiographs, although the initial films may also demonstrate these features, thus providing an early indication of the extent and degree of nodal involvement.

Malignant lymphomas initially produce a diffuse infiltration of the lymph

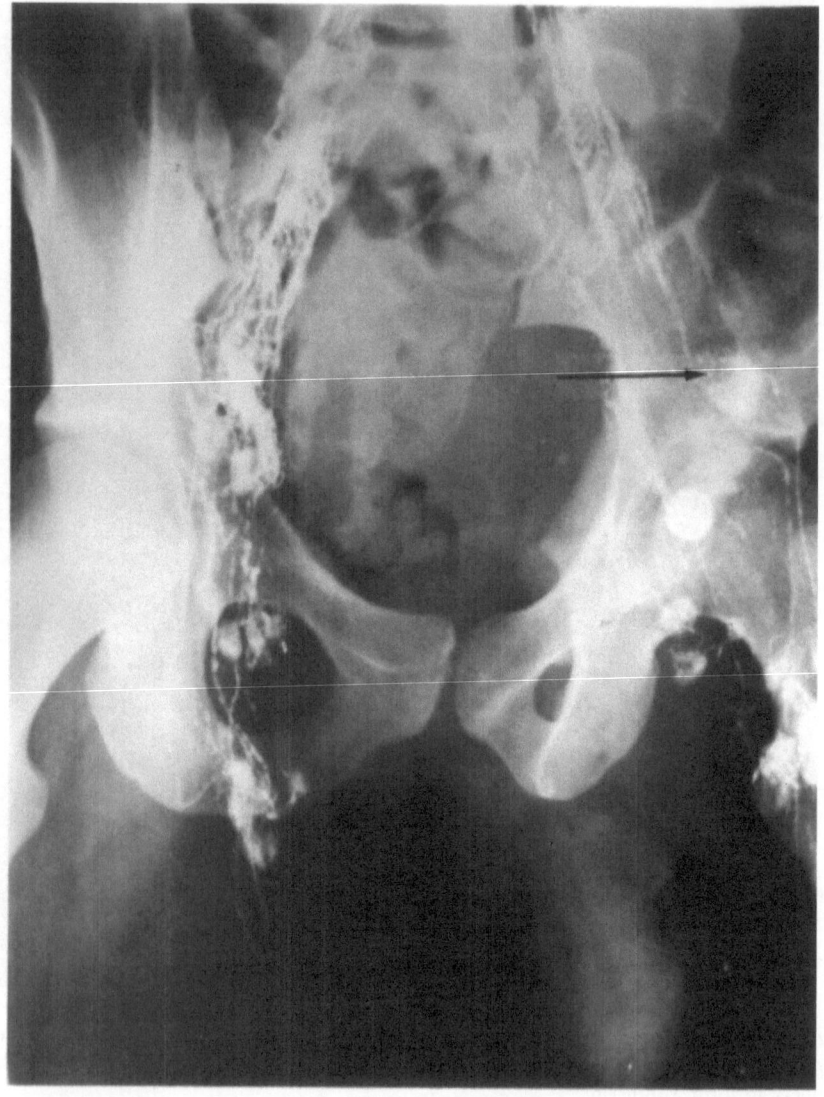

Figure 6. (a) Normal lymphangiogram during the filling phase: note vessels leaving from hilum of external iliac node on the left (arrow). (b) Nodal filling 24 hours later. The defect in the same left external iliac node is again seen and should not be mistaken for a metastatic deposit.

nodes and this can frequently be differentiated from the more sharply defined, irregular filling defects produced by metastatic involvement arising from other malignancies such as pelvic carcinomas.

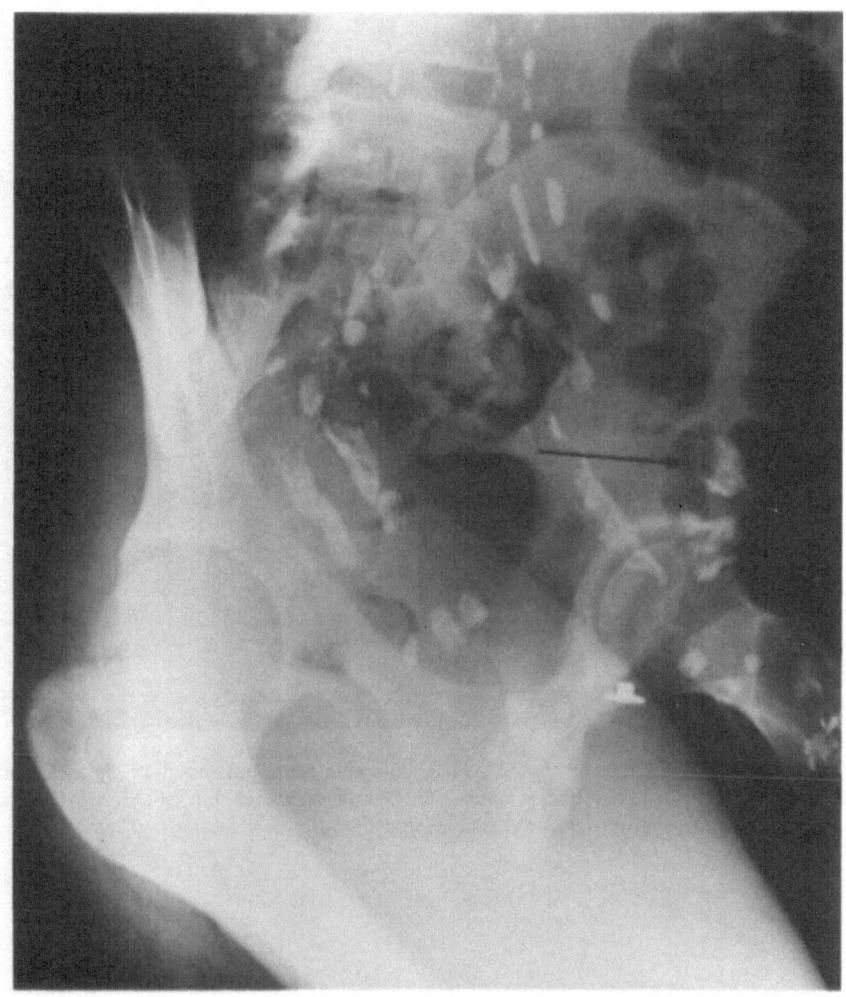

b

Early lymphomatous replacement of normal nodal tissue results in a coarsening of the granular texture of the lymph node (Figure 3). As the disease progresses, a more characteristic 'foamy' or reticulated pattern develops in the involved nodes (Figure 4). The opaque contrast medium is later displaced out towards the periphery of the node to form a thin rim (Figure 5). Incomplete, patchy filling is seen in larger nodal masses and may be associated with displacement, and delayed emptying of adjacent lymphatic vessels, with or without the development of collateral channels and other signs of lymphatic obstruction.

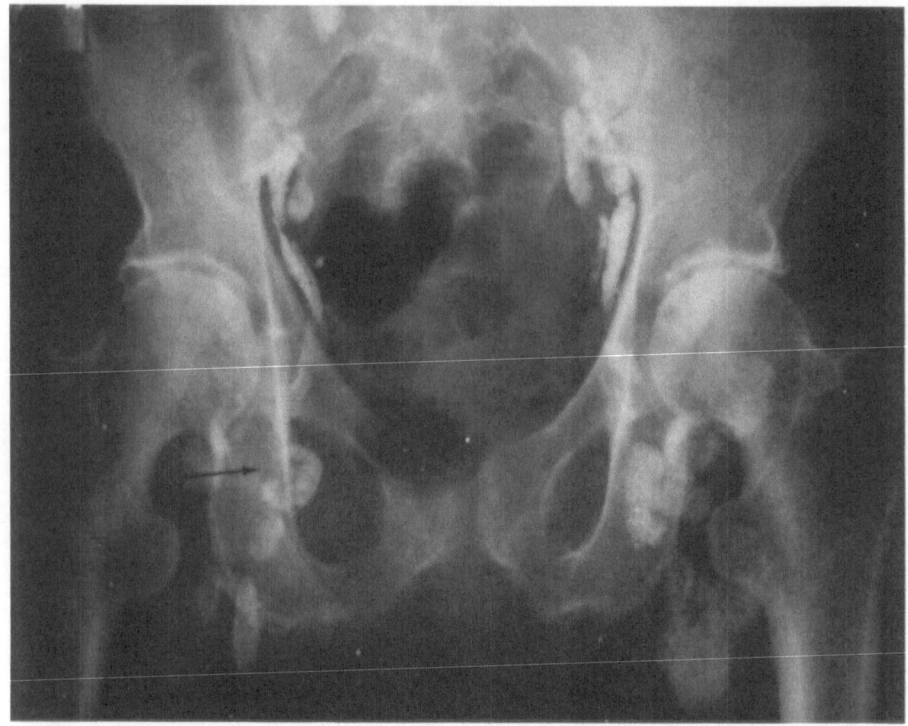

Figure 7. Diabetic patient with abscess of left foot: note acute inflammatory changes causing enlargement of left inguinal nodes which are slightly coarsened but not destroyed. Note: fibrolipomatosis on right (arrow) producing central filling.

In addition to the architectural abnormalities discussed above, other diagnostic criteria used to evaluate the nodal phase of the lymphangiogram include filling defects, irregularity of node margins, lymph node enlargement, discontinuity of the lymph node chains, and displacement of nodes. Filling defects due to nodal replacement by tumor (Figure 5) must be differentiated from the lymph node hilum (Figure 6), and poor filling due to prior inflammation.

Fibrolipomatosis, a manifestation of the normal physiologic involution of the lymphatic system, must be differentiated from nodal replacement by tumor. Typically, these nodes are characterized by large central filling defects (Figure 7). Other benign conditions, such as hyperplastic inflammatory changes (Figure 7) must be differentiated from malignant infiltration.

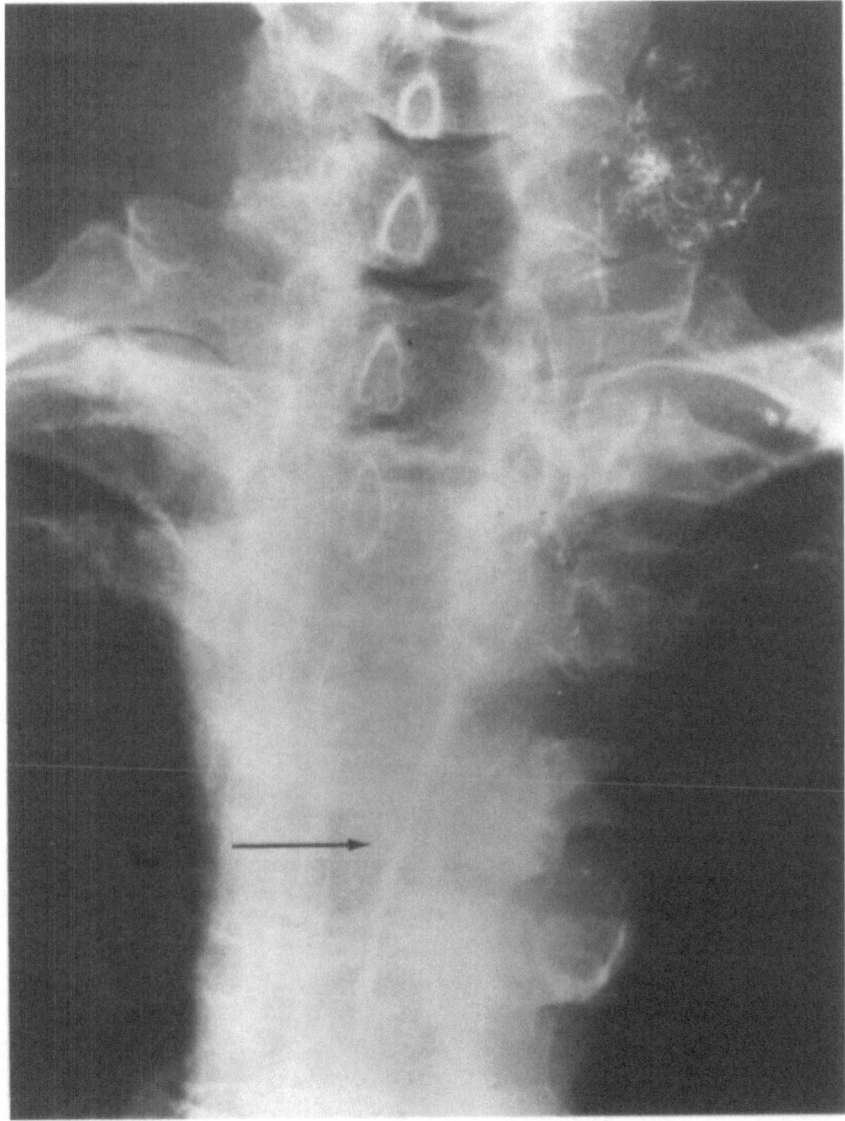

Figure 8. Visualization of the thoracic duct (arrows) with opacification of abnormal left supraclavicular lymph nodes.

The thoracic duct is usually visualized during the lymphangiographic procedure and occasionally opacification of abnormal supraclavicular lymph nodes may result (Figure 8). Also, the cisterna chyli may be demonstrated as

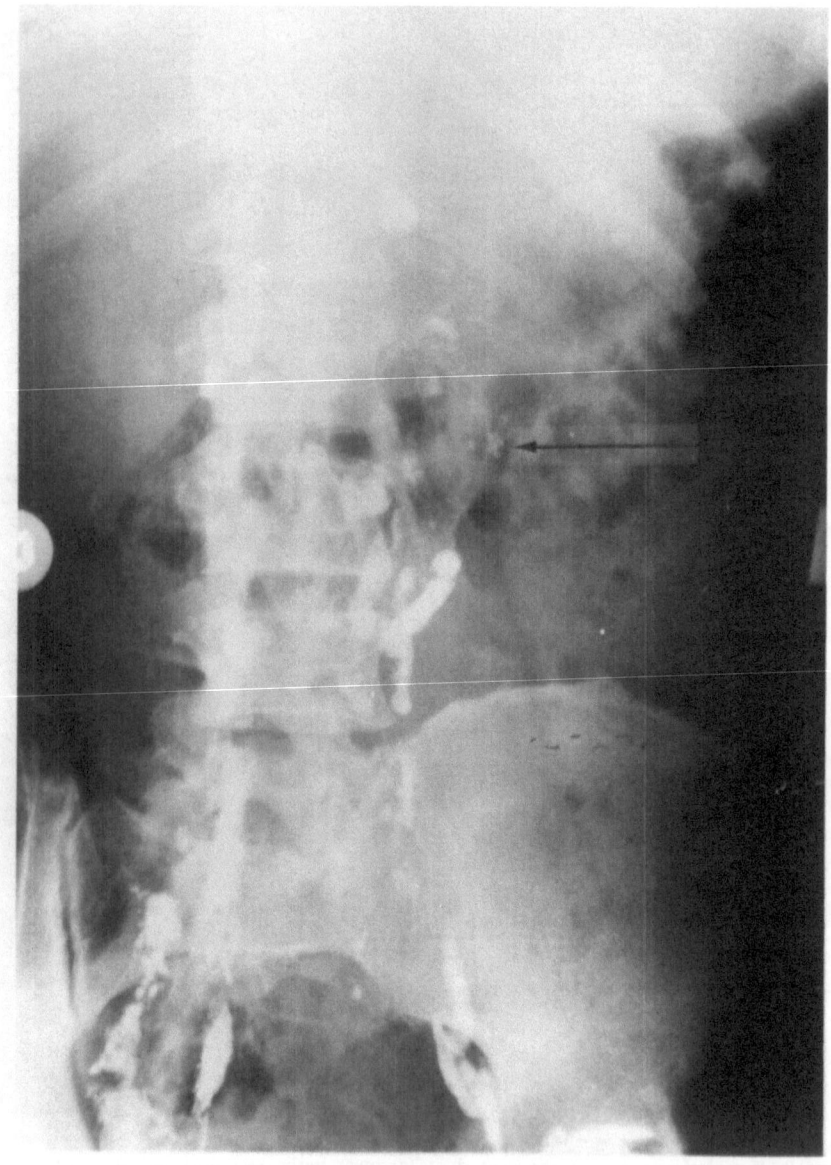

a

Figure 9. (a) Left para-aortic lymph node enlargement is seen in this patient with Hodgkin's disease (arrow). Displacement of nodes away from the vertebral bodies is present and best seen on this slightly oblique view. (b) Same Patient 4 months later following chemotherapy. Significant decrease in size of lymph nodes seen on oblique and AP views. Patient also had mediastinal lymph node involvement which also responded well (Figure 33).

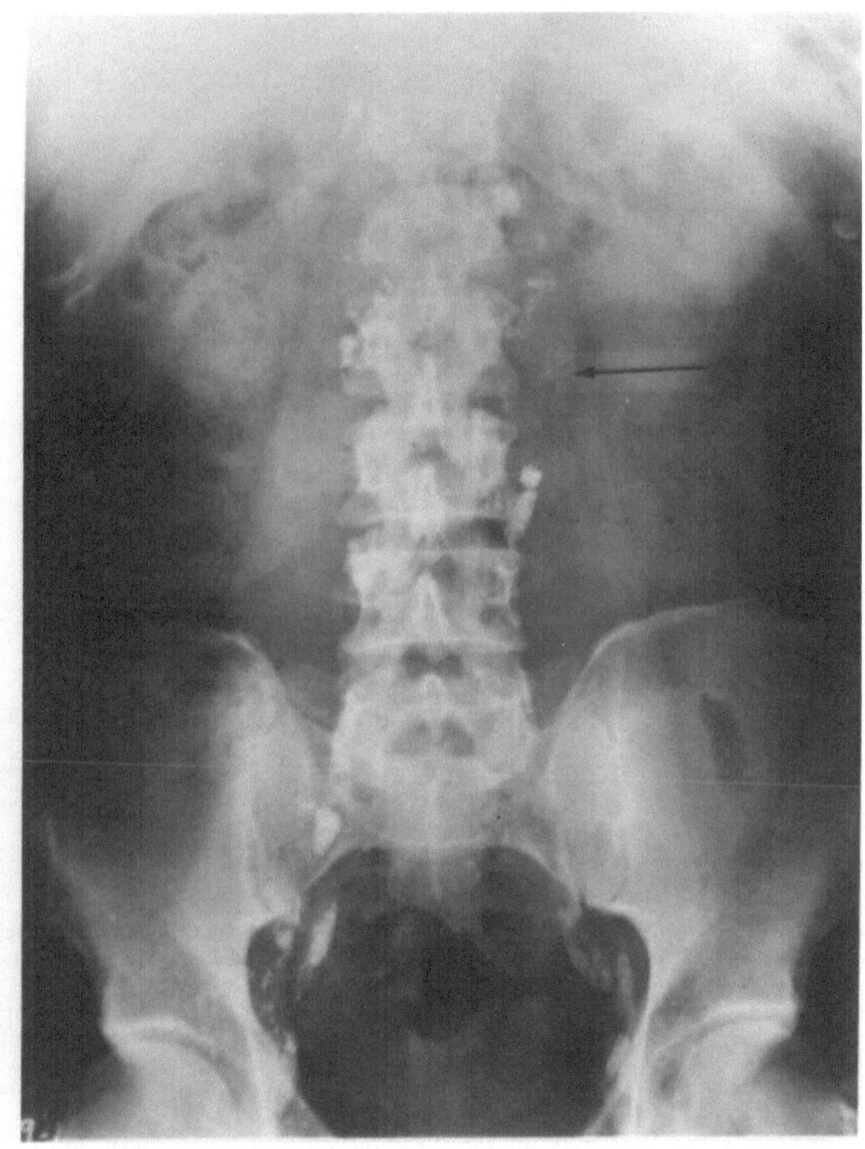

b

a tortuous, dilated structure, with other features of lymphatic obstruction (Figure 2).

Lymphographic contrast agent slowly empties from opacified lymph nodes. The rate of emptying is variable and may take from several months to

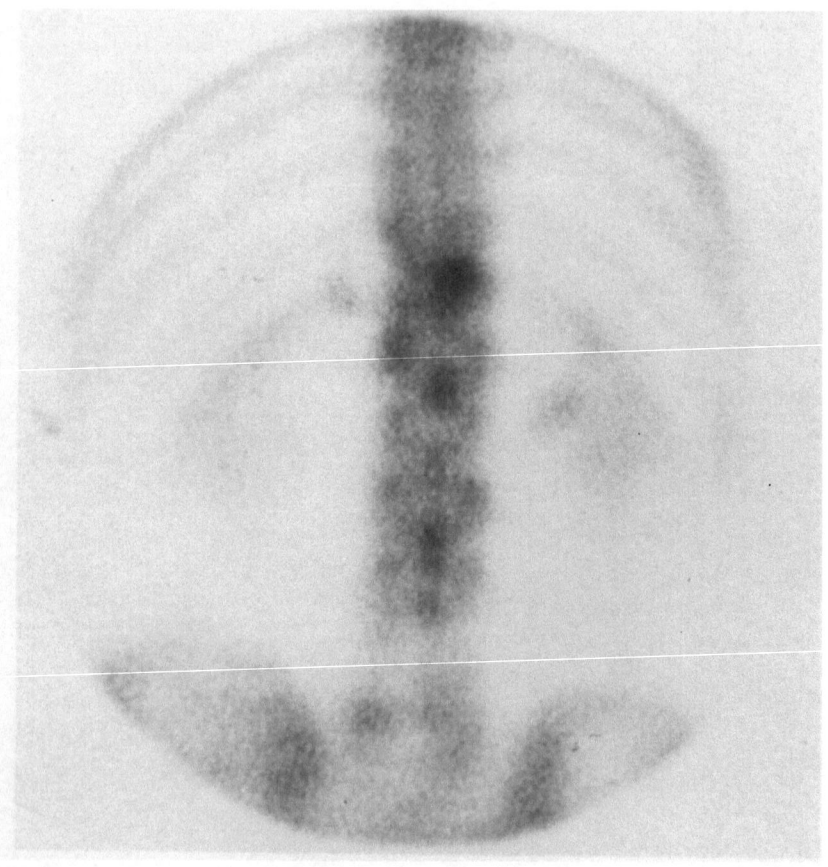

a

Figure 10. Phosphonate colloids of radioactive technetium (^{99m}Tc) can demonstrate relatively early lymphomatous bone changes such as in this patient with several areas of increased uptake in T12 vertebral body and several lumbar vertebrae due to diffuse histiocytic lymphoma.

two or more years, thus enabling serial radiographs during the early course of the disease to be used to assess the results of treatment (Figure 9).

With the advent of routine staging laparotomy came a means of correlating the lymphangiographic appearances of normal and abnormal lymph nodes with surgical and pathological data. Several studies reveal an overall diagnostic accuracy in Hodgkin's disease of over 90% utilizing lower extremity lymphangiography [5, 6]. This high degree of accuracy, plus the fact that 31–46% of pathologically staged patients with Hodgkin's disease have involvement of abdominal lymph nodes [5, 7–9], has lead to lymphangiography being considered an essential feature in the diagnostic workup of patients

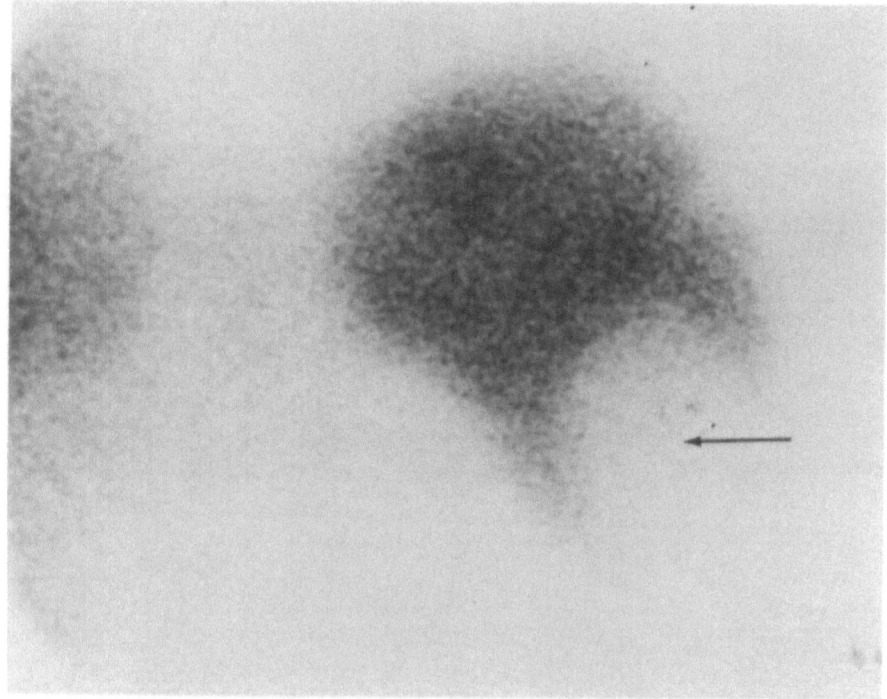

Figure 11. Clearly visible focal filling defect in the spleen of this patient with Hodgkin's disease.

with this disease except where specific medical (such as extensive pulmonary disease) and allergic contraindications exist [10].

3. LYMPHANGIOGRAPHIC FINDINGS IN HODGKIN'S DISEASE AND NON-HODGKIN'S LYMPHOMA

Under optimal conditions, the lymphangiogram can detect focal involvement by Hodgkin's disease only a few millimeters in diameter within a lymph node [11]. This degree of accuracy in the depiction of internal architectural change is of particular importance in the case of lymph nodes which are abnormal but not obviously enlarged. Computed tomography is now able to demonstrate lymph nodes of the order of 3–10 mm but even using modern scanners with improved image resolution architectural abnormalities in normal sized nodes are not revealed.

A similar high degree of accuracy is obtained in the evaluation of

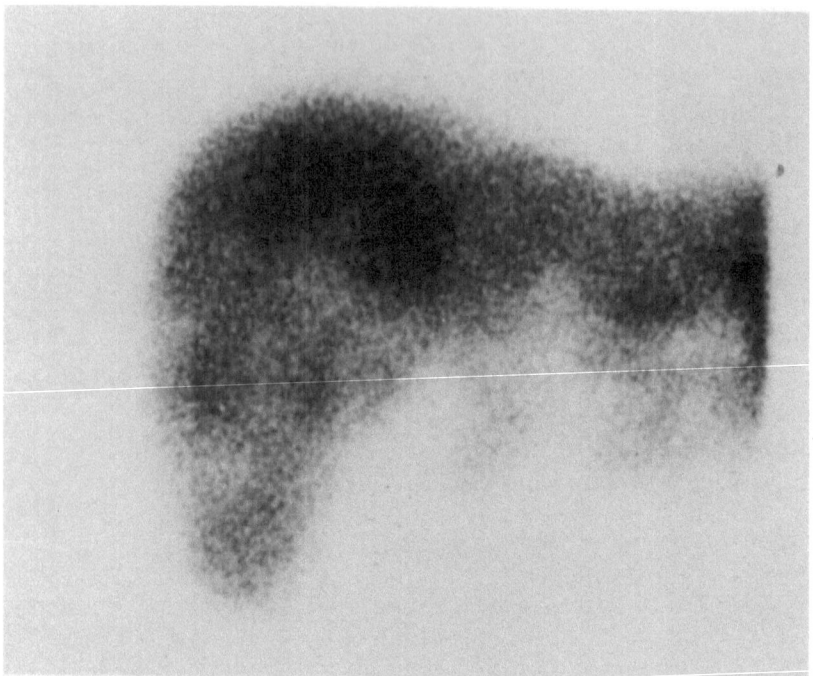

Figure 12. Diffuse lymphomatous involvement, with hepatomegaly, in this 28-year-old patient with Hodgkin's disease. Patchy uptake particularly noted in the right lobe of the liver.

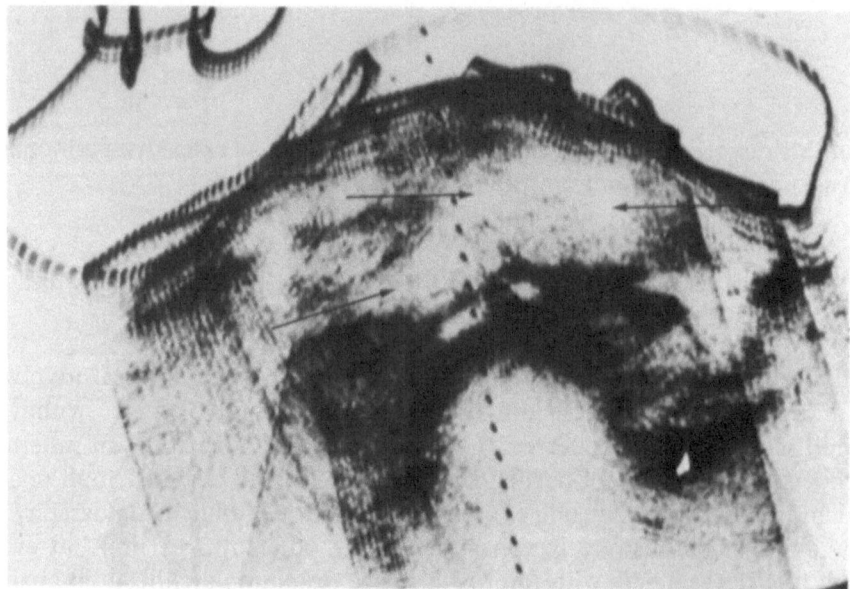

Figure 13. Ultrasonography reveals the presence of mesenteric lymph node masses (arrows) anterior to aorta and vena cava.

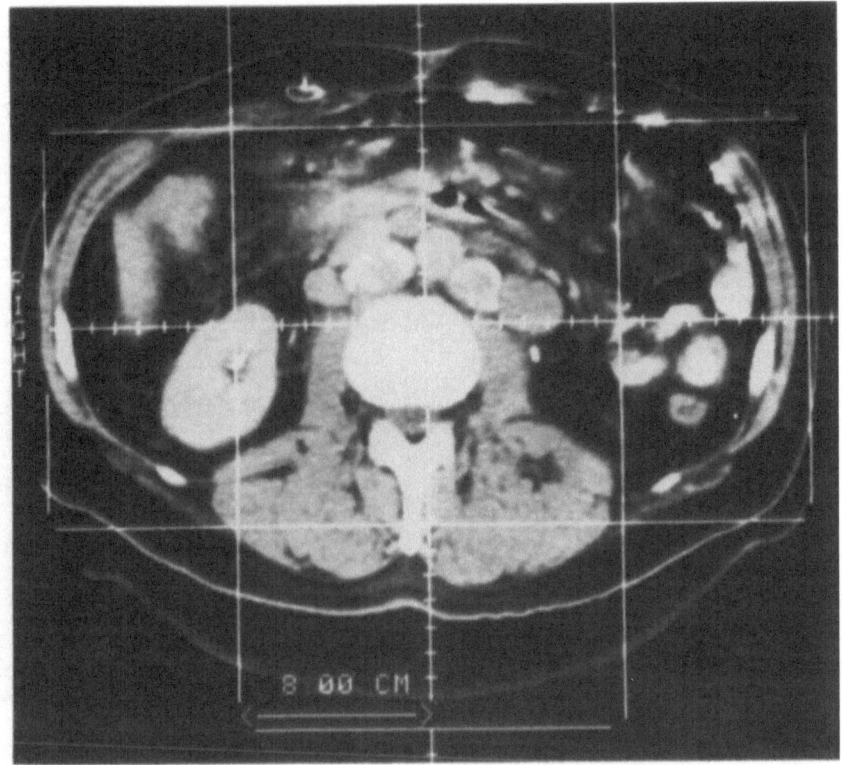

Figure 14. (a) Partially filled para-aortic lymph nodes following lymphangiogram are revealed on this CT scan. (b) Partial filling of iliac nodal groups in this patient with Hodgkin's disease. The true extent of the lymphomatous replacement is better shown on the CT scan than lymphangiogram (Figure 5).

non-Hodgkin's lymphomas by lymphangiography as is achieved with Hodgkin's disease. A study of 69 untreated patients with non-Hodgkin's disease subjected to laparatomy following lymphangiography revealed an accuracy of 92% [12].

Evaluation of a larger series of patients (423) staged between 1971 and 1976 confirmed an accuracy rate in normal and abnormal para-aortic lymph nodes of 88% and 87% respectively [13]. However, this series revealed that a negative lymphangiogram does not reliably predict absence of disease below the diaphragm, particularly in patients with nodular lymphomas. Lymphoma was found in almost 50% of the resected spleens and mesenteric lymph nodes in these patients. Where para-aortic lymph node involvement was seen

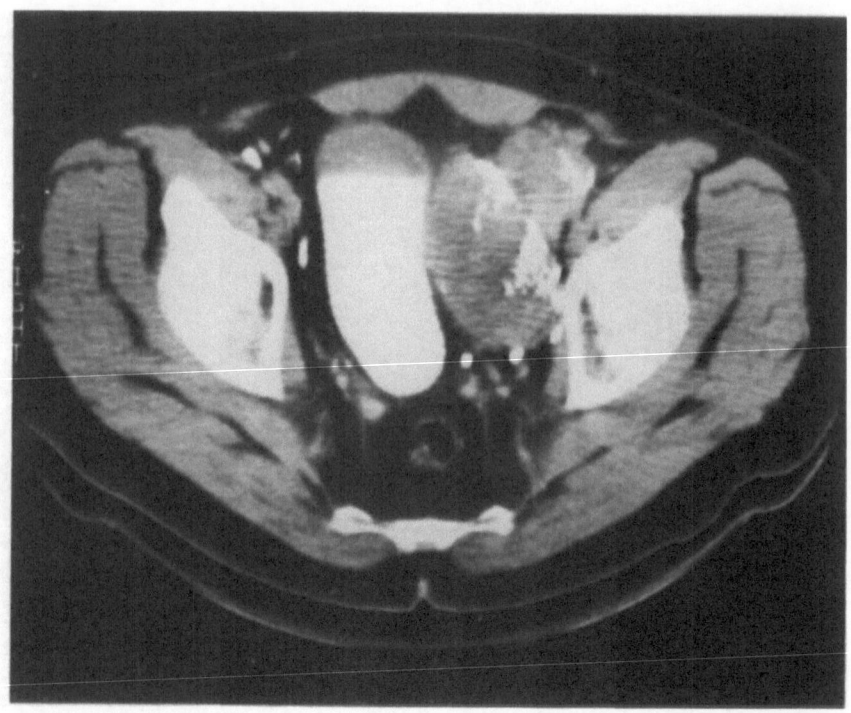

b

on the lymphangiograms of patients with nodular lymphomas, a very high frequency of mesenteric lymph node involvement (79%) was noted. Sub-diaphragmatic hepatic and mesenteric lymph node involvement ranged from 20% to 50% in the case of patients with diffuse lymphomas and positive lymphangiogram. The other findings of interest were that in contrast to Hodgkin's disease, there is an increased incidence of gastro-intestinal, mesenteric, hepatic and pulmonary involvement in patients with non-Hodgkin's lymphoma. Due to the inaccessibility of these regions to LAG, computed tomography has been suggested as the preferred initial staging modality in patients with biopsy-proven lymphoma (extra-abdominal) when abdominal involvement is suspected [14].

Potential problems in the CT evaluation of enlarged mesenteric lymph nodes in patients with non-Hodgkin's lymphoma and negative LAGs were noted at the time of a laparatomy series of 68 patients with lymphangiogram-staged I and II NHL [15]. Only one patient had a mesenteric node larger than 2.5 cm which was considered by the investigators as the upper limit of

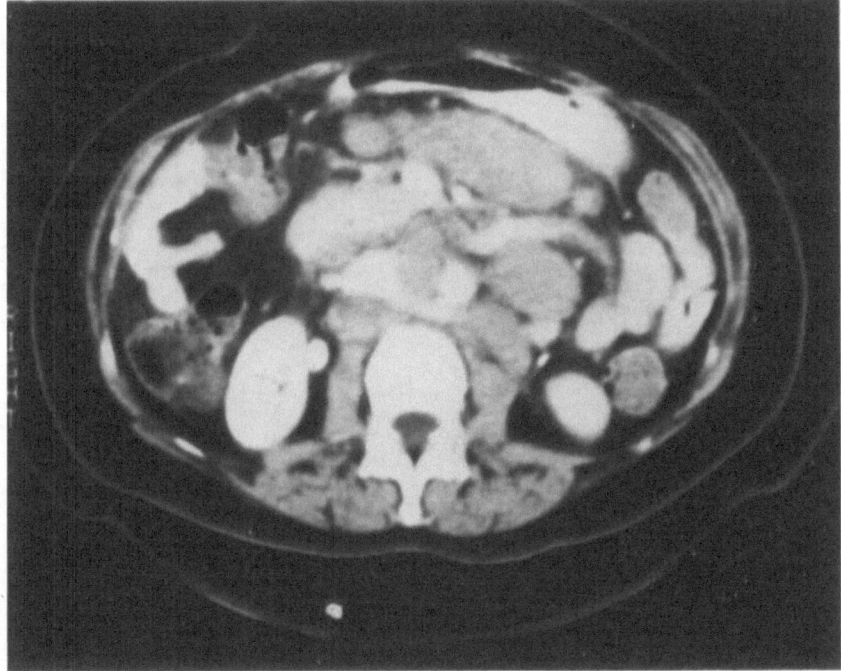

Figure 15. CT scan showing extensive mesenteric lymph node enlargement in a patient with diffuse histiocytic lymphoma.

normal and only one patient had a spleen sufficiently large to have been abnormal by size criteria on CT scan.

In addition to mesenteric lymph nodes, other nodal groups noted to be inaccessible to evaluation by lymphangiography include high retroperitoneal nodes, plus retrocrural, and splenic and hepatic hilar lymph nodes. Computed tomography is particularly useful in delineating involvement of these nodal groups.

The inaccuracy of lymphangiography in demonstrating disease in these sites has resulted in the use of a variety of non-invasive imaging techniques in further attempts to avoid the need for staging laparotomy. Most of the LAG errors are 'false positives', usually due to reactive changes in lymph nodes or to sampling error by the surgeon: The error rate varies considerably, from 2% [16] to 21% [17]. Nevertheless, in Hodgkin's disease, LAG remains an important staging examination and guide to the surgical sampling of lymph nodes in addition to aiding the delineation of radiation therapy ports, documenting the effects of therapy and detecting relapse.

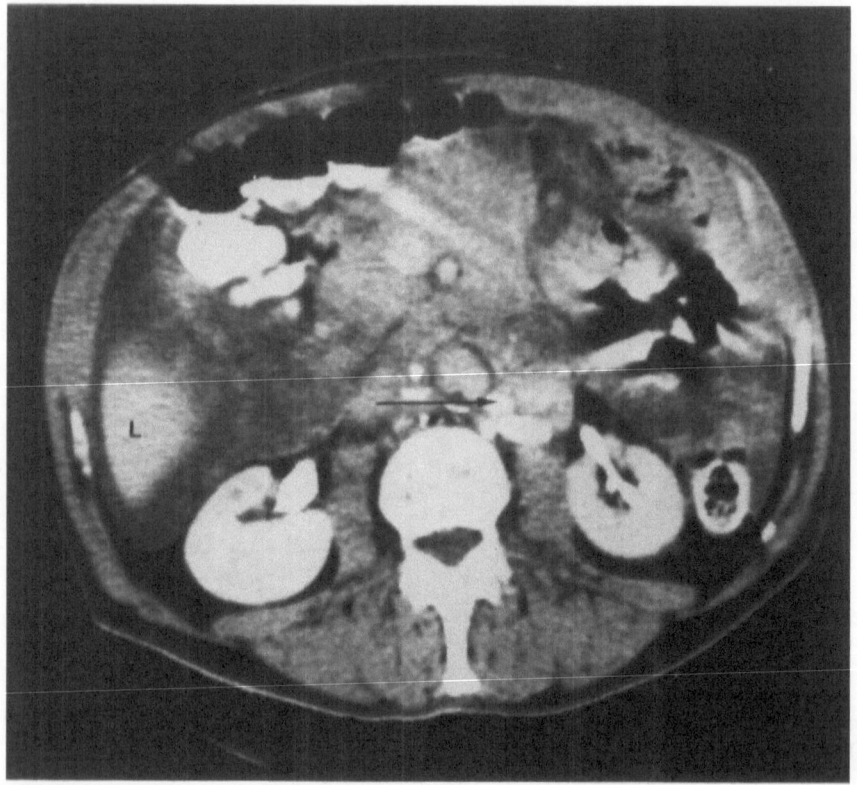

Figure 16. Another patient with mesenteric nodal masses. Also high left para-aortic nodal disease only partially filled with contrast after lymphangiogram (arrow). Patient also has ascites around liver (L).

4   RADIO-NUCLIDE SCANNING

4.1. Gallium-67 Imaging

Radioactive gallium (Ga-67) citrate localizes selectively in lymph nodes involved by malignant lymphoma [18] and many studies have been performed in an attempt to assess the role of Ga-67 scanning in the evaluation of lymphomas. Interpretation of many of these studies has been difficult due to variability in Ga-67 dose administered and techniques of measurement of uptake. Also, proof of disease in suspected tumor areas frequently was judged clinically rather than by biopsy or radiologic examination. Early hopes were that this method of assessment of disease with Ga-67 would eventually

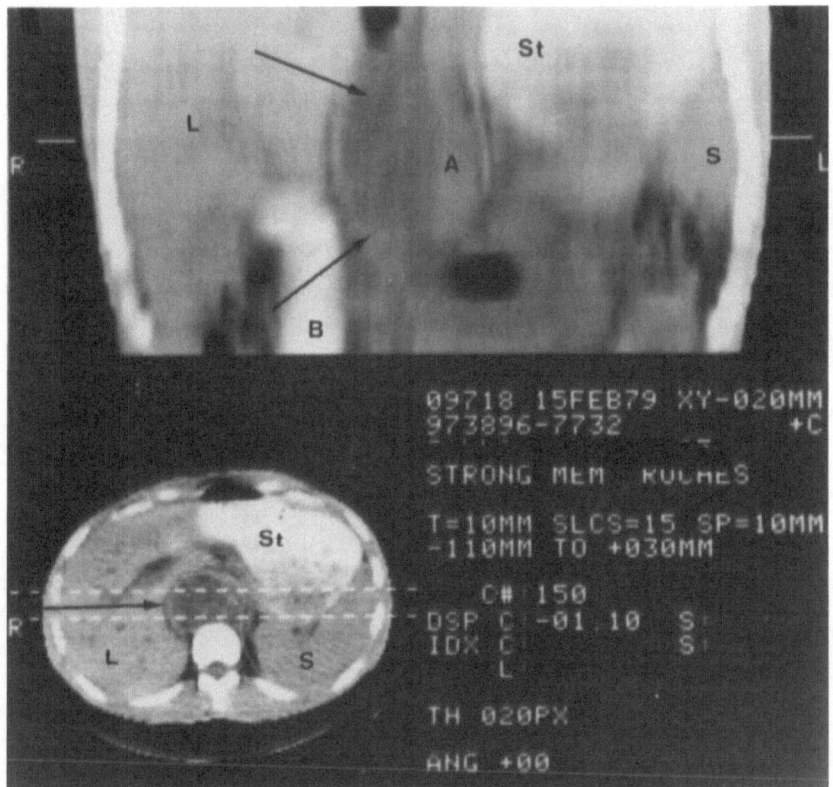

Figure 17. Reconstructed CT image in the coronal plane shows true extent of right retrocrural lymph node masses (arrows) including cranio-caudal dimension. Aorta (A) is labeled, also stomach (St), spleen (S) and liver (L). Oral contrast agent is present in the small bowel (B). The corresponding axial section is shown below.

decrease the need for lymphangiography in the detection of subdiaphragmatic lymphoma. Unfortunately, although Ga-67 remains useful in evaluating subdiaphragmatic lesions, interpretation of abdominal scans is often difficult due to interference from uptake of the isotope in liver and large bowel [19, 20].

The role of Ga-67 imaging in Hodgkin's disease was evaluated by Johnston *et al.* [21] utilizing a group of 668 patients of whom 240 were untreated and 420 treated. Sixty-nine percent of the patients studied had a positive scan (88% of the untreated and 56% of the treated groups). A slightly lower accuracy of detection was found in the lymphocyte predomi-

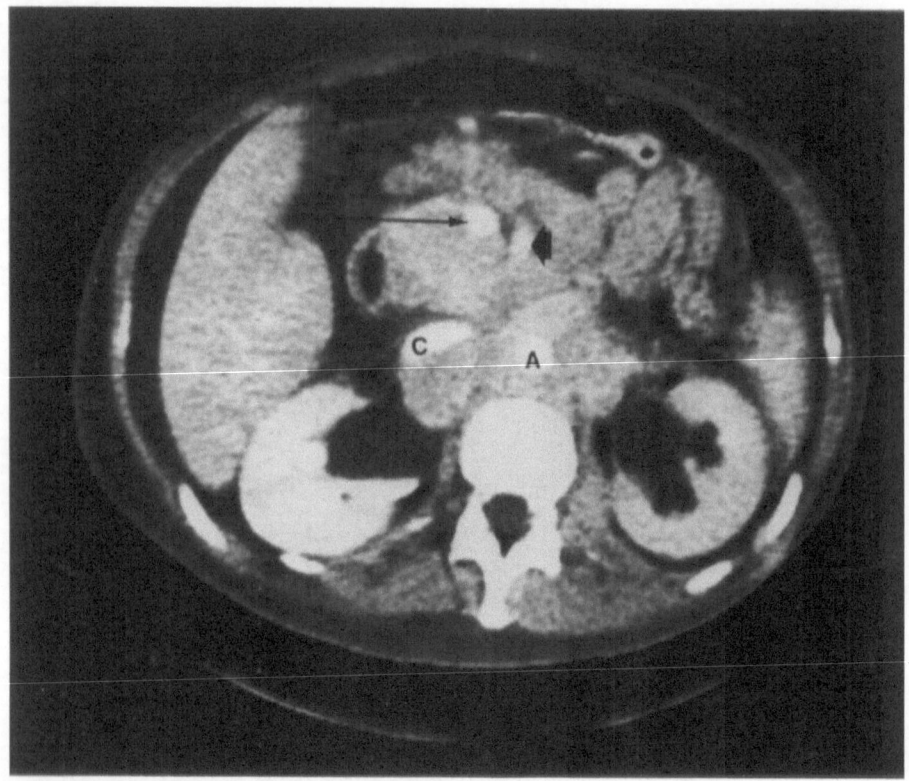

Figure 18. Para-aortic and mesenteric lymphadenopathy with anterior displacement and partial compression of inferior vena cava (C). Aorta (A) is well seen. Superior mesenteric vein (arrow) and artery (arrowhead) are also clearly identified.

nant group. A 15% incidence of false positive scans occurred in the abdominal area. The size of the lesion appeared to be important. One centimeter lesions were the smallest that could be detected, and accuracy improved considerably with the larger lesions up to a 90% detection rate for 5 cm lesions. When lymphangiography and Ga-67 scans were performed in the same patient, the results of the two studies were comparable. However, once chemotherapy or radiotherapy was administered, the lymphangiogram was the superior tool. Analysis of data from Stanford University Medical Center revealed that Ga-67 scintigraphy correctly detected 61% of supra-diaphragmatic sites, and only 40% of the infradiaphragmatic sites [20].

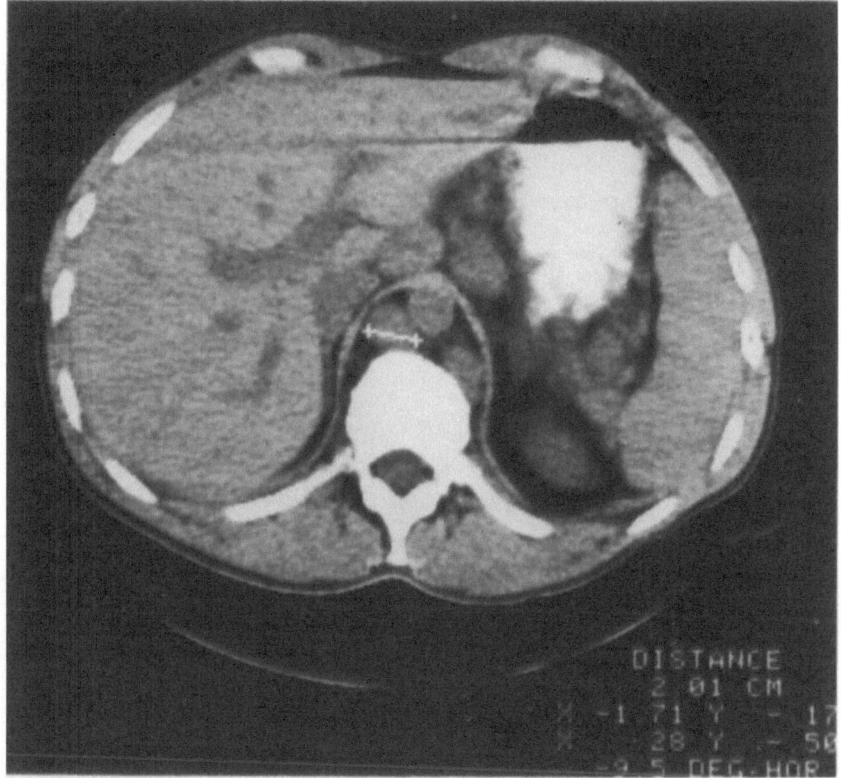

Figure 19. Enlarged retrocrural lymph nodes.

In terms of the evaluation of accuracy of Ga-67 citrate imaging in patients with non-Hodgkin's lymphoma, the cooperative group assessed 296 patients with untreated non-Hodgkin's lymphoma plus 394 treated patients, with 2994 sites undergoing examination [22] 76% of the untreated cases were positive, with 3% being equivocal. In the treated group, 57% were positive, with 6% being equivocal. The histiocytic cell type was positive in 89% of the untreated cases. Lymphocytic well-differentiated cases had a significantly lower positive rate of 59%. In untreated cases where histological confirmation was available for specific sites a true positive figure of 52% was obtained, with a false negative rate of 42% and a false positive rate of 2%. Thus, the overall detection in non-Hodgkin's lymphoma was considerably less than in Hodgkin's disease. In addition, therapy and chemotherapy

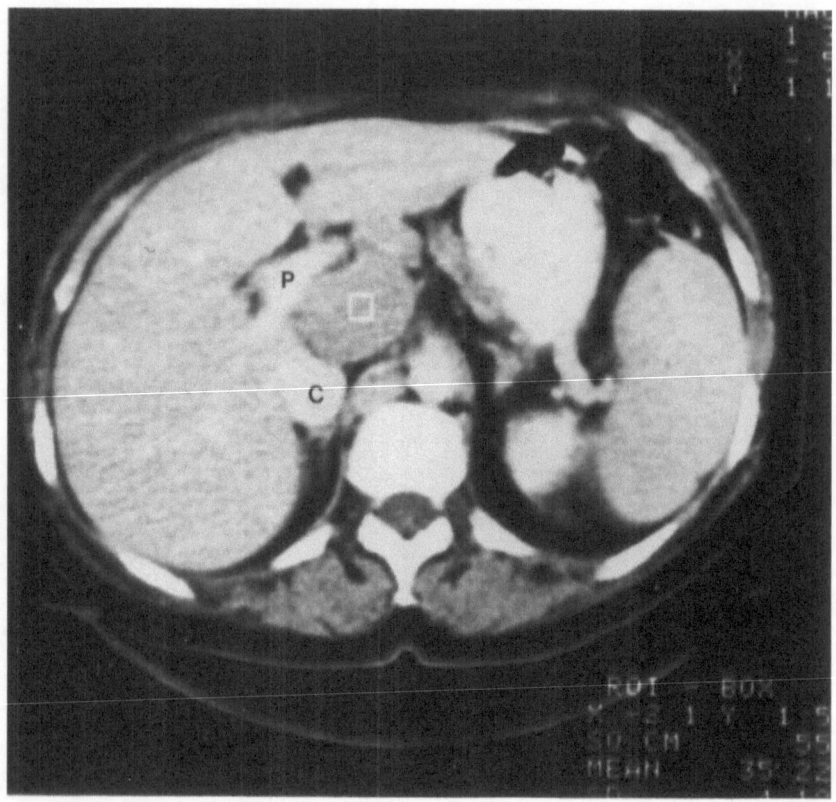

Figure 20. Patient with Hodgkin's disease and large, solid lymph node mass in porta hepatis displacing portal vein (P) anterolaterally and inferior vena cava (C) postero-laterally. IV contrast agent clearly differentiates vessels from the mass which has a lower CT attenuation value.

decreased the uptake of Ga-67 in previously positive sites frequently rendering them undetectable. As with Hodgkin's disease the areas poorly evaluated were the axillary, abdominal, pelvic and inguinal regions. Lymphangiograms appeared to be more sensitive in detecting disease in the abdomen and pelvis than Ga-67.

4.2. Other Radionuclide Procedures

Significant advances in radionuclide bone imaging have been made since the introduction, in the early 1970s, of ^{99m}Tc-labeled polyphosphonate and disphosphonate.

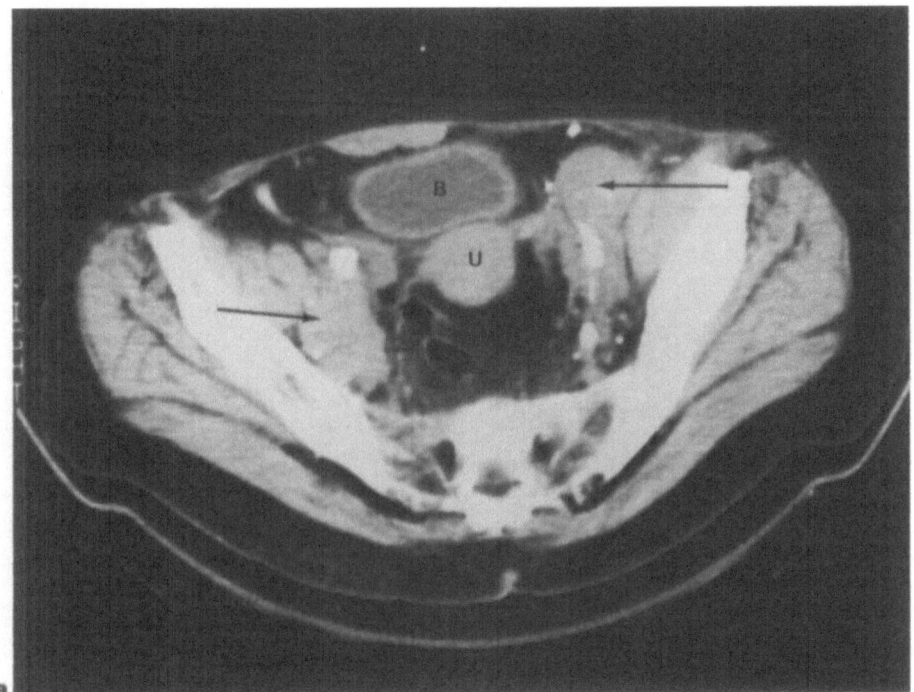

Figure 21. (a) Extensive involvement of external and internal iliac lymph nodes (arrows) were only partially demonstrated by lymphangiogram. CT is particularly useful in identifying disease in internal iliac groups. Bladder (B) and uterus (U) are labeled. (b) Iliac lymph node groups involved by diffuse histiocytic lymphoma in this 32-year-old patient presenting with low grade fever of unknown etiology. Patient originally considered to have possible pelvic abscess.

Early bone lesions due to lymphomatous infiltration are now able to be located and evaluated using this procedure [23] (Figure 10).

Unfortunately, liver and spleen scans employing various radionuclides have yielded disappointing results [24–26], although frequently performed in newly diagnosed patients with Hodgkin's disease. Only infrequently is a clearly visible filling defect present in patients with Hodgkin's disease (Figure 11, 12). When using technetium-99m sulfur colloid, heterogeneous uptake and hepatomegaly are more common scintigraphic abnormalities but these are non-specific. Liver biopsy at laparoscopy or laparotomy is the most specific method of detecting hepatic Hodgkin's disease [26]. Percutaneous biopsy techniques have been utilized, sometimes under CT guidance, but the yield has been low [28] and tissue fragments obtained may be difficult to interpret [29].

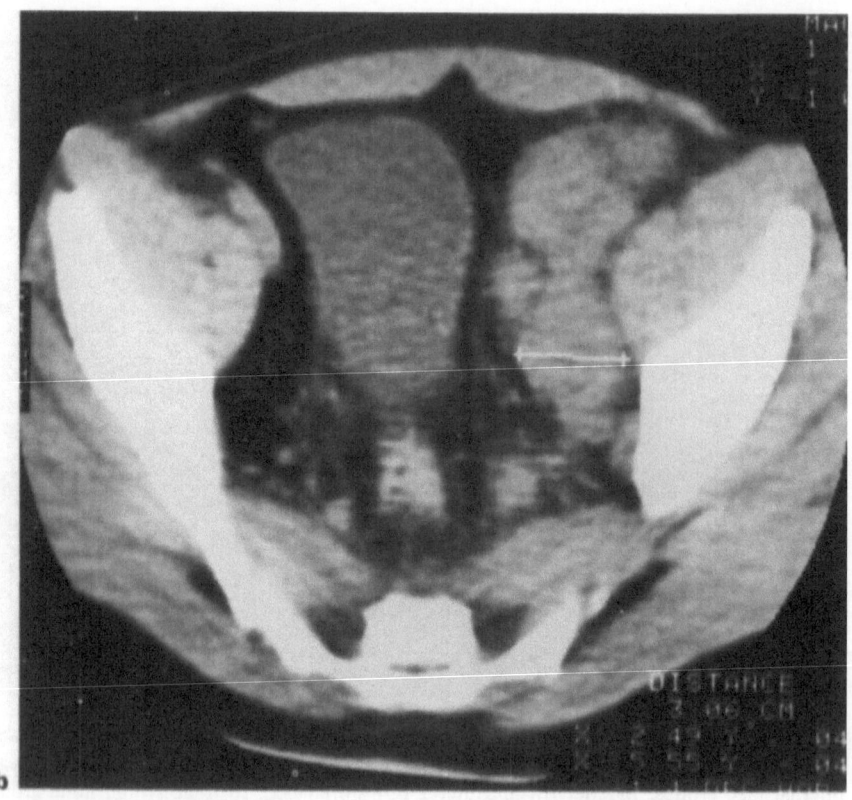

5. ULTRASONOGRAPHY

Diagnostic ultrasound has been described as a useful imaging technique for assessing involvement in the abdomen, pelvis and retroperitoneal area by Hodgkin's disease and NHL [30]. Ultrasound was found to be accurate in demonstrating retroperitoneal and para-aortic lymph node involvement in 88% of 56 patients with Hodgkin's disease and non-Hodgkin's lymphoma where histological confirmation was available [31]. Ultrasound was 98% accurate in predicting node size of 2 cm or greater. However, ultrasound (as with computed tomography) cannot depict architectural abnormalities in normal sized nodes which contain malignant disease. Ultrasound is particularly useful in demonstrating nodes in the upper abdomen (porta hepatis, splenic hilum, peripancreatic). Involved lymph nodes appear as smoothly

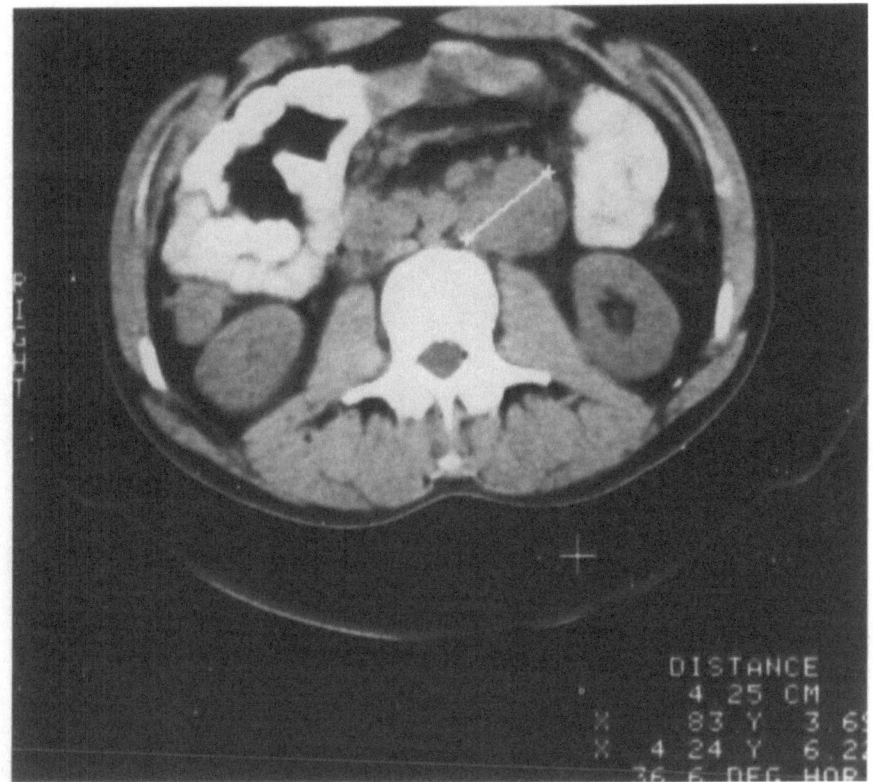

Figure 22. (a) Extensive lymph node enlargement in para-aortic regions in patient with diffuse non-Hodgkin lymphoma. (Maximum node size is 4.25 cm.) (b) Following chemotherapy same patient seven months later now has normal sized lymph nodes. (c) Different patient initially with left external and internal lymph node disease shows good response to therapy (right).

lobulated sonolucent masses. If located in the para-aortic region, these masses tend to obliterate the anterior margin of the aorta creating an 'echo silhouette' [32]. Mesenteric nodes may also be demonstrated (Figure 13).

Limitations in the technique include inability to detect nodes less than 1.5 cm in size plus problems in differentiating other causes of node enlargement [33]. False positive results may result from hyperplasia, non-caseating granuloma and lymphangiogram reaction. Therefore, it has been suggested [27] that ultrasonography be performed prior to LAG so as to avoid false positives secondary to reactions to the LAG contrast agent. Grey scale ultrasonography, with its ability to characterize lesions, was considered to be

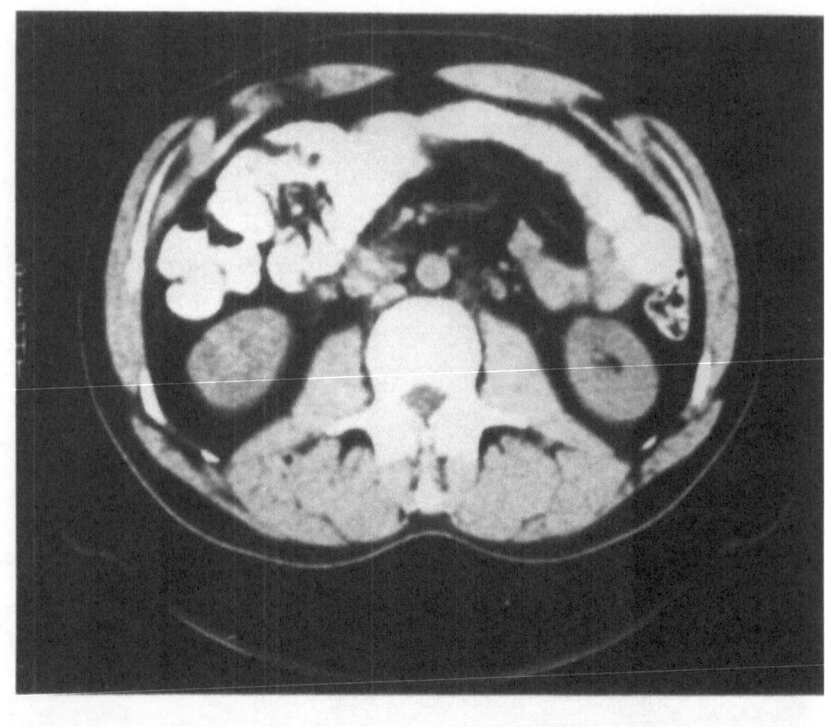

b

c

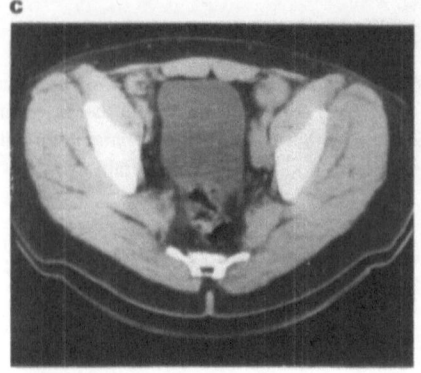

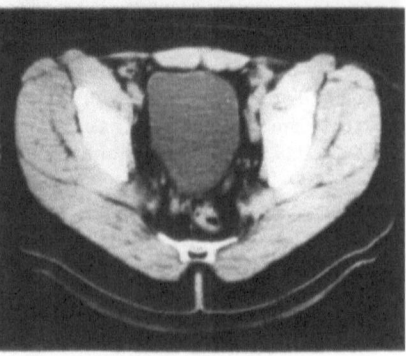

potentially useful in the assessment of diffuse splenic involvement [34]. In addition to the demonstration of abnormal lymphadenopathy in retroperitoneal, celiac, porta hepatis and mesenteric lymph nodes and the delineation

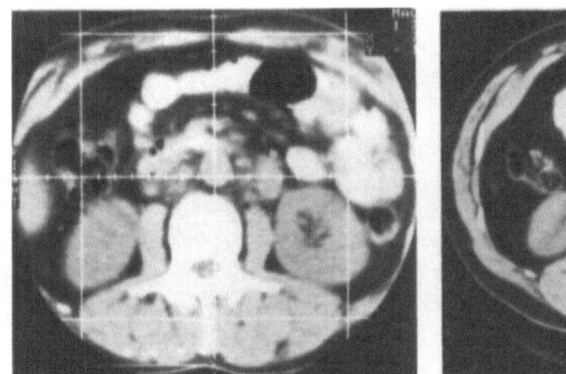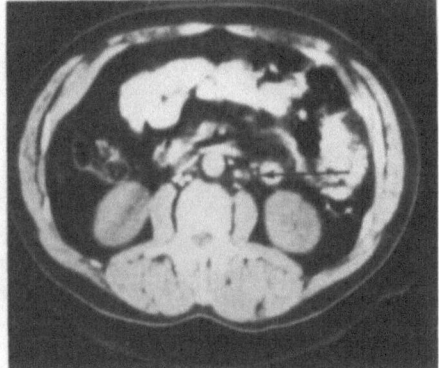

Figure 23. Patient with Hodgkin's disease prior to treatment (left) and following therapy (right). Para-aortic lymph nodes decreased in size. Possible small area of fibrous tissue (arrow) in left para-aortic area after therapy.

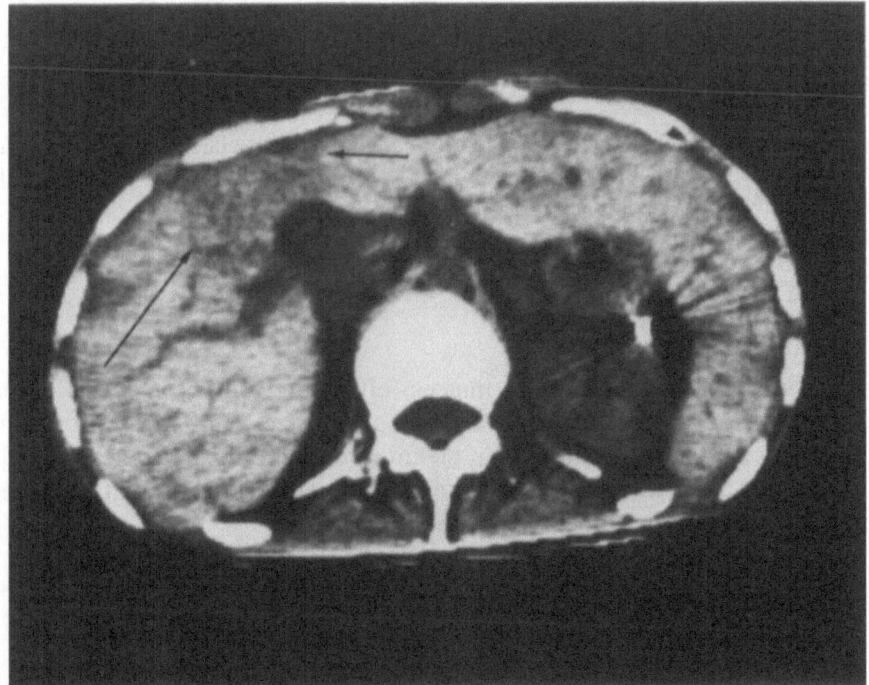

Figure 24. Diffuse Hodgkin's involvement of part of right lobe of liver (arrows). This was best seen before contrast enhancement in this patient.

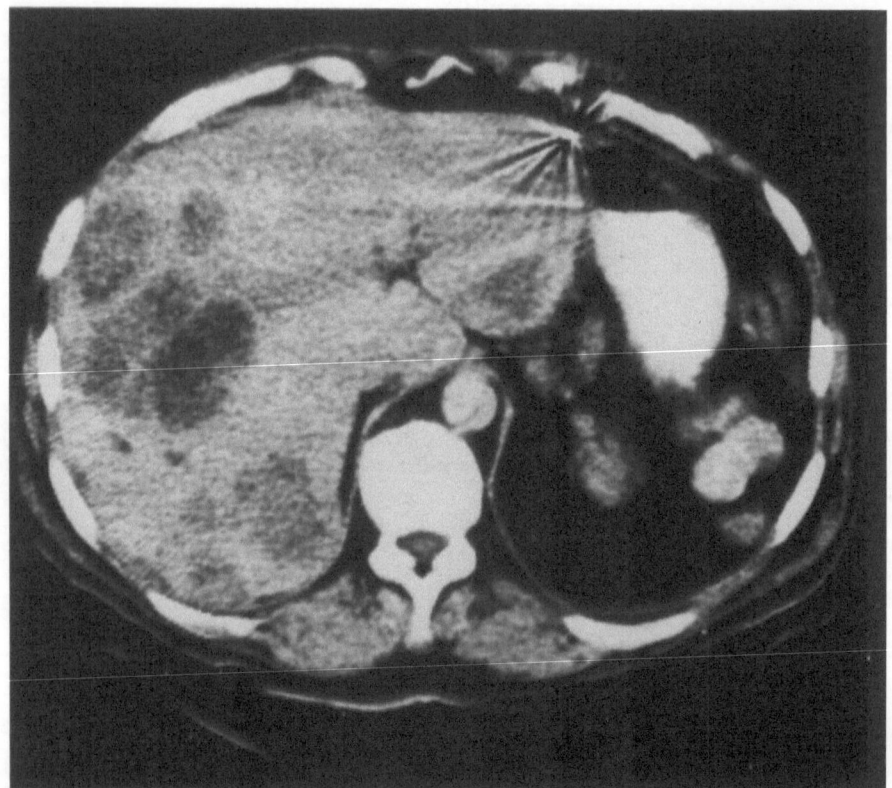

Figure 25. Focal areas of hepatic infiltration by diffuse histiocytic lymphoma were best seen in this patient following contrast enhancement which is recommended in those patients with suspicious findings pre-contrast enhancement.

of intra-abdominal lymph node masses, ultrasound has been found to be helpful in the evalution of the liver and splenic size, renal masses, ureteral and biliary obstruction and in the planning of radiotherapy ports [35, 36]. However, its resolution appears to be substantially less than that of either lymphangiography or computed tomography [30, 37].

6.   THE ROLE OF COMPUTED TOMOGRAPHY (CT) IN THE STAGING AND
      MANAGEMENT OF THE LYMPHOMAS

6.1. Introduction
   The introduction of computed tomography (CT) of the body has provided

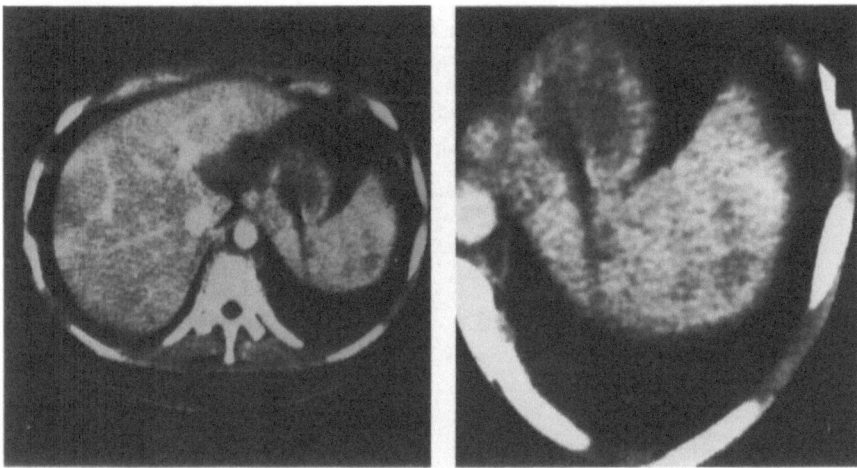

Figure 26. Diffuse hepatic and splenic involvement is best seen on this CT scan following intravenous contrast enhancement. Magnification on right better demonstrates splenic infiltration.

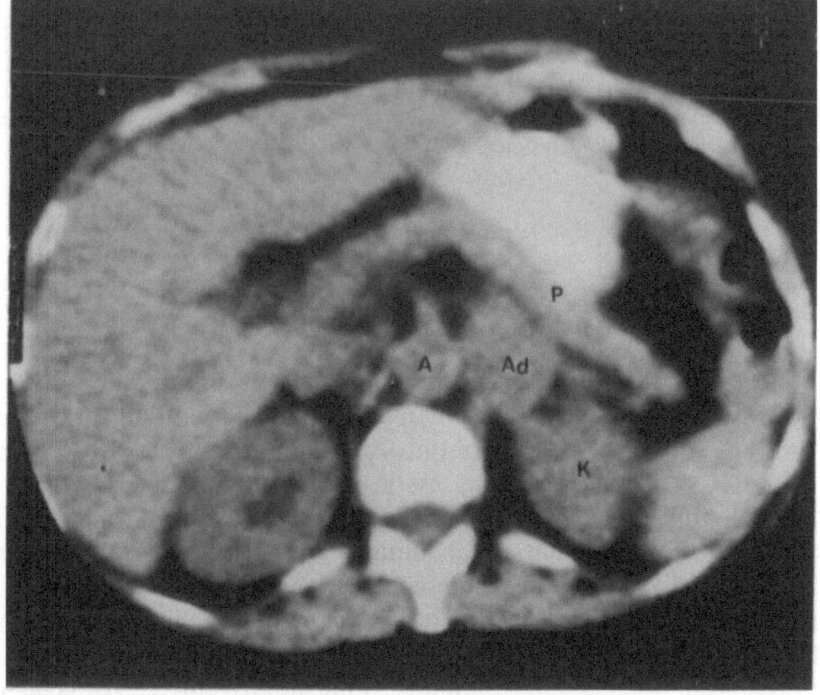

Figure 27. Hodgkin's disease metastatic to left adrenal gland (AD). Pancreas (P), left kidney (K), aorta (A) are labeled.

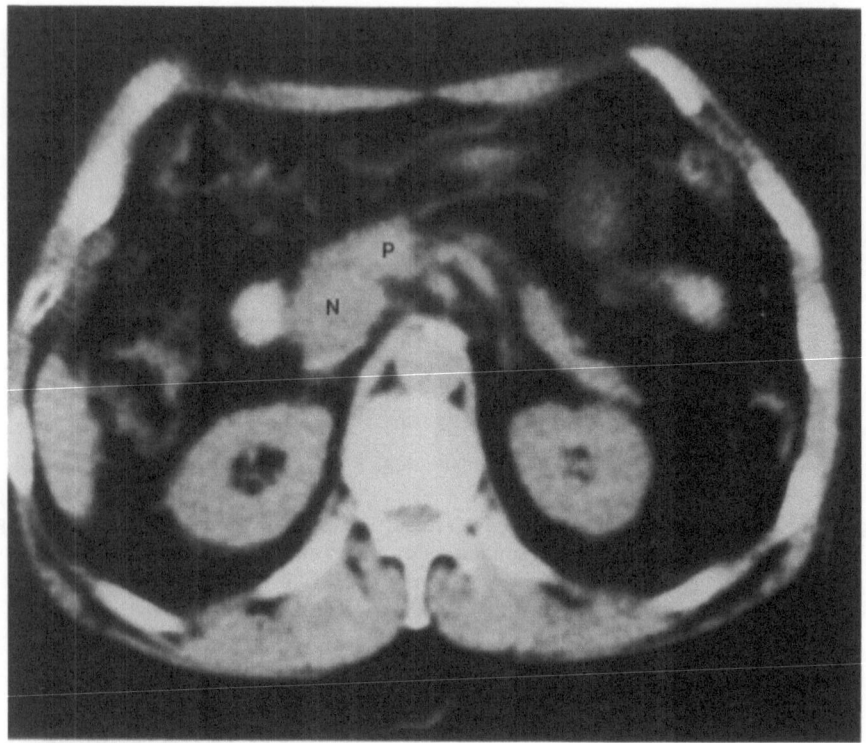

Figure 28. Diffuse histiocytic lymphoma with parapancreatic lymph node mass (N) posterior to head of pancreas (P). Differentiation from primary pancreatic carcinoma was made by percutaneous skinny needle biopsy under CT guidance.

a means for easy, non-invasive assessment of the retroperitoneal lymph nodes and for simultaneous evaluation of lymph nodes and organs elsewhere in the body. In general, enlarged retroperitoneal nodes are clearly depicted by CT due to the adjacent fat of markedly lower attenuation value. The exception to this usual state of affairs is produced by cachectic and emaciated patients where recognition of abdominal and pelvic structures is more difficult. Usually, CT readily differentiates between lymphadenopathy and other retroperitoneal masses but on occasion nodal enlargement may be simulated by retroperitoneal fibrosis, primary retroperitoneal tumors and retroperitoneal hematoma. Computed tomography, therefore, is able to provide a clear delineation of retroperitoneal lymph nodes in most patients and differentiate nodal enlargement from other retroperitoneal lesions. CT

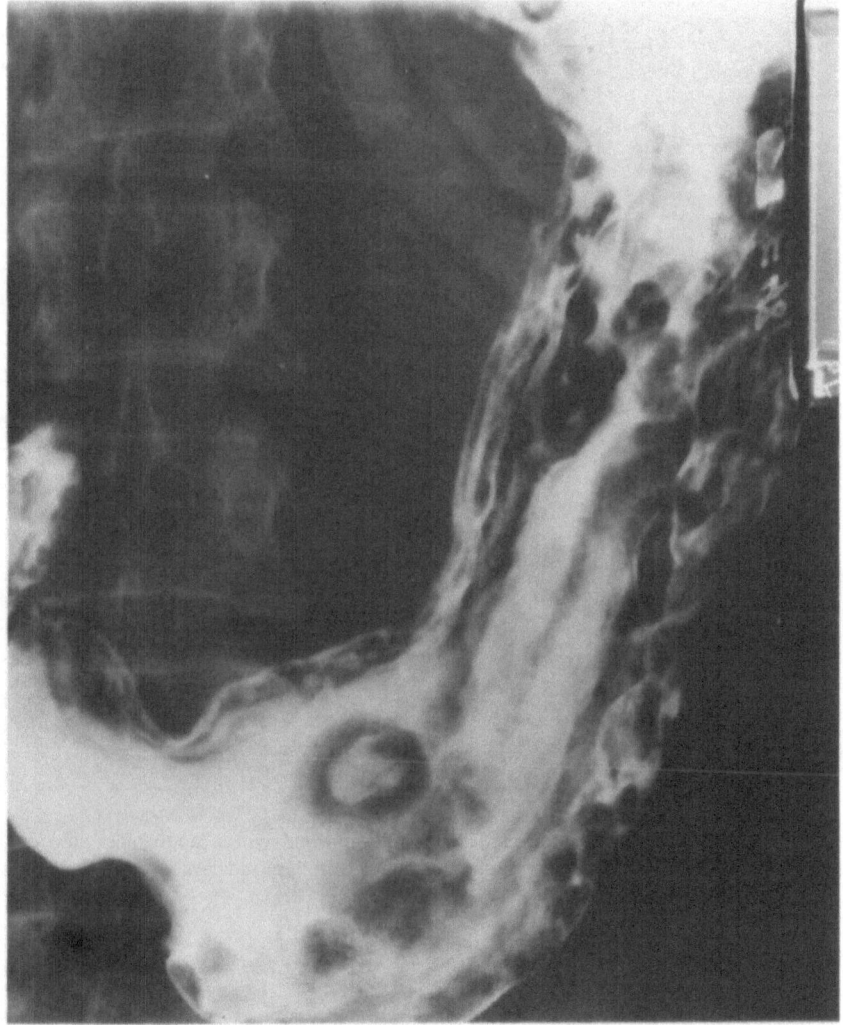

Figure 29. Diffuse histiocytic lymphoma producing characteristic coarse, thickened gastric folds. A large nodular defect with ulcer is also present.

does not, however, differentiate between benign and malignant causes for lymph node enlargement. This is due to a similarity in attenuation values of benign hyperplasic lymph nodes and lymphomatous nodes [14].

No data are currently available concerning the possible use of intravenous contrast enhancement techniques to aid the differentiation of benign from

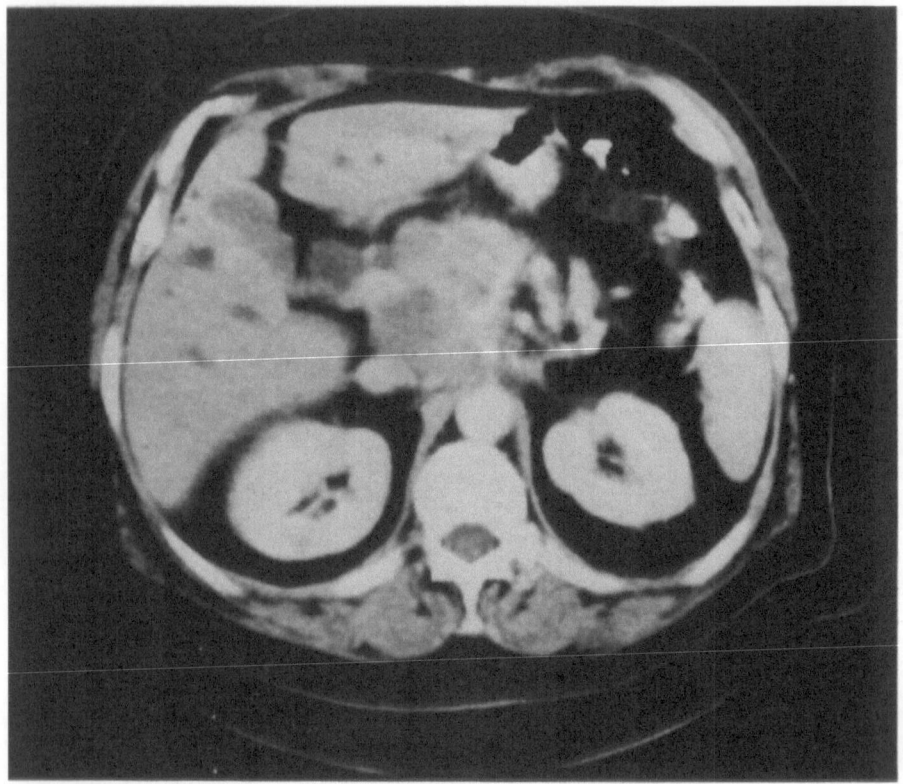

Figure 30. Patient with diffuse non-Hodgkin lymphoma and lymph node mass surrounding celiac axis in jaundiced patient with dilated intrahapatic biliary radicals.

malignant nodes. We have on occasion seen marked enhancement of abnormal nodes. The reason for this enhancement is not clear and may be related to the histological type of lymphoma present, the rate of advancement of the disease, and/or the effects of treatment.

6.2. Criteria for Abnormality on CT

Normal lymph nodes 3–10 mm in diameter are readily demonstrated by CT, particularly with the advent of the third and fourth generation fast scanners with considerably less artefact due to motion.

Abdominal lymph nodes are considered by some to be abnormal if they

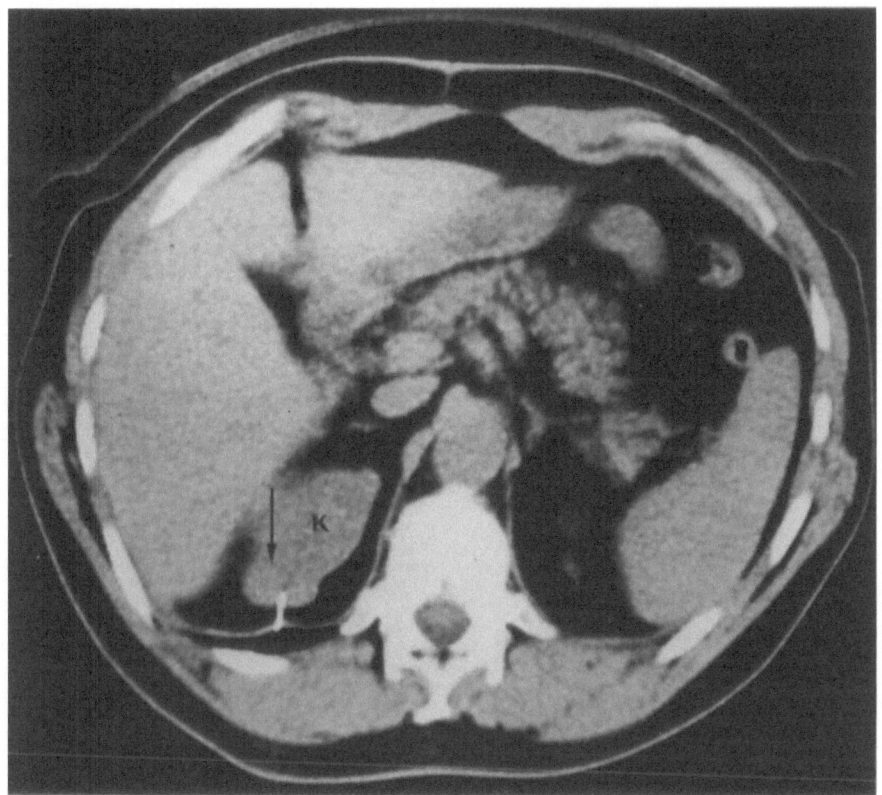

Figure 31. Right renal mass (posteriorly) was biopsied under CT guidance. Part of the needle is seen in the mass (the remainder is not seen on this CT image). Diffuse histiocytic lymphoma.

exceed 2 cm in diameter and isolated nodes 1–2 cm in size are considered suspicious. The presence of numerous lymph nodes of this size is considered pathologic [14].

Others [38] consider those nodes over 2 cm in diameter as abnormal and those over 1.5 cm in cross-sectional diameter as suspicious and in terms of lymph node disease in cervical, axillary and mediastinal areas abnormal nodes may be considered present if extra, rounded structures more than 1.5 cm in diameter are demonstrated. The same investigators, assessing the role of CT in the initial staging and subsequent management of 160 patients with HD and NHL, accepted a previously stated figure of 6 mm [39] to be the upper limit of normal node diameter in the retrocrural region.

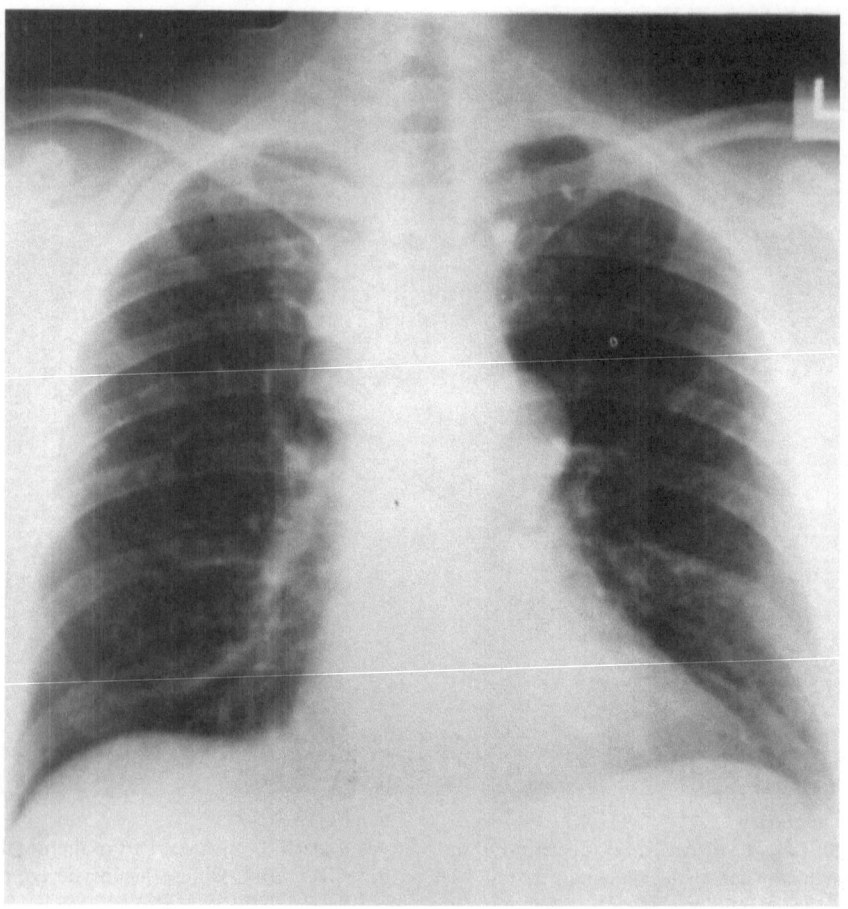

Figure 32. Patient with Hodgkin's disease and right paratracheal and left hilar adenopathy on conventional chest PA radiograph.

6.3. Advantages and Disadvantages of CT and Lymphangiography in the Staging of Lymphoma

In general, CT compares favorably with lymphangiography as a method of detecting intra-abdominal and pelvic lymph node involvement [40–43]. Ellert and Kreel [38] state that in 95 % of 63 patients with Hodgkin's disease and non-Hodgkin's lymphoma in whom LAG was omitted and CT performed as the investigation of choice, CT was judged to have been successful enough to make LAG unnecessary. In particular, CT appeared to be equally

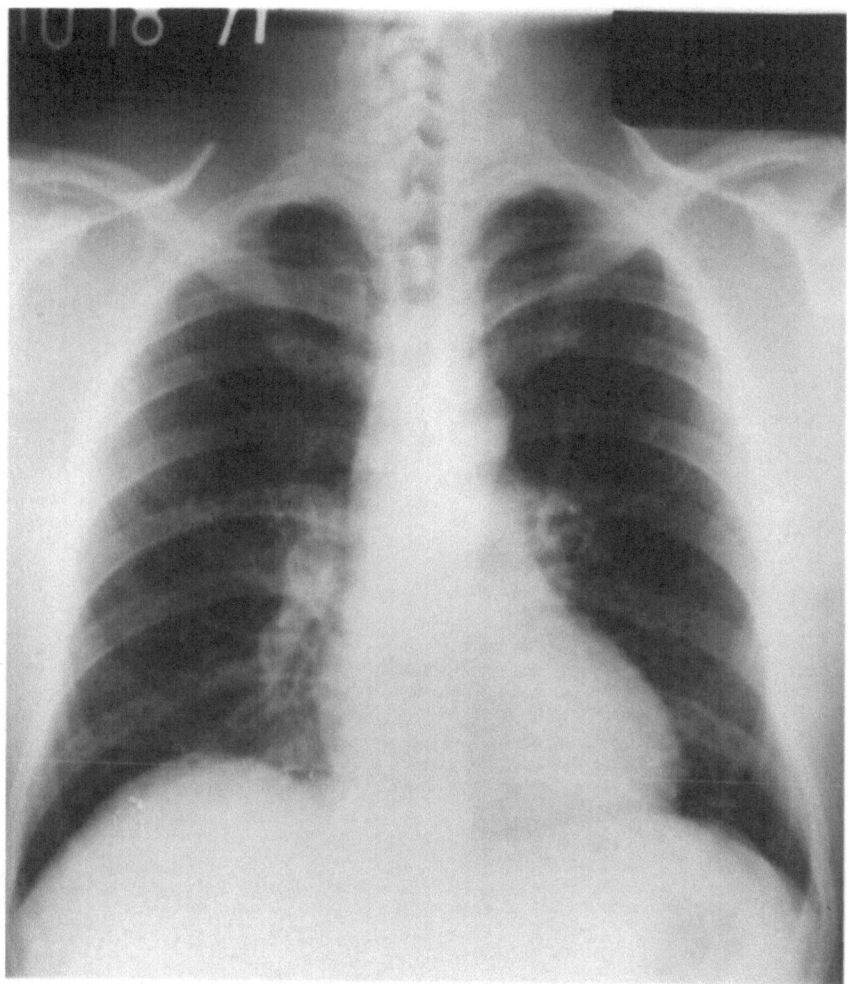

Figure 33. Another patient with Hodgkin's disease. (a) Normal chest in 1977. (b) **Right** paratracheal adenopathy seen January 1979. (c) These abnormal nodes were opacified by contrast following lymphangiogram 5 days later. (d) One year later, following therapy, nodes now normal in appearance.

sensitive to LAG in depicting minimal or early lymph node involvement. These authors recognize, however, that in the case of normal-sized, but involved nodes, CT is currently unable to demonstrate the characteristic foamy appearance due to lymphomatous infiltration, particularly in the Hodgkin's lymphomas.

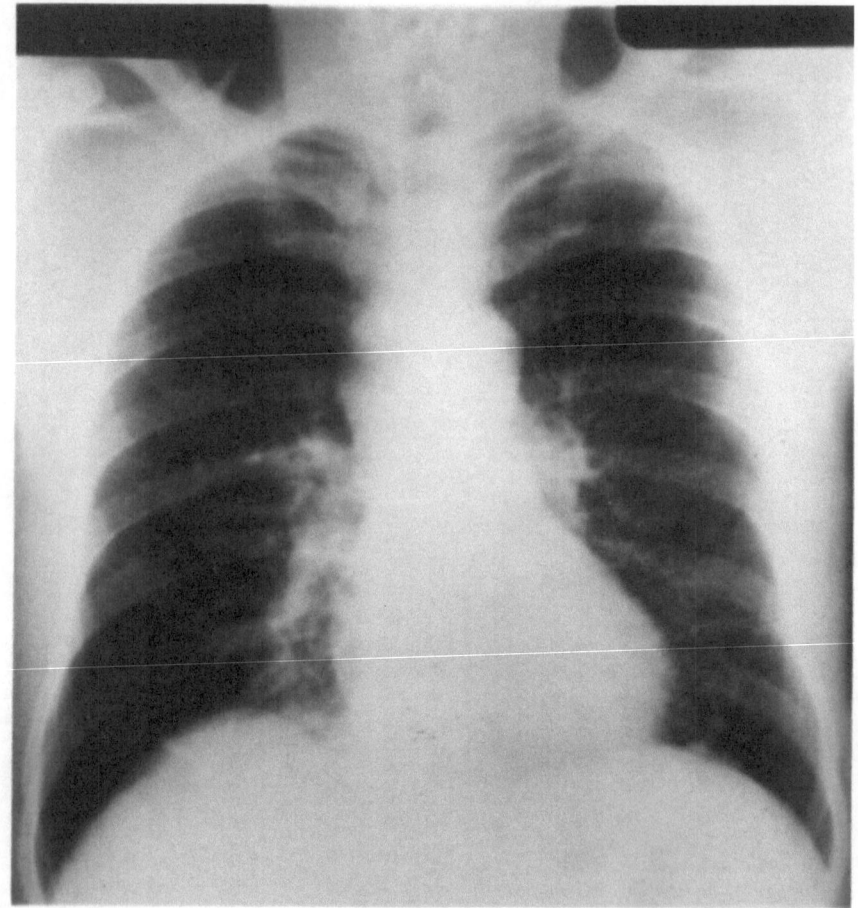

b

A major advantage of CT over LAG is its ability to more completely delineate the true extent of the disease process. CT frequently demonstrates the true extent of the disease process. CT frequently demonstrates involved nodes only partially filled with lymphographic contrast. (Figures 14 (a) and (b)). The CT examination, therefore, frequently provides more reliable information concerning the overall amount of tumor replacement in *nodes which are accessible to LAG.*

Perhaps the most valuable contribution of CT to the staging and management of lymphoma, however, is its ability to successfully demonstrate nodal areas and *sites inaccessible to LAG.* CT has been seen to be particularly useful

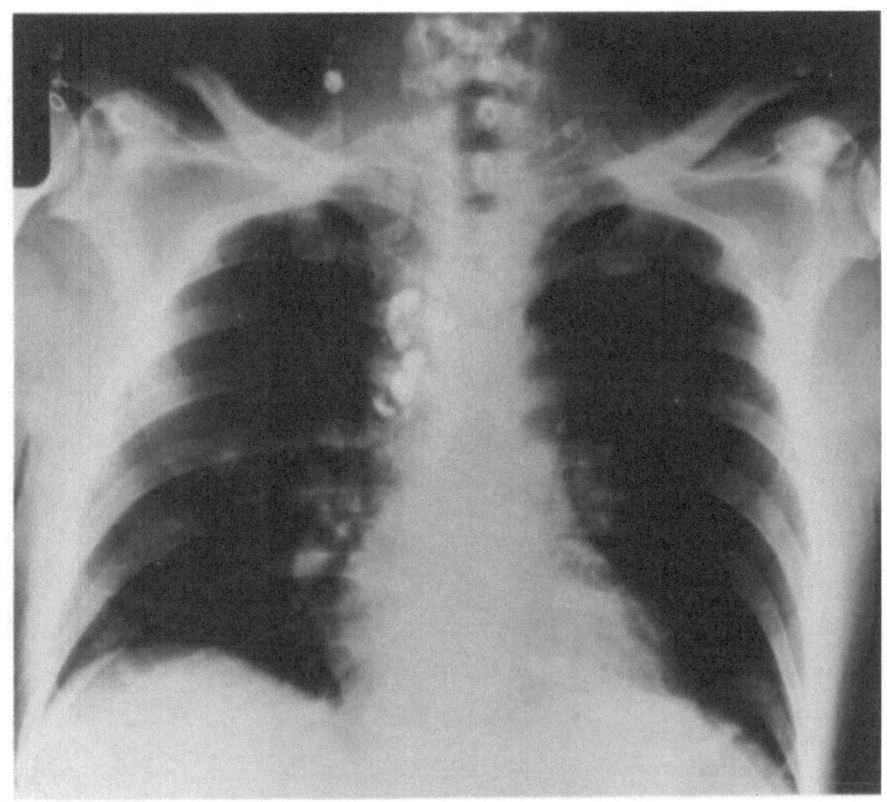

c

in the evaluation of spread of lymphoma to involve mesenteric nodal groups [38, 44–46] (Figures 15 and 16). The incidence of mesenteric node involvement has been found to be particularly high (40%) in the follicular type of non-Hodgkin's lymphomas [38]. A large series of non-Hodgkin's patients evaluated at laparotomy was found to have a similarly high incidence of mesenteric node involvement by follicular lymphoma [13]. Since up to 61% of all NHL have been shown to have positive mesenteric nodes at the time of presentation, the true extent of disease will be missed if LAG alone is used for diagnosis and staging [12]. This contrasts with Hodgkin's disease in which only 5% will have mesenteric involvement. Although CT is capable of demonstrating mesenteric nodal disease, it is essential to opacify the entire small bowel with contrast agent to successfully delineate abnormal areas [47]. Adequate bowel opacification facilitates the recognition of intra-abdominal disease when utilizing conventional axial

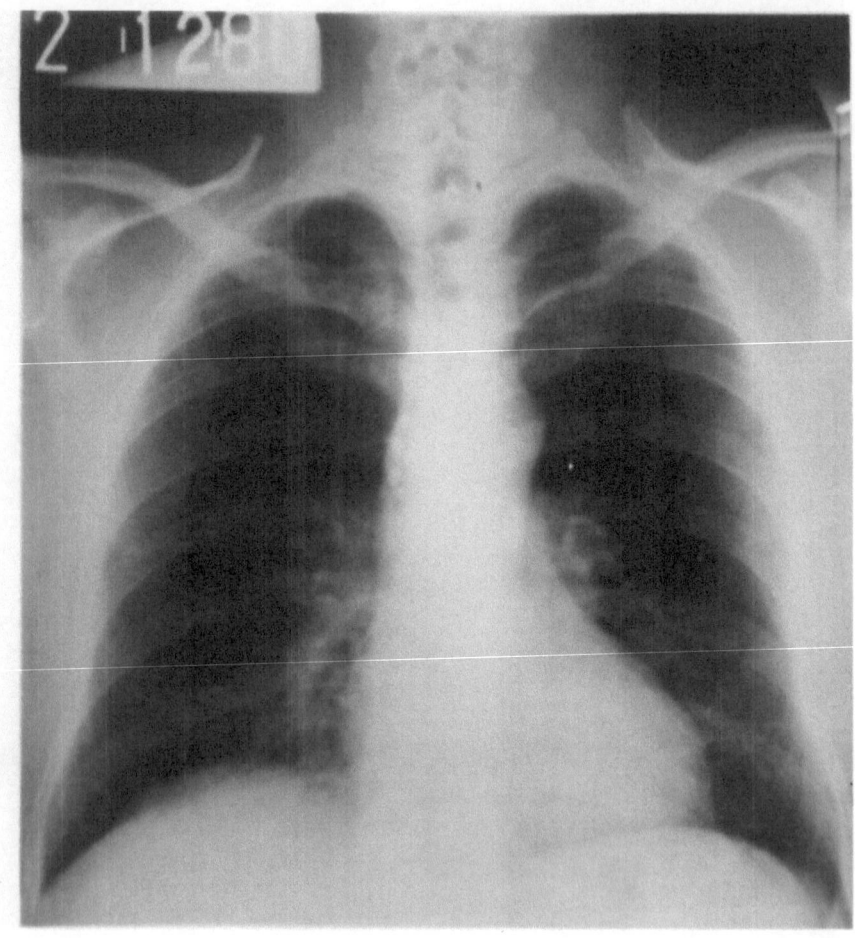

d

transverse CT images and reconstructed images which have been shown to
be useful in obtaining a better overall demonstration of cranio-caudal tumor
extent and in achieving improved three-dimensional anatomic orientation [48] (Figure 17).

Other inaccessible areas where CT is superior to LAG in the evaluation of
lymphomatous nodal involvement include nodal areas in the upper abdomen [42, 49–51]. The extra information gained by CT in the evaluation of
high para-aortic and mesenteric nodal groups, including displacement and/or
compression of major blood vessels (Figure 18) plus other inaccessible areas
such as retrocrural nodes, splenic and hepatic hilar nodes, and the internal

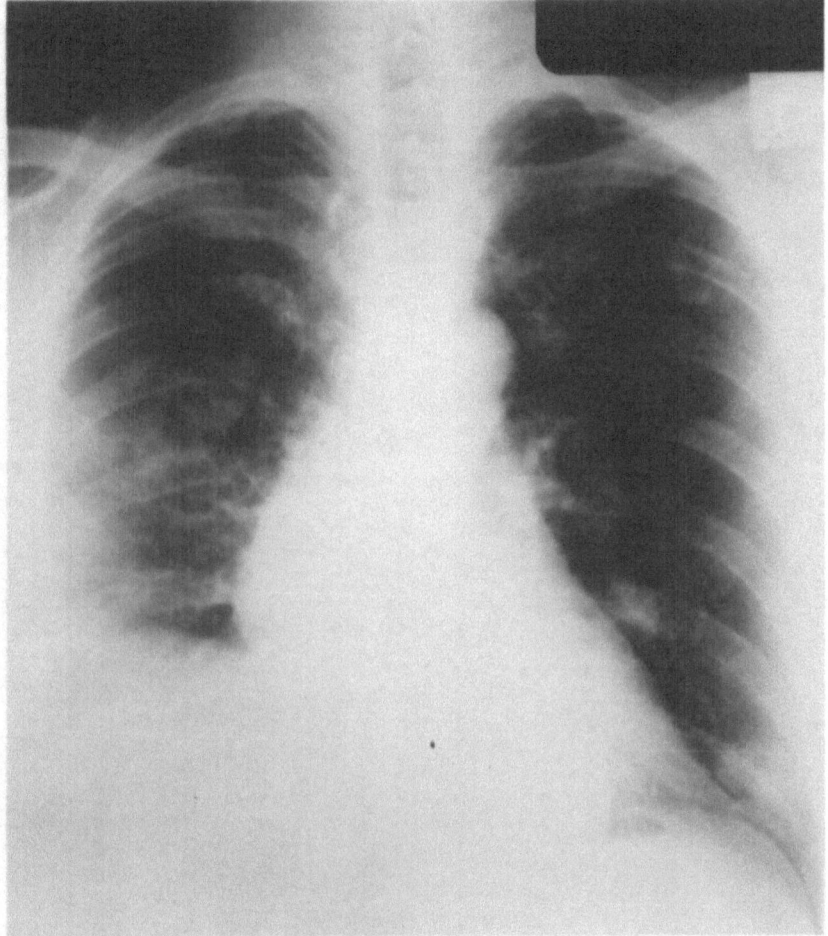

a

Figure 34. (a) and (b) Diffuse histiocytic lymphoma with parenchymal masses best seen on the lateral radiograph..

iliac groups in the pelvis has an important bearing on subsequent treatment planning (Figures 19–21). In terms of the detection of occult infradiaphragmatic disease, CT plays a vital role in that disease below the diaphragm frequently goes undetected when LAG alone is used in the evaluation of patients with lymphoma. This may explain why, in a study by Rubin [52], a significant number of patients with HD developed disease below the

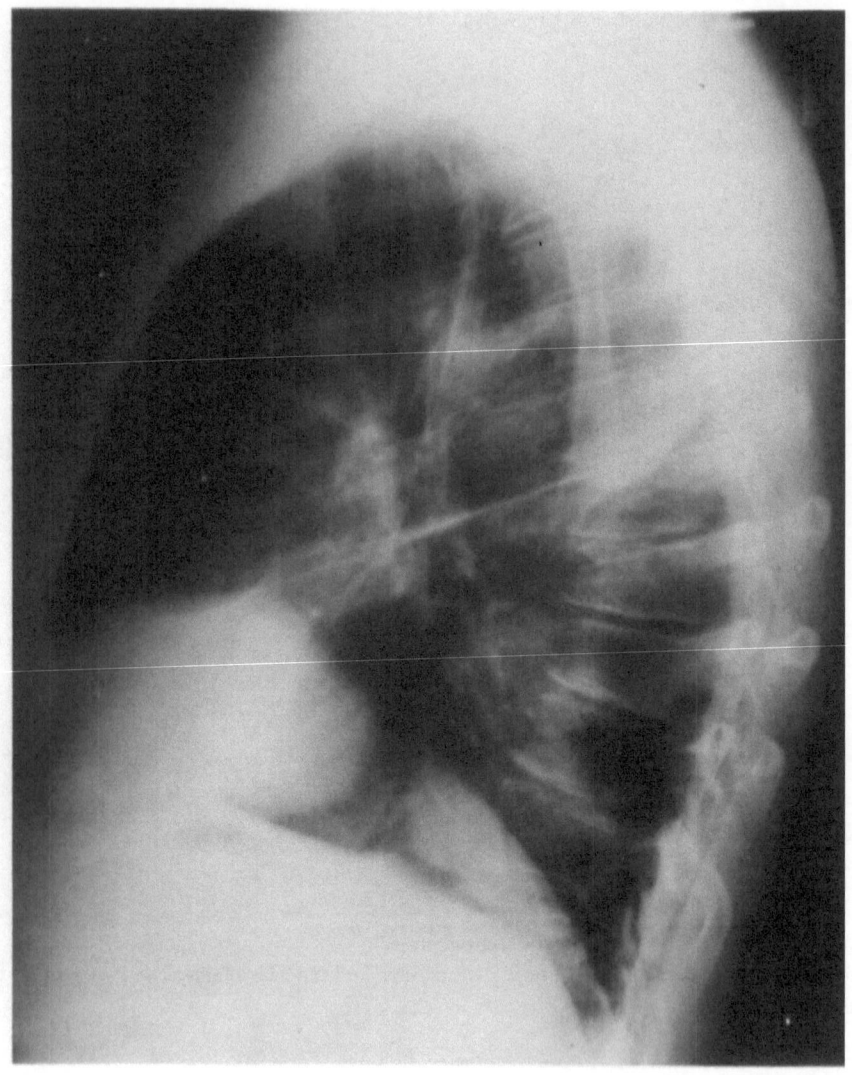

b

diaphragm following radiation therapy for supradiaphragmatic disease. Another worker [53] discovered a 25% incidence of abdominal disease within 2 years of upper hemi-body radiation therapy for disease considered to be confined to the supradiaphragmatic region. In addition, it has been shown that in the case of the follicular lymphomas a normal LAG does not

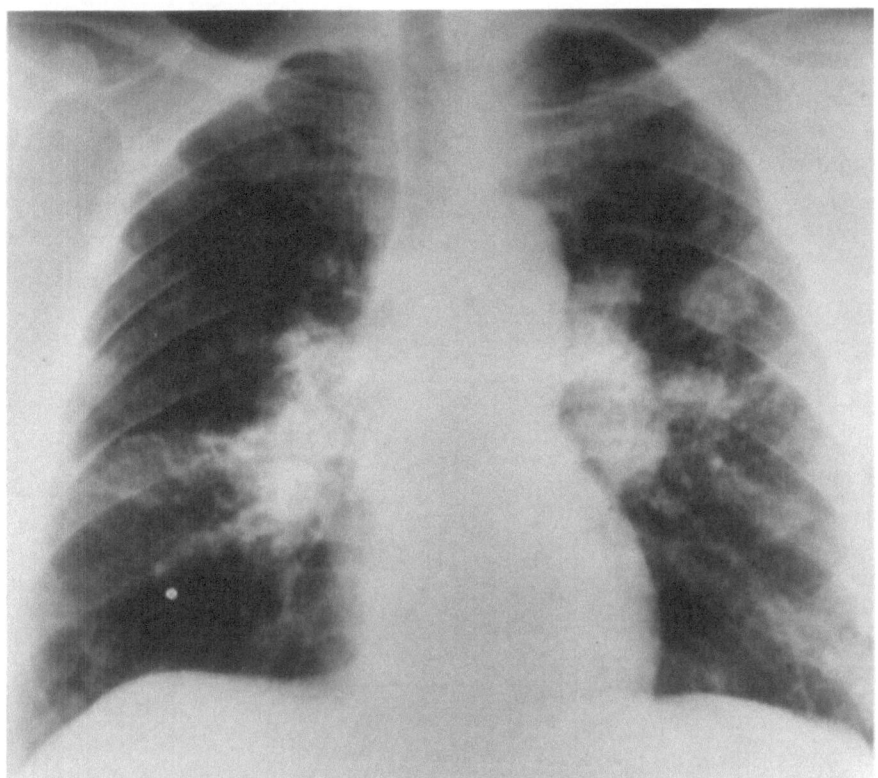

Figure 35. Parenchymal masses, reticulo-nodular pattern and bilateral hilar lymphadenopathy in patient with diffuse histiocytic lymphoma.

constitute a reliable prediction of absence of disease below the diaphragm, with mesenteric lymph node and splenic involvement observed in approximately 50% of the patients at laparotomy [12]. In these patients, CT would most likely have been able to demonstrate the presence of additional non-contrast filled nodes (particularly in the upper abdomen), depict partial filling of nodes, and delineate areas inaccessible to LAG.

Other advantages of computed tomography over LAG, apart from the above, are mainly concerned with the depiction of extranodal disease, including spread to abdominal organs, bone and soft tissue.

CT is well suited to provide a means for accurately assessing the results of therapy (Figures 22 (a), (b) and (c)) and to evaluate tumor progression. Large lymphomatous masses frequently do not disappear completely but are

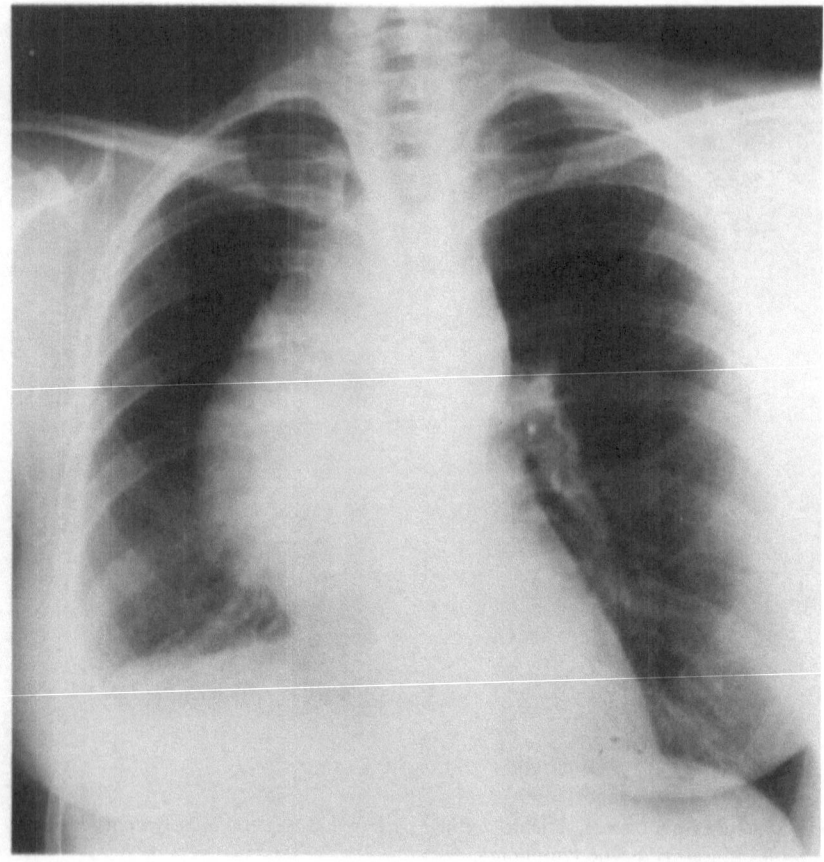

Figure 36. (a) Female patient with Hodgkin's disease and large right mediastinal mass. Right pleural effusion seen also on this PA chest radiograph. (b) CT scan shows true extent of this mass which involves the soft tissues of the anterior chest wall (arrow). Bilateral pleural effusions are present.

reduced to small, persistent foci of fibrous tissue (Figure 23). Recurrent lymphomatous disease, often clinically unsuspected, may be identified by CT scanning. The economic implications of repeat CT scanning and the necessary intervals between scan examinations still have to be assessed and compared with the use of less costly plain film radiographs after LAG in the detection of recurrent retroperitoneal disease. The variable rate of disappearance of contrast from lymph nodes following LAG often results in a negative plain radiograph in patients shown on CT to have residual disease.

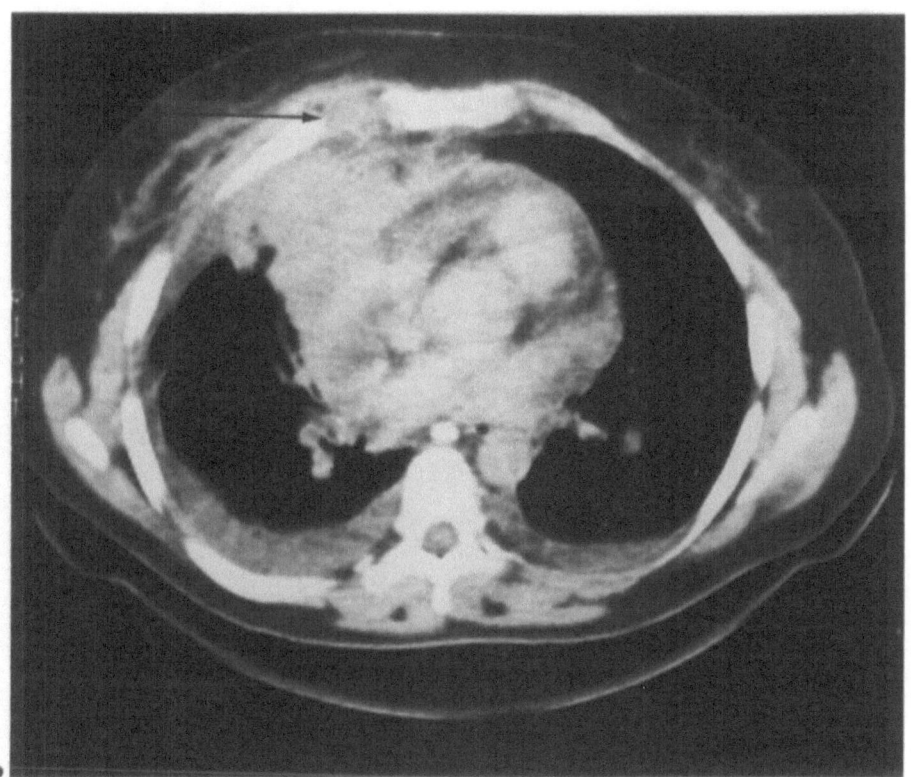

b

6.4. Disadvantages of CT

Computed tomography is more expensive than other imaging modalities such as ultrasound. The false negative CT examination is usually due to non-recognition of lymphomatous involvement of normal-sized nodes. Fortunately, in most instances, particularly with the NHLs, lymphomatous nodes are enlarged, but in 5–10% of patients with Hodgkin's disease para-aortic and para-caval nodes will be involved with tumor but not enlarged, i.e. these nodes will be 'normal' on CT. Thus, sound clinical judgement must enter into the interpretation of a 'normal' CT scan and, where needed, the nodal architecture should be evaluated by an LAG procedure.

In emaciated patients and in young patients with a paucity of intra-abdominal fat, the evaluation of retroperitoneal nodal groups by CT is frequently difficult. Mesenteric nodes in particular are poorly delineated and in these patients, ultrasonography is often advantageous in assessing the extent of the disease.

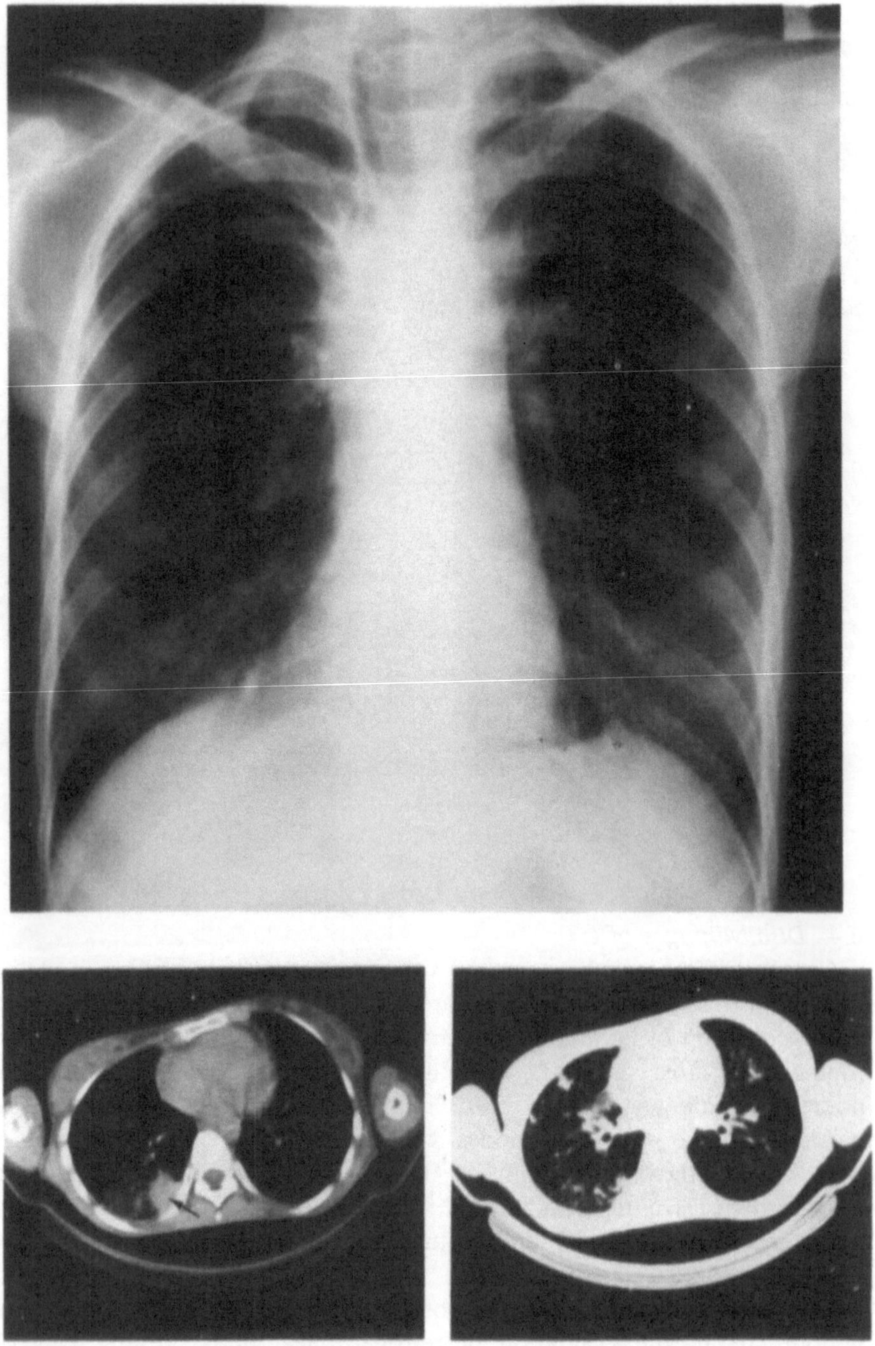

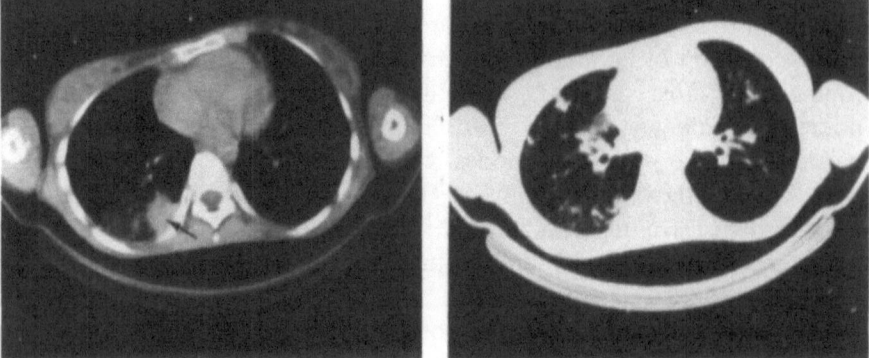

Figure 37. (a) Twenty-eight-year-old female with Hodgkin's disease: mediastinal fibrotic changes. (b) CT scan better demonstrates small peripheral parenchymal lesions plus pleural-based lesion (arrow) posteriorly in right lower lobe.

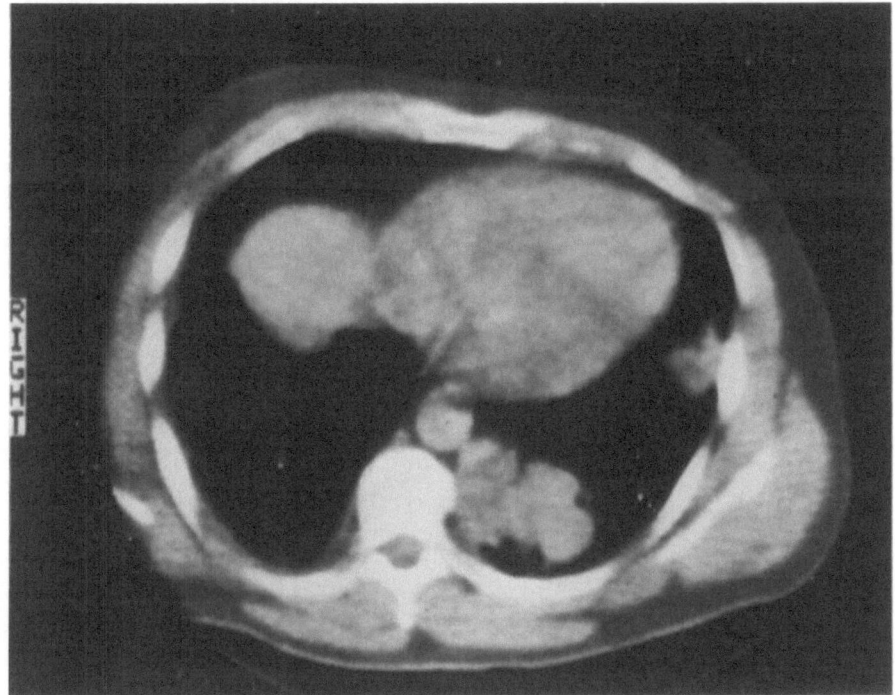

Figure 38. Parenchymal masses plus pleural based disease in Hodgkin's disease again well shown by CT.

6.5. The Assessment of Extranodal Lymphoma by CT

6.5.1. Liver and Spleen. In an analysis of 814 consecutive, unselected, previously untreated patients with HD, involvement of the surgically resected spleen was demonstrated in 38% of cases and was most prevalent in those patients with lymphocyte depletion [54]. Liver and bone marrow involvement documented by biopsy at the time of staging laparotomy were detected in 43 and 23 instances, respectively, and were invariably associated with involvement of the spleen. The study also showed that the para-aortic and splenic hilar nodes were each involved in approximately 50% of the patients with involved spleens. In a further review by Kaplan of 335 patient with untreated HD [55], the probability of association and eventual hepatic involvement in the presence of splenic disease is at least 63%. Therefore, in those patients with HD and obvious splenic involvement, the liver should be

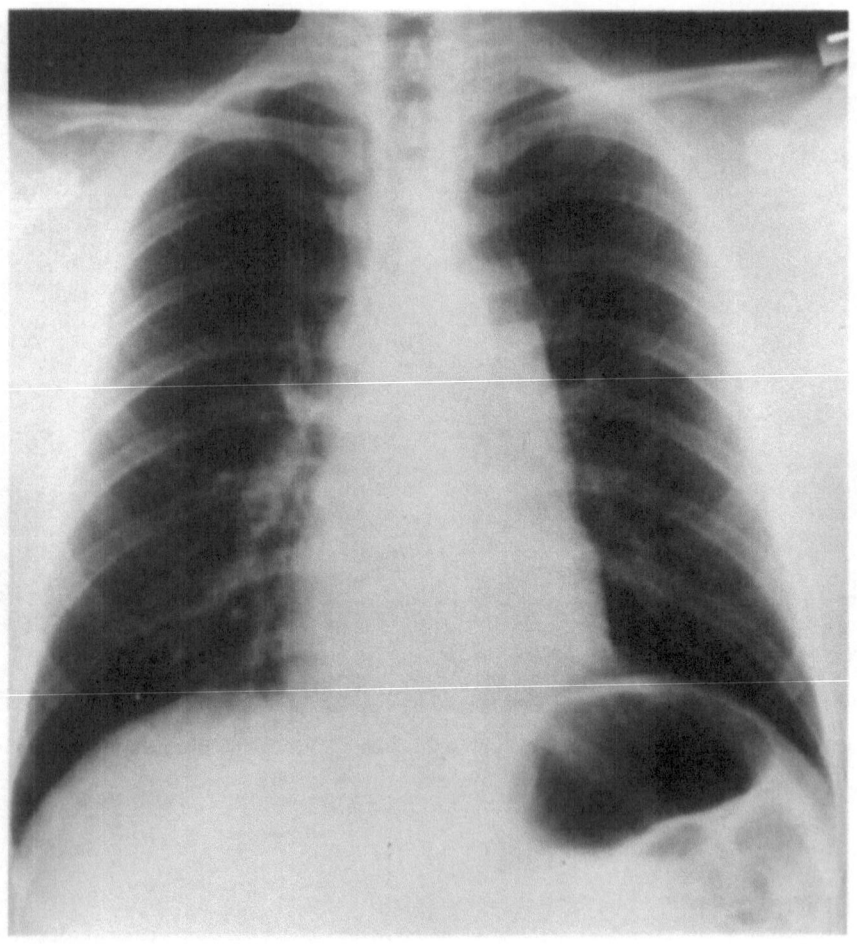

Figure 39. (a) Anterior mediastinal mass silhouetting aorta. (b) CT scan shows solid mass with necrotic center in anterior mediastinum adjacent of the aortic arch. Hodgkin's disease of thymus gland was found at surgery.

carefully studied for lymphomatous infiltration. Liver function tests have been found to have little predictive value for the presence of hepatic involvement by HD, nor have radionuclide scans been valuable in the detection of small foci of involvement in the liver [11].

In terms of the CT evaluation of liver involvement, Ellert and Kreel [38] stress the use of contrast enhancement in addition to precontrast CT scans

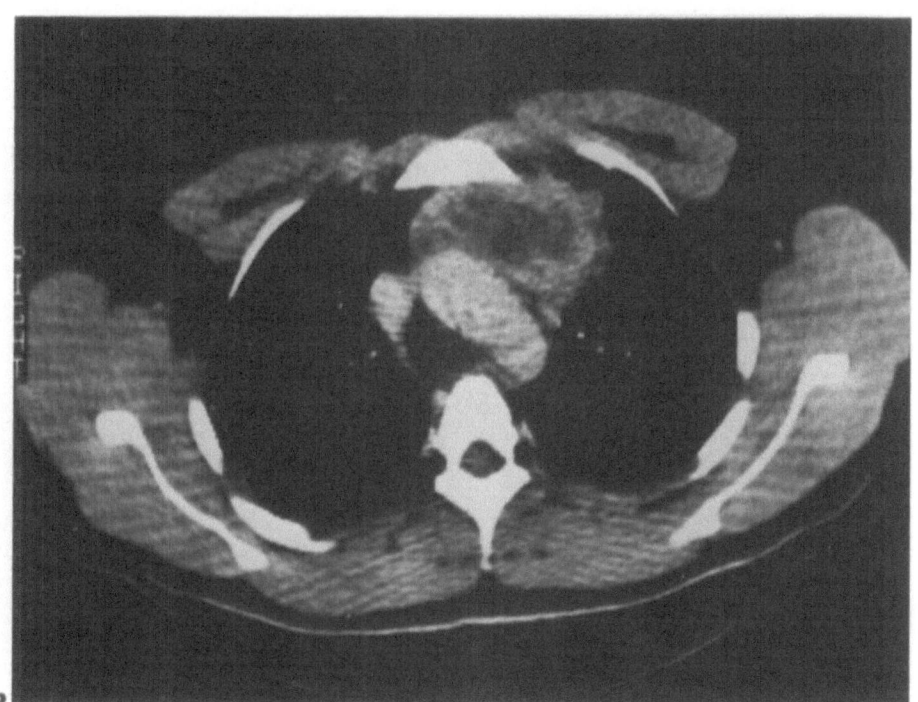

b

which frequently show focal lesions measuring 34–50 Hounsfield Units (HU) within the normal liver parenchyma (60–70 HU) (Figure 24). Improved demonstration of the vascular anatomy of the liver, together with opacification of the parenchyma and enhanced visualization of the bile ducts has been found to occur with an experimental contrast agent [56]. Currently, however, the emphasis is on quantitative measurements of attenuation values using conventional iodinated contrast agents administered intravenously (Figures 25 and 26) in spite of a report stating that attenuation values are unreliable indications of lymphomatous involvement of liver and spleen by lymphoma [57].

In addition to infiltration of the liver and spleen, other intra-abdominal organs may be involved. Involvement of these organs, including adrenal glands (Figure 27) kidney and the parapancreatic area (Figure 28) is frequently demonstrated at the time of the CT examination. Also, matted loops of bowel and lymphomatous masses related to the bowel may be delineated. However, in the evaluation of intrinsic bowel involvement, barium studies

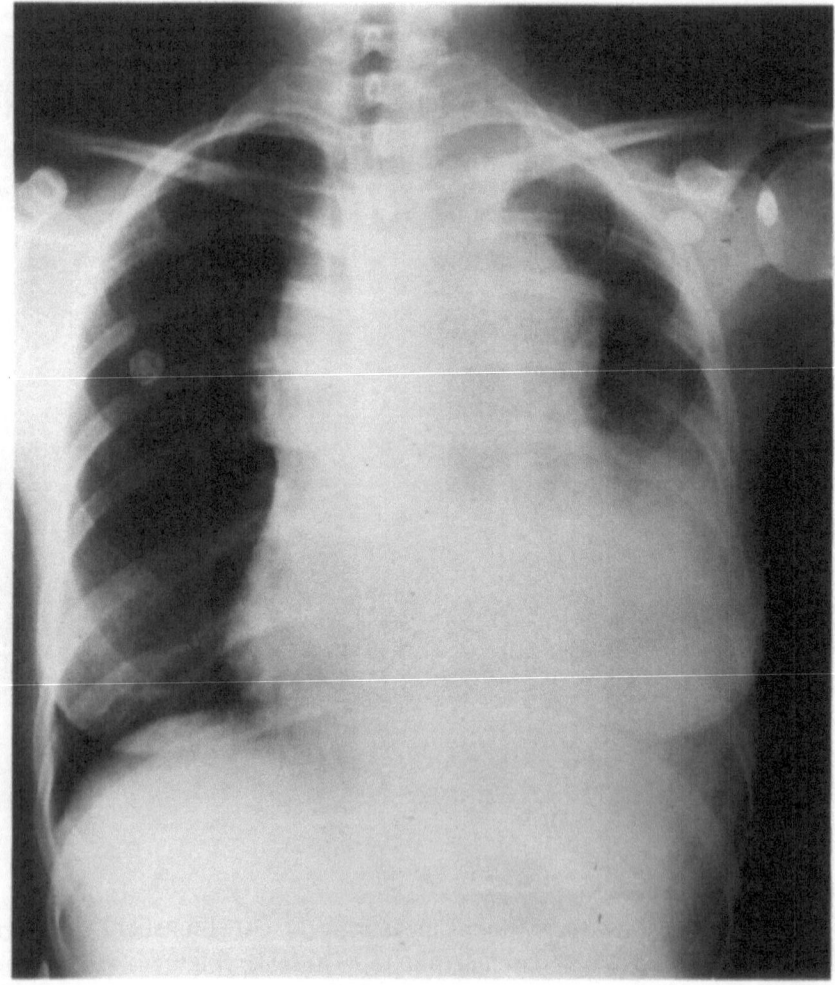

a

Figure 40. (a) Young female patient with Hodgkin's disease admitted with shortness of breath. PA chest radiograph shows mediastinal mass plus left pleural effusion. (b) CT scan showed huge anterior mediastinal mass compressing superior vena cava (at a higher level), plus large pericardial effusion (arrows) and left pleural effusion (PE).

remain important radiological procedures (Figure 29). Localized abdominal histiocytic lymphoma may be encountered (Figure 30) and the true extent of disease is frequently shown to best advantage utilizing ultrasound, CT or a combination of these imaging modalities depending on the size and site of

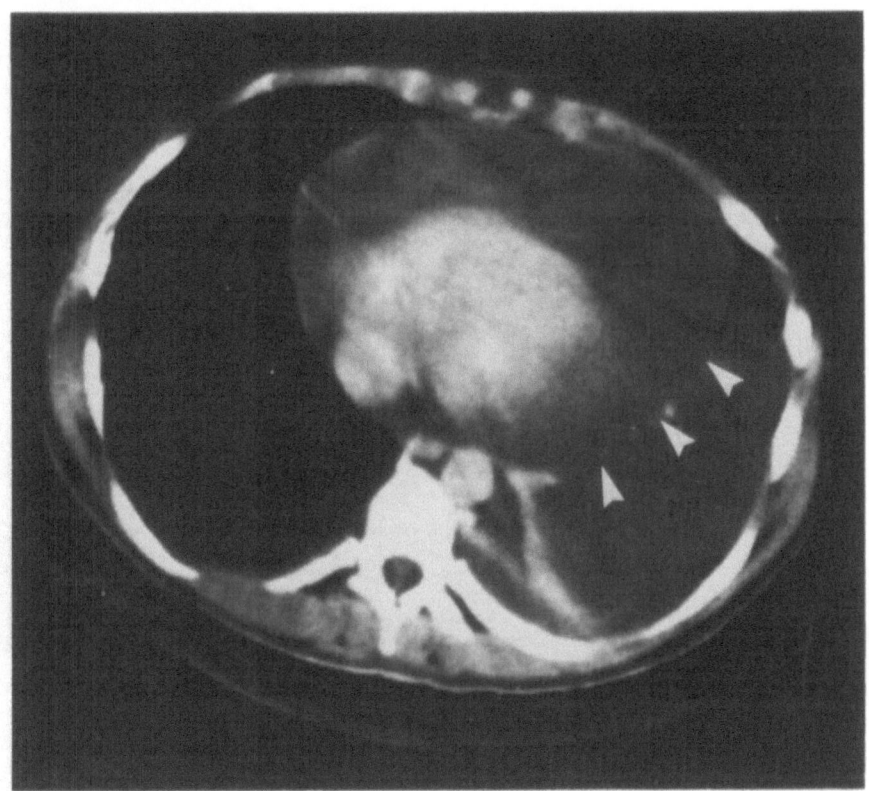

b

the lesion, the presence or absence of gas, and the size of the patient (intra-abdominal fat facilitates improved CT identification of structures but decreases the ease of demonstration of the abnormality by ultrasound). On occasion, extranodal involvement of intra-abdominal organs is an incidental finding at the time of the CT examination and in view of the potential need to modify therapy because of this additional area of involvement, percutaneous needle biopsy has been utilized to verify the CT findings. Where the lesion is inadequately demonstrated by other imaging modalities, biopsy under CT guidance may be utilized (Figure 31).

6.5.2. Radiographic Evaluation of Intrathoracic Lymphomas. Routine high kVp PA and lateral chest radiographs define most of the intrathoracic sites of the lymphomas [58] (Figures 32–35) and are of major use in assessing response to therapy and progression of disease. Shallow oblique views aid in

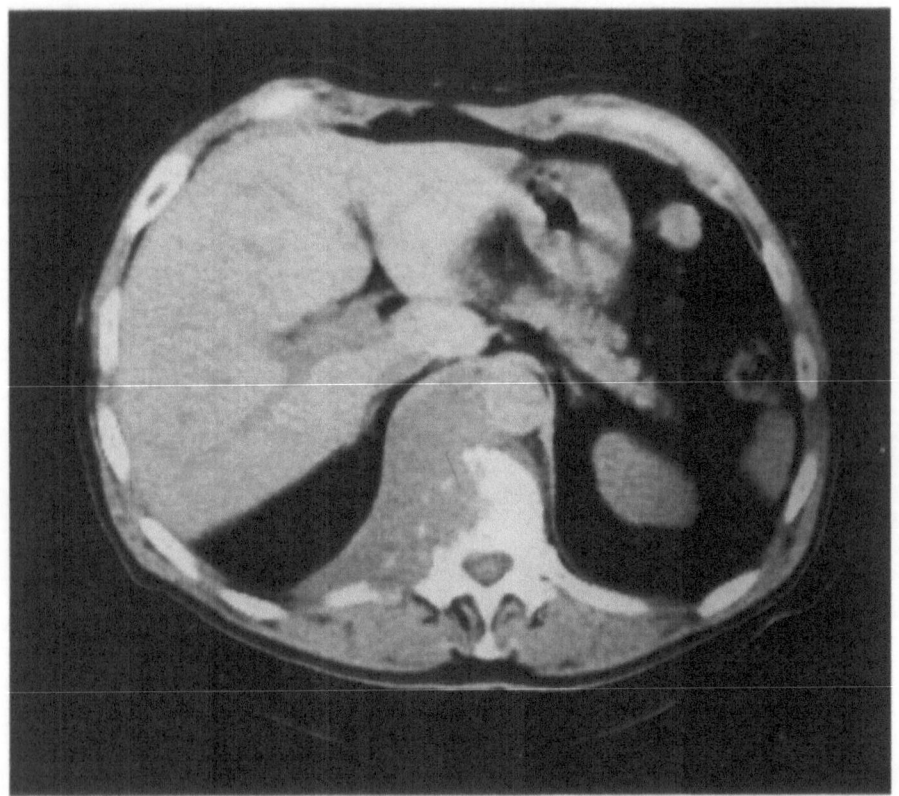

Figure 41. Patient with diffuse histiocytic lymphoma: T12 vertabral body partially destroyed plus large retrocrural soft tissue mass.

the demonstration of mediastinal adenopathy and are of use in the evaluation of the lung hilum. Radiographic assessment of hilar involvement is particularly important in HD. Low dose radiation therapy is advocated to the lung fields [59] if the hilar nodes are radiologically involved. This important area is also well shown by oblique hilar tomography [60]. Routine full-lung, AP tomography in all lymphoma patients was shown to have a yield of only 1–2% in changing a patient's stage and 3.3% in providing new information which affected the treatment plan. Lateral tomography of the hilum and lung was found useful when this area was obscured by mediastinal disease or equivocal on routine films [61].

Radionuclide procedures are only occasionally helpful in defining additional sites of disease or in detecting persistent lymphoma following treatment [58].

CT evaluation of the chest has proved to be extremely sensitive in detecting early or minimal disease, both nodal and extranodal. These changes include mediastinal involvement (Figure 36) and small peripheral, pleural and subpleural nodules and plaques [38, 62], subclinical pleural effusions, and early lymph node enlargement [38, 63]. In particular, small peripheral lesions are frequently difficult to detect by conventional radiography but are easily demonstrated by CT [64, 65] (Figures 37 and 38). Ellert and Kreel found in their series [38] that in those cases of Hodgkin's nodular sclerotic lymphoma with pulmonary nodules, there was an increased association between hilar and paratracheal adenopathy and obvious involvement of the thymus. The CT demonstration of localized pulmonary infiltrates adjacent to involved mediastinal nodes is important in that these infiltrates may be treated by radical mantle irradiation yielding a prognosis comparable to nodal involvement alone [66]. Utilizing CT, radiation fields can be accurately planned to include all involved areas. The full potential of CT in detecting localized pulmonary infiltrates becomes all the more obvious when involved tissue is not evident on the plain film radiographs, particularly in the paravertebral and paramediastinal areas [38].

Involvement of the *thymus gland* by lymphoma may also be well demonstrated on conventional radiographs (Figure 39 (a)) but for smaller lesions and for accurate pre-surgical evaluation, including overall tumor extent and degree of involvement of adjacent major mediastinal vessels, CT is of great use (Figure 39 (b)).

In addition, pericardial involvement with pericardial effusion may be demonstrated by CT (Figure 40) as well as by ultrasonography. In general, ultrasonography is the imaging modality of choice in these cases.

6.5.3. Radiology of Lymphomas Presenting with Osseous Lesions. At initial presentation, radiologically demonstrable bone involvement has been estimated as being present in approximately 2% of patients with HD, with an additional 2% developing overt lesions during the course of the disease [67]. In NHL, slightly more patients develop osseous involvement during the course of their disease, with adults (15.6%) [68] having a slightly lower incidence than children (24.3%) [69]. In patients with bone pain, radionuclide bone scans employing ^{99m}Tc-diphosphonate have been reported to detect bone involvement by HD with greater sensitivity than conventional radiographic skeletal surveys [23].

In terms of the role of CT in detecting osseous involvement by HD and NHL, no large series is forthcoming but it would appear that significantly more bone involvement in the non-Hodgkin's lymphomas is present (and can be depicted by CT scan) at initial presentation (up to 14%) [38] than the previously documented figure of 3.8% [38] of patients presenting with an osseous lesion would suggest (Figure 41).

230   D.J. HAMLIN

REFERENCES

1. Kinmonth JD: Lymphangiography in man. Method of outlining lymphatic trunks and operation. Clin Sci 11:13–20, 1952.
2. Bruun S, Engeset A: Lymphadenography. A new method for the visualization of enlarged lymph nodes and lymphatic vessels (preliminary report). Acta Radiol 45:389–395, 1956.
3. Baum S, Bron KM, Wexler L, Abrams HL: Lymphangiography, cavography, and urography. Comparative accuracy in the diagnosis of pelvic and abdominal metastases. Radiology 81:207–218, 1963.
4. Lee BJ, Nelson JH, Schwarz G: Evaluation of lymphangiography, inferior vena cavography, and intravenous pylegraphy in the clinical staging and management of Hodgkin's disease and lymphosarcoma. N Engl J Med 271:327–337, 1964.
5. Castellino RA, Billingham M, Dorfman RF: Lymphographic accuracy in Hodgkin's disease and malignant lymphoma with a note on the 'reactive' lymph node as a cause of most false-positive lymphograms. Invest Radiol 9:155–165, 1974.
6. Ferguson DJ, Allen LW, Griem ML, Moran ME, Rappaport H, Ultmann JE: Surgical experience with staging laparotomy in 125 patients with lymphoma. Arch Intern Med 131:356–361, 1973.
7. Desser RKEM, Ultmann JE: Staging of Hodgkin's disease and lymphoma. Med Clin N Am 57:479–498, 1973.
8. Mitchell RI, Peters MV: Lymph node biopsy during laparotomy for the staging of Hodgkin's disease. Ann Surg 178:698–702, 1973.
9. Ultmann JE: Current status: the management of lymphoma. Semin Hematol 7:441–453, 1970.
10. Kaplan HS: Hodgkin's lymphomas – role of intensive radiotherapy in the management of Hodgkin's disease. Cancer 19:356–367, 1966.
11. Kaplan HS: Hodgkin's disease: unfolding concepts concerning its nature, management and prognosis. Cancer 45:2439–2474, 1980.
12. Goffinet DR, Castellino RA, Kim H, et al.: Staging laparotomies in unselected previously untreated patients with non-Hodgkin's lymphomas. Cancer 32:672–681, 1973.
13. Goffinet DR, Warnke R, Dunnick NR et al.: Clinical and surgical (laparotomy) evaluation of patients with non-Hodgkin's lymphomas. Cancer Treat Rep 61:981–992, 1977.
14. Sagel SS: CT of the retroperitoneum: nodes, masses, and vessels. Computed tomography 1979: interpretation of facts and artefacts, Second Annual Postgraduate Course, Harvard Medical School, Cambridge, Massachusetts, Sept. 17–20, 1979.
15. Heifetz LJ, Fuller LM, Rodgers R, et al.: Laparotomy findings in lymphangiogram-staged I and II non-Hodgkin's lymphomas. Cancer 45:2778–2786, 1980.
16. Sutcliffe SJB, Wrigley PFM, Smyth JF, et al.: Intensive investigation in management of Hodgkin's disease. Br Med J ii:1343–1347, 1976.
17. Sandusky WR, Jones RCW, Shelton Horsley J, et al.: Staging laparotomy in Hodgkin's disease. Ann Surg 187:485–489, 1978.
18. Edwards CL, Hayes RL: Tumor scanning with ^{67}Ga citrate. J Nucl Med 10:103–105, 1969.
19. Hoffer PB, Turner D, Gottschalk A, Harper PV, Ultmann JE: Whole-body radiogallium scanning for staging of Hodgkin's disease and other lymphomas. Natl Cancer Inst Monogr 36:277–285, 1973.
20. Horn NL, Ray GR, Kriss JP: Gallium-67 citrate scanning in Hodgkin's disease and non-Hodgkin's lymphoma. Cancer 37:250–257, 1976.
21. Johnston G Go M, Benua R, Larson S, Andrews G, Hubner K: Gallium-67 citrate imaging in Hodgkin's disease. Final report of cooperative group. J Nucl Med 692–698, 1977.
22. Andrews G, Hubner K, Greerlaw R: Ga-67 citrate imaging in malignant lymphoma: final

report of cooperative group. J Nucl Med 19:1013–1019, 1978.

23. Schecter JP, Jones SE, Woolfenden JM, Lilien DL, O'Mara RE: Bone scanning in lymphoma. Cancer 38:1142–1148, 1976.

24. Lipton MJ, DeNardo GL, Silverman S, Glatstein E: Evaluation of the liver and spleen in Hodgkin's disease. I The value of hepatic scintigraphy. Am J Med 52:356–361, 1972.

25. Silverman S, DeNardo GL, Glatstein E, Lipton MJ: Evaluation of the liver and spleen in Hodgkin's disease. II. The value of splenic scintigraphy. Am J Med 52:362–366, 1972.

26. Ell PJ, Britton KE, Parker-Brown G, Keeling DH, Jelliffe AM, Wood TP: An assessment of the value of spleen scanning in the staging of Hodgkin's disease. Br J Radiol 48:590–593, 1975.

27. Sweet DL, Kinncaley A, Ultmann JE: Hodgkin's disease: problems of staging. Cancer 42:957–970, 1978.

28. Bagley CM, Roth JA, Thomas LB, DeVita VT: Liver biopsy in Hodgkin's disease. Ann Intern Med 76:219–225, 1972.

29. Thomas LB: Summary of informal discussions on the histologic criteria for diagnosis of the extent of Hodgkin's disease. Cancer Res 31:1799–1800, 1971.

30. Filly RA, Marglin S, Castellino RA: The ultrasonographic spectrum of abdominal and pelvic Hodgkin's disease and non-Hodgkin's lymphoma. Cancer 38:2143–2148, 1976.

31. Brascho DJ, Durant JR, Green LE: The accuracy of retroperitoneal ultrasonography in Hodgkin's disease and non-Hodgkin's lymphoma. Radiology (in press).

32. Asher WM, Freimanis AK: Echographic diagnosis of retroperitoneal lymph node enlargement. Am J Roentgenol 105:438–445, 1969.

33. Brascho DJ, Green LE, Durant JR: The accuracy of diagnostic ultrasound in detecting retroperitoneal lymph node enlargement in malignant lymphoma and Hodgkin's disease. J Clin Ultrasound 2:224A, 1974.

34. Taylor KJW, Milan J: Differential diagnosis of chronic splenomegaly by grey-scale ultrasonography: clinical observations and digital A-scan analysis. Br J Radiol 49:519–525, 1976.

35. Brascho DJ: Diagnostic ultrasound in radiation treatment planning. J Clin Ultrasound 1:320–329, 1974.

36. Taylor KJW, Carpenter DA, McXreary VR: Grey scale echography in the diagnosis of intrahepatic disease. J Clin Ultrasound 1:285–287, 1974.

37. Asher MW, Freimanis AK: Echographic diagnosis of retroperitoneal lymphnode enlargement – ultrasonic scanning technique and diagnostic findings. Am J Roentgenol 105:438–445, 1969.

38. Ellert J, Kreel L: The role of computed tomography in the initial staging and subsequent management of the lymphomas. J Comput Assist Tomogr 4(3):368–391, 1980.

39. Callen PW, Karobkin M, Isherwood I: Computed tomographic evaluation of the retrocrural and prevertebral space. Am J Roentgenol 129:907–910, 1977.

40. Schaner EG, Head GL, Doppman JL, Young RC: Computed tomography in the diagnosis, staging and management of abdominal lymphoma. J Comput Assist Tomogr 1:175–180, 1977.

41. Schaner EG, Head GL, Kalman MA, Dunnick NR, Doppman JL: Computed tomography in the diagnosis of abdominal and thoracic malignancy: review of 600 cases. Cancer Treat Rep 61:1537–1560, 1977.

42. Lee JKT, Stanley RJ, Sagel SS, Levitt RG: Accuracy of computed tomography in detecting intra-abdominal and pelvic adenopathy in lymphoma. Am J Roentgenol 131:311–315, 1978.

43. Earl HM, Sutcliffe SBJ, Fry IK, et al.: Computerised tomographic (CT) abdominal scanning in Hodgkin's disease. Clin Radiol 31:149–153, 1980.

44. Breiman RS, Castellino RA, Harell GS, Marshall WH, Glatstein E, Kaplan HS: CT-

pathologic correlations in Hodgkin's disease and non-Hodgkin's lymphoma. Radiology 126:159–166, 1078.

45. Marshall WH, Jr, Brieman RS, Harell GS, Glatstein E, Kaplan HS: Computed tomography of abdominal paraaortic lymph node disease: preliminary observations with a 6 second scanner. Am J Roentgenol 128:759–764, 1977.

46. Redman HC, Glatstein E, Castellino RA, Federal WA: Computed tomography as an adjunct in the staging of Hodgkin's disease and non-Hodgkin's lymphomas. Radiology 124:381–385, 1977.

47. Bernardino ME, Jing BS, Wallace S: Computed tomography diagnosis of mesenteric masses. Am J Roentgenol 132:33–36, 1979,

48. Hamlin DJ, Wandtke JC: CT correlation of axial, coronal and sagittal abdominal disease. CRC Crit Rev Diagn Imaging (in press).

49. Kreel L: The EMI whole body scanner in the demonstration of lymph node enlargement. Clin Radiol 27:421–429, 1976.

50. Kreel L: Computerised tomography in the diagnosis of lymph node disease. In: Computer assisted tomography, Proceedings of a Symposium held on the Occasion of the Tenth Anniversary of St. Lucas Hospital, Dec. 10, 1976, Kuhler WJ, ed. Amsterdam: Excerpta Medica, 1977, pp 105–120.

51. Kreel L: C.A.T. scanning in lymph node disease. In: The first European seminars on computerised axial tomography in clinical practice, du Boulay GH, Mosely IF eds. New York: Springer-Verlag, 1977, pp 396–405.

52. Rubin P, Haluska G, Poulter CA: The Basis for segmental sequential irradiation in Hodgkin's disease; clinical experience of patterns of recurrence. Am J Roentgenol 105:814–829, 1969.

53. Smithers DW: Spread of Hodgkin's disease. Lancet 1:1262, 1970.

54. Kaplan HS: Hodgkin's disease, 2nd edn. Cambridge, Mass.: Harvard University Press, 1980.

55. Kaplan HS: On the antural history of Hodgkin's disease. Harvey Lecture, 1970.

56. Alfidi RJ, Laval-Jeantet M: A promising contrast agent for computed tomography of the liver and spleen. Radiology 121:491, 1976.

57. Alcorn FS, Mategrano VC, Petasnick JP, Clark JW: Contributions of computed tomography in the staging and management of malignant lymphomas. Radiology 125:717–723, 1977.

58. Bragg DG: The clinical, pathologic and radiographic spectrum of the intrathoracic lymphomas. (Progress in clinical radiology). Invest Radiol 13:2–11, 1978.

59. Parker BR, Castellino RA, Kaplan HS: Pediatric Hodgkin's disease I. Radiographic evaluation. Cancer 37:2430, 1976.

60. McLeod RA, Brown LR, Miller WE, DeRemee RA: Evaluation of the pulmonary hila by tomography. Radiol Clin N Am XIV 1:51–84, 1976.

61. Castellino RA, Filley R, Blank N: Routine full-lung tomography in the initial staging and treatment planning of patients with Hodgkin's disease and non-Hodgkin's lymphoma. Cancer 38:1130, 1976.

62. Stolberg HO, Patt NL, MacEwen KF, Warwick OH, Brown TC: Hodgkin's disease of the lung. Roentgenologic-pathologic correlation. Am J Roentgenol Radium Ther Nucl Med 92:96–115, 1964.

63. Jones SE, Tobias DA, Waldman RS: Computed tomographic scanning in patients with lymphoma. Cancer 41:480–486, 1978.

64. Kreel L: Computed tomography of the lung and pleura. Semin Roentgenol 13:213–225, 1978.

65. Muhm JR, Brown LR, Crowe JK: Detection of pulmonary nodules by computed tomography. Am J Roentgenol 128:267–270, 1977.

66. Peckham MJ: Lung involvement. In: Hodgkin's disease, Smithers DW, ed. London:

Churchill Livingstone, 1973, pp 120–127.

67. Macdonald JS: Bone involvement. In: Hodgkin's disease, Smithers DW, ed. London: Churchill Livingstone, 1973, pp 128–136.

68. Rosenberg SA, Diamon HD, Jaslowitz B, Craver LF: Lympho-sarcoma: a review of 1269 cases. Medicine (Baltimore) 40:31–84, 1961.

69. Sherman RS, Wolfson SL: Roentgen diagnosis of lymphosarcoma and reticulum cell sarcoma in infancy and childhood. Am J Roentgenol 86:693–701, 1961.

4. The Role of Radiation Therapy in Malignant Lymphomas, Including Hodgkin's Disease *

GUNAR ZAGARS and PHILIP RUBIN

1. THE ROLE OF RADIATION THERAPY IN HODGKIN'S DISEASE

1.1. Basic Concepts: Past to Present

The two decades spanning 1960 to 1980 have been witness to a remarkable expansion in knowledge concerning the nature, management, and prognosis of the malignant lymphomas including Hodgkin's disease. This rapid gain in understanding, which is reflected in the outstanding therapeutic achievements of today, owes much to the painstaking investigation of several generations of radiation oncologists. Their efforts, often thwarted by primitive technologies, limited by patient referral patterns, and oftentimes opposed by a hostile medical opinion which deemed these disease fatal by definition, passed through many of the vicissitudes – the blind alleys, the frustating sidetracks – that many great scientific endeavors have had to negotiate. Finally, in the mid 1960s, the modern conceptions emerged. Before presenting these fundamental principles a brief journey through the annals of history will be undertaken to outline some of the milestones along the road to the present position.

In 1902, William Pusey of Chicago published [1] the first report of malignant lymphoma and Hodgkin's disease subjected to X-ray therapy [2, 3]. He noted the dramatic radioresponsiveness so characteristic of the lymphadenopathy in these diseases and one year later, a fine parallel to this clinical observation was reported by Heineke from Leipzig who documented the very marked response of healthy lymphoid tissue of mice and guinea pigs exposed to ionizing radiation [2, 3]. However, these were not auspicious beginnings. Very soon it was obvious that just as they melted away, so too the irradiated nodes soon regrew and the treatments had no influence on the

* Supported in part by the Clinical Radiation Research Center Grant, CA-11053. We acknowledge our gratitude to Miss Laurie Quinn for typing the manuscript.

course of the disease [2]. Up to the introduction of high voltage X-ray tubes in the early 1920s [3], the technical constraints were enormous. Much of radiation therapy between 1900 and 1922 was administerd with local radium applicators [2–4]; the Coolidge tube operating at 140 KV was manufactured in 1913 [3] but, at best, it might deliver 50% of the skin dose at a depth of 4 cm. Gilbert [2] has left us a brief summary of some of the observations made in Continental Europe during this early period, and it is clear that little significant was accomplished in the field of lymphomas.

With the advent of the orthovoltage deep therapy (200 kV) unit in 1922 [3], the delivery of realistic tumor doses became a possibility. The 1920s were a time of great clinical experimentation on different radiation dose fractionations with opinions polarizing between the 'single massive dose' concept – the Erlangen technique – and protracted daily treatments, more or less as used today – the Coutard School. A number of disastrous results encountered by the Erlangen practitioners soon established daily fractionation as empirically the best method [3]. In regard to the malignant lymphomas, we must appreciate that the prevailing wisdom in these days deemed these diseases to be disseminated in the majority, if not in all patients, and while Hodgkin's disease had been regarded as a distinct clinicopathologic entity, since the review by Reed in 1902 [5], confusion abounded when it came to the non-Hodgkin's lymphomas. Giant follicle lymphoma was often regarded as merging with reactive lymphadenopathy and therefore not as a true malignant lymphoma [6]; lymphosarcoma was at times difficult to distinguish from reticulum cell sarcoma [7], but this hardly mattered since both had an appalling prognosis – as late as 1937 Jackson noted [8] that patients with lymphosarcoma rarely survived three years and never ten. In the face of apparent dissemination at inception, it made little sense to stage these diseases apart from a broad subdivision into 'early' and 'late' cases to serve as some guide to the likely time of death [7, 9]. The notion that spread might be orderly was non-existent and Reed had made the intriguing statement: 'Hodgkin's disease seems not to metastasize by cellular transplantation but by causing a proliferation in pre-existing lymphoid tissue, *apparently anywhere* in the body' [5]. It was against this background that the earliest radiotherapeutic inroads into the malignant lymphomas began in the mid 1920s.

The concept of vigorous regional irradiation with systematic, sequential coverage of all involved sites seems to have originated simultaneously in a number of centers. As early as 1921, the Mayo Clinical procedure for Hodgkin's disease was outlined as follows by Bowing [4]: 'The two great body cavities and all possible superficial glandular enlargements should be treated ... at the onset of the disease in order to ward off the impending mediastinal and abdominal enlargements...'. Accordingly, a combination of local radium applications to involved superficial nodal regions followed by wide-field multiple portal Coollidge tube irradiation to the thorax and abdomen was recommended. It was Gilbert, however, who must clearly perceived the problems in Hodgkin's disease. He emphasized the need to continue irradiation to an involved node beyond the point of complete regression if response was to be durable. Having observed many times '... recurrences developing in the immediate vicinity of a field too narrowly irradiated' [2], he developed his 'sequential roentgen therapy' which required *wide* irradiation of involved regions and adjacent clinically normal sites. The para-aortic nodes and spleen were to be treated in those patients whose systemic symptoms had not abated after conclusion of comprehensive supradiaphragmatic treatment. Significant as they were, these ideas did not bear dramatic results. Gilbert could only achieve a freedom-from-relapse in 16% of his patients followed for 5 years, though his overall survival figure of 38% was a considerable improvement over earlier series [2]. His own position was that segmental irradiation was not a curative procedure, but that it was significant in that it reduced the rate of evolution of disease in patients so treated. A brief review of the physical treatment parameters available at that time reveals the problem: the technology simply could not meet the biologic demands. Gilbert's basic tumor dose was about 500 rads for deep lymph nodes, to be only cautiously raised for massive or refractory disease.

In a 1934 review of the role of a variety of irradiation techniques in lymphosarcoma and Hodgkin's disease, Leucutia [9] could show only a prolongation of median survival and a palliation of symptoms, but little, if any, effect on ultimate survival. Curiously, he recommended prophylactic irradiation in lymphosarcoma but not in Hodgkin's disease. As late as 1947, investigators were reporting that on account of the unpredictable pattern of future relapse, prophylactic irradiation was contraindicated in Hodgkin's disease [10]. However, as was soon to become evident, a number of centers had already adopted the wide-field high-dose concept for the lymphomas including Hodgkin's disease. Refinements in dosimetry and technique yielded significant improvements in depth-dose even with orthovoltage equipment and the 1950s saw the first detailed analysis of a significant number of Hodgkin's disease patients treated 'radically' [11, 12]. These reports by Vera Peters from Canada represented a clear advance and showed that 25% of patients with Hodgkin's disease treated by radiation alone were alive at 20 years [12]. A number of prognostic factors were delineated, including the importance of a newly introduced staging system. Prophylactic irradiation to adjacent uninvolved sites was estimated to have increased survival by about 20% and the feasibility and safety of 2500–3000 rads in 2 weeks to involved regions followed by 1000 rads to adjacent uninvolved fields was established. In 1963, the Manchester group reported their results on localized Hodgkin's disease treated between 1934 and 1956 by wide-field techniques to doses of 2500–2700 rads in 3 weeks and concluded that about 40% of these patients were cured [7]. Early lympho- and reticulosarcomas appeared to do as well.

Even as these reports were appearing, a giant quantum step had already been taken at Stanford University – this was to rapidly transform the field of lymphology. With the recent availability of megavoltage beams, Kaplan took the bold course of encompassing all major lymphatic structures above the diaphragm in one large field by shielding out the majority of both lungs [13]. Furthermore, without the restriction of excessive skin dose, the Stanford group explored higher midplane doses and rapidly showed that 4000 rads was tolerable. The early results of this approach were impressive indeed [13] and a number of investigators adopted this 'mantle' field. Armed with this therapeutic technique and reassured by the recently introduced bipedal lympangiogram, the radiation oncologist of the early 1960s finally seemed assured of success in early Hodgkin's disease. It was, therefore, astonishing to observe retroperitoneal nodal relapse in many of these lymphangiogram-negative patients [14–17]. This transdiaphragmatic mantle failure had a number of significant repercussions. It would have been so easy to conclude that Hodgkin's disease even though apparently localized was indeed a disseminated disease, spread beyond the diaphragm implying very advanced disease (as it did in Peters' original staging system). Fortunately, the Stanford group boldly continued their adherence to the contiguity concept and postulated that the para-aortic nodes were contiguous with those in the left supraclavicular region by virtue of the thoracic duct [18]. This now required that in addition to the mantle field one should also include the para-aortic region. For completeness, the lateral pelvic nodes and spleen were also included and total lymphoid (TLI) or total nodal (TNI) irradiation was born. The almost complete elimination of transdiaphragmatic nodal failures and a corresponding gain in freedom from relapse and survival fully vindicated the contiguity concept. A no less remarkable evolution that followed in the wake of retroperitoneal nodal relapse was the staging laparotomy and splenectomy [19]. An invasive procedure of this magnitude purely for diagnostic purposes had not been the rule in medicine and yet by the early 1970s, many centers throughout the world were more or less routinely using it [20–22].

Radical radiation therapy is critically dose-volume dependent for its results. Quite obviously, two requirements must be fulfilled for a radiotherapeutic cure to result: an adequate 'tumoricidal' dose must be delivered; and the volume treated must contain all the disease, macroscopic and microscopic. The interplay between dose and volume, in this sense, is illustrated in Figure 1, and we refer to this as the 'basic radical radiation therapy equation.' In deriving this simple expression, use is made of the multiplication theorem in probability calculus, i.e. the likelihood that two or more mutually non-exclusive stochastic events occur together is the product

THE RADICAL RADIATION THERAPY EQUATION

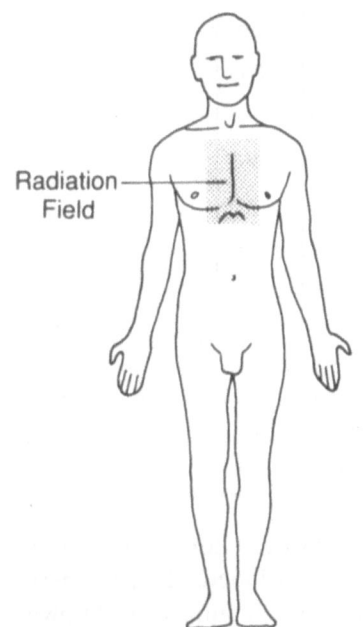

Radiation Field

$$P_C = P_{LC} \times P_{DF}$$

P_C: probability for cure.
P_{LC}: probability that cancer in-field is eradicated.
P_{DF}: probability that all cancer is in-field.

Figure 1. The conceptual relation between tumor cure and radiation dose-volume factors. P_{LC}: determined by the dose chosen from the usually sigmoid radiation dose-response curve, modulated by tumor volume, tumor sensitivity, time, fractionation, pharmacologic modifiers and limited by tolerance of in-field normal structures. P_{DF}: determined by staging procedures used and by field sizing, shaping, positioning according to retrospectively recognized high risk sites of involvement that cannot be delineated by current staging procedures.

of their respective probabilities. Stochastic events (events that individually cannot be predicted with certainty but that occur with statistical regularity in populations) are ubiquitous in medicine and in the treatment of malignant lymphomas both local control and tumor localization are inescapably probabilistic. That local control is stochastic is a radiobiologic fact [23]; the stochastic character of tumor localization was expressed by Kaplan in the following way: '... no matter how careful the workup, there will be an irreducible residue of cases in which occult metastasis to distant areas had already occurred' [13]. Figure 2 shows the theoretic relation between cure probability (P_C) and its two determinants, local control probability (P_{LC}) and accuracy of tumor localization (P_{DF}). Since it is now possible to deliver radiation doses achieving very high local control probabilities (>90%) even

$$P_C = P_{LC} \times P_{DF}$$

P_{LC} \ P_{DF}	0.25	0.50	0.75	0.85	0.95
0.85	0.21	0.43	0.64	0.72	0.81
0.90	0.22	0.45	0.68	0.77	0.86
0.95	0.24	0.48	0.71	0.81	0.90

Figure 2. Theoretic relationship between cure probability and its two determinants: radiation dose (P_{LC}) and accuracy of field placement (P_{DF}). Accuracy of field placement increases as staging improves and as high-risk clinically uninvolved sites are recognized. With the high local control now achieved, the cure probability is a critical function of P_{DF}..

to large volumes such as in conventional total nodal irradiation (TNI), only the upper range of local control probability is included. Under these circumstances it is the certainty with which one can encompass all known and presumed disease which largely determines the outcome. Let us now consider the two elements, local control and volume design in more detail.

'The concept of an "all or none cancericidal dose" had dominated radiotherapy since the discovery of radium and X-rays' [24]. Often this supposed tumor-lethal dose was linked to the dose needed to damage the tissue of origin of the neoplasm and Gilbert [2], for example, laid great emphasis on the correspondence between the radiosensitivity of normal lymphoid tissue and of the lymphomas. While there is more than a measure of truth in this correspondence, there is no truth in the supposition that a given tumor type has one unique 'all or none tumoricidal dose' [24]. For tumors in general and malignant lymphomas in particular, there is a relation between dose and local control such that the percentage (or probability) of local control increases with absorbed dose [25–28]. In most experimental systems, this curve has a sigmoid shape [23] quite like the drug-concentration-response curves familiar in clinical pharmacology [29, 30]. Though the exact shape of the radiation dose-response curves for malignant lymphomas is a subject of some controversy [25, 27], there appear to be no compelling arguments against the sigmoid shape. Figure 3 illustrates in principle such local control curves and a corresponding toxicity curve. There is no unique tumoricidal dose; instead there is a range of doses (the 'therapeutic window')

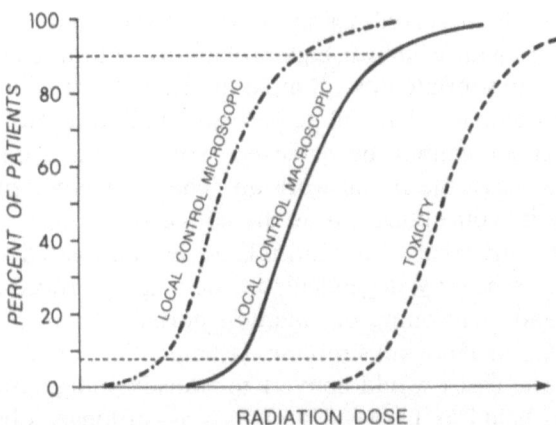

Figure 3. Theoretic radiation dose-response curves for local control of macroscopic and microscopic disease and for local toxicity. For the malignant lymphomas, the local control curve for macroscopic disease is relatively to the left of the toxicity curve for many, but not all organs, thereby assuring a positive therapeutic ratio. There is clearly no unique tumoricidal dose; instead we can, in theory, choose any dose to achieve a certain probability of local control associated with some probability of toxicity.

over which variable proportions of patients experience local control with acceptably low complication risks. However, there are doses (4000–4500 rads) that achieve very high local control rates in the malignant lymphomas (>90%), and one may loosely refer to this dose region as tumoricidal. Apart from dose, a number of factors modifying local control have been identified in Figures 1 and 3 and will be discussed in later sections.

Figure 3 also shows a typical dose-toxicity curve and while the local control curves for malignant lymphomas are positioned relatively to the left of the complication curves for many organs, this is not true for a number of critical structures. The inclusion of substantial volumes of any of the radiation class I organs [31] (lungs, kidneys, liver, bone marrow, bowel, pericardium, spinal cord) within a radiation field may be a limiting factor to the permissible dose and to local control. The very marked dependence of radiation toxicity on volume irradiated made it *a priori* unlikely that very large fields could ever be treated to effective doses. It was, therefore a major advance in the radiotherapy of malignant lymphomas when the Stanford group first demonstrated the toxicologic feasibility of irradiation to large volumes such as in their TNI to high doses by careful shielding of vital structures [13, 32].

The ideal radiation volume in any given case of cancer is the one which includes all disease (macroscopic and microscopic) but excludes all uninvolved normal structures. Clearly if a Stage I patient were truly Stage I, then local irradiation to the involved region (or ideally, only to the involved node) would assure a cure with whatever high probability of local control we desire by delivering the appropriate dose. Simple in principle, this idea is not at all easy to execute in practice. The full delineation of all locations of lymphoma in any given patient cannot be achieved with certainty no matter how extensive and intensive the initial work-up. The error inherent in any stage designation may be conceptualized as the conversion ratio: the fraction of cases which, following local treatment, relapse in non-treated sites first [33]. Conversion ratio is heavily dependent on the staging procedures used and on the volume and positioning of radiation portals. Prior to the advent of staging laparotomy in Hodgkin's disease, at least 1/3 of apparently localized supradiaphragmatic cases would convert to transdiaphragmatic failures following a mantle field [16, 17, 34–37]. This was strikingly observed in the first Stanford trial where lymphangiogram (LAG) stage IA and IIA patients fared no better with a mantle field than with 'involved field' radiation. The high incidence of transdiaphragmatic nodal failure (TDNF) in both groups led to similar relapse rates with no advantage to the mantle field [38, 39]. The LAG was clearly inadequate to rule out disease below the diaphragm. More recently, even a negative laparotomy does not guarantee immunity against TDNF though the probability is reduced [40, 41]. Similar phenomena have been observed in the non-Hodgkin's lymphomas (NHL). Whereas the nodular variants had been more often regarded as localized than the diffuse histologic subtypes [6, 9], recent intensive sequential staging procedures have shown the facts to be in the reverse – it is only the exceptional nodular lymphoma that is truly localized [42, 43]. The conversion ratio following radiation therapy has been high in clinically staged apparently localized diffuse histiocytic lymphoma [44], but recent studies on intensively staged patients treated for localized disease show a marked reduction in beyond-field relapse [45].

Conversion ratio has, apart from its quantitative magnitude, also a qualitative aspect: the pattern of relapse. Patterns of relapse following local treatment have been among the strongest guides to the design of radiation portals. Clearly, a disease that relapses in a variety of sites with a largely random frequency is not amenable to 'prophylactic' irradiation. On the other hand, where relapses follow a pattern with statistical regularity, prophylactic irradiation may play a part. Analysis of relapse patterns following localized irradiation has contributed as much, if not more, to our understanding of the spread of malignant lymphomas, than any other investigational approach. The early demonstration of long-term survivors among those irradiated for localized extranodal lymphoma suggested that a significant proportion of diffuse histiocytic lymphomas is localized [8] – an observation confirmed by intensive investigation of new cases [45]. Similarly the frequent relapse of nodular lymphomas in distant sites and bone marrow is based on their initially disseminated nature. The rather sharp polarization of cases of NHL between those truly localized and those disseminated has limited the value of wide prophylactic fields as employed in Hodgkin's disease. In regard to 'prophylactic' fields, it is perhaps worth repeating Gilbert's statement: '... the question is not to protect prophylactically groups of normal lymph nodes against future invasion [but rather to] include in one large field portions already involved, if only histologically' [2].

To optimize the *predictive value* of conversion ratios, in both their quantitative and qualitative aspects, use is made of 'prognostic factors'. Prognostic factors are symptoms, signs, demographic data, or laboratory results that either alone or in some combination correlate statistically with a particular clinical outcome. Prognostic factors are linked not only to the biology of the underlying disease, but indeed are affected by our interventional maneuvers. Probably no field in medicine has witnessed such profound changes in prognostic factors as have occurred in the malignant lymphomas over the past decade. To cite one example, we read in 1973 that '... the young female with nodular sclerosing [Hodgkin's] disease, mediastinal involvement, and other favourable signs is particularly fortunate' [46]. In 1980, we find that either '... the few deaths due to Hodgkin's disease in this series occurred in the group of patients who presented with mediastinal disease' [47], or that '... the extent of mediastinal Hodgkin's disease was not of prognostic importance' [48]. Such changing values are a legacy of the rapid advances in therapy and require the oncologist to remain in immediate contact with all the fine nuances, the apparent contradictions and the unending complexity that now characterize the field of lymphology. For the faint-hearted, there is a theoretical limit, since it is reasonable to suppose that once easily curable, a disease loses all its prognostic factors!

Rapid advances in the chemotherapy of Hodgkin's disease are yielding curative results in a substantial proportion of patients with late stage disease. Accordingly, there is a rationale for introducing chemotherapy into earlier stages as an adjunct to radiation therapy. However, the use of two such super-radical modalities in *all* patients when one modality alone already produces a high incidence of long-term freedom-from-disease is not optimal medicine, but leads to significant overtreatment of the majority of patients to potentially benefit only a few. Cure rates may increase slightly, but toxicity escalates greatly and for the patients as a whole, therapeutic ratio declines. A sounder philosophy is to seek out those subgroups of patients who have a high propensity for relapse and to subject only these to an initial multimodal approach.

1.2. Radiation Oncology Treatment Principles

1.2.1. Dose-Control Factors. Increasing the dose of radiation to a site involved by Hodgkin's disease produces an increasing likelihood of permanent local control [25–27, 49–52]. There is, however, some controversy as to the exact shape of the dose-control curve [25, 27, 52] and in particular, on the optimal dose routinely indicated for an acceptably high rate of local control of macroscopic or microscopic disease [25, 27, 52–55]. The likelihood of local radiation control in cancers is generally determined by a large number of factors [23, 56], chief among which are: the total dose administered, the number of fractions used, the time interval between the first and last doses, the relative biologic effectiveness of the radiation used, the number of clonogenic tumor cells present, the radiosensitivity of these stem cells, the status of oxygenation in the tumor, and the presence or absence of pharmacologic modifiers of the radiation response. The past decade has produced much quantitative data to guide us in the choice of an appropriate dose in this disease. Local control is defined as the likelihood of permanent control for *each* involved site irradiated. This is somewhat different to the local control rates we have assembled in Table 1, based on patient assessment, where each patient may have had *several* sites of initial involvement and true recurrence may have occurred in more than one site in a patient who recurred. The data for the curves in Figure 4 were first assembled by Kaplan [25] and subsequently re-analyzed by Fletcher and Shukovsky [27]. The latter authors discarded what they regarded as 'erratic control rates' [27] from some of the original publications and used small dose intervals (e.g. 2000 ± 100) for each 'percent control point' [25]. Clearly the two curves

Table 1. Incidence of true recurrence in Hodgkin's disease following 4000–4500 rads to involved regions.

Dose/fractionation *		Patients **	Patient with true recurrence †	Investigators
4400:	210–275	462	10 (2.2)	Spittle *et al.*, 1973 [34]
4000:	200	155	6 (3.9)	Werf-Messing, 1973 [61]
4000:	200	82	4 (4.9)	Johnson *et al.*, 1976 [54]
4000:	split	54	1 (1.9)	Johnson *et al.*, 1976 [54]
4000:	180–200	116	4 (3.4)	Mill *et al.*, 1977 [62]
4000:	200	67	2 (3.0)	Levi *et al.*, 1977 [63]
4000–4500:	150–200	111	6 (5.4)	Mauch *et al.*, 1978 [60]
4000:	150–200	62	1 (1.6)	Mintz *et al.*, 1979 [64]
4000–4500:	160–200	131	5 (3.8)	Prosnitz *et al.*, 1980 [65]
4000–4500:	200	90	1 (1.1)	Fuller *et al.*, 1980 [47]
		1330	40 (3.0)	

* Total dose: dose per fraction.
** >90% were Stages I or II.
† ( ) percentage true recurrence.

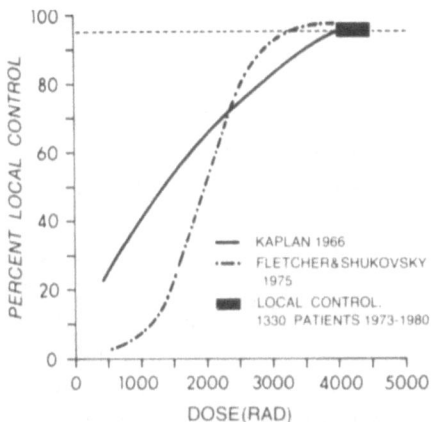

Figure 4. Local control curves for Hodgkin's disease according to the data of Kaplan [25] and Fletcher and Shukovsky [27]. Both analyses used the same data and defined local control as

$$\frac{\text{number of involved fields recurring}}{\text{number of involved fields treated}}$$

Also shown are the rates of local control reported in 10 series over the past 7 years with 4000–4500 rads (see Table 1).

differ significantly in both the low- and high-control probability regions. These differences have implications for the selection of an appropriate dose for macroscopic disease and for 'prophylaxis' of microscopically involved regions.

The sigmoid curve crosses 95% control at about 3500 rads and by its shape in this region suggests that very little would be gained by increasing the dose even to 4500 rads. Indeed, a number of workers have recently championed the use of doses between 3500 and 4000 rads, arguing that more than 4000 rads to involved regions is wasteful in terms of relative benefit and toxic in absolute terms [27, 52–54, 57–59]. On the other hand, the majority of recent large series on Hodgkin's disease treated by radiation report the use of 4000–4500 rads to involved regions and stress the importance of this dose range for adequate control [47, 60]. Table 1 is a compilation of local recurrence rates reported in 10 series over the past 7 years. In each series a minimum of 4000 rads was delivered to every involved area, and in fact, sites of involvement were often boosted up to 4500 rads [34, 47, 54, 60–65]. More than 90% of the 1330 patients represented were in stages I or II. Local control rates, with 4000–4500 rads to involved regions, are excellent: in each series, local control fell in the range of 94.6% to 98.9% with an overall average of 97% in the whole group of 1300 patients. It is also evident from these same reports that such doses can be delivered with relative safety

providing that attention is paid to technical details such as off-axis dose
calculations for irregular fields in each patients [52], selective and adequate
shielding of critical structures such as lungs, heart, kidneys, spinal
cord [52, 57], and frequent verification of treatment set-ups with port
films [66]. A review of these technical factors will be presented in the next
section, but here it is emphasized that the 'cone down' or 'boost' concept is
critical if one plans to go above 4000 rads.

The question as to whether lower doses, in the range of 3500 to 4000 rads,
without attempting to boost bulk disease above 4000 rads, are equally
effective and perhaps therapeutically advantageous in producing fewer complications cannot be answered presently. Ultimately, it will need a large
number of patients, treated to these lower doses, to be analyzed for local
control and toxicity before definitive recommendations can be made. In the
meantime, there is another reason to recommend the use of that dose which
offers highest local control probabilities within an acceptable toxicity framework [55]. If we use probability of control for each involved site as the basic
yardstick, then it follows that the likelihood of at least one true recurrence
increases as the number of involved sites per patient increases [55, 67]. This
is illustrated in Figure 5 where the theoretic risk of at least one site failing is
plotted against increasing numbers of initially involved sites and for different
control probabilities (doses) per site. As expected, the likelihood of failure in
at least one site increases as the number of involved sites increases, but more
importantly, the rate at which this risk rises increases dramatically as the
probability of local control per site (dose) decreases. There is clear evidence

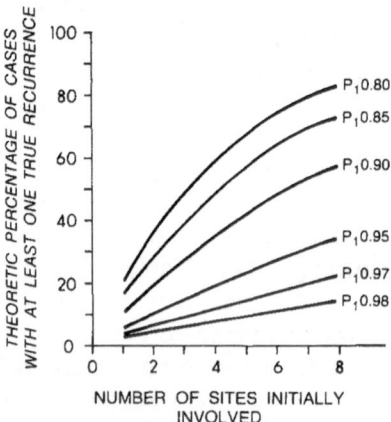

Figure 5. Theoretic relation between the likelihood of at least one recurrence and number of
sites initially involved for radiation doses achieving various control probabilities per site. Note
the increasingly steep rate of rise of this relation as control probability per site (P_1)
decreases.

in the literature that this phenomenon is a clinical reality [68, 69]. Carmel and Kaplan [68] published a curve relating the incidence of supradiaphragmatic relapse to the number of supradiaphragmatic sites initially involved and treated by the mantle technique to 4400 rads. The relation was linear, with no relapses in patients with only one involved site to 45% relapses in patients with seven involved sites. In pathologic stage IIIA patients, the true recurrence in three recent series [62, 67, 70] was 12/99 patients (12%) and of the nodal failures encountered, 60% were judged to be true in-field failures – this is higher than in the early stages presented above. It is of course likely that inadvertent shielding of gross disease contributes to these trends, since a larger number of involved sites amplifies the likelihood that at least one will be over shielded. Nevertheless, these data hardly encourage the use of lower doses especially when multiple sites are involved.

One of the major determinants of local control for cancers generally is tumor volume at the site in question – the larger the volume, the greater the dose needed to achieve a certain control probability [23, 24, 56]. Increasing numbers of clonogenic stem cells and deficient vascularity are the major factors accounting for the dose increments required [23, 56]. This phenomenon has been given relatively little attention in the literature on Hodgkin's disease. The early report by Seydel and co-workers [49] indicated that such a relation could be relevant, but subsequent reports have largely neglected any volume relation, concentrating more on 'tumoricidal dose' independent of volume. Indeed some recent reports have failed to document any relation between in-field recurrence and nodal volume for doses in the range of 4000-5000 rads [65]. However, a number of reports do suggest that volume is an important factor in local control even at or above 4000 rads [47, 51, 60, 68, 69]. One report [60] showed that massive mediastinal adenopathy measuring more than one-third of the chest diameter, and receiving at least 4000 rads, recurred in 6/18 patients, while mediastinal masses measuring less than this were locally controlled in all patients (33/33). Combining the results of two reports [62, 69] which specified node volume in terms of the largest diameter of a mass, we find that for lesions <6 cm, local control with >3000 rads was achieved at all sites (159/159); for masses >6 cm given >3000 rads, failure to control occurred in 11/48 sites (23%). Clearly, these data do not permit more than the most tentative and general conclusions, and the quantitative aspects of any relation between volume, dose and local control are presently poorly defined. The date suggest that 3500 rads is adequate for small volume disease (<6 cm largest diameter) and that local recurrence may be problematic for large volume disease even at 4500 rads. However, in the face of a rather large body of information (Table 1) attesting to the efficacy of a minimum of 4000 rads to involved sites irrespective of their measurable volume, we consider it premature to recommend the routine use of lower doses to clinically evident, though small, nodal masses. Future analyses of additional data may change this view.

From time to time attempts have been made to assess the radiosensitivity of individual lesions by observing their rate of regression during treatment, or their completeness of response immediately upon conclusion of treatment [71]. In Hodgkin's disease, there is no consistent relation between rate of regression and likelihood of permanent local control [55], and residual lymphadenopathy immediately on completion of 4000 rads is not an adverse factor [54]. Two recent series show that of 103 patients having some bulk residue, 25 (25%) relapsed in these sites compared to relapse of 51 patients out of 201 immediate complete responders (25%) [68, 69]. Residual masses are more common with nodular sclerosis histology but there is no evidence for the need to use different doses for different histologies.

A closely allied and conceptually related problem is that of the dose required to control microscopic disease. An analysis of this issue is complicated by a number of factors, chief of which is the requirement for a denominator in the equation defining percentage local control – this elusive parameter has never been quantified for microscopic disease. Moreover, 'subclinical' is not synonymous with microscopic; there are numerous anatomic sites where involved nodes 1–3 cm in diameter would be subclinical even after extensive staging workup. Therefore, even if it were shown that prophylactic doses as low as say 1500 rads were adequate for truly microscopic Hodgkin's disease, it would not, *ipso facto,* follow that these same doses are adequate as prophylaxis for 'blind' areas such as the mediastinum or the para-aortic region. Despite all these difficulties, a number of workers have attempted to specify the minimal adequate prophylactic dose [26, 49, 51, 69]. Seydel reported no failures in prophylactic sites given more than 2500 rads, but only six such sites were documented; there were four sites failing out of 40 given less than 2500 rads [49]. Thar and Million [69] report no relapses in areas receiving 3000 rads or more prophylactically while Ibrahim and co-workers report 2/24 areas failing with prophylactic doses of 3000–3500 rads and 1/23 such areas failing after 4000 rads [51]. The prophylactic doses reported in the series summarized in Table 1 were all at, or in excess of, 3500 rads and relapses in previously uninvolved regions as a first manifestation of failure was reported in only one patient. Clearly, 3500 rads to prophylactic fields is adequate; whether this can be safely lowered to 3000 rads as recently suggested [52] awaits further experience.

A problem that now faces the radiation oncologist with increasing frequency in this multi-modal era, is the question of radiation dose in combination with chemotherapy [29]. A number of different clinical situations are typically encountered. Those patients who fail to achieve complete remission following adequate chemotherapy (say, 6 cycles of MOPP) require radical radiation if they are to be salvaged at all. Low dose irradiation (1500–2000 rads) converted only 1/18 partial chemotherapy responders to complete remission [72]; better salvage was achieved with doses of 3000–3500 rads to nodal sites and 2000 to 2500 rads to involved organs: 6/7 partial chemotherapy responders became complete responders after this radiation regimen [73]. Those patients who achieve a complete remission after adequate chemotherapy presumably require lower radiation doses, if they are to be irradiated at all [72]. We will consider this question later and now merely indicate that two series [72, 73] support the use of low doses to sites of previous involvement. One study utilized 1500–2000 rads [72] and the other, 2000–3500 rads [73], with very comparable results. Another, and an increasingly more common situation, arises in earlier stages with bulky lymphadenopathy when 2 or 3 cycles of combination chemotherapy are given prior to radiation therapy [74–76]. Under these circumstances, full doses of radiation must be given. One study employing 2 cycles of MOPP prior to a minimum of 4000 rads for stage III disease reported eight true recurrences in 88 patients (9 %) [77] – an incidence not significantly lower than that reported by others using radiation alone in stage III [62, 67, 70]. All these data therefore suggest that full doses of radiation are needed if treatment is to be radical in patients who either fail to achieve complete remission or who, irrespective of their remission status, received suboptimal chemotherapy.

Finally, we will address the question of radiation fractionation and overall treatment time in relation to local control of Hodgkin's disease. The malignant lymphomas and Hodgkin's disease are exceptional among neoplastic diseases in that they show little, if any, dependence of local control on dose per fraction and overall time, at least with reasonable limits [26, 27, 49, 50, 52, 54, 57]. Accordingly, there is no need to deliver 4000 rads in 4 weeks at the rate of 200 rads per fraction. A common practice is to use 150–170 rads per fraction, delivering 4000 rads in 5 weeks [62, 64]. Additional boost doses can be delivered at the same rate. This finesse has important implications for the therapeutic ratio; normal tissues respond in the 'classic' way to fractionation – time alterations and whereas 4000 rads in 4 weeks produces a significant incidence of bothersome complications in some organs [32, 68, 78], the same total dose given in 5 weeks is significantly less toxic [52, 54, 79].

1.2.2. Volume and Shielding Techniques. The predictable patterns of relapse and the contiguous character of regional lymph node involvement have led to the development of reasonably standardized radiation fields for the treatment of Hodgkin's disease. This standardization is reflected in the use of widely recognized terms such as 'mantle', 'inverted Y', and 'spade' to describe various field configurations. The term 'extended field', on the other hand, has no consensus meaning and should be defined when used. 'Involved field' is usually taken to imply irradiation of the whole lymph

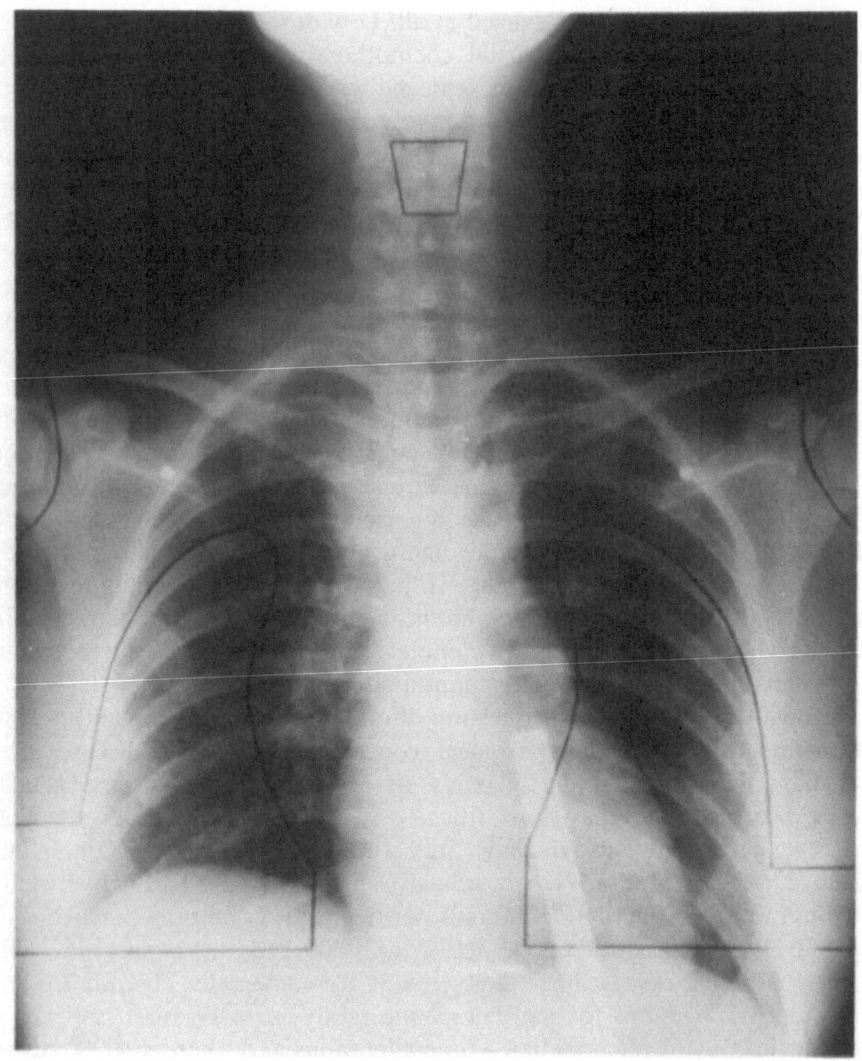

Figure 6. Typical anterior (A) and posterior (B) mantle fields. The lateral edge of the lung shield is drawn along the inner aspect of the rib cage. Mediastinal structures, except the heart, are given a 1 cm margin. The posterior lung blocks (B) rise higher than the anterior ones (A). The larynx is shielded anteriorly and the cervical cord is shielded posteriorly usually after 2000 rads.

node site involved by Hodgkin's disease, though to some it might mean an even smaller field and the term should be defined explicitly whenever it is used. Despite this apparent standardization there are significant differences in the actual techniques used in various centers, often reflecting certain convictions about the particular merit of some technical point [47, 52, 55, 57, 80–82]. However, there is no convincing evidence to

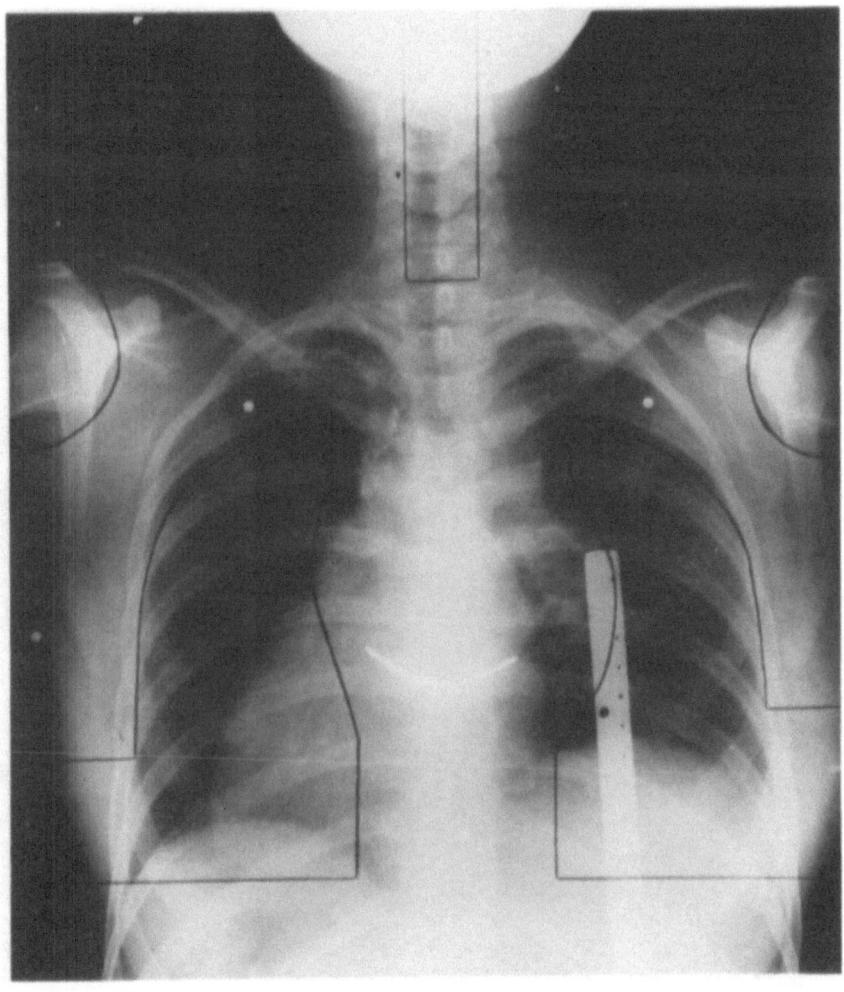

b

single out one particular technique as distinctly superior to the others. Indeed, the comparable regional control rates reported by many large centers imply that such technical finesses are not of themselves important providing that one is familiar with one's own technique and eliminates any systematic errors that could produce complications or failures. Accordingly, the radical radiation treatment of Hodgkin's disease can only be performed by those experienced in wide-field megavoltage techniques, possessing full physics and dosimetric facilities and attuned to the often subtle technical peculiarities of their particular method. There really is no system that can be directly borrowed from the literature and implemented without considerable prior phantom evaluation with the therapy unit to be used. Thus, the actual technical parameters will vary from center to center; what remains constant

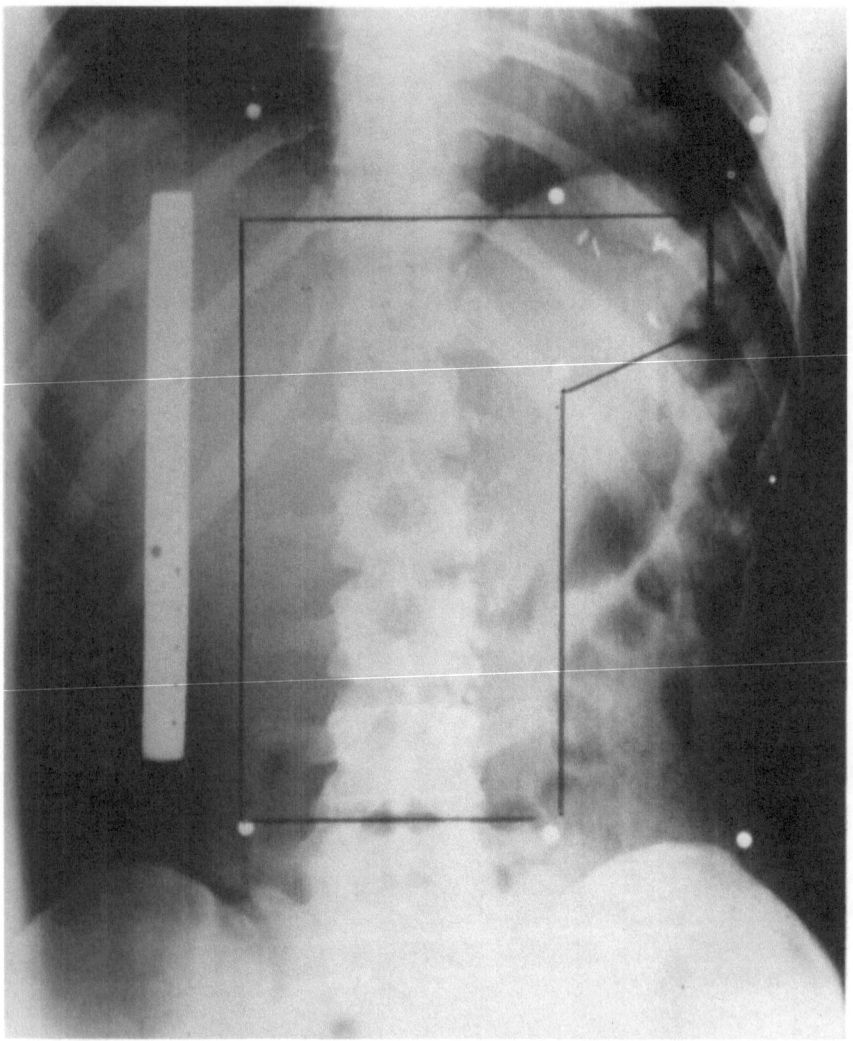

Figure 7. Peri-aortic-splenic pedicle field. The upper end is in the lower posterior mediastinum with an appropriate gap to the mantle. Laterally the field encompasses lymph nodes visualized by lymphangiogram and includes the transverse processes of the lumbar vertebrae. The splenic pedicle is indicated by surgical clips.

is the aim: to deliver an adequate dose via appropriate fields to those areas involved or at risk, with minimal irradiation of critical normal structures. A number of recent publications have described the various wide-field techniques used by their authors in extensive detail [52, 55, 57, 81, 82] and a general method for irregular-field dose calculation in Hodgkin's disease has also been published [83]. We will not present any particular method in all its

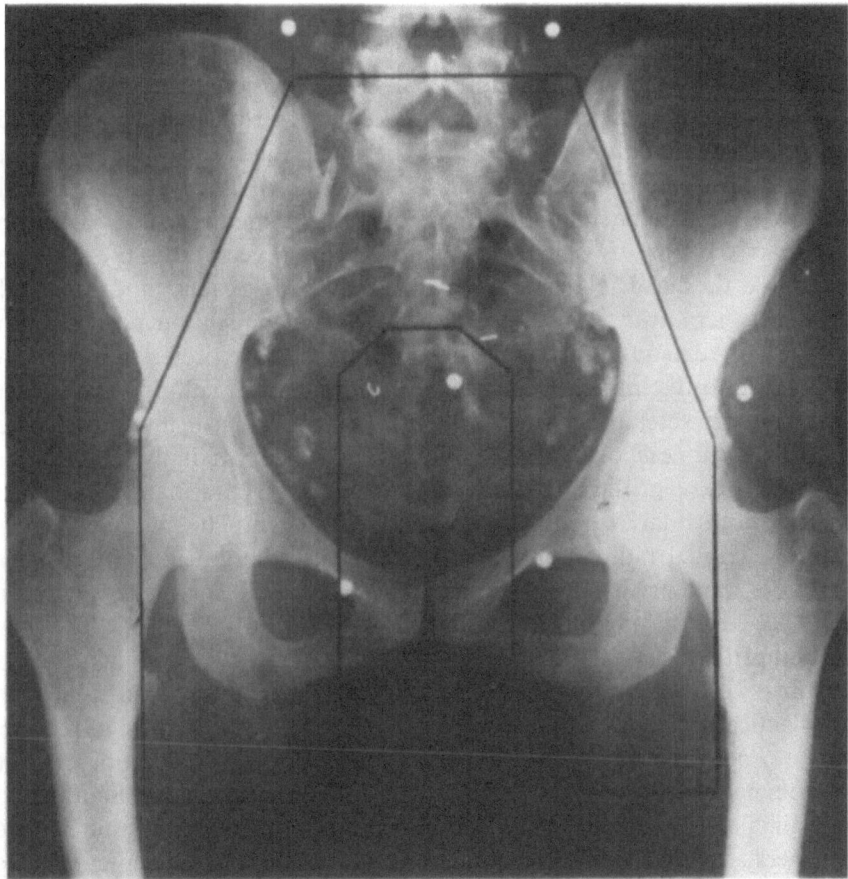

Figure 8. Pelvic-inguinal-femoral field. Posteriorly this field may be cut off at the inguinal ligament and two anterior electron fields are then used to boost the dose to the anteriorly located inguinal and femoral nodes.

detail, but will illustrate the fields typically employed in our practice and highlight problem areas and pitfalls commonly encountered in field design and dosimetry.

Figures 6, 7, and 8 illustrate typical field designs used at the University of Rochester. We share the views recently expressed by Million [52] that the mantle field is the single most complex field generally employed in radiation oncology, requiring explicit attention to each of the lymph node sites to be included in every patient and consideration of a number of normal structures that need maximal shielding. The key to a good mantle lies clearly in the lung blocks which must avoid shielding macroscopic and microscopic disease while protecting as much lung and heart as is compatible with low failure risks. We routinely bring the lateral edge of our blocks to the medial surface of the lateral rib cage as visualized on simulation film, and for the anterior field, sweep this lateral margin medially to include the infraclavicular region for about 2 cm below the medial end of the clavicle (Figure 6A). Others draw this lateral margin at the middle of the rib cage or even include a 2 cm strip of lateral lung in the field [52]. The critical issue here is whether the axillary nodes are adequately dosed. Certainly if the axilla is clinically involved, we take the lateral edge of our shield medially and check the adequacy of coverage by placing lead shot over involved nodes. Elevating the arms above the head is a maneuver that may shift axillary nodes laterally and project them away from the chest wall [84]. Although our posterior lung blocks usually extend higher than the anterior ones, we prefer to have some transmission to the infraclavicular region from behind. 'Fall-off' to the chest wall laterally is shielded below a line level with the fourth intercostal space anteriorly [57] unless low axillary nodes are involved. Medially, any mediastinal shadow (except the heart) or any masses are given a margin of at least 1 cm and both hilar regions are routinely irradiated. The hilum is not an accurately defined radiographic structure and its anatomical designation as the 'root of the lung' is hardly specific. There is therefore, much variation in the medial edge of lung blocks as shaped by different oncologists. There are even authorities who doubt the necessity to irradiate radiographically negative hila [47]. One study however, suggested that there is a benefit in prophylactically treating these regions and that the lateral extension required to do so produces no added pulmonary morbidity [85]. We do not irradiate the whole pericardium to low prophylactic doses as practiced at Stanford for mediastinal disease [68, 81], and we rarely use a subcarinal block [68] – never if the mediastinum is involved. We do not shield the thoracic spinal cord at all in the presence of mediastinal disease and posterior cervical cord shielding is limited to levels above the thoracic inlet. Thin lung blocks [60, 86] transmitting 50% of the dose are employed if whole-lung irradiation is given. Large mediastinal masses are treated with a shrinking field technique by progressively enlarging the lung blocks medially. We have not employed the 'split course' technique [54, 68] for large mediastinal disease, preferring continuous irradiation or pre-irradiation chemotherapy. The upper edge of the field includes the submental nodes and the angle of the mandible. For mid and high cervical nodal presentations our prophylaxis had been delivered with a lateral electron beam to each parotid region. This avoids irradiating the oropharynx, nasopharynx, and posterior oral cavity since it is unnecessary to treat Waldeyer's ring. Doses delivered to mantle fields in literature reports range from 3500 to 4500 rads [52–55, 65, 80]. We deliver 4000 rads at 150 rads per fraction, 5 days a week, for supradiaphragmatic presentations and follow this with cone-down fields to raise involved sites to 4500 rads. For subdiaphragmatic presentations, the mantle receives a prophylactic dose of 3500 rads in 23 or 24 fractions.

The classic subdiaphragmatic portal for Hodgkin's disease is the 'inverted Y' [82], which covers the axial para-aortic nodes, the spleen or splenic pedicle and the nodes of the pelvic brim including inguinal, in one large field. However, a number of different techniques are used by many authorities. The use of a separate para-aortic splenic pedicle portal followed by pelvic irradiation, if indicated, is an increasingly common approach [52, 57, 65, 79]. A typical para-aortic field is illustrated in Figure 7. In planning this portal a bipedal lymphangiogram and an IVP are essential; abdominal CT scanning may add additional information. As a rule, the lateral margins are drawn to include the widest lumbar transverse process, usually L3. The splenic pedicle is localized by surgical clips and the spleen, if present, can be delineated by radionuclide or CT scanning. An appropriate gap is calculated for the mantle–para-aortic interface and the lower border is typically placed at the L4-5 junction. This field may require modification under certain conditions. If there is subdiaphramatic disease then assurance of adequate coverage requires careful evaluation of the lymphangiogram, IVP, abdominal CT scan and preferably laparotomoy. Involvement of the porta hepatic nodes requires lateral extension of the right field border in the upper lumbar region. The pelvic filed is placed to include the common and external iliac nodes and is extended down to include both inguinal and femoral regions below the inguinal ligaments. The central pelvic nodes and those in the presacral region are low risk areas and the bladder and rectum can be safely shielded, reducing testicular and ovarian irradiation – the ovaries having been moved medially to lie under the block or laterally to lie outside the field during staging laparotomy. In the absence of oophoropexy, the ovaries will be in the primary radiation field.

A number of variations in abdominal field design have been reported. The 'extended mantle' [80] is designed to cover in one field all the high risk nodal sites from the upper neck down to the lower para-aortic region. This is said to have the advantages of firstly avoiding a gap in regions where disease may be present and where the spinal cord may be overdosed, and secondly of assuring coverage to all likely involved sites from the very first day of treatment [87, 88]. However, there seems to be a significant acute morbidity with this large field [80]. The Stanford group have explored a thin liver block technique for patients with splenic disease, staged II or III. Here, in addition to the standard inverted Y, the upper end of the field is enlarged to include the liver beneath attenuating blocks to deliver prophylactic irradiation. The M.D. Anderson group, on the other hand, favor irradiation to the entire upper abdomen with one half value layer (HVL) of shielding over the liver anteriorily and 2 HVL over each kidney posteriorily [89, 90]. Whether these modifications produce significantly different results is unclear and for the present most investigators adhere to the inverted Y or some modification that confines irradiation to the axial lymphatics [40, 55, 65, 70, 79, 88].

The accurate implementation of any wide-field technique is strictly dependent on the use of megavoltage irradiation and while cobalt beams can certainly be used [57, 78], it is technically considerably simpler to employ linear accelerators in the range 4 to 10 MeV. The cobalt beam for a mantle, for instance, almost invariably requires the use of tissue compensators, boosting fields and other technical maneuvers [57], that are seldom necessary with linear accelerators. High energy beams beyond 6 MeV have the disadvantage that significant sparing of the first few centimeters of tissue occurs so that subcutaneous nodes may receive less than the prescribed dose. Bolus applied every other day allows for skin sparing while delivering the desired dose a few millimeters below the epidermis. Whatever beam is actually used, dose calculations for irregular fields using exact methods must be done for each patient. Rules of thumb and approximations are inadequate; often in retrospect regions of significant under or overdosing are found [52, 62, 83]. A general method for performing these calculations has been published [83]. Finally, no matter how careful the planning, errors in daily set-up are not rare [52, 66, 68]. The frequency with which verification port films are taken varies, some institutions doing this daily [52]. We regard two beam films per week as adequate for the case which shows no significant variation. Where reproduction of the set-up appears fragile it is best to replan the whole procedure.

1.3. Radiation in Early Stages of Hodgkin's Disease: I and II

1.3.1. Pathologic Stages IA and IIA. With the availability of toxicologically feasible tumoricidal doses that assure high control rates for localized deposits of Hodgkin's disease, the radiation oncologist is required to define, in each patient, the optimal volume needing irradiation to achieve a high cure rate with acceptably low complication risks. In terms of our 'radical radiation therapy equation' this problem can be reformulated thus: utilizing a dose that assures a high local control probability (P_{LC}), we must delineate that volume having the highest reasonable likelihood of containing all disease, macroscopic and microscopic (P_{DF}), realizing that as volume increases, so do radiation complications. Just as we accept a certain low risk of local failure, so also we must accept some risk of beyond-field failures. To irradiate all early-stage patients with the widest possible fields to the highest possible doses, in the hope of eliminating every possible relapse is not only forbiddingly toxic and doomed to failure, but is totally irrational in an era where salvage chemotherapy is proving increasingly effective. On the other hand, we do not concur with radiation techniques that leave large numbers of failures in the hope that chemotherapy will salvage these. Quite apart from the fact that survival rates of patients failing initial therapy are not yet equal to those of the previously treated group [91–93], the psychologic effects of any relapse can be devastating. Whatever radiation shields are used, the likelihood that all disease will be encompassed by any given field, increases as the extensiveness of staging workup intensifies. In laparotomy-negative patients the results of various radiation therapy techniques can be most unequivocally analyzed and inferences made regarding optimal treatment for less intensively staged patients.

In analyzing the results of radical radiation treatment, it is essential to present the patterns of failure in Hodgkin's disease according to some consistent classification scheme, to facilitate the development of appropriate corrective therapeutic measures [17, 55]. There is no universally agreed-upon terminology, but we use a modification of that initially proposed by Kaplan [25]. Table 2 defines various terms as we employ them and though the categories may appear clear and distinct, it is not always easy to separate the true recurrence from an extension or a prophylaxis failure. The 'marginal recurrence' is variously defined by different authors [63, 68]; we regard it as essentially an extension. Some extranodal relapses, notably in the lung, have characteristics of regional contiguity spread rather than hematogenous dissemination.

Two patterns of relapse are unquestionably amenable to potential elimination by radiation therapy: the regional relapse and the transdiaphragmatic nodal failure (TDNF). Recognition of this fact has played the major role in developing the currently standard radiation portals for early-stage Hodgkin's disease. The effectiveness of prophylactic irradiation in reducing regional relapse was documented by Peters in 1950 [11] and 1958 [12] and by Kaplan in 1962 [13]. Since then a number of reports on clinically or lymphangiographically (LAG) staged I and II patients have revealed a substantial incidence of regional relapse when prophylactic regional radiation was not employed and a dramatic reduction in this failure pattern when extended fields were employed [16, 34, 94–96]. For example, one study shows a 28% initial regional relapse rate in 18 clinical stage (CS) I and II patients receiving the

Table 2. Classification of patterns of failure in Hodgkin's disease.

RELAPSE: Any reappearance of disease following treatment.
REGIONAL RELAPSE: Relapse within lymph node regions on the same side of the diaphragm;
    (i) True recurrence: relapse within an irradiated, initially involved lymph node region.
    (ii) Prophylaxis failure: relapse within a prophylactically irradiated regional site.
    (iii) Extension: regional relapse in a site not irradiated.
TRANSDIAPHRAGMATIC NODAL FAILURE (TDNF): Relapse within an initially negative lymph node region on the opposite side of the diaphragm (may be prophylaxis failure).
EXTRANODAL RELAPSE: Relapse in viscera such as lung, liver, bone marrow, or bone.

Table 3. Regional relapse rates in PS IA and IIA Hodgkin's disease treated by IF or EF radiation.

Technique *	Patients	Total number relapsed	Regional relapse only	Investigators
IF	15	6	4	Chan *et al.*, 1976 ** [95]
IF	19	4	2	
M/STN	17	0	0	Miller *et al.*, 1976 *** [96]
IF	21	10	7	
M/STN	12	2	0	Fuller *et al.*, 1980 † [47]

*   IF: Involved field; M/STN: Mantle or subtotal nodal.
**   Median follow-up <2 years.
*** Median follow-up 53 months.
†   5-year follow-up, non-mediastinal cases only.
13/55 (24%) IF had regional relapse as sole failure.
0/17 EF had regional relapse as sole failure.
Table 6 indicates in a large series that 20/242 (8%)
PS IA/IIA had regional relapse with EF and long follow-up.

mantle field [16]. A much larger study [94], though with a short median follow-up of 27 months, reported 38 regional relapses in 224 CS I and II patients randomly assigned to IF therapy, compared to only two regional failures in 243 patients randomized to receive at least a mantle field. Although laparaotomy staging seems unlikely, *a priori,* to influence regional supradiaphragmatic relapse patterns, there may be some confounding of the issue by potential reseeding from unrecognized initial para-aortic disease in CS or LAG.staged patients. Moreover, in these earlier studies, asymptomatic (A) patients were not separated from symptomatic (B) patients [16, 93, 94]. A more decisive demonstration of the superiority of regional prophylactic treatment is found in pathologically staged (PS) IA and IIA patients treated either by IF or mantle therapy. Table 3 is a summary of some recently reported regional relapse rates in PSIA and IIA Hodgkin's disease treated with IF or at least a mantle. Regional relapses are common following IF therapy, occurring in about 1/4 of these patients. Regional prophylactic irradiation reduces this hazard substantially. Similar findings were reported in the randomized Stanford trial comparing IF and TNI in PS IA and IIA patients [35, 39]. As we shall review later, the regional supradiaphragmatic relapse rate in PSIA and IIA cases receiving at least a mantle field and followed for many years, is less than 10%.

It has been suggested that there may be some PS IA patients who do not require irradiation beyond the region involved to achieve high FFR rates [46, 47, 51, 97, 98]. The high cervical or solitary inguinal presentation are most often said to belong to this favorable group. These two subgroups account for less than 17% of all PS IA and IIA patients [20, 36, 47, 96], a small subset that makes significant evaluations of different approaches difficult. Early reports on the high cervical presentation indicated a favorable outcome with IF therapy, providing that this histologic subtype was either lymphocyte predominant (LP) or mixed cellularity (MC) [21, 51, 53, 59, 97, 99]. Nodular sclerosis (NS) disease in this location appeared relatively unfavorable with a strangely high propensity to TDNF [46, 93, 97, 99]. Thus one study on CS IA high cervical presentations reported that 21 of 24 patients (88%) receiving 'IF' therapy remained disease-free with follow-up of more than 5 years in most [51]. More than 3/4 of these patients had LP or mixed cellularity (MC) histologies, but two of the three relapsing patients had NS disease. All three relapses were TDNF. In fact, about half of all the high cervical presentations this series did *not* receive true IF treatment, prophylaxis having been given to the mediastinum [51]. Another study reports an FFR of about 75% in LP high cervical cases receiving IF therapy [59] – this is not an especially good result for IA, LP Hodgkin's disease. The E.O.R.T.C. trial in CS I and II patients could find no prognostic basis for distinguishing the upper cervical presentation [93], noting the high preponderance of LP and MC subtypes and the tendency to TDNF. The fact that mediastinal irradiation was employed allows no conclusions to be reached on the true propensity for regional relapse. Recent studies on laparotomy-staged IA high cervical presentations shed little light on the question of optimal radiation fields [47, 96, 100]. One recent report included two upper cervical presentations in PS IA treated by IF, with one recurring in the ipsilateral and contralateral neck [95]. There is also a significant risk of failure in the ipsilateral parotid nodes estimated to approach 10% if prophylactic irradiation is not given to that region [55, 68]. In the absence of firm evidence to the contrary, it appears that irradiation to the mantle and parotid region remains the treatment of choice for the high cervical presentation.

The solitary inguinal or iliac presentation is even rarer than the high cervical pattern. In the pre-laparotomy era, lower torso presentations of Hodgkin's disease were unfavorable [93, 97], but laparotomy-staged patients have a prognosis no different to corresponding supradiaphragmatic stages [47, 101]. One recent study reports that of six patients with PS IA inguinal or iliac involvement, none relapsed following IF *or* inverted Y treatment and it was suggested that IF fields may be adequate [47, 90]. This is a small number of cases on which to base any treatment recommendation and in the face of the generally true contiguous spread pattern of Hodgkin's disease, it seems prudent to utilize the inverted Y as the minimal subdiaphragmatic field in these cases.

In summary, it remains the consensus of available evidence, that *for laparotomy-staged patients the minimal regional fields for Hodgkin's disease are the mantle for supradiaphragmatic irradiation and the inverted Y for subdiaphragmatic presentations.*

The occurrence of occult para-aortic node involvement in Hodgkin's disease has been recognized for decades and, as we have indicated, Gilbert considered it essential to irradiate these nodes in all patients whose systemic symptoms had not resolved following full supradiaphragmatic treatment, even in the absence of unequivocal demonstration of disease below the diaphragm [2]. In 1962 when the first Stanford trials in Hodgkin's disease were launched, the prevailing view was that mediastinal nodes were contiguous with those in the upper para-aortic region. Accordingly for Stages I and II, the 'extended field' in mediastinal cases included the para-aortic region, but in non-mediastinal presentations a mantle was regarded as adequate [55]. The success of this approach seemed even more assured by the use of bipedal lymphangiography as a staging procedure. However, by 1966 [14] and more so by 1968 [18] it was clear that contiguity needed redefinition and the concept of retrograde transdiaphragmatic spread was introduced [34, 41]. This TDNF following mantle irradiation of CS or LAG-staged I and II patients was soon confirmed by a number of investigators [16, 17, 46, 53, 59]. The reported incidence of this relapse pattern under these circumstances varied from 17% to 50% of all I and II patients [16, 17, 41, 59, 94], the variations probably reflecting different frequencies in the use of the lymphangiogram both in staging and in follow-up and differences in the duration of follow-up.

The TDNF has a number of unique features that require emphasis. Perhaps the most remarkable feature is the conversion of a previously normal LAG to a distinctly abnormal one, occasionally after many years of apparent freedom from disease. Not uncommonly, several follow-up LAGs performed over some years after mantle irradiation remain normal, only to convert to a distinctly abnormal pattern at later date [41]. This evolution from occult to gross suggested to Kaplan [18, 102] a retrograde spread mechanism from initially involved left supraclavicular nodes to the upper para-aortics via the thoracic duct. An alternative hematogenous spread concept was favored by others [103] and more recently the spleen has been implicated as the first subdiaphragmatic site generally involved [87]. Whatever the exact mechanism, the TDNF is characterized by a relative delay in manifestation [41, 59]. Whereas 80% of relapses in Hodgkin's disease are evident by 2 years following treatment with very few first failures beyond 5 years [47, 55, 59, 60, 65], the TDNF is evident in only 2/3 of those destined to have it by 2 years and up to 13% will develop it after 5 years [41, 59]. We have seen this failure occur 16 years after apparently successful mantle irradiation. Another important feature of the TDNF is its poor outcome when managed by radiation alone. Although it is quite easy to encompass this relapse by an inverted-Y field in most patients, very few achieve long-term control following radiation alone. Two series treating a total of 45 TDNF patients with subdiaphragmatic irradiation could report long-term control in only seven (13%) [17, 29, 41]. The majority of the 45 patients either disseminated to extranodal sites or reseeded into previously irradiated lymphatic regions and required chemotherapy. The addition of MOPP to radiation achieves a 50–60% 5-year salvage [41, 91]. Clearly, the TDNF is better prevented than treated.

TDNF might be prevented by more intensive staging employing laparotomy or by routinely irradiating the axial lymphatics below the diaphragm or by doing both. Although laparotomy detects occult abdominal disease in about 1/3 of LAG-stage IA and IIA patients [20, 22, 36, 37, 55], it cannot be relied upon to exclude microscopic disease in all abdominally negative patients. The true incidence of a false negative laparotomy in IA and IIA patients will depend on the actual lymph node sampling technique and some abdominal sites such as the peripancreatic and high lumbar regions are not easy to evaluate even by laparotomy [37]. Unequivocal data on the false negative laparotomy are difficult to cull from the literature, but many authors have reported significant TDNF rates following supradiaphragmatic irradiation only, in PSIA and IIA [40, 47, 59, 94, 96]. In their classic review of the TDNF, the Stanford Group [41] reported that out of 40 TDNFs, seven had initial negative laparotomies. Stoffel and Cox [59] report that laparotomy did not reduce the incidence of TDNF in their patients treated with supradiaphragmatic ports and the Royal Marsden Hospital Group decided to include the para-aortic region in their fields in laparotomy negative patients, following a 'small proportion' of relapses in this area [40]. More recently, the M.D. Anderson Group report three TDNF in 25 (12%) PSIA and IIA patients who had no mediastinal disease at diagnosis [47]. These investigators again re-affirmed the difficulty of salvage of this pattern of failure. On the other hand, whether laparotomy is employed or not, prophylactic irradiation below the diaphragm virtually eliminates the TDNF. In the University of Rochester series [17]there was no TDNF in 50 clinically or lymphangiographically staged I and II patients who received TNI, compared to a 40% incidence (33/83) in a similar group given only mantle therapy. The Stanford Group report seven TDNF in 272 stage I and II patients (about 1/3 were LAP-staged) (2.5% incidence) receiving prophylactic para-aortic irradiation, compared to 33 TDNF in 134 similar patients (25% incidence) receiving no infradiaphragmatic treatment [41]. The negligible incidence of this failure pattern has also been clearly demonstrated in PSIA and IIA patients treated with STN irradiation [60, 64, 65, 104, 105]. Finally, we find no firm evidence that any subgroup of PSIA and IIA can safely avoid TDNF without prophylactic para-aortic irradiation; the TDNF in high cervical presentations has already been noted.

Considerations such as the above have led many radiation oncologists to

Table 4. Results of extended field radiation therapy in PS IA and IIA Hodgkin's disease.

Patients	Technique *	FFR (5 year)	Survival (5 year)	Investigators
111	STN	85%	95%	Mauch *et al.*, 1978 [60]
41	STN	81%	91%	Mintz *et al.*, 1979 [64]
131	STN	77%	95%	Prosnitz *et al.*, 1980 [65]
199	TNI/STN	78%	95%	Hoppe, 1980 [104]
482	TNI/STN	77–85%	>90%	

* STN: Subtotal nodal irradiation (mantle + para-aortics).
* TNI: Total nodal irradiation (mantle + inverted Y).

consider either TNI or STN irradiation as the optimal treatment for PSIA and IIA Hodgkin's disease [40, 64, 65, 79, 104]. In reviewing the results achieved with this approach, the freedom-from-relapse (FFR) and survival at 5 years in four recent series of PSIA and IIA patients treated by STN or TNI is summarized in Table 4 [60, 64, 65, 104]. The 482 patients treated in four centers achieved FFR of 77–85% at 5 years and salvage therapy increased the overall survival to more than 90%. FFR projected beyond 5 years drops by only a few percentage points [55, 65, 104]. Clearly in a disease with as long a natural history as Hodgkin's, many more years of follow-up will be needed to give a final verdict on cure rates but in the meantime we can conclude that radiation to extended fields is a highly effective modality in at least 3/4 of PSIA and IIA Hodgkin's patients. As Table 5 demonstrates, the likelihood of pelvic node extension in supradiaphragmatic PSIA and IIA patients receiving mantle and para-aortic irradiation is less than 5% and does not justify the use of prophylactic pelvic fields in such cases [105]. However, up to 1/4 of PSIA and IIA Hodgkin's disease patients will relapse following STN irradiation – a fact in need of analysis, explanation and prevention. We will first consider the patterns of relapse and prognostic factors in this patient group.

Table 5. Incidence of pelvic extension as a first site of relapse in PS IA and IIA Hodgkin's disease treated by STN irradiation.

Patients	Pelvic relapse	Investigators
86	4 (5%)	Weller *et al.*, 1977 [41]
111	0	Mauch *et al.*, 1978 [60]
131	5 (4%)	Prosnitz *et al.*, 1980 [65]
328	9 (3%)	

Table 6. Relapse patterns in PS IA and IIA Hodgkin's disease treated with STN irradiation.

Patients	Relapses	Supradiaphragmatic * relapse only	Other ** relapse sites	Investigators
111	14	14	0	Mauch *et al.*, 1978 [60]
131	26	16	10	Prosnitz *et al.*, 1980 [65]
242	40	30	10	

* 11/30 had more than one supradiaphragmatic site: lung 12; axilla 8; mediastinum 7; neck 3; hilum 2; other nodal sites 3.
** Pelvic nodes 5; liver 2; bone marrow 1; brain 1; skin 1.

1.3.2. Patterns of Relapse and Prognostic Factors in PSIA and IIA. Two recent reports on a total of 242 PSIA and IIA patients treated with STN irradiation provide details on relapse patterns [60, 65]: Table 6 shows the observed relapse patterns. The majority of the relapses were above the diaphragm in what might be regarded as 'mantle territory' and the lung emerges as an especially common site for relapse, occurring in 12 of the 40 relapsing patients (30%). Similar relapse patterns have been recorded by a number of investigators over the past 5 years. Levi and co-workers [63] reported 11 relapses of 40 PSIA and IIA patients and noted 8/11 (73%) above the diaphragm only, with lung being the single commonest site. Thar and co-workers [69] reported that 11/16 failures in CSI and II patients were surpadiaphragmatic with lung or pleura accounting for five. The M.D. Anderson results on PSIIA and IIB mediastinal presentations reveal that following irradiation (mostly STN) 15 of 16 patients failing did so above the diaphragm only and lung was a relapse site in 11 patients [47]. The Stanford Group has also reported a predominantly supradiaphragmatic relapse pattern in PSI and II patients receiving TNI or STN radiation [48]. Lung relapse in the vast majority of cases having this failure pattern takes the form of single or multiple, unilateral or bilateral peripheral nodules [47, 60, 106]. Thus, of a total of 21 lung relapses reported in two recent series [47, 106], 19 had a peripheral nodular pattern, suggesting either lymphogenous or hematogenous spread rather than direct tissue invasion.

The rather well-defined regular types of relapse observed in PSIA and IIA patients receiving STN radiation have prompted a search for prognostic factors to allow recognition of high risk cases prior to institution of treatment. A number of classic prognostic indices delineated in non-Laparotomy staged patients have faded and largely lost their relevance in PSIA and IIA Hodgkin's disease. Sex, an important factor favoring females in the pre-laparotomy era [38, 46, 51, 93, 99], has no relevance in PSIA and IIA patients [47, 48, 55, 60, 65]. Certain patterns of presentation such as the axillary, the stage II non-mediastinal, the multiple small node type and the subdiaphragmatic early stage – all associated with a relatively poorer prognosis in CSI and II patients [21, 46, 51, 97, 99, 107, 108] – are no longer demonstrably adverse in recent series. Histology, the single most important factor just one decade ago, has lost significance in PSIA and IIA [47, 48, 65, 79, 90, 102]. However, a number of potentially significant prognostic factors have been identified in recent years for PSIA and IIA patients: number of nodal regions involved [40, 68, 69]; mediastinal status [47, 48, 60, 65, 68, 69, 76, 109]; and limited extranodal (E stage) disease [63, 110]. It should be understood that the major correlation between these prognostic factors and subsequent outcome refers almost solely to the likelihood of supradiaphragmatic relapse, including lung failure. The low incidence of TDNF and non-pulmonary extranodal relapse precludes the definition of any meaningful relation between this type of relapse and pre-treatment features in these early patients treated with STN.

The influence of the number of initially involved lymphatic sites on prognosis has been recognized in a broad sense since the reports by Peters in the 1950s which revealed a better survival in stage I (58% at 10 years) than in stage II (35% at 10 years), stage I being defined as 'involvement of a single site or lymphatic region' and stage II as involvement of 2 or 3 proximal lymphatic regions' [12]. The Ann Arbor system also recognizes this and the committee authoring that system gave, as an optional recommendation, the use of a subscript to indicate the number of node regions involved in stage II [111]. Most recent reports combine the PSIA and PSIIA cases into one group (PSIA/IIA), and some reports show no difference in FFR following STN radiation in the two stages [48]. However, there does seem to be enough evidence to say that post-radiation relapses are substantially less frequent in PSIA than in PSIIA (Table 7). Indeed, relapse in PSIA is extremely rare and one study achieved FFR at 5 years in 97% of such patients given STN irradiation [60]. PSIIA, on the other hand, is a heterogeneous group with regard to extent of disease. There are 12 major anatomic lymph node regions above the diaphragm: Waldeyer's ring, preauricular (two), cervical-supraclavicular (two), axillary (two), epitrochlear (two), mediastinal (one), hilar

Table 7. Incidence of relapse in PS IA versus PS IIA treated by STN irradiation *.

	Ref. [40]	Ref. [63]	Ref. [60]	Ref. [64]	Total
IA	1/14	0/8	1/35	1/13	3/70 (4%)
IIA	5/25	11/32	13/76	10/43	39/176 (22%)

* Duration of follow-up variable, but similar for IA and IIA within any one series.

(two), not including the internal mammary or pericardial nodes. There is a corresponding diversity in the extent of supradiaphragmatic Hodgkin's disease in PSIIA patients, and a number of authors have emphasized the prognostic significance of this variable [52, 60, 68, 69]. In 1975, the Royal Marsden Hospital results showed that no patients with PSIIA having two or three regions initially involved relapsed, while 5/7 PSIIA cases with more than three sites relapsed [40]. Thar and coworkers [69] report a very significantly rising risk of supradiaphragmatic failure as the number of involved sites increases: for two involved sites surpadiaphragmatic failure occurred in 2/14 patients (14%), with three to four sites such failure occurred in 5/15 (33%) and with five or more sites 4/6 failed. In a much larger series, though mostly LAG-staged and including stages I to IIIB, the Stanford Group revealed a linearly increasing risk of supradiaphragmatic failure as the number of involved sites above the diaphragm increased. going from no relapses for one involved region to 60% relapse for nine involved sites [68].

A number of mechanisms underlie the increasing risk for regional relapse as extent of disease advances. We have already discussed the stochastic nature of the radiation-response curve and shown that this alone will account for a higher relapse rate as the number of involved sites rises (section 1.1). Furthermore, the need to protect critical normal tissues while yet assuring adequate coverage to each of several macroscopically involved sites creates a circumstance where marginal misses are more likely. Finally, adverse biologic factors associated with widespread regional disease will also contribute to proximal failure. Thus, accepting contiguous lymphatic spread as valid, numerous sites of involvement imply extensive lymphatic permeation even to areas usually not irradiated such as pulmonary parenchyma.

With regard to subcategorizing patients, the apparently linear nature of the relation between relapse probability and number of involved sites in IIA Hodgkin's disease, precludes any sharp demarcation between 'favorable' and 'unfavorable' using this criterion alone. In making any subgroup of patients 'unfavorable' with the implication that this requires more intensive treatment, one must balance the degree of unfavorability and the probability of salvage against the toxicity and potential efficacy of the new treatment program. We will take up this problem in a later section and only note here that PSIIA with two regions involved, other things being equal, would have to be regarded as very favorable, with relapses occurring in fewer than 15% following radiation alone.

The mediastinum has been a region of interest to students of Hodgkin's disease for almost half a century both in terms of etiology-pathogenesis and of prognosis. During the 1940s and 1950s the idea that Hodgkin's disease had a thymic histogenesis was explored by several investigators, with Ewing [112] favoring the view that the sarcomatous variant arose in thymic epithelial cells and Thompson [113] postulating a universal thymic origin with ectopic thymic tissue in the cervical region accounting for primary neoplasms in the neck. Autopsy studies soon disclosed a substantial fraction of patients having no evidence of thymic involvement and a surgical series found that 19 of 40 early stage mediastinal patients had no thymic disease [114]. More recently, etiologic theories implicating the thymic lymphocyte have been elaborated [55]. The prognostic significance of mediastinal disease was first recognized in 1966 by a group of French workers who observed that among long-term survivors, a large proportion had initial mediastinal disease [93]. This idea was further developed by Peters [21, 46, 97] who reported median survivals of 16–17 years for stage II patients with mediastinal disease, compared to 2.5–7.5 years median survival for all other stage II cases [21]. A similarly favorable outlook for the mediastinal case was reported by the M.D. Anderson Group [99, 107]. With the recognition of a relation between mediastinal disease and nodular sclerosis (NS) histology, a number of workers addressed the question of whether the favorable outcome of mediastinal cases was entirely due to this relatively favorable, slowly progressing histologic subtype. It appears that site, in its own right and quite independent of histology, was significant. Peters [21, 46, 97] found that NS in peripheral sites, such as axilla or mid to upper neck, without mediastinal involvement was unfavorable. The E.O.R.T.C. study reported a favorable outcome for mixed cellularity (MC) with mediastinal involvement. In this study a total of 274 CSI and II patients received mantle radiation and, with a short period of follow-up, 27 (10%) experienced TDNF [61, 93]. In those with mediastinal disease, a 5% incidence (5/101) of TDNF was observed; in those without mediastinal disease, a 13% incidence (22/173) was found. In MC histologies, those with mediastinal disease had only 4% TDNF (1/24) compared to 23% (15/66) without mediastinal disease. The subsequent introduction of staging laparotomy has confirmed the expected lower incidence of occult para-aortic and splenic disease in mediastinal presentations [36, 90], but there is no clear explanation for the apparent protective effect against infradiaphragmatic spread which mediastinal involvement provides.

The elimination of TDNF by staging laparotomy and prophylactic subdiaphragmatic irradiation has resulted in a most dramatic reversal of the implications of mediastinal disease in PSIA and IIA patients. Table 8 summarizes the incidence of mediastinal involvement in early stage Hodgkin's disease. Approximately 2/3 of stage II patients have disease within the mediastinum; mediastinal involvement as the sole site of disease (PSIA) is relatively uncommon. Hilar lymphadenopathy occurs in about 30% of mediastinal cases but is exceptionally uncommon with a normal mediastinum. The anatomic sites of nodal disease within the mediastinum are predominantly the anterior superior nodal groups, the paratracheal nodes

Table 8. The incidence of mediastinal and hilar disease in PS IIA Hodgkin's disease.

Patients	Mediastinum involved *	Hilum involved **	Investigators
76	50 (66%)	14	Mauch *et al.,* 1978 [60]
85	56 (66%)	15	Prosnitz *et al.,* 1980 [65]
66	42 (64%)	14	Fuller *et al.,* 1980 [47]
227	148 (65%)	43	

* ( ) percentage of all PS IIA patients.
** Hilar disease without involved mediastinum exceptionally rare 110 PS IA patients in same series had mediastinal disease in 17 (15%).

and the superior tracheobranchial nodes [115]. Much less frequently involved are the subcarinal, the lower posterior, the paracardiac and the internal mammary groups. More than 3/4 of mediastinal cases have NS histology and of all patients with this histology about 3/4 have mediastinal disease [46, 47, 60, 108].

Relapses in PSIA and IIA disease are now relatively uncommon and differences in relapse rates among various subgroups often do not reach statistical signficance in individual reports. Moreover, direct comparisons between apparently similar patients groups treated in different institutions may not always be valid. Nevertheless, it is difficult to dismiss as spurious the numerous observations on the untoward prognostic implication of

Table 9. Incidence and pattern of relapse according to mediastinal status in PS IA and IIA Hodgkin's disease treated with STN irradiation.

Incidence of Relapse According to Mediastinal Status		
Mediastinum negative	Mediastinum positive	
1/51	13/60	Mauch *et al.,* 1978 [60]
10/69	13/62	Prosnitz *et al.,* 1980 [65]
11/120 (9%)	29/122 (24%)	

Incidence of Relapse According to Bulk of Mediastinum		
Mass Absent or <1/3 *	Mass >1/3 *	
5/84	9/18	Mauch *et al.,* 1978 [60]
17/107	9/24	Prosnitz *et al.,* 1980 [65]
22/191 (12%)	18/42 (43%)	

* 1/3 of maximal chest width

mediastinal involvement, especially the bulky lymphadenopathy in PSIA and IIA. Even before the routine use of laparotomy, a relation between mediastinal involvement and subsequent lung relapse was noted [34, 107, 116]. Two series reporting a total of 35 patients developing lung relapse indicated that the mediastinum was involved in 30 of these at diagnosis [34, 116]. Later, a Stanford report showed that only 18/271 (7%) patients with minimal mediastinal disease sustained intrathoracic relapse, while 25/106 (24%) patients with bulky mediastinal disease had an intrathoracic failure [68]. Two recent reports on PSIA and IIA patients treated with STN radiation specifically address the question of relapse versus mediastinal disease [60, 65] and the patterns of relapse are given in Table 6. Table 9 presents the relapses according to mediastinal status. Clearly. there appears to be an increase in relapse rate with mediastinal involvement and for bulky disease, measuring more than 1/3 of the of the maximal chest width on chest X-ray, failures occur in 38–50%. As shown in Table 6, the majority of relapses were in supradiaphragmatic structures with lung being the single most common site. The M.D. Anderson report [47] on PSIA and IIA disease treated by a variety of radiation techniques also revealed a high pulmonary relapse rate among those with mediastinal disease. Of 33 PSIA and IIA patients without mediastinal disease, none sustained pulmonary relapse, while seven of 34 (21%) with mediastinal disease relapsed in lung. In this latter group the likelihood of lung relapse was greater in those with large (greater than 7.5 cm) mediastinal disease (6/17 failed in the lung). Two other papers describe a similar relapse pattern [69, 109] and a recent Stanford report [48] revealed a significantly worse FFR in patients with large mediastinal disease (39% FFR at 5 years). Finally, Table 10 summarizes the incidence of lung relapse in three series according to mediastinal status. With an initially negative mediastinum, the likelihood of pulmonary relapse is very small; with mediastinal disease pulmonary failures occur in about 17%

Table 10. The incidence of pulmonary relapse in early stages of Hodgkin's disease according to mediastinal status. All patients received radiation therapy without prophylactic lung irradiation.

Stage	Mediastinum negative	Mediastinum positive	Investigators
CS I and II	2/54 (4%)	16/37 (22%)	Peckham, 1973 [116]
PS IA and IIA	2/69 (3%)	6/62 (10%)	Prosnitz *et al.*, 1980 [65]
PS IA and IIA	0/33	7/34 (21%)	Fuller *et al.*, 1980 [47]
	4/153 (2.6%)	29/169 (17%)	

of early cases treated with STN radiation. More than 80% of pulmonary failures have NS histology [47, 116]. The role of hilar node involvement, as distinct from mediastinal disease, in predisposing to lung relapse in unclear [47, 60, 65, 68, 85, 86] and there are no firm data on which to base definitive conclusions. Some radiation oncologists prefer to give prophylactic radiation to lungs having radiologic evidence of hilar disease [60, 68], others do not [47, 65].

If we consider just those PSIA and IIA patients who have either no mediastinal disease or a mass less than 1/3 chest width, then following STN irradiation alone, this group which accounts for over 80% [60] of early cases achieves long-term FFR in more than 90% [60]. We are then left with a small subgroup, less than 20% of PSIA and IIA, which is distinctly unfavorable when irradiated with STN fields alone, experiencing a relapse rate in excess of 40% (Table 9). The relapses tend to be confined to supradiaphragmatic structures with lung being the single most common site. The pulmonary relapses occur either as peripheral nodular opacities – the most common pattern [106] – or as direct extensions from recurrent mediastinal nodes [116]. These lung failures probably represent retrograde lymphatic spread from mediastinal structures.

The role of limited extranodal spread – the E stage – in limiting the results of regional radiation has been controversial. Following the report by Musshoff in 1971 that the transgression of a mediastinal node capsule by Hodgkin's disease with limited direct lung involvement did not adversely influence prognosis for localized presentations receiving regional radiation [117], the Ann Arbor system introduced the E concept [111]. Since then the majority of reports on PSIA and IIA with limited extranodal pulmonary disease (IEA or IIEA) have not found this to be an adverse factor [64, 65, 79, 93, 102, 104]. There is, however, a logically necessary relation in most cases between IIEA and mediastinal disease and this correlation possibly accounts for the adverse influence of E stage reported by some workers [63, 110].

In summary, the major prognostic factor in PSIA and IIA Hodgkin's disease is mediastinal status. About 80% of these early-stage patients fall into a favorable group with either no mediastinal disease or lymphadenopathy smaller than 1/3 of the thoracic width. These patients enjoy an FFR at 5 years of about 90% when treated with STN radiation alone [48, 60]. Those with bulky mediastinal involvement fare rather badly with STN alone and 40–60% relapse mainly above the diaphragm and especially in the lung. Increasing numbers of involved lymph node regions above the diaphragm also decrease FFR, but the linear nature of this relation and the association between large mediastinal disease and more numerous sites of involvement [60], preclude a sharp definition of prognostic groups on this criterion alone. Finally, it is now established that PSIA and IIA subdiaphragmatic

Table 11. Relapse rates in PS IIB Hodgkin's disease following various radiation therapy techniques. Corresponding relapses in PS IIA are given for comparison.

Patients	Technique	Median follow-up Months	IIB Relapses	IIA Relapses	Investigators
9	STN	Not given	3/9 (33)	5/25 (20)	Peckham *et al.*, 1975 (40)
7	M/STN	>40	4/7 (57)	11/32 (34)	Levi *et al.*, 1977 [63]
11	STN/TNI	32	2/11 (18)	5/56 (9)	Goodman *et al.*, 1977 [74]
11	IF/M/TNI	>30	2/11 (18)	7/33 (21)	Mill *et al.*, 1977 [62]
6	IF/M/TNI	50	5/6 (83)	10/43 (32)	Mintz *et al.*, 1979 [64]
14	IF/M/TNI	>60	8/14 (57)	8/34 (24)	Fuller *et al.*, 1980 [47]
58			24/58 (41)	46/223 (21)	

( ) percentage

disease has a prognosis no different to that of corresponding supradiaphragmatic stages [47, 101].

The implications of these prognostic factors for therapeutic intervention will be considered after we review stages IB and IIB.

Pathologic Stages IB and IIB. Systemic symptoms are relatively uncommon in laparotomy-staged I and II patients. A review of seven recent series on PSI and II Hodgkin's disease [20, 40, 47, 62–64, 79] shows that of 612 PSI/II patients, 135 (22%) had systemic symptoms and only seven were PSIB (1%). Clearly, systemic symptoms in PSI occur with almost negligible frequency. About 1/4 of PSII cases are symptomatic. This small number of cases hampers any evaluation of treatment results and prognostic factors. A number of early reviews demonstrated the adverse influence of B symptoms on prognosis in CSI and II patients [12, 34, 46, 53, 61, 93, 97, 108], though perhaps surprisingly some investigators failed to find such a correlation [94, 99, 107]. The untoward influence of B symptoms was nowhere more dramatically displayed then in the first Stanford trial launched in 1962 [38]. Involved field therapy for CSIB and IIB patients produced a 2-year FFR in less than 20%, and this compared to the 70% FFR with mantle or TNI fields in B patients, led Kaplan to abandon the use of limited fields in these patients. Since then reports from a number of institutions have concluded that radiation alone is inadequate for early B-stage disease. However, the radiation techniques used appear to be surprisingly inadequate, as shown in Table 11. The Stanford group have continued to use TNI for PSIB and IIB and report 5-year FFR of 75% with overall survival fo 86% in 53 patients treated [104]. In 1980, they could find no difference between results for PSIB and IIB treated with TNI and PSIA and IIA given STN radiation [48]. In a randomized study, the addition of MOPP to TNI produced no FFR or survival advantage [118].

The patterns of relapse for PSIB and IIB patients receiving radiation have not been well defined, but there is some evidence that they correspond to those seen in PSIA and IIA. Fuller and co-workers [47] report that 8/13 mediastinal IIB patients relapsed following radiation therapy, five failing within the thorax, and lung was the most common relapse site. Lung relapses following radiation to mediastinal IIB disease were also reported by Peckham [116].

Evidently, the data on this group of patients are small and inconclusive, but there appears to be sufficient evidence to regard TNI as appropriate treatment and that the prognostic factors identified in PSIA and IIA in all likelihood also apply to the IIB group.

1.3.4. Therapeutic Challenges in Stages I and II. The demonstration of a high long-term FFR in patients with early Hodgkin's disease treated with modern megavoltage radiation techniques has set the stage for a systematic endeavor to optimize the whole management of these patients. In this process of optimization, a number of issues are involved related to both diagnosis and staging on the one hand, and therapeutic intervention on the other. The question of therapy cannot be totally isolated from problem of staging particularly with a volume restricted modality such as radiation, but as a point of departure we will begin with laparotomy staged patients and follow with such inferences as may be safely made regarding non-laparotomy cases.

The goal of treatment optimization is to achieve the highest cure probability with lowest complication risk. Following any therapeutic intervention, four categories of outcome are possible: I. FFR with no complication; II. FFR with complication; III. Relapse without therapy-related complications; and IV. Relapse with residual treatment complication. At a time when alternative therapies are emerging and when salvage treatment is proving increasingly effective, a clear distinction between these various categories of outcome is crucial. A category I result is the ideal, and even a category III outcome (relapse without complication) may ultimately be salvaged, but, depending on the nature of the residual toxicity, a category IV patient may be unsuitable for any serious salvage effort. Combined modalities even sequentially administered some time apart are often additive and sometimes supra-additive in their toxicities; their effect on Hodgkin's disease, when one modality is used for salvage, is at best non-additive and at worst antagonistic. It should be clear that many complications have a significance over and above any direct inconvenience to the patient – they may significantly compromise salvage, should relapse occur. However, it is impossible with any single modality to achieve a high success without some toxicity. What we desire is a high frequency of category I outcomes with only occasional category II results and few, if any, category IV cases. In principle, the administration of concerocidal therapy to a tumor alone, without exposure of normal tissue, would offer the highest likelihood for an uncomplicated cure. With any cytotoxic modality, the more normal tissue that is exposed, the higher the risk of toxicity; accordingly, we subscribe to the philosophy that purely local or regional disease is better treated with a local-regional modality, reserving systemic treatment for disseminated disease.

If we consider all PSI and II patients, without attempting any subcategorization according to prognostic factors, STN irradiation or TNI will produce prolonged FFR in more than 75% of the patients. The administration of chemotherapy in addition to radical radiation could be of no benefit to the 75% that are apparently cured by radiation alone and the long-term toxicity of such combined modality programs will not be fully defined without several decades of observation. Moreover, the 25%, or so that are destined to relapse following radiation cannot be guaranteed to avoid this fate by the addition of chemotherapy. As the Stanford trails on combined modality therapy show, the 8-year FFR for stage I and II patients receiving both modes is about 85% [118] – a gain of only 10 patients for every 100 given chemotherapy an adjunct to radiation. It seems a high price to pay to submit 100 people to an additional protracted and toxic therapy to benefit only 10, especially when an overall survival improvement cannot be shown [48, 60, 63, 65, 119]. What is at stake here is the well-known and theroretically appealing argument that a modality having significant effect against macroscopic disease should be even more effective against microscopic disease. Unappealing as it may seem, there is no evidence that this holds for the chemotherapy of stages I and II as a whole. To establish the validity of this theoretic concept one needs to demonstrate that freedom-from-*first*-relapse in a combined treatment arm is statistically superior to freedom-from-*second*-relapse in a radiation only arm, or to find a clear long-term survival advantage with combined modes. Data from the randomized Stanford trials [118, 119] show no such phenomena. Of course, it is possible that there are subgroups among early-stage patients within which such differences are observable, but it can hardly be construed that the universal administration of radical combined modes in early Hodgkin's disease is a step toward treatment optimization.

The alternative combined approach of reducing radiation volume with systemic therapy to compensate has been explored by a number of investigators [55, 63, 110, 118–120] with somewhat conflicting results. Where less than optimal volumes were irradiated in those receiving radiation only, significant improvement in both FFR and survival were shown in the combined approach group [63, 110, 118]. Studies employing optimal radiation fields (STN or TNI) in the radiation-only arm have revealed little, if any, advantage for FFR in the combined modality group, and no advantage in survival [55, 118, 119]. Any implication that involved-field therapy combined with chemotherapy may be less toxic than STN irradiation is unlikely to be true. The major toxicities of STN irradiation are related to the mantle field and will be reviewed later, but in brief, two recent reports clearly document the relative safety and complication-freedom of well-administered radiation therapy [65, 79]. Of a total of 340 patients receiving at least a mantle field, significant complications occurred in 29 (8.5%). In these 29 cases, spontaneous resolution occurred in nine and seven resolved after steroid therapy leaving only 16 patients (5%) with persistent problems, three of whom died. While IF radiation will reduce some of the complications of wide-field treatment, about 1/2 of these PSIA and IIA patients will need mediastinal and cervical radiation and would remain at significant risk for pulmonary and pericardial toxicity. Additionally, there is the problem of steroid withdrawal pericarditis and pneumonitis [121], the possibility of increased second malignancies, and the fact of sterility in most males and many females [122].

Finally, one might argue to delete radiation altogether and rely solely on chemotherapy in early-stage disease. The fact that 40–60% of advanced patients achieve long-term disease-free status following multiple agent chemotherapy [122–126] is a good theoretic argument for moving chemotherapy into earlier stages. It would require, however, the demonstration of considerably better cure rates than are currently achieved with radiation and chemotherapy salvage programs (in excess of 85% survival at 8 years), to justify the toxicity of this approach for regionalized disease. The program initiated by Ziegler in Ugandan children has revealed a 78% FFR (greater than 5-year median follow-up) among 18 IA-IIA cases treated with MOPP alone [127]. This relatively good result may to some extent reflect the fact that only three of these 18 children had NS disease, a subtype that occurs in about 60% of early-stage patients in the Western world [55, 128–130] and which has a tendency to relapse after chemotherapy.

The challenges to radiation therapy in early-stage disease outlined above are indeed based on genuine problems that the radiation oncologist must face. Optimally delivered radiation therapy does fail in about 1/4 of fully-staged early patients and radiation fields cannot be safely extended much beyond the standard TNI set-up. However, the patterns of relapse and associated prognostic factors delineate two groups of early patients, one having an extremely favorable outlook and the other destined to relapse in up to 1/2 of its patients. Both groups raise questions regarding optimal therapy.

The favorable group which includes PSI and II patients without bulky mediastinal disease and accounts for over 80% of all early cases, achieves FFR at 5 years in about 90% when treated with STN irradiation or TNI, and salvage of the few failures raises 5-year survival to greater than 95 % [48, 60]. There can be no justification for treatment intensification in this group and it is doubtful whether any malignancy intrinsically as dangerous as Hodgkin's disease can ever achieve results better than these. A more immediate question is whether the radiation dose and/or volume can be reduced without a significant compromise of the excellent results already achieved. One's immediate instinct would be to refrain from meddling with any treatment program as effective as that outlined, but in the quest for even further optimization, a number of possiblities need consideration. As already stated, we do not consider it established that there are clearly definable early-stage patients who can be safely treated with less than STN fields. However, a a number of authorities do hold that the unilateral upper neck case can be managed with sharply limited fields [46, 47, 51, 55, 98]. Similarly, the isolated inguinal or iliac presentation has also been claimed to do well with involved fields therapy [47]. Whether such approaches are indeed optimal remains to be seen. It is, however, doubtful that prophylactic para-aortic irradiation will be avoidable for the foreseeable future in the majority of early cases, since the TDNF continues to present .significant salvage problems [47].

An alternative to volume reduction may be dose decrease. It is possible that early-stage patients without bulky disease and with fewer than three or four involved regions may be safely treated with doses of 3500–4000 rads to involved sites as recently suggested by several investigators [27, 52, 54, 59, 69]. Prophylactic doses, too, might be reducible to 2500–3000 rads [52]. However, while such dose reductions are likely to reduce the incidence of complications, they would not be acceptable if control rates drop appreciably. Patient tolerance of currently employed STN techniques is superior to the MOPP regimen and it would be illogical to reduce the effectiveness of a well-tolerated treatment in lieu of salvage with a considerably more taxing schedule. The question of dose reduction will not be resolved until many more patients receiving this form of treatment have been reported.

A more significant radiotherapeutic challenge is posed by the early patient with bulky mediastinal adenopathy and/or multiple sites of involvement. This presentation comprises a small subset of PSI and II cases and the clearest adverse influence is related to mediastinal disease greater than 1/3 of the chest width. The high frequency of supradiapragmatic failure, in particular the lung relapse, suggest that the shielding employed in a typical mantle field may be excessive in this presentation. Salvage therapy for pulmonary relapses has proved to be difficult. The M.D. Anderson group report very few durable second remissions [47, 131] and the Stanford report suggests a borderline decrease in survival in this group [48].

A number of investigators have explored various techniques for prophylactic lung irradiation [60, 68, 86, 132], though only one preliminary report has specifically addressed the problem of whole-lung irradiation for large mediastinal disease [132]. There is little doubt that prophylactic irradiation does reduce lung relapse. Carmel and Kaplan [68] report five lung failures in 103 lungs (5%) judged to be at high risk and therefore given prophylactic irradiation; a smaller number of 35 high-risk lungs did not receive prophylaxis and three relapsed (8%). While not statistically significant, these differences were regarded as clinically important since the treated cases were those with the bulkier disease [68]. The report by Mauch and co-workers [60] reveals no lung relapse among 12 patients receiving pulmonary prophylaxis for mediastinal or hilar disease, while Fuller and co-workers [47], not employing lung prophylaxis, had pulmonary relapse in seven of 34 patients (21%) stages IA and IIA with mediastinal disease. Another report [132] also shows substantial reduction in pulmonary relapse in patients with bulky mediastinal disease receiving prophylactic whole-lung irradiation. Whether this approach achieves better overall FFR awaits further investigation, but the thin-lung-block-technique (TLBT) has proven to be safe [55, 68].

An alternative to lung irradiation may be the use of adjuvant chemotherapy [47, 48, 52, 76, 120]. This approach could have the potential for avoiding laparotomy, a potentially hazardous procedure for patients with large mediastinal masses [133]. However, the elimination of pulmonary relapse by this method seems to require full courses of chemotherapy. Two cycles of MOPP do not adequately reduce this pattern of relapse as the M.D. Anderson results on PSIII patients show: with a median follow-up of 45 months, six of 47 patients (13%) with large mediastinal disease treated with two MOPP cycles followed by radiation relapsed in the lung [77]. This same group of investigators also report that three cycles of MOPP are insufficient [77]. The SWOG trial on combined modalities for stage I and II shows that six MOPP cycles do substantially reduce pulmonary relapse inthis group of patients [120]. Similarly a recent Stanford report shows that the addition of intensive chemotherapy to radiation has a significant effect in diminishing relapses in this unfavorable group [48].

Which of the two approaches, whole-lung irradiation or adjuvant chemotherapy, is in fact optimal, awaits further study, but for the radiation oncologist it is worth remembering that thin lung block whole lung prophylaxis has produced encouraging results and in theory, at least, has some advantages over the combined approach: avoidance of sterility and a lessened chance of second malignancy.

Finally, we need to discuss the role of staging laparotomy and splenectomy, but since the arguments here depend strongly on the treatment options for PSIIIA disease, we will defer the discussion to the end of the next section.

1.4. The Intermediate Stage of Hodgkin's Disease: IIIA

1.4.1. Results of Radiation Thearpy in Pathologic Stage IIIA. No group of Hodgkin's disease patients has created more controversy regarding optimal therapy than the PS IIIA category with views ranging from radiation alone [55, 118, 134–136], through combined modalities [67, 70, 77, 137–139] to chemotherapy alone [126, 136, 140]. Among laparotomy series, PS III constitutes about 1/3 of all Hodgkin's cases [20, 22, 37, 55] and as shown in Table 12 about 2/3 of these are PS IIIA. Therefore, fewer than 25 % of all PS Hodgkin's patients fall into this group – a small number that has hampered statistical analysis.

Prior to the mid 1960s patients with disease on both sides of the diaphragm were regarded as essentially incurable and as suitable only for palliative treatment. The first curative attempt was launched in 1962 at Stanford, where a trial comparing low-dose palliation against high-dose TNI was launched [14]. Quite apart from demonstrating the toxicologic feasibility of the TNI plan, this study revealed a dramatic improvement for those receiving radical therapy. At 2 years the FFR for the palliative group was 20 % compared to a 50 % FFR among radically irradiated CS IIIA and B patients [38]. Accordingly, palliation was abandoned and a subsequent 5-year follow-up reported that 42 % of the TNI treated group were disease-free and 61 % were alive. Fifteen years later, 40 % of those patients initially receiving TNI are alive and disease-free [102]. As a token to the large-volume concept, it is worth noting that this group of CS III patients fared better than a simultaneous group of CS IB and IIB patients receiving IF therapy [38]. Soon however, it became evident that IIIB patients had an exceptionally poor outlook following radiation alone with 5-year FFR rates below 10 % [39], and with the advent of multi-agent chemotherapy, stage III

Table 12. Relative proportion of asymptomatic patients (IIIA) among laparotomy-proven stage III cases.

Total PS III	Number IIIA	Investigators
79	52 (66)	Kaplan *et al.,* 1973 [20]
46	31 (67)	Piro *et al.,* 1973 [22]
23	15 (65)	Stein *et al.,* 1978 [141]
51	34 (67)	Desser *et al.,* 1977 [87]
104	60 (58)	Rosenberg *et al.,* 1978 [118]
58	37 (64)	Mauch *et al.,* 1979 [70]
361	229 (63)	

( ) percentage.

Table 13. Results of radiation therapy on PS IIIA Hodgkin's disease.

Patients	Technique	FFR (5 year)	Survival (5 year)	Investigators
42	TNI	65%*	85%	B.N.L.I., 1976 [134]
48	TNI	35%	80%	Prosnitz *et al.*, 1978 [67]
37	TNI	51%	90%	Mauch *et al.*, 1979 [70]
86	TNI ± HRT	66%	86%	Hoppe, 1980 [104]
85	TNI/STN	49%	76%	Stein *et al.*, 1980 [88]
20	TNI	74%	88%	Timothy *et al.*, 1980 [136]
318		35–74%	76–90%	

* 4-year figures
HRT: hepatic radiation therapy

became sharply divided into IIIA for radiation therapy (TNI) and IIIB for chemotherapy (MOPP ×6 or its equivalent).

A significant number of reports utilizing TNI in PS IIIA have now been published and Table 13 outlines some recent results. FFR rates show a striking variation between 35 and 74% at 5 years; overall survival shows smaller fluctuations between 76 and 90%, with most series achieving greater than 80% at 5 years. Not only are these results a quantum step below those for PS I and II (Table 4), but the remarkable variations in results are in need of analysis.

1.4.2. Patterns of Relapse and Prognostic Factors in PS IIIA. Patterns of relapse among 96 PS IIIA patients relapsing after TNI are presented in Table 14. Purely nodal failure accounts for about 40% of all relapses and, interestingly, about 2/3 of these are true in-field recurrences (see our theoretic curves in Figure 5). Extranodal relapse accounts for 60% of failures

Table 14. Patterns of relapse in PS IIIA Hodgkin's disease treated with TNI.

Patients	Relapses	Nodal*	Extranodal**	Lung	Liver	Bone	Marrow	Ref.
14	6	4	2	2	–	–	–	[62]
48	26	13	13	3	4	1	2	[67]
37	17	3	14	5	5	3	–	[70]
85	42	16	25	8	7	4	3	[88]
20	5	2	3	2	1	–	–	[136]
204	96	38	57	20	17	8	5	

* Nodal only.
** Extranodal ± nodal.

with lung and liver making up 2/3. Other extranodal sites of relapse (bone, bone marrow, muscle, skin) are considerably less common making up about 20% of all failures. Clearly, there is a pattern to radiation therapy failures in PS IIIA and each of three major escape mechanisms, the true recurrence, the pulmonary relapse and the liver failure raise questions regarding mechanism, antecedent predisposing factors and new therapeutic approaches. Together the three patterns account for about 2/3 of relapses in PS IIIA treated with TNI.

A number of authors have presented analyses of putative prognostic factors that might correlate with a high relapse propensity. Unfortunately, in no stage of Hodgkin's disease are the data so conflicting and the conclusions so diametrically opposed as here. We will therefore begin by presenting each of the many variables that have been considered significant by different authorities.

Perhaps the most obvious parameter to consider first is the LAG result. In any series there are two groups of PS IIIA patients: (a) CS IA and IIA but PS IIIA (LAG negative), and (b) CS IIIA and PS IIIA (LAG positive). It might be anticipated that the prognosis would be sharply different for these groups. However, two recent series could find no statistically significant differences in relapse rates between subgroups [55, 70]. Another recent report revealed that among III_2-A patients, there was no difference in outcome whether the LAG was positive or negative [88]. These are surprising results, implying as they do that the bulk of disease within *each* lymph node involved in the node groups visualized by lymphography plays no prognostic role. *A priori*, this is extremely unlikely and the observations probably imply instead that some other factor(s) exerts such strong prognostic influence as to overshadow the role of purely bulk lymph node disease.

A recently proposed theory has made use of the idea that Hodgkin's disease spreads to the abdomen, not by way of the thoracic duct, but mostly hematogenously into the spleen and from there into abdominal lymphatics [87]. To take into account this proposed pathway of spread, subdiaphragmatic disease has been classified in terms of the extent of spread from spleen to splenic nodes, to celiac nodes, to portal hepatis nodes and to para-aortic nodal sites. Stage III_1-A includes cases with an involved spleen, splenic nodes, celiac nodes and porta hepatis nodes in various combinations, but without para-aortic nodal disease. III_2-A includes any case with para-aortic disease irrespective of upper abdominal status [47, 87, 88, 141]. A variation of this scheme defines III-AS as disease confined to spleen or splenic nodes and III S+N+A as more extensive abdominal nodal disease [131]. A numerical tally of the substaging reported in four series [67, 88, 104, 136] shows that exactly equal numbers fall into III_1-A and III_2-A (130 vs 129 cases respectively). A number of investigators have reported their experiences with this systems [87, 138, 141, 142], but due to

Table 15. The incidence of splenic involvement in PS IIIA Hodgkin's disease.

PS IIA patients	Positive spleen	Investigators
28	20 (71)	Shipley *et al.*, 1974 [143]
30	21 (70)	Peckham *et al.*, 1975 [40]
48	33 (69)	Prosnitz *et al.*, 1978 [67]
130	105 (81)	Stein *et al.*, 1980 [88]
42	42 (100)	Fuller *et al.*, 1980 [77]
86	72 (84)	Hoppe, 1980 [104]
364	293 (80)	

( ) percentage.

small patient numbers their conclusions have been tentative. Recently a collaborative four-institution report on 48 III_1-A and 37 III_2-A patients receiving TNI showed a highly significant difference in FFR and survival between these subgroups [88]. For III_1-A, 5-year FFR was 63% with 91% survival, while for III_2-A, FFR was only 32% and 5-year survival 56%. Two other recent reports show similar trends [67, 142] but significantly two other studies failed to corroborate the above concepts [104, 136]. In particular, the Stanford results on 46 III_1-A and 40 III_2-A patients reveal no differences in FFR (about 60% at 5 years) or survival (about 80%) between these groups [104]. Since the majority of Stanford patients received prophylactic liver irradiation and since this technique totally eliminated hepatic failure, one might argue that therapeutic differences account for the disparate results. This argument, however, would only be true if III_2-A had a higher propensity to hepatic failure then III_1-A – in fact, the collaborative study reported five liver failures in III_1-A and only two in III_2-A. For the present, this dilemma must remain as another of the many controversies in PS IIIA Hodgkin's disease.

Splenic involvement is another possible prognostic factor in Stage III disease. Following the early laparotomy experience at Stanford [19] where occult splenic disease was first clearly described and the virtually universal relation between hepatic and splenic involvement first defined, the significance of the spleen in Hodgkin's disease has created considerable debate and speculation [143]. In fact, the spleen is involved in the vast majority of PS IIIA patients (Table 15). The Stanford group decided to regard splenic involvement as an unfavorable sign even in the absence of demonstrable liver involvement and elected for prophylactic hepatic irradiation in all spleen-positive patients [35, 144]. Others continued to regard the spleen as a lymph node. A relation between initial splenic disease and subsequent hepatic relapse was indeed noted in one study [143] and it was suggested that about 15% of spleen-positive patients fell into an adverse group that sustained early hepatic relapse. Over the past 5 years, a number of other publications have revealed trends suggesting an adverse outcome for spleen-positive patients receiving TNI compared to the much smaller subgroup of spleen-negative cases [70, 76, 136, 138, 141]. Such trends were noted by Prosnitz and co-workers: 22/23 spleen-positive cases relapsed compared to 6/15 relapses in spleen-negative patients [67]. A similar trend was observed by Stein and co-workers who report a 47% FFR for spleen-positive versus a 61% FFR for spleen-negative patients following TNI [88]. A specific relation between splenic involvement and hepatic relapse is suggested by two reports wherein 7/53 spleen-positive patients experienced hepatic relapse as a first failure, compared to only 1/24 such relapses in spleen-negative cases [40, 67]. However, these data are only suggestive at best and the preponderance of splenic involvement in PS IIIA makes it difficult to discriminate subgroups in terms of a positive or a negative spleen. However, quantification of the extent of splenic involvement within the large group of PS IIIA patients having splenic disease, may be a more discriminating approach. Indeed, it was noted in 1977 that patients with splenic disease, but without para-aortic nodal disease, in general, had less extensive splenic disease (fewer nodules and each of smaller size) than patients with para-aortic disease [138]. It was also reported that extranodal relapse was more likely in those with multiple splenic nodules [138]. This approach has been further refined by the Stanford group and they have subdivided their splenic cases into those with minimal involvement (less than five nodules) and those with extensive involvement (greater than or equal to five nodules). Their latest statement on PS IIIA is that the extent of splenic disease is overwhelmingly the single most important prognostic index for PS IIIA treated with TNI and hepatic prophylaxis [104]. The 5-year FFR for minimal splenic disease is 78% compared to 50% FFR for extensive splenic involvement. This finding that the extent of splenic disease correlates with prognosis among patients who experienced *no* hepatic relapse implies a relation between extensive splenic involvement and widespread extranodal dissemination, especially to marrow [139]. Extending radiation fields in these circumstances is unlikely to improve results.

So far we have considered prognostic factors in terms of subdiaphragmatic disease. There is no reason to suppose, however, that supradiaphragmatic factors relevant in PS I and II lose all significance in stage III. In fact, the lung is a very common site of first relapse following TNI and we might anticipate that bulky mediastinal disease is a strong determinant of this failure pattern. The M.D. Anderson group have presented evidence that this is so [77]. Their study involved two cycles of MOPP followed by extensive irradiation to a mantle, an upper abdominal field and a pelvic field, and both IIIA and IIIB stages were included. Of 16 relapses, five were nodal, seven were pulmonary, and four hepatic [77]. Of the seven lung failures, six had initial mediastinal disease. The only significant prognostic factors with this approach were age and mediastinal status. Mediestinal-negative patients achieved an 84% FFR at 5 years; mediastinal-positive patients had a 57% FFR. However, extent of splenic involvement does not appear to have been evaluated.

Histology has not been found to have any influence on relapse rates for PS IIIA following TNI [67, 70, 88, 104].

Clearly, PS IIIA is a complex stage and no final statement on prognostic factors following TNI can be given. Three major predicators have been isolated by different observers as possibly important, though none is devoid of controversy: (i) substage, III_1 versus III_2; (ii) extent of splenic involvement; (iii) mediastinal status. We will consider the therapeutic implications of each in the next section.

1.4.3. Therapeutic Challenges in PS IIIA. It is almost universally agreed that PS IIIA disease represents a highly heterogeneous group of Hodgkin's disease patients [55, 67, 70]. The quest to isolate various prognostically distinct subgroups has only begun and the major challenge facing the radiation oncologist in this stage is to clearly define those patients who will achieve high FFR rates following irradiation alone. Such delineation will almost certainly entail a multivariate analysis, defining those constellations of findings that are favorable and contrasting these to the unfavorable groupings. In view of the data presented above, it appears unlikely that any one factor alone is of such overwhelming significance as to dominate the outcome. At present it is not possible to define clearly the various prognostic groups, but we might hazard the guess that the patient without mediastinal disease, with upper abdominal lymphadenopathy only, and with limited splenic involvement falls into an extremely favorable group and might expect an FFR rate equal to that of a favorable stage I or II case. This group, however, probably accounts for no more than 1/4 of all PS IIIA cases. At the other extreme is the patient with mediastinal adenopathy, para-aortic disease and extensive splenic involvement – he could well have a relapse risk in excess of 70% following TNI alone. Again, this unfavorable group is unlikely to make up more than 20% of the PS IIIA populations. Between these extremes lies a spectrum of prognostically variable patients some of whom may well do poorly enough following TNI to merit some alternative approach.

The criticality of identifying such subgroups is highlighted by considering the various radiation techniques that might be employed to minimize the different relapse patterns. It is clear that prophylactic lung irradiation can reduce the incidence of pulmonary relapse in patients with mediastinal disease. Similarly, prophylactic liver irradiation reduces hepatic failures, as shown by the Stanford experience where no initial hepatic failures occurred in 86 PS IIIA patients [104]. Accordingly, the optimal radiation needed for a high-risk 'lung relapser' is different to that for a high-risk 'hepatic relapser.' However, it is unlikely that patients would regularly tolerate both forms of prophylaxis in addition to TNI and patients at risk for relapse in both lung and liver are beyond the realm of regular cure by radiation alone. Patients at low risk for either of these relapse patterns need only TNI.

In the absence of any clear definition of various subgroups, a rather unsatisfactory multiplicity of therapeutic approaches has emerged for PS IIIA disease, with opinions divided between radiation alone [55, 134, 136], chemotherapy alone [140], or combined modes [67, 79]. Following irradiation alone, about 1/2 of the patients can be expected to relapse (Table 13) and subsequent salvage therapy will rescue some of these for an overall 5-year survival of about 80%. The proponents of this radiation and salvage chemotherapy approach argue that perhaps 1/2 of the patient population is spared unnecessary chemotherapy and, in some series at least, there is no clear survival advantage to adjuvant chemotherapy [55, 88, 118]. On the other hand, some reports do show a survival advantage for those IIIA patients receiving adjuvant therapy [138]. In the randomized Stanford study on 60 PS IIIA patients [118, 119], those receiving radiation alone had an 81% 5-year survival compared to 90% in the adjuvant group ($P = 0.22$). In a non-randomized comprison of radiation alone versus radiation and chemotherapy [138], the single modality group had a 5-year survival of 76%, compared to 89% ($P < 0.02$) in the combined therapy group. Controversies such as these will probably never be settled unless explicit account of prognostic factors is taken into consideration. We will discuss various combined modality approaches later but the implications of two recent studies for IIIA patients will be considered here. It has been argued that if radiation is accepted as the basic modality for PS IIIA disease, then less than radical chemotherapy (say, only three cycles of MOPP) is adequate [52, 75, 77]. The M.D. Anderson study utilizing two cycles of MOPP which gives '... more complete response than is usually gotten with one cycle...' [77], followed by extensive radiation including liver prophylaxis, resulted in a 5-year FFR in 68% of 62 stage IIIA patients [77] – a result identical to that achieved by radiation alone at Stanford [104]. It is difficult to see what benefit the two cycles of MOPP really gave to the IIIA patients. On the other hand, a planned course of six cycles of MOPP in the Stanford trial resulted in a 96% FFR at 5 years. Three cycles of MOPP, however, are apparently superior to two in this context and a SWOG study [75] implied that six cycles were not necessary if full-dose radiation is given.

Finally, it can be argued that radiation has little place in PS IIIA disease which should be managed by chemotherapy from the start [140]. Two studies on a total of 40 PS IIIA patients have reported very satisfactory results following chemotherapy alone [136, 140]. With prolonged follow-up, 38 (95%) have not experienced a relapse. On the other hand, a randomized trial comparing TNI against MOPP revealed a statistically significant superiority to radiation in PS IIIA patients [134]. At 4 years, the FFR in those receiving TNI was 65% compared to a 38% FFR in the chemotherapy group. Overall survival was the same in both groups.

Clearly, an optimal treatment for PS IIIA Hodgkin's disease cannot be presently defined. We believe that only by further observation and analysis of prognostic factors and patterns of relapse, will the understanding of this small, but complex stage reach levels where optimal treatment approaches can be confidently defined.

1.4.4. Laparotomy in Hodgkin's Disease. Staging laparotomy for Hodgkin's disease had its origins deeply rooted in a radiotherapeutic background. The finding that radiation hepatitis limited the dose possible for hepatic irradiation [145] and the observation of the characteristic TDNF following mantle irradiation, prompted the use of exploratory laparotomy to better define the extent of abdominal disease [19]. In recent years, the majority of large centers treating Hodgkin's disease have adopted laparotomy-splenectomy as a more or less routine procedure for patients without otherwise demonstrable stage IV disease [60, 64, 65, 104]. As we have emphasized (section 1.1), accurate field placement corresponding to all disease, macroscopic and microscopic, is essential in radiation oncology and the staging laparotomy has done much to define optimal fields for various circumstances and for particular patients. However, it is legitimate to ask whether the understanding of involvement sites and of spread patterns achieved over the past 20 years is now such that laparotomy can be safely avoided in some, perhaps most, cases of Hodgkin's disease. It would be an undisputed step toward optimal treatment if laparotomy could be dispended with, without compromising therapeutic results, and there seems little doubt that during the 1980s the value of this procedure will be increasingly questioned.

First, some of the issues for those patients who are LAG-negative, CS IA or IIA need to be considered. On the whole, without looking at separate patterns of supradiaphragmatic disease, this group will have abdominal involvement in 20–40%, but only a negligible number will be LAP-staged to IV [20, 22, 36, 37, 55, 79, 90]. As we have summarized (1.3.1), negative laparotomy does not dependably exlude microscopic disease and PS IA and IIA does need para-aortic prophylaxis. These laparotomy negative patients have, however, gained the assurance that omission of a pelvic field will not significantly compromise their outlook. Accordingly, they can be spared the added marrow depression and gonadal irradiation unavoidable with pelvic treatment. On the other hand, what has the CS IA or IIA, LAP-positive group gained by having had a laparotomy? Could it be treated by STN fields rather than TNI? If it could, then this argument gives no rational basis for the laparotomy. As clearly as this problem can be formulated, so equally difficult is it to answer. Very few PS IIIA patients have been treated with STN fields, though one report had seven patients with 'early' PS IIIA (spleen and/or splenic nodes only involved) treated this way and one relapsed by pelvic extension as a first failure [88]. Given the small size of the PS IIIA group, it is unlikely that direct resolution of this question will emerge. However, there is indirect evidence that at least for MC and LD subtypes, pelvic irradiation in non-laparotomy staged patients cannot be safely avoided. Of a total of 27 MC patients mostly clinically staged (73%), six relapsed first in pelvic nodes following a treatment program that involved STN irradiation in the majority [59]. On the other hand, another report on CS I and II NS disease treated by STN fields reported on one pelvic node extension in 46 patients treated [58]. These data suggest that in terms of the need for a pelvic field, laparotomy is important for MC, but perhaps not for NS.

Another possible advantage of laparotomy in CS IA and IIA patients is that splenectomy reduces the volume of kidney that needs irradiation. However, a recent investigation of delayed renal damage following splenic irradiation revealed some fibrosis of the upper pole of the left kidney in most patients but with no demonstrable physiologic abnormality either in renal function, renin production or hypertension [146]. It should be noted that splenic atrophy following radiation can lead to the syndrome of fulminant septicemia [147] and therefore radiation is not necessarily a safer alternative to splenectomy in this regard.

For the CS IB or IIB patient, laparotomy probably remains an unchallengeable necessity. Those patients who are truly PS IB and IIB do extremely well following TNI; those who are PS IIIB have a very poor outlook and need chemotherapy. The only way that a distinction between these groups can be regularly made is by laparotomy.

Finally, the PS I or II patient can receive lower doses below the diaphragm; the CS I or II patient must receive radical treatment in this region.

Patients who are LAG-positive with B symptoms are very rarely restaged to PS IB or IIB following laparotomy [55] and more often in fact are increased to IVB. There is no justification for laparotomy in this group. However, the CS IIIA patient has potentially much to gain from laparotomy if the treatment is planned to be radiation. Some 10–20% of these patients are changed to PS IA or IIA [20, 22] and if use is to be made of the prognostic and therapeutic implications of splenic disease, then laparotomy is the only way to achieve this.

There are a number of patterns of supradiaphragmatic disease for which the yield of staging laparotomy is very low and where treatment alterations from the STN layout virtually never eventuate following laparotomy. Lymphographically negative CS IA high cervical LP or MC cases or cases with NS disease sharply confined to the mediastinum [20, 36, 95] probably do not benefit from laparotomy.

1.5. Advanced Hodgkin's Disease: Stage IIIB and IV

Multiple drug chemotherapy is the only acceptable primary approach to the management of stages IIIB and IV of Hodgkin's disease. Following a flexible cycle number approach which gives a minimum of six MOPP cycles, but more if necessary, with two cycles following carefully documented complete response (CR), an FFR can be expected in about 55% of advanced patients at 5 years and 51% at 10 years [123]. Complete remission occurs in 66–80% of previously untreated patients [124–126], with asymptomatic cases responding significantly better than symptomatic ones. Of the complete responders, between 1/3 and 1/2 will relapse usually within the first 2 years following induction [123–126]. It is against this background that radiation has been employed as an adjunct, principally with the aim of reducing relapses, but also to increase the CR rate. A number of radiation approaches have been suggested for optimal integration into a chemotherapy program and conceptually, at least, a sharp distinction can be made between stage IIIB and IV. For a PS IIIB patient it is radiotherapeutically possible to deliver tumoricidal doses to all sites of bulk disease; for a stage IV patient this is almost never possible. Accordingly, attempts have been made to integrate full TNI into chemotherapy programs for PS IIIB [55, 77, 118, 119, 148–150] while stage IV requires a 'consolidation' radiation approach [72, 73].

Stage IIIB cannot be adequately managed by radiation alone since FFR at 5 years is below 10% [55]. Chemotherapy alone produces about 50% FFR at 5 years [123, 124]. The demonstration by two groups of investigators that relapses following MOPP chemotherapy tend to initially manifest at sites of initial involvement, especially in pre-treatment bulky lymphadenopathy [125, 151], adds a further rationale for integrating radiation into therapy programs for IIIB disease. The earliest systematic investigation of this approach commenced in 1968 at Stanford where advanced patients were randomized to receive either TNI alone or TNI followed by six cycles of MOPP [35]. Patients receiving both modes had their radiation first and after an interval of 1 to 2 months, cyclic chemotherapy was commenced. Following the observation that steroid withdrawal at the end of a MOPP cycle occasionally unmasked radiation pneumonitis or pericarditis, prednisone was deleted [121]. This approach produced a 50% FFR at 8 years, while the TNI alone group achieved only a 7% result [118]. The hematologic toxicity of the combined program proved to be acceptable with no serious hemorrhagic or infective problems but a high incidence of herpes zoster was encountered [111]. An alternative approach was explored by the NCI group [148]. A series of 28 patients, mostly IIIB, was given a minimum of six cycles of MOPP with the intention of full dose TNI to follow. Twenty-seven of these patients achieved CR, but five relapsed before radiation could be commenced and a surprisingly high incidence of morbidity was associated with the radiotherapy. Fifteen of 28 patients experienced a variety of radiation complications not ordinarily observed after radiation therapy. Four patients died and two had persisting life-threatening morbidity. Hematologic toxicity was also profound with 12 patients having persistent thrombocytopenia (less than $50,000/mm^3$). The overall FFR with a median follow-up of 48 months was 61%. A high rate of local-marginal relapse (14%) was attributed to the use of fields that did not cover the full extent of pre-treatment bulk [148]. It may be fairly concluded from these two experiences that the combination of radical chemotherapy with radical radiation therapy is best sequenced with the radiation first. When the Stanford group first initiated their H-7 protocol for stage IV disease, the initial aim was to deliver six cycles of MOPP followed by TNI, but after experiencing major problems in the delivery of radiation to their first eight patients, a sandwich technique, of two or three pre-irradiation chemotherapy cycles followed by TNI and then by completion of six courses, was introduced [118]. Goodman and co-workers reported on the use of such a sandwich technique in 21 PS IIIB and although hematologic tolerance was diminished, 75% of the anticipated dose of nitrogen mustard and procarbazine and 90% of the vincristine dose were administered to patients receiving TNI [74]. No serious complications were encountered and with a median follow-up of 50 months, 19/21 IIIB patients were in remission (90%).

Recently the Stanford group have introduced what appears to be the least toxic way for combining radical chemotherapy with radical radiation therapy for IIIB Hodgkin's disease – the so-called 'ping-pong' technique [149]. Treatment begins with two cycles of MOPP followed by full dose irradiation to the region most involved (mantle, para-aortic or pelvic field), then a further two cycles of MOPP followed by irradiation to the lesser involved region, then two more cycles of MOPP and a final irradiation to the least involved region. This approach allowed for the administration of 78% of the optimal alkylating agent and 75% of the optimal procarbazine doses. Hematologic toxicity with leukopenia and thrombocytopenia was observed in about 1/2 the patients. With limited follow-up, FFR at 45 months was 79% and survival 84% [149] – results considerably superior to those hitherto reported.

Finally, the M.D. Anderson group have approached IIIB from a somewhat different angle. While accepting the poor outcome following radiation alone, they nevertheless chose to emphasize this modality reserving chemotherapy for an adjuvant. A total of 38 IIIB patients were planned to receive two cycles of MOPP followed by TNI including the whole upper abdomen [77].

Thirty-three completed the full treatment and achieved a 78% FFR at 5 years. Five patients did not complete therapy principally because of disease progression yielding an overall FFR for the group of 68% at 5 years and survival of 74% [77]. Hematologic toxicity was not a major problem but radiation hepatitis occurred in six patients receiving 3000 rads in 4 weeks to the upper abdomen. Prior experience without chemotherapy had revealed no cases of this complication utilizing the same technique and it was attributed to the two cycles of chemotherapy [77]. A thin lead shield reducing hepatic dose to 2300 rads eliminated this problem.

Unfortunately, none of the above studies compare MOPP alone against MOPP with radiation and in the absence of such a direct comparison, it is uncertain whether anything is gained by the addition of radiation. One recent trial on IIIB and IV patients has addressed this question in a randomized comparison. Following three cycles of MOPP, patients in CR or 'adequately controlled' were randomized to receive either three further cycles of MOPP or irradiation to whole abdomen and mantle field to doses of 2000–3000 rads. Those receiving six MOPP and remaining in CR or 'adequate control' were then further randomized to receive radiation, more MOPP or no further treatment [150]. The full results have not been published but no group fared better than another. The addition of radiation reduced nodal relapse but since this relapse pattern was successfully salvageable, no survival advantage was evident [150]. It has been established that about 60% of relapsed following MOPP can be reinduced again with same combination [152].

An alternative concept for integrating radiation into the chemotherapy of advanced disease has been proposed by Prosnitz [72, 153]. The observations that following chemotherapy relapses tend to first appear in sites of previous involvement and that chemotherapy can probably replace prophylactic irradiation in early stages, imply that six cycles of MOPP can adequately deal with microscopic disease but leave a residue of clonogenic cells in areas of prior bulk. It seemed logical to employ low radiation doses limited strictly to sites of pre-chemotherapy involvement in an effort to eradicate the microscopic disease. One might have been tempted to pick orthodox prophylactic doses, but Prosnitz and co-workers chose 1500–2000 rads, the great advantage of this being that virtually every organ could be irradiated. In an early report on 80 advanced or relapsed patients, chemotherapy produced CR in 75%. Following 'consolidation' radiation to areas of pre-chemotherapy involvement only, 92% of the complete responders were projected to be alive at 5 years, and the survival of the whole group was 68% [72]. An update on this experience reveals that of 125 patients given chemotherapy, 84% achieved CR and following consolidation radiation, 90% of these are disease-free at 5 years. For the whole group, FFR at 5 years is 73% and survival 80% [154]. Two cases of acute non-lymphocytic leukemia occurred.

Bonadonna and co-workers [73] have applied this concept to MOPP and ABVD chemotherapy, though their radiation doses are a little higher with 2000–2500 rads to organ sites of involvement and 3000–3500 rads to nodal regions. These higher doses may have had some advantageous effect in that many partial responders to chemotherapy became CR following radiation; this was not the case in Prosnitz's series. The Milan study has achieved a FFR of greater than 90% at 4 years in those who achieve CR [73]. Currently, the ECOG is conducting a randomized trial to compare this form of radiation in chemotherapy treated IIIB and IV patients against ABVD consolidation [155]. The study is still in progress and results are unavailable.

Of all the combined approaches investigated, the consolidation approach seems the most logical, least toxic and most promising.

1.6. Relapsing Hodgkin's Disease

Prior to the advent of multi-agent chemotherapy, the outcome for patients sustaining a relapse was poor and the vast majority were destined to farily rapid death [17, 41, 92, 93, 99, 156]. Relapse apparently limited to nodal regions (regional or TDNF), and seemingly adequately covered by radiation fields, was rarely followed by sustained remission. The majority of such patients sustained hematogenous dissemination or reseeding into previously irradiated volumes [17, 41]. Regional relapses fared somewhat better than TDNF [17, 41, 92] while extranodal relapses, especially in liver or marrow, were rarely salvaged [92]. With the availability of chemotherapy, radiation alone has little role as the primary salvage modality no matter how localized the relapse appears. However, radiation may have a significant role as an adjunct to chemotherapy.

The incidence of CR for relapsing disease treated by chemotherapy varies between 50 and 85% in different reports [124–126, 154]. Patients who received chemotherapy as part of their initial treatment seem to have lower CR rates than those treated by radiation alone [91, 124, 125] and patients initially staged IIIB or IV also respond less often [91, 157]. A second relapse occurs in the complete responders in about 40% by 50 months [124]. The Stanford group have reported an FFR of 40% for 64 PS I–III patients relapsing following initial treatment, and the overall 5-year survival for these patients was 50% [91] compared to the 80% achieved in the whole group of 244 I-III patients [118]. As effective as it is, salvage therapy is in need of further improvement. Unfortunately, a proportion of relapsing patients, especially those failing early after initial treatment, has significant marrow compromise and may be untreatable with radical chemotherapy [77], let alone combined modes. However, in those achieving a CR, the consolidation radiation approach of Prosnitz has apparently been successful [72, 153, 154, 158].

The role of radiation in salvage programs clearly needs further investigation, but the view that salvage therapy is universally successful is untrue, and this underscores the need to employ optimal radiation techniques initially and to seek out those patients at high risk so that their primary treatment may be modified to reduce the incidence of failure.

1.7. Pediatric Hodgkin's Disease

Hodgkin's disease in pediatric patients ($\leq$15 years of age) is an uncommon neoplasm, accounting for 4–5% of all childhood cancers [159]. The incidence increases sharply with age, and at least 1/2 of all cases are in the 10–15 years age group, occurrence below age 5 is extremely rare [128, 130, 159–161]. In terms of its patterns of presentation and natural history, the disease is not significantly different to that observed in adults [159–161]. Stage IV cases are, however, infrequent [159, 160, 162]. In parallel with the improved results experienced by adults with this disease, the pediatric population has undergone an equal, if not a greater, gain in survival. However, increasing awareness of various long-term therapy-related complications to which the immature, actively growing and progressively longer surviving pediatric cancer patient is especially prone, has led to a re-evaluation of treatment approaches with particular attention to detoxification of therapeutic programs.

The evolution of therapeutic strategies for the child with Hodgkin's disease has passed through all the phases trespassed by adults over the years. Early experiences utilizing localized radiation fields for 'early' clinically staged cases revealed a high rate of contiguous regional failure. Two series reveal that of 39 children staged without LAG and receiving involved field therapy, 32 (82%) relapsed, mostly in nodal areas [129, 161]. Following the introduction of LAG staging and mantle fields, the TDNF emerged as a problem [129]. In one report, of 11 LAG-negative children receiving mantle irradiation, four experienced TDNF [129]. As laparotomy became acceptable for the adult population, so too, children were subjected to this procedure with results not substantially different to those reported for adults [128, 130, 162]. Clearly, from the viewpoint of disease control alone there is no reason to approach the child with Hodgkin's disease any differently than the adult and a number of investigators have applied exactly this philosophy to the management of pediatric Hodgkin's disease [162–164].

The Boston group [162] have presented perhaps the most uniformly staged and treated group of children to date. Their approach was identical to Hellman's program for adults [79]. Fifty-two CS I-III children underwent staging laparotomy. Six had their stage increased with two becoming PS IV because of occult liver disease; five were decreased in stage to PS II. All IA and IIA children received STN irradiation alone; PS IIIA received TNI;

PS IIB and IIIB had TNI followed by six cycles of MOPP. Radiation doses were a little lower than for adults and mostly ranged between 3600 and 4000 rads. The results of this program are remarkable. With a median follow-up of 36 months, 90% of the PS I-III children remain disease free, with a projected 5-year survival of 98% [162]. Apart from a high incidence of herpes zoster, two cases of transient pneumonitis and one of hypothyroidism, no particular toxicity was encountered. Clearly any growth delay problems will need longer follow-up to delineate. A similar program at the Mayo Clinic also resulted in a 90% FFR at 4 years in PS IA and IIA children [164]. It has been stated [128] that such good results could not be duplicated by other investigators – and that is true, but only because clearly suboptimal radiation techniques and staging methods were employed.

The Stanford results [165], for example, reflect varying staging and treatment policies as employed by that group in their different trials and one could hardly conclude that their results in say the L-1 protocol are representative of the current achievements in this disease. Of the 79 children they reported in 1976, only 41 (52%) had staging laparotomy and of 18 nonlaparotomized CS IIA patients, 11 did *not* receiving subdiaphragmatic irradiation – it is not at all surprising that the FFR at 7 years in IIA children was oly 40%! Overall, the 79 children achieved FFR at 5 years of 66% and survival of 89%. A more conclusive finding in this report was the high incidence of radiation-induced complications with 47% of the children experiencing one or a number of significant problems including thyroid dysfunction in 27, pericarditis in 12, pneumonitis in four, bone growth retardation in four and soft tissue hypoplasia in three. Five fatal therapy complications occurred (one pneumonitis and four infective). In viewing these complication problems, the radiation techniques employed must be recalled. Doses of 3500–4400 rads were delivered at the rate of 1100 rads per week treating only *one* field per day (220 rads midplane per field). These doses are substantially higher than most pediatric radiation oncologists would employ. Nevertheless, this experience [166] led Kaplan and his team to explore alternative approaches that will be considered later.

Another study, in attempting to avoid the potential hazards of radiation, explored the use of IF therapy in laparotomy negative I and II children [95]. As we have already indicated, a negative laparotomy does not assure protection against TDNF unless para-aortic prophylaxis is given – this was stressed by one report on pediatric Hodgkin's disease from the Princess Margaret Hospital, Toronto. Three of sixteen relapses were first detected in laparotomy-negative unirradiated para-aortic nodes [129]. Moreover it is very difficult to imagine why a negative laparotomy should alter the risk for regional relapse above the diaphragm. Therefore, the results of this recent IF study are no surprise. Of 20 children treated, eight have relapsed, all within nodal regions (six regional, two TDNF). Actuarial FFR at 2 years was 57%.

All but one of the relapses achieved a second CR producing a 2-year survival of 89% [95]. It is difficult, however, to justify an approach so contrary to established principles, so ineffective as to assure relapse in about 1/2 and relying so heavily on a salvage concept which hasn't been shown to be more than 60% effective.

In an attempt to avoid the potentially adverse effects of irradiation, many investigators have explored the use of chemotherapy in conjunction with low dose radiation [55, 128, 167,168]. There is now no doubt that this approach is extremely effective in terms of FFR and survival. The Toronto series of 41 CS I-IV children receiving three cycles of MOPP followed by low-dose (about 2500 rads) irradiation to areas of disease and then a final three MOPP cycles, shows a FFR at 5 years of 85% and a survival of 89% [128, 168]. Since chemotherapy is the mainstay of treatment, laparotomy was not utilized (the technique of 'treatment with low dose radiation and MOPP without staging laparotomy'). Another series utilizing MVPP chemotherapy following IF therapy to 3000 rads, revealed a FFR in 32/34 (94%) stage I-IV children followed for at least 2 years (24, for more than 3 years) [167]. Kaplan has also utilized this approach, with IF radiation therapy to 1500–2500 rads followed by six cycles of MOPP. In stage IV, two or three MOPP cycles are given first and in stage I, the first cycle coincides with radiation. Of 35 children treated in this way, at 9 years the FFR is 90% and survival 94% [55]. The full long-term toxicologic implications of this bimodal approach remain to be defined, but apart from gonadal dysfunction principally in males [55], specific problems have not been identified. Abnormalities in bone growth do not follow chemotherapy [127].

In view of the exceptionally good results with this combined approach, it seems most unlikely that any pure radiation regimen will have a significant role in pediatric Hodgkin's disease. Investigators are attempting to define favorable subcategories that may not need chemotherapy [55, 128, 161, 168], but with the small number of cases available a clear definition of such a subgroup may never occur. The deletion of staging laparotomy has the added potential advantage of avoiding fulminant post-splenectomy septicemia.

Finally, the program initiated by Ziegler in Uganda, wherein children with Hodgkin's disease received only MOPP chemotherapy, supports the need for some radiation even in early stages. Of a total of 48 stage I-IV children, 42 achieved CR (88%), but 11 have relapsed and overall survival at 5 years was 73% [127]. A high incidence (21%) of herpes zoster was reported showing that this is not specifically related to radiation therapy.

1.8. Radiation Complications

The occurrence and incidence of radiation-induced complications are determined by the anatomic region irradiated, the relative volumes of various tissues and organs included, and the dose-fractionation regimen employed. The critical roles of volume and fractionation in generating complications have repeatedly been demonstrated with the wide-field techniques employed for Hodgkin's disease [27, 32, 53, 54, 68, 80]. Doses of up to 4000 rads in 4 weeks (200 rads per fraction) to mantle fields produce less than a 10% incidence of significant complications, but increasing this dose to 4400 rads in 4 weeks, at least doubles the risk [53]. Since there is no evidence that rapid fractionation is essential for good local control in this disease, there is no need to employ radiation fractions in excess of 200 rads, and both the anterior and posterior fields should be treated daily to avoid high dose 'lateral effects'. The major complications following radical irradiation of Hodgkin's disease are related to the mantle field and Table 16 summarizes the common and more major problems encountered. The incidences quoted are derived from reports utilizing a maximum of 200 rads daily, treating both fields [52–54, 65, 79, 136–171].

Symptomatic pulmonary radiation reaction is the commonest clinically evident abnormality following mantle irradiation. The reported incidence varies from less than 3% [79] to more than 49% [169] and is dependent on volume-dose factors. The Stanford group had 45 cases out of 274 treated without lung irradiation [68] at doses of 4400 rads in 4 weeks; Hellman and co-workers report only five cases out of 209 treated with 4000 rads in 4–5 weeks [79]. Fazekas and co-workers [53] had a 32% incidence at 4400 rads, which dropped to only 4% with 3800 rads in 4 weeks. Whole-lung irradiation

Table 16. Major complications following mantle irradiation with 4000 rads in 4–5 weeks (<200 rads per fraction).

Complication	Usual time of onset months following complication	Incidence	Major manifestations
SPRR *	1–4	<10%	Dry cough; dyspnea chest pain; fever. CXR: opacification confined to radiation field
Pericarditis	4–12	<5%	Usually an asymptomatic pericardial effusion; sometimes a classic acute pericarditis; dyspnea
Myxedema **	>6	3%	Weight gain; cold intolerance; lethargy
Xerostomia	<2	<5%	Dry mouth; decreased taste
Myelopathy	>6	<1%	Paraplegia; myelogram to exclude cord compression

* SPRR: Symptomatic pulmonary radiation reaction.
** The incidence of subclinical thyroid depression is much higher (30–50%).

using a rapid fractionation technique (1650 rads in 10 fractions) produces a 35% incidence of pneumonitis, while the thin lung block technique (1650 rads in 20 fractions) gives only a 15% incidence [68]. An increased incidence is likely in the patient with large mediastinal disease and a shrinking field technique should be employed [60, 68]. Prior or concomitant bleomycin treatment has been documented to enhance symptomatic pneumonitis but the radiation oncologist must be vigilant for such adverse reactions with other chemotherapeutic agents as well.

Radiation induced pericarditis has been reported in 0–35% of patients and the incidence is very closely related to pericardial dose. The Stanford technique of low dose pericardial prophylaxis to 1500 rads in conjunction with their standard 4400 rads in 4 weeks produces a 13% incidence [68]. Another technique utilizing heavily weighed anterior fields and delivering in excess of 4500 rads in 4 weeks to the anterior pericardium gave a 35% incidence [169]. On the other hand, slower fractionation and lower dose virtually eliminate this problem. Two recent series utilizing ≤200 rads per fraction for a total dose of 4000–4500 rads, without whole pericardial irradiation reveal five cases out of 209 (1.5%) treated [65, 79]. A number of authors have noted the very occasional myocardial infarction in relatively young patients [47, 79] and these anecdotal reports may indicate some myocardial damage following radiation. Again, the risks of combined modality will need fuller assessment, but adriamycin does have an untoward interaction with radiation in terms of cardiac toxicity [55].

The incidence of overt myxedema following radiation is about 3% in most reports [170–172]; however, subclinical thyroid depression with elevated TSH has been reported in up to 44% of patients [171]. Whether this is a permanent abnormality is uncertain and it does raise the problem of potential thyroid carcinogenesis due to both radiation and TSH stimulation [169]. We prefer to treat elevated TSH with exogenous thyroxine.

Other complications following supradiaphragmatic irradiation are very uncommon and spinal cord myelopathy is entirely avoidable by protracting the dose, and by off-axis dose calculation to assure that treatment is within tolerance.

Subdiaphragmatic irradiation is in general well tolerated without major complications. Intestinal, hepatic and renal problems can generally be eliminated by careful technique. For para-aortic irradiation only, the gonadal dose is low and normal testicular or ovarian function is retained. With pelvic irradiation, substantial doses are received by the ovaries or testes. Aspermia is usual in males following pelvic-inguinal irradiation, but recovery occurs in many [169, 173]. Testicular doses can be minimized by testicular shielding [52]. Following oophoropexy and ovarian shielding, about 2/3 of females given pelvic irradiation will experience normal menstrual function and fertility has been documented in a number [32, 55].

Bone marrow depression is a common and increasingly important side effect as multi-modal approaches are introduced [174, 175]. With irradiation alone the peripheral blood count does not fall substantially during mantle irradiation; depression often occurs toward the end of para-aortic treatment and is universal if a pelvic field is added [55]. Recovery of blood counts is usually rapid within the first 6 months [176] but this does not reflect marrow regeneration. In-field marrow regeneration following 4000–4500 rads does not begin until 1 year after treatment, though by 4–5 years about 3/4 of these patients will show some regeneration [176]. The factors determining marrow regeneration and extension are complex [175–178] and will not be reviewed, but there is no doubt that the bone marrow is a very critical structure for some patients who suffer early relapse and are unable to receive adequate salvage therapy [77, 175]. Autologous marrow preservation and transplantation may play some role in the future management of Hodgkin's disease [175, 179].

An increasing number of reports of second malignancy in patients successfully treated for Hodgkin's disease has awakened considerable interest and concern [55, 180–184]. In particular, acute nonlymphocytic leukemia (ANLL) has emerged as a unique complication with few remissions resulting from therapy of this disease. In view of the known carcinogenicity of radiation and of many of the chemotherapeutic agents employed in therapy, the widely accepted view is that the increased incidence of second malignancies is iatrogenic. The exact risks with various treatment approaches have not been defined but radiation alone or chemotherapy alone have only been modestly implicated. Radiation may increase the risk of second malignancy by up to 4-fold [184] though some series have failed to report any risk enhancement [180]. The major risks are linked with combined modality therapy where the actuarial risk of leukemia may be higher than 7% by 8 years and still increasing [180, 184]. This risk, more than any other factor, will require a careful analysis of patients receiving combined modes in order to achieve an optimal balance between relapse-free survival and second malignancy.

1.9. Summary of Treatment Policies

Radiation therapy is the primary treatment modality for laparotomy-staged, stage I, II and IIIA patients with Hodgkin's disease. Lymph node regions on the involved side of the diaphragm receive 4000 rads at 150–180 rads per fraction and involved sites are boosted to 4500 rads. Uninvolved sites on the disease-free side of the diaphragm are treated to a prophylactic dose of 3500 rads. Rest periods of 2–4 weeks are allowed between successive phases of radiation therapy. Unfavorable presentations of stages I, II and III receive combined modality treatment with emphasis in radiation therapy. In this setting, three cycles of MOPP followed by full dose radiation therapy

Table 17. Treatment policies for Hodgkin's disease according to stage and pattern of presentation.

Stage	Presentation	Treatment
1) PS IA and II	a) Supradiaphragmatic, mediastinal nodes <1/3 CD, lymphangiogram and laporotomy negative, hilar nodes negative.	Mantle, para-aortic-splenic pedicle (STN) irradiation.
	b) As in 1a, but hilar nodes positive.	STN with thin lung blocks over ipsilateral lung. Lung dose 2000 rads.
	c) Subdiaphragmatic presentations, laparotomy staging.	Inverted Y, mantle irradiation (TNI).
2) CS IA or IIA	Supradiaphragmatic presentation with massive mediastinal lymphadenopathy (>1/3 CD). No laparotomy, negative LAG and abdominal CAT scan.	3 MOPP followed by STN-splenic irradiation. Three further cycles of MOP(P).
3) PS IB or IIB	As in 1a, 1b, or 1c.	As in 1a or 1b, but use TNI.
4) CS IB or IIB	As in 2.	As in 2, but use TNI-splenic irradiation.
5) PS IIIA	a) Mediastinal nodes <1/3 CD, fewer than 5 splenic nodules and negative lower para-aortic nodes.	TNI.
	b) Mediastinal nodes >1/3 CD. No laparotomy.	3 MOPP followed by TNI and 3 further cycles of MOP(P).
	c) Mediastinal nodes <1/3 CD, or more than 5 splenic nodules and/or positive lower para-aortic nodes.	3 MOPP followed by TNI and 3 further cycles of MOPP.
6) IIIB or IV	Any.	Full chemotherapy followed by consolidation radiation to *all* sites of initial disease except marrow. 1500–2000 rads.
7) I, II or IIIA	Pediatric patients.	Involved-field radiation therapy, 2000 rads, followed by 6 MOP(P).
8) IIIB or IV	Pediatric patients.	6 MOPP followed by consolidation radiation therapy.
9) Relapsing disease	Any.	6 MOPP followed by consolidation radiation depending on prior radiation dose to critical structures.

and finally three further cycles of chemotherapy is the recommended approach.

Advanced stages of Hodgkin's disease, IIIB or IV, receive full chemotherapy followed by low-dose consolidation radiation therapy to all sites of initial disease (nodal and extranodal) without, however, any systematic attempt to treat bone marrow. A similar chemotherapy-consolidation radiotherapy approach is recommended for pediatric patients.

Table 17 is a summary of the treatment policies.

2. THE ROLE OF RADIATION THERAPY IN THE NON-HODGKIN'S LYMPHOMAS

2.1. Histology

Although the histopathologic controversies surrounding the non-Hodgkin's lymphoma (NHL) group of diseases have been considered in a separate chapter, the overwhelming importance of this issue in relation to the outcome of radiation therapy merits some comment in this section too. As Bonadonna has so aptly termed it, the 'histopathology maze' [44] continues to confound and confuse our understanding of the natural history, clinical presentation and response to treatment of the various different entities encompassed by the designation of NHL. The previously widely used terminology of lymphosarcoma, reticulum cell sarcoma and giant follicular lymphoma fails to distinguish prognostically distinct subcategories within the lymphosarcoma-reticulum cell sarcoma groups especially by its failure to recognize lesser degrees of nodularity than is implied by the term giant follicle lymphoma [185, 186]. With the rediscovery of the Rappaport concept [6] in the early 1970s, a number of investigators have documented the distinct lack of correlation between the older system and that utilizing the criteria proposed by Rappaport [185–187]. Unfortunately, even the latter system is open to more than a desirable level of subjectivity [185, 186] and has needed some modification over the years [89, 185, 187]. A large number of alternative classification systems has also emerged [187, 188], each purporting to be biologically more correct than the others, though their clinical relevance remains unsettled. This extraordinary profusion of nomenclature has resulted in a fragmentation of case material into innumerable and largely incomparable nosologic categories, rendering any comparative analysis difficult.

Since the largest body of recent and apparently homogeneous case material is being reported under the Rappaport system (or some modification), we will principally adhere to this as summarized in Table 18. A number of other entities require separate analysis: lymphoblastic lymphoma, Burkitt's lymphoma, mycosis fungoides. Within the Rappaport system a widely recognized distinction is made between favorable types (NLPD, NM, NH) and unfavorable types (DLPD, DM, DHL, DU). The prognostic implications of such a subdivision have been repeatedly verified [28, 186, 189–194], though it is no longer clear that NH can be regarded as favorable [190, 194] and

Table 18. Histopathologic classification of non-Hodgkin's lymphoma according to a modified Rappaport system.

Nodular		Diffuse	
NLPD:	Nodular lymphocytic poorly differentiated	DLPD:	Diffuse lymphocytic poorly differentiated
NLWD: *	Nodular lymphocytic well differentiated	DLWD: **	Diffuse lymphocytic well differentiated
NM:	Nodular mixed lymphocytic-histiocytic	DM:	Diffuse mixed lymphocytic-histiocytic
NH:	Nodular histiocytic	DHL:	Diffuse histiocytic
		DU:	Diffuse undifferentiated

* Extremely rare, existence doubted by some.
** Rare, often regarded as variant of chronic lymphocytic leukemia.

DHL is increasingly yielding to curative therapy [195–197]. While the rate of progression of disease (prognosis) is related to nodularity, evidence is emerging to indicate that extent of involvement at presentation (stage) is more related to cytology, with lymphocytic and mixed variants having extensive disease and histiocytic types being more often localized [42, 43, 198]. The radiation oncologist also needs to be aware of the generally greater radiosensitivity of deposits of nodular lymphoma than of diffuse types, realizing, however, that some evidence suggests that sensitivity is more closely related with lymphocytic and mixed cell make-up than with nodularity *per se.*

2.2. Dose-Control Factors

The definition of a clear dose-response curve for the group of diseases classified under the heading of non-Hodgkin's lymphoma (NHL) has proved exceedingly difficult. Many factors serve to confound any analysis of the relation between probability of local control and radiation dose. The non-Hodgkin's lymphomas are a heterogeneous group of disorders both in terms of their natural history and their relative radioresponsiveness. The past and present controversies regarding classifications, the differing criteria among pathologists for naming the various subgroups and the rapidly changing nomenclature make data evaluation over several decades impossible to compare amongst different institutions. Moreover, in a group of disease where occult systemic dissemination is so common, the possibility of reseeding into a treated field always exists. Nevertheless, the specification of what is an appropriate dose is so crucial to radiation oncology (see section 1.2) that every effort must be made to define it.

In her classic report on the radiotherapy of NHL, Peters noted that there was some difference in dose needed to achieve consistent control in different histologic subtypes. For giant follicular lymphoma the dependable dose seemed to lie between 2500 and 3000 rads given over 2 to 4 weeks; for lymphosarcoma 1500–4500 rads in 1 to 4 weeks seemed appropriate, and for reticulum cell sarcoma a high 5000 rads in 4 weeks was necessary [199]. Since then a number of authors have addressed the question of optimal dose for NHL. Friedman in 1970 analyzed 76 lesions of reticulum cell sarcoma treated with doses between 500 and 7500 rads [200]. No dose-response relation was evident, with approximately 80% of lesions remaining locally controlled at all dose levels between 1000 and 6000 rads. Site of involvement, however, seemed important with nodal or gastrointestinal lesions responding to lower doses (all controlled at or above 3500 rads), head and neck lesions needing 5000 rads and bone being most resistant (20% recurring after >5000 rads). The time-dose isoeffect curve for control was flat. In 1971, Seydel reported on 105 lymphosarcoma and 40 giant follicle lymphoma lesions [201]. A dose-response curve was found for both. Lymphosarcoma lesions receiving less than 2000 rads recurred more than 80% of the time; at 2000–4000 rads less than 50% recurred, and with more than 4000 rads no recurrences were noted. Giant follicle lymphoma receiving more than 2800 rads did not recur, but with 1000–2500 rads, 60% recurred. Fuks and Kaplan reported their experience in 1973 [190] and utilizing the Rappaport classification showed an increasing control rate as dose increased for the lymphocytic lymphomas (nodular and diffuse) and for nodular histiocytic, but not for diffuse histiocytic lymphoma (DHL). Their data indicated a need for 4000–4500 rads for >90% control of the lymphocytic subtypes. Doses up to 4400 rads achieved only 75% control of DHL. Cox in 1974 [202] reviewed his experience with 273 lesions and concluded that for nodular histologies no relapse occurs above 2200 rads, while diffuse histologies require in excess of 4000 rads to assure control. His data suggested too, that for diffuse subtypes the size of the mass affected control probability. Lesions <3 cm achieved >90% control with 3500–4000 rads, while those >3 cm required in excess of 4000 rads for similar control [202]. Overall time had no effect on local control.

In a large review of dose-response data at the Princess Margaret Hospital, Toronto, Bush and co-workers elicited a dose-response relation in all histological subtypes [28]. For all the lymphocytic and mixed lymphohistiocytic subtypes and for nodular histiocytic disease, doses in excess of 2500 rads controlled more than 90%. For DHL, 4000–5000 rads produced 90% control, while doses <2500 rads controlled only 25%. Raising doses beyond 5000 rads did not improve control of DHL and it was suggested that a small subgroup of this cell type was indeed totally refractory to current radiotherapeutic approaches [28]. The Chicago group reported a 95% control rate for DHL with 4000–5000 rads [203] and the latest Stanford data on

Waldeyer's ring lymphomas reveal a 97% control with 4400-5000 rads [204].

Summarizing these data, it seems fair to recognize three subgroups within NHL, each having slightly different radiosensitivies: (1) Nodular poorly differentiated lymphocytic lymphoma (NPDL) (and, possibly other nodular cytologic types), where all data [28, 199-202, 205] except those from Stanford [190], suggest that 3000 rads is an adequate dose for >95% local control; (2) Diffuse lymphocytic or mixed lymphohistiocytic, where doses of 4000 rads will produce >95% control; (3) DHL, where most studies have failed to reveal a clear dose-response, but where 4000 rads or more produces 83-97% control [28, 190, 201, 203, 204] and where an appropriate level might be 5 000 rads. There is general agreement that the time-dose isoeffect relation is flat [27, 200-202] and that fractions of 150-200 rads are adequate.

There are no data to ascertain the dose required for microscopic disease and with the generally unpredictable pattern of relapse and high incidence of systemic dissemination it is not certain that an attempt to control microscopic disease is relevant for NHL. Most studies employing combined radiation and chemotherapy for early-stage disease have used full-dose radiation and it is unknown whether radiation can be reduced under these circumstances. The unique low dose total body irradiation approach to advanced lymphomas will be considered separately.

2.3. Staging NHL - the Relation to Radiation Volume

In many respects, the NHL have been regarded as caricatures of Hodgkin's disease, perhaps distorted, but nevertheless displaying some similarity and hopefully more than just a passing semblance in therapeutic response. In point of fact, there is little biologic or clinical basis for any such parallels and nowhere are the differences between the two lymphoma groups more evident than in their respective patterns of presentation and extent of involvement. The delineation of optimal staging procedures, and even the very definition of what would be a good staging system in NHL, have lagged considerably behind those for Hodgkin's disease and only the last 5 years have witnessed the beginnings of a crystallization of staging approaches appropriate to NHL as distinct from Hodgkin's disease. In this regard, we again emphasize that no matter how precise the execution of a radiotherapy technique, the result will at best be only palliative if all the disease is not encompassed.

The Ann Arbor staging system for Hodgkin's disease has generally been adopted for NHL and a number of reports have shown its relative value in this regard [28, 189, 191, 193, 206, 207]. Some investigators, however, report that the utility of this system in 'early' NHL is suboptimal especially in relation to stage II. There is no doubt that CS I patients fare consistently better than CS II (see Table 20) but the outcome for stage II has often been indistinguishable from that for CS III [28, 207] and some investigators have sought to subdivide CS II into a 'true' II and an advanced II. This issue is by no means settled but there is evidence that stage II can be subdivided into II *localized* (only two contiguous nodal regions involved) and II *advanced* (greater than two nodal regions on the same side of the diaphragm), with the localized subgroup having FFR and survival expectations similar to stage I following radiation therapy [28, 52, 199, 203, 208]. A 75% cure rate has been reported for CS I and II *localized* following involved field radiation and salvage chemotherapy, while CS II *advanced* had a survival curve which failed to reveal evidence for cure up to 6 years following treatment [28]. Another report found that PS II DHL could be divided into those with fewer than four sites involved, where none relapsed and those with four or more disease sites where all relapsed following irradiation [203]. However, no generally accepted modification of the Ann Arbor system for NHL has emerged.

Another aspect of uncertainty surrounding the Ann Arbor system reflects the diversity of 'sites of origin' for NHL. Whereas Hodgkin's disease almost universally presents as nodal disease, mostly supradiaphragmatic, the NHL manifest initially in a variety of sites, nodal and extranodal. Most investigators find that localized extranodal disease has either the same [185, 190, 191, 193, 203, 206, 207, 209, 210] or a somewhat better prognosis [211] than correspondingly localized nodal disease. Similarly a distinction is not often made between supradiaphragmatic and subdiaphragmatic presentations. However, these diverse disease sites present the radiation oncologist with significantly different technical problems both in terms of irradiation volume and permissible dose. Evidence is available that diffuse lymphomas in some sites such as mediastinum or abdominal nodes are not readily controllable by toxicologically safe doses [212, 213, 214]. The radiotherapeutic implications of different sites involved by apparently localized NHL will be discussed later.

The development of a uniform staging procedure for NHL has been complicated by the diverse sites of presentation, by the generally older age of the patients and by unwarranted parallels drawn with Hodgkin's disease. In particular, the question of laparotomy seems to have been emphasized out of proportion to its relative importance as a staging procedure in NHL. The majority of NHL patients can be shown to have advanced disease (PS III or IV) by interventions short of laparotomy and a number of centers have reported their experiences with a sequential staging approach utilizing sequences such as: physical exam → LAG → bone marrow biopsy → liver biopsy → laparotomy [42, 43, 198, 203, 215]. A number of conclusions are warranted: (i) the detection of occult disease rises in proportion to the intensiveness of work-up; (ii) nodular lymphoma is rarely localized as PS I or II, 6% [42], 12% [215], 20% [43], 25% [198]; (iii) DHL is more commonly truly localized, 30% [42], 31% [203], 60% [43], 62% [198]; (iv) fewer than 1/2 of all patients [43, 198] and perhaps fewer than 20% [42, 215] need laparotomy to document advanced disease; (v) primary extranodal presentations do not differ significantly in their extent to corresponding nodal presentations [42]. However, a number of unexplained discrepancies remain between the various series and the optimal work-up pattern remains to be defined. Some of the staging controversies as they are relevant to the radiation oncologist who wishes to avoid potential pitfalls in the staging and field design for NHL need consideration.

The two largest sequential staging series are from the NCI [42] and Stanford [43], reporting a total of 593 consecutive, unselected patients. Both series are very similar in their initial patient characteristics including histologic subtyping. Both series agree that the LAG is an important diagnostic procedure and is more often positive with the nodular variants (70–90%) than with diffuse histologies (40–66%). Patients with a positive LAG have a high incidence of mesenteric node involvement (80% for nodular and 50% for diffuse) and a substantial risk of splenic and hepatic disease as well. Patients with negative LAG and unfavorable histology (diffuse) have, surprisingly, a low incidence of subsequently detectable abdominal disease (less than 10%). However, major conflicts are found in comparing nodular LAG-negative patients in the two series. The NCI investigators report a low incidence of subsequently documented abdominal disease for nodular LAG-negative patients (15%), while the Stanford group found close to a 50% incidence of subdiaphragmatic involvement in such cases. Mesenteric nodes (47%) and spleen (41%) were the most common sites. The M.D. Anderson investigators found an even higher incidence of occult abdominal disease in LAG-negative nodular lymphomas with a 57% incidence mainly in spleen, celiac nodes and mesenteric nodes [198]. This latter report also noted that only one nodular lymphoma patient with occult abdominal disease had an involved node measuring more than 3 cm in diameter; the majority of involved nodes in these patients were 2 cm or less in diameter and, presumably, would not have been detected as abnormal by CT scan [198]. In contrast to these findings, the University of Chicago team [215] had results largely in agreement with the NCI. The issue of occult abdominal disease in nodular LAG-negative lymphoma patients remains unsettled. The inverted Y field, however, is not an appropriate field for subdiaphragmatic irradiation, definitive or prophylactic, in NHL [213, 216, 217].

The incidence of documented liver disease also shows major variations between various series. The NCI documented hepatic disease in 43% of their patients while Stanford found only an 8% incidence. The University of Chicago report [206] had a 22% incidence of hepatic disease in lymphocytic and mixed lympho-histiocytic lymphomas. Perhaps the high detection rate

tomy is the only accurate method for its detection. The omission of percutaneous biopsy, laparoscopy-directed biopsy and finally laparotomy liver biopsy. The incidence of hepatic involvement seems to correlate with cytologic subtype: lymphocytic and mixed have the highest involvement rates in all series, 67% [42], 38% [215], while DHL has a lower incidence, 7% [43], 23% [42].

All investigators agree that marrow involvement is common in lymphocytic and mixed lymphohistiocytic subtypes, and that more than one marrow *biopsy* may be necessary to detect involvement [42, 43, 215]. One series reported that about 1/3 of patients with a negative first biopsy were found to have marrow involvement on a second or third repeat biopsy [215]. Virtually all patients with DLWD lymphoma have marrow involvement [42, 43, 215] and some authorities regard this cell type to be identical to that described in chronic lymphocytic leukemia [89]. Poorly differentiated lymphocytic or mixed lymphohistiocytic (nodular or diffuse) lymphomas have marrow disease with a frequency variously reported at 25% [43], 44% [42] or 65% [215]. DHL has a less than 15% incidence of marrow involvement at presentation [42, 43].

Following the various ante-laparotomy procedures, more than 1/2 of all NHL patients will have documented stage III or IV disease. The cases remaining as I or II are potentially candidates for laparotomy, though some will have had this procedure as a diagnostic measure. The advanced age of many NHL patients and associated cardiopulmonary disease will render a significant proportion unsuitable for staging lapartomy. Some investigators routinely exclude those aged 65 or over, while others require more specific surgical contraindications such as cardiopulmonary disease. Reflecting these different views as to what constitutes a contraindication to staging surgery, as many as 87% of sequentially staged patients have been considered as laparotomy candidates [203, 215], while others have felt that as few as 33% were reasonably acceptable for this procedure [198]. Whatever criteria are used for selecting sequentially staged I and II patients for laparotomy, all investigators agree that positive findings are relatively uncommon with DHL: less than 10% in the Stanford report [43]; 18% in the NCI series [42] and 24% at the M.D. Anderson [198]. Despite this low laparotomy yield, surgery appears to remain the only method for detecting those with occult abdominal disease, and for delineating those patients with truly stage I or II disease. Two recent reports have found FFR in about 3/4 of PS I and II DHL patients treated by IF radiation therapy and attribute this good result to the accuracy of staging [45, 212]. The argument for laparotomy seems even more cogent with the availability of potentially curative chemotherapy for advanced DHL.

The LAG-negative nodular lymphoma patients present a controversy and dilemma. Whatever the true incidence of occult abdominal disease, laparo-

found by the NCI workers reflects their aggressive approach involving laparotomy will hinder the accumulation of accurate data on the natural history of these diseases, but it is by no means clear the particular patient in question loses anything by forgoing laparotomy. Currently there is no curative therapy for advanced nodular lymphomas [196, 215, 218, 219] and there is much evidence to suggest that adequate disease control, if not complete remission, can be induced in the majority of those who relapse following radiation therapy [44, 215, 218]. Accordingly, even if we accept a laparotomy conversion ratio in these patients, laparotomy would not be expected to change the chances for cure of an ante-laparotomy staged I or II patient with today's therapy. The choice for or against staging laparotomy in

Table 19. Heuristic summary of sequential staging in diffuse and nodular DHL. The patient numbers quoted are not meant to imply precise results, but rather, best estimates of yields by the different staging procedures. The sequence of pre-laparotomy investigation may not be optimal and CT scanning may be preferable to an initial LAG. For nodular lymphomas bone marrow biopsy is preferable prior to LAG.

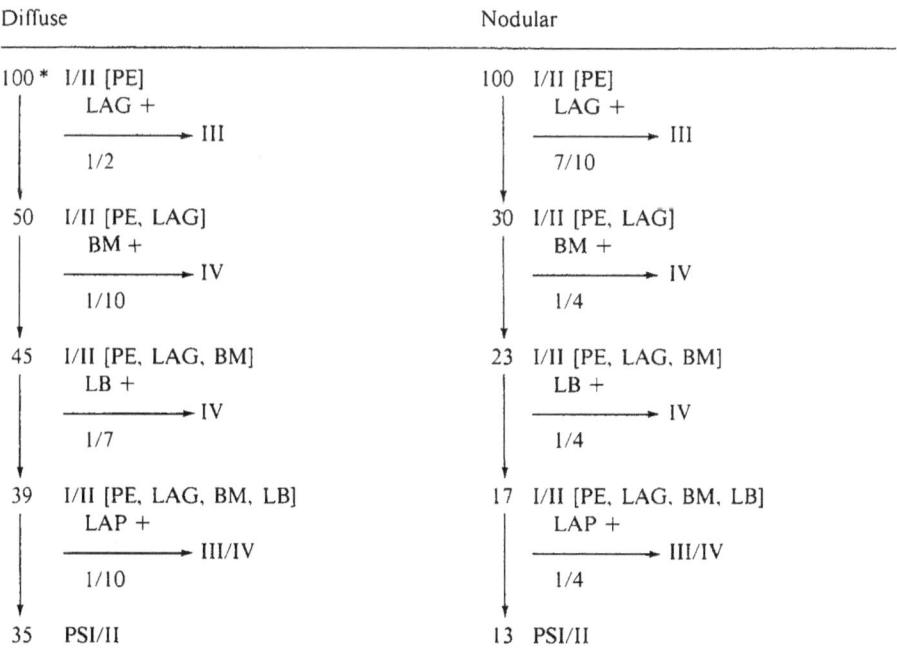

Diffuse	Nodular
100 * I/II [PE] LAG + ──────→ III 1/2	100 I/II [PE] LAG + ──────→ III 7/10
50 I/II [PE, LAG] BM + ──────→ IV 1/10	30 I/II [PE, LAG] BM + ──────→ IV 1/4
45 I/II [PE, LAG, BM] LB + ──────→ IV 1/7	23 I/II [PE, LAG, BM] LB + ──────→ IV 1/4
39 I/II [PE, LAG, BM, LB] LAP + ──────→ III/IV 1/10	17 I/II [PE, LAG, BM, LB] LAP + ──────→ III/IV 1/4
35 PSI/II	13 PSI/II

*   : number of patients
PE   : physical exam
LAG : lymphangiogram
BM   : bone marrow biopsy
LB   : liver biopsy
LAP : laparotomy

these patients will depend upon the oncologist's philosophy and the studies in which he is engaged.

Table 19 is a heuristic presentation of the flow of patients along the sequential pathway; it is intended to emphasize the need for a deliberate, sequential staging approach, reserving laparotomy as the last measure for the majority of patients. The role of newer techniques such as ultrasound and CT scanning will need further evaluation.

2.4. Early Stages of NHL: I and II

2.4.1. The Results of Radiation Therapy. Prior to the recent demonstration of long term disease-free survival in advanced DHL patients treated by multiple agent chemotherapy, radiation was the only potentially curative mode available for NHL and appropriately it became the treatment of choice for early stage disease. The early report by Peters in 1960 disclosed an overall 50% 5-year survival following high dose radiation therapy and revealed an apparent lack of benefit from prophylactic irradiation [199]. Since then, radiotherapeutic approaches to localized NHL have been considerably more varied in radiation volume than is the case in Hodgkin's disease. Consider-

Table 20. Results of radiation therapy in CS I and II NHL *.

Patients	Stage	FFR (5 year)	Survival (5 year)	Investigators
51	I + II	—	63%	Peckham *et al.*, 1975 [210]
65	I	—	55%	Tubania *et al.*, 1975 [223]
88	II	—	30%	
52	I	—	72%	Musshoff *et al.*, 1975 [211]
68	II	—	37%	
65	I	60%	83%	Hellman *et al.*, 1977 [209]
	II	<20%	83%	
140	I	—	70%	Bush *et al.*, 1977 [28]
153	II	—	60%	
54	I	55%	77%	Reddy *et al.*, 1977 [191]
38	II	30%	46%	
12	I	50%	50%	Hoppe *et al.*, 1978 [204] **
22	II	25%	25%	
84	I + II	52%	72%	Chen *et el.*, 1979 [193]
47	I	—	50%	Fraser *et al.*, 1979 [206] **
43	I	49%	61%	Mill *et al.*, 1980 [224] **
33	II	39%	53%	
413	I	49–60%	50–83%	
423	II	20–39%	25–83%	

*   Involved field or regional irradiation.
** Exclusively extranodal presentations.

Table 21. Results of radiation therapy in CS I and II NHL according to nodularity.

Patients	Nodularity	FFR (5 year)	S (5 year)	Investigators
62	Nodular	—	65%	Fuller *et al.*, 1975 [214]
152	Diffuse	—	26%	
21	Nodular	—	75%	Peckham *et al.*, 1975 [210]
30	Diffuse	—	50%	
	Nodular	55%	100%	Hellman *et al.*, 1977 [209]
65	Diffuse	0	<50%	
23	Nodular	55%	90%	Reddy *et al.*, 1977 [191]
67	Diffuse	40%	55%	
26	Nodular	83%	100%	Chen *et al.*, 1979 [193]
58	Diffuse	37%	59%	
132	Nodular	55–83%	65–100%	
307	Diffuse	0–40%	26–59%	

able indirect evidence has accumulated to suggest that extended field techniques such as TNI or STN offer little advantage compared to more localized approaches [191, 193, 206, 208, 209, 220], though some authorities have made a plea for the systematic evaluation of large volume approaches [221, 222]. Evaluation of radiation therapy results is also hampered by non-uniform and incomplete staging approaches. Even in many recent series, significant fractions of patients have not had an LAG or a bone marrow biopsy, led alone staging laparotomy [28, 191, 193, 204, 206, 223, 224]. In view of the now recognized propensity of these diseases for early dissemination, the somewhat disappointing results achieved in what seemed to be localized processes are perhaps not too surprising. However, there is no doubt that significant numbers of 'early' patients with NHL have been cured by radiation alone.

Table 20 is a summary of 20 series reported during the past 5 years on CS I and II NHL patients treated by high dose (3500–4000 rads), local or regional fields. For CSI, FFR at 5 years varies between 50% and 60% with an overall survival in 1/2 to 2/3 of the patients. Results are distinctly poorer in CS II, with FFR at 5 years in only 1/5 to 1/3 and a survival, in general, less than 50%. The influence of nodularity is summarized in Table 21 which documents the favorability of nodular disease (5-year FFR greater than 55%, survival up to 100%) compared to diffuse variants (5-year FFR less than 40%, survival mostly less than 50%). The influence of specific histologic subtype according to the Rappaport scheme is more difficult to analyze. Table 22 summarizes the outcome for localized DHL, where FFR is less than 50% and survival occurs in fewer than 2/3. Stage II DHL has a distinctly worse prognosis than stage I in all series where this distinction is

Table 22. Results of radiation therapy in CS I and II DHL.

Patients	Stage	FFR (5 year)	S (5 year)	Investigators
13	I	45%	65%	Jones *et al.*, 1973 [207]
35	II	25%	25%	
91	I + II	−	26%	Fuller *et al.*, 1975 [214]
43	I + II	−	60%	Peckham *et al.*, 1975 [210]
16	I	35%	46%	Reddy *et al.*, 1977 [191]
12	II	18%	35%	
31	I + II	<36%	59%	Chen *et al.*, 1979 [193]
38	I + II	45%	57%	Mill *et al.*, 1980 [224]
279	I + II	18–45%	25–65%	

made [45, 191, 207] and it is doubtful whether IF therapy for CS II DHL can achieve better than 25% FFR at 5 years. DLPD lymphomas seem to have an outcome not much different to DHL of corresponding stage when treated by radiation [207]. The favorable survival results of the nodular categories are largely a direct reflection of the outcome for NLPD and NM lymphoma. NH is a rare variant and there is evidence that its prognosis falls between the classic nodular and diffuse variants, tending more toward the unfavorable than the favorable [189, 194, 207].

It has been recognized for some time that the time course of relapse is quite distinct for nodular as compared to diffuse subtypes. In their original analysis Rappaport and co-workers noted the relatively indolent and slowly progressive nature of nodular lymphomas, with an acceleration in disease tempo often corresponding to a transition in histology from nodular to diffuse [6, 225]. This long natural history is reflected in a slow relapse rate. Since 1973 [207] it has repeatedly been documented that relapses from apparent CR continue to appear over many years [28, 187, 217, 218, 227] with resultant survival curves that do not become parallel to those of a corresponding normal population for at least 7 years [28, 196]. Consequently, 10, 15, or even 20 year follow-up may be necessary to fully evaluate the impact of treatment on nodular type disease. There is nevertheless sufficient evidence to regard approximately 60% of stages I and II (localized) nodular NHL patients as curable by involved-field or regional therapy [28, 207]. The high continuing relapse rate of nodular lymphomas following localized radiation therapy is not surprising in view of the recent, perhaps paradoxical, finding that it is the favorable subtype which is most often disseminated at presentation. Disappointing, however, is the finding that chemotherapy, too, is unable to totally eradicate this form of disease.

Table 23. Patterns of relapse following localized radiation therapy for *nodular* NHL, CS I and II.

Number relapsed	Nodal relapse only	Contiguous nodal relapse	Investigators
40	25	*	Fuller *et al.,* 1975 [214]
10	6	*	Peckham *et al.,* 1975 [210]
30	24	10	Fuks *et al.,* 1975 [221]
8	6	9	Chen *et al.,* 1979 [193]
88	61 (69%)		

* Not stated.

In contrast, diffuse lymphomas have a rapid tempo of progression and relapse, if it is to occur, will usually (in more than 85%) be evident by the end of the second year following treatment [28, 45, 195, 196, 207]. Thus, the patient with a diffuse lymphoma, though less likely to survive 2 years than the one with nodular disease, once passing this time point free from disease, has a very high chance of permanent disease freedom. Clearly, if the achievement of CR in localized DHL is made more likely either by accurate staging [45] or by adjuvant chemotherapy [192, 228], this 'unfavorable' histology may well become 'favorable'.

Patterns of relapse following radiation to CS I and II NHL are presented in Tables 23 and 24. For nodular NHL a high incidence of subsequent nodal failure has been reported by most investigators. The majority of such failures have been noncontiguous and often involved a number of nodal sites. For upper torso presentations, subsequent abdominal nodal failure is common [214, 221] and a similar transdiaphragmatic pattern is encountered for

Table 24. Patterns of relapse following localized radiation therapy for *diffuse* NHL, CS I and II.

Number relapsed	Nodal only *	Investigators
71	17	Fuller *et al.,* 1975 [214]
45	22	Peckham *et al.,* 1975 [210]
63	43	Fuks *et al.,* 1975 [221]
21	8	Hoppe *et al.,* 1978 [204]
38	14	Chen *et al.,* 1979 [193]
76	14	Mill *et al.,* 1980 [224]
314	118 (38%)	

* Two series report 24/57 (43%) nodal relapses as contiguous [193, 221].

lower torso presentations [214]. Contiguity, however, does not apply to the majority since patterns such as mid cervical → inguinal or central abdominal → right axillary are not unusual. Apropos of our earlier discussion on the staging of these diseases, such patterns of relapse are not unexpected but do preclude the delineation of prophylactic fields short of virtually whole-trunk irradiation. Moreover, the recognition of a high incidence of marrow involvement at presentation makes it likely that systematic evaluation of relapsed patients will disclose a similar pattern. Indeed, the most commonly reported sites of extranodal relapse of nodular lymphoma have been marrow and liver [193, 210, 221].

Diffuse NHL subtypes have a higher propensity for obvious extranodal relapse than do nodular lymphomas. Nodal relapse as an only initial site of failure occurs in about 1/3 of all patients (Table 24). Contiguous nodal relapse accounts for fewer than 1/2 of all these nodal failures [193, 221]. However, true recurrence is virtually confined to the diffuse subtype, especially DHL [28, 44, 221]. The most common sites of extranodal failure are lung, gut, skin, and bone [204, 210, 221, 224]; marrow and liver are less frequently involved. Again, these findings appear to preclude any significant gains by extending radiation fields beyond sites of involvement.

A number of prognostic factors, apart from histology and Ann Arbor stage, have emerged from the studies of CS I and II NHL treated by irradiation, though the influence of any one of these on ultimate outcome is perhaps less dramatic than anticipated. Many series have documented the adverse influence of increasing *age,* with patients over 65 years faring consistently worse than younger individuals [191, 193, 214, 221, 223]. This is probably a reflection of the less intense work-up which elderly patients can withstand and of their lesser ability to tolerate aggressive chemotherapy when relapse occurs. The presence or absence of *systemic symptoms* appears to have little influence on the outcome of early NHL and most series have failed to find a significantly worse prognosis for the early B patient [191, 193, 206, 207, 211, 214]. B symptoms are, however, uncommon in stage I and II [185, 210, 214]. Likewise, *mediastinal disease* is relatively uncommon in NHL occurring in fewer than 24% of all patients [42, 43], but its presence seems to have an adverse effect on outcome; in one series 31/51 (61%) patients without an involved mediastinum were reported to be disease-free following irradiation, while only 1/8 was free from disease in those with mediastinal involvement [210]. The M.D. Anderson investigators have also presented data showing high failure rates for mediastinal disease, especially DHL, managed by radiation alone [212, 214], with true recurrence and dissemination being very common. It is crucial to distinguish the clinicopathologic entity of lymphoblastic lymphoma [229] which often, though not always, has mediastinal disease. This entity, though often apparently localized initially, has such a high conversion ratio to leukemia and CNS involvement that it must be regarded as disseminated from the beginning [229, 230]; radiation alone has only a palliative effect. *Lower torso* presentations have an overall prognosis similar to LAG-negative upper torso disease, but local control is problematic and progressive abdominal disease is a common failure pathway [89, 212–214]. As the staging for supradiaphragmatic disease improves one may anticipate that abdominal lymphadenophy will become an adverse factor since radiation tolerance is limited by structures below the diaphragm. Indeed, the M.D. Anderson group regard abdominal nodal presentations as unfavorable and treat such patients with combined radiation and chemotherapy. The significance of *disease extent* within stage II has already been considered (section 2.3).

2.4.2. Extranodal Presentations. NHL has an extranodal presentation in about 25% of patients in North America [231, 232]. That such presentations are not always merely local manifestations of a widespread process is evident by long-term cure of significant proportions of patients irradiated for apparently localized disease. Most series report little difference in prognosis, stage for stage, between early nodal and early extranodal NHL [185, 189, 191, 203, 206, 207, 209, 210]. However, the radiotherapeutic problems posed by different anatomic sites of disease require separate consideration. It will not be possible to review all potential sites of presentation, since every structure within the body has on occasion been reported as a primary focus, and we will restrict our discussion to certain more common regions of origin.

Prior to the introduction of the Rappaport classification, many reports documented the predilection of reticulum cell sarcoma for extranodal sites [211, 223, 231–233], though lymphosarcoma accounted for about 40% of cases [231, 323]. According to the Rappaport scheme, investigators now report that 70–98% of extranodal presentations have diffuse histology and that DHL accounts for 40–55% of all cases [204, 206, 224, 234, 235]. The second most common histologic variant is DLPD, accounting for 10–44% of all cases in these series. The most common anatomic sites of involvement in extranodal cases are Waldeyer's ring, the gastrointestinal tract, skin, and bone which together account for 2/3 to 3/4 of all extranodal presentations [231, 232]. It should be noted that although Waldeyer's ring is defined as a nodal site in the Ann Arbor system [111], most reports regard it as an extranodal site for NHL.

Waldeyer's ring: The radiation oncologist traditionally regards the upper aerodigestive tract as a region involved by carcinomas having many features in common. This approach is reflected in the tendency of literature reports on NHL, to separate out those involving the upper respiratory and digestive tract and to report these as a whole [208, 236, 237]. Waldeyer's ring (tonsil, nasopharynx, base of tongue) accounts for about 75% of all primary

Table 25. Survival following radiation therapy to CS I and II NHL involving Waldeyer's ring.

Stage	Patients	Survival (5 year)	Investigators
I	24	79%	Wang, 1969 [238]
II *	23	48%	
I	56	54%	Banfi *et al.,* 1972 [208]
II *	156	30%	
I + II	51	46%	Wong *et al.,* 1975 [237]
I	12	50%	Hoppe *et al.,* 1978 [204]
II	22	20%	

* II = Involvement of Waldeyer's ring and contiguous nodes only.

aerodigetive NHL [231, 232, 237] and is associated with features that distinguish it from other head and neck presentations. The most common site of disease within Waldeyer's ring is the palatine tonsil, involved in 37–62% of all cases, followed by nasopharynx (27–36%), and least often, base of tongue (5–15%) [204, 208, 237–239]. Involvement of multiple sites within Waldeyer's ring is common and massive lesions are not unusual [208, 238]. Base of skull and cranial nerve involvement is possible, though unusual [238]. More than 1/2 of all patients have palpable cervical lymphodenopathy, most often upper cervical and unilateral. Careful examination and biopsy of Waldeyer's ring in all NHL patients with localized cervical lymph node enlargement is essential to detect occult disease in this area.

Table 25 presents the results of irradition for localized, clinically-staged NHL of Waldeyer's ring. The single most important prognostic factor is cervical node status [204, 208, 236, 237]. Patients with negative cervical nodes can be expected to have long-term survivals in excess of 50%; with node involvement the outlook is poor and low neck disease is particularly ominous; fewer than 15% survive 5 years [239]. Tonsillar involvement appears to have an adverse effect, with lesions confined to nasopharynx or base of tongue faring somewhat better [208, 239]. Patterns of relapse are similar to those encountered in nodal diffuse histology disease (Table 24), with a high incidence of extranodal failure in the gastrointestinal tract, liver, lung, skin, and marrow [204, 208, 236]. Mediastinal involvement at presentation is very unusual and relapses also show a remarkable tendency to avoid this site [204, 208, 236]. Failure to irradiate initially negative neck nodes is associated with a substantial risk for contiguous failure in this region [206, 208] and most authorities recommend that prophylactic cervical radiation be used in stage I cases. There is no benefit in treating a negative mediastinum [204, 208].

In parallel with recommendations for the staging of nodal NHL, all investigators are increasingly emphasizing the need for adequate evauation of apparently localized aerodigestive NHL patients with LAG, marrow biopsy, liver biopsy and even laparotomy. LAG has been found to be positive in 12–39% of apparently localized patients [208, 236] and laparotomy was positive for occult disease in 4/13 LAG-negative patients explored at Stanford [204]. The apparently special association between NHL of Waldeyer's ring and gastrointestinal involvement reported by Banfi [208] and corroborated by the French workers [236] has not been found by North American investigators [204, 224, 237], suggesting that a geographic variable may be involved.

Paranasal sinuses: Involvement of the paranasal sinuses and/or nasal cavity by NHL, though rare, needs to be recognized. Most commonly the maxillary sinus is the apparent primary site and, in their clinical presentation, NHL in this site are indistinguishable from squamous cell carcinoma [240, 241]. In contrast to Waldeyer's ring disease, cervical lymph node involvement is uncommon (less than 30%) [224, 237, 239, 241] and LAG is less frequently positive [241]. Cervical node relapse is uncommon even in the absence of prophylactic irradiation [240, 241]. The use of wedge-field techniques similar to those employed for squamous carcinomas in this site has resulted in 5-year survivals of about 70% [241].

Thyroid: Primary malignant lymphoma of the thyroid has received increasing attention in view of its association with Hashimoto's thyroiditis, its higher incidence in females than in males and the problem of distinguishing it from so-called anaplastic small cell carcinoma [242–244]. It is important to appreciate the rarity of small cell carcinoma [245, 246] – some pathologists even doubt its existence [244, 245], and the distinction may require electron microscopy [246]. Lymphomas of the thyroid commonly present as a rapidly enlarging goiter or as a thyroid nodule, cold to isotopic scanning [242, 244]. The diagnosis is rarely made prior to surgery, but surgery has little place in its management apart from biopsy [247]. The vast majority are histiocytic lymphomas [242, 244] mostly diffuse, but nodular variants are perhaps more common than in other extranodal sites [244]. Following regional irradiation, patients with disease initially localized to the neck experience a 50% 5-year survival [247]. One recent study reports an 89% 5-year survival if neck nodes are negative, compared to a 27% survival for stage II cases [244]. Patterns of failure following local therapy reveal a high incidence of extranodal relapse and some authors have emphasized gastrointestinal relapse as especially common [242, 243]. The need to adequately stage these patients is evident.

Less commonly affected head and neck sites such as oral cavity [240] and orbit [248] have also been managed by local-regional radiation with results not dissimilar to those presented above.

Gastrointestinal tract: Primary lymphoma of the gastrointestinal tract (GIT) is among the most common of extranodal NHL presentations [231, 232]. It is also among the most difficult to analyze and to define optimal therapeutic approaches. Recent histopathologic controversies assure further uncertainties in the classification of these diseases especially with the reports of plasmacytomas, true histiocytic malignancies and variants such as Mediterranean-type lymphoma masquerading as 'typical' GIT NHL [249–251]. Furthermore the not uncommon presentation of this group of diseases as abdominal emergencies requires laparotomy in a setting not conducive to optimal evaluation of extent of intra-abdominal disease. The urgency of defining therapeutic aproaches is accentuated by recent reports that DHL of the GIT is surprisingly refractory to multi-agent chemotherapy [252].

NHL of the GIT is most common in the stomach, followed by distal small bowel and ileo-cecal region with colonic and rectal disease being uncommon [234, 253–257]. Lymphoma is the most common malignant neoplasm of the small bowel [258] and in that site is occasionally associated with celiac disease or dermatitis herpetiformis [251]. The vast majority of lesions are solitary [253, 254, 258], though multiple sites of mucosal involvement sometimes occur [253]. Recent series report that the majority of lesions are of diffuse histology, especially DHL [235, 252]. Regional node involvement (gastric or mesenteric nodes) occurs in about 1/2 of all patients [235, 253] but the true incidence of para-aortic and celiac involvement is poorly documented. A recent Stanford report found that 45 % of GIT NHL were stage IE or IIE [235], while the NCI could find only 28 % to be in these early stages [252]. There is, however, uncertainty on the applicability of Ann Arbor stages to GIT lymphoma and attempts have been made to utilize staging systems developed for carcinoma by taking into account depth of penetration [259]. There is good evidence that disease spread to para-aortic nodes or spleen, even though staged as II, decreases survival considerably [255, 260].

In a review of the predominantly surgical experience with GIT NHL spanning the years 1932 to 1959, Nicoloff *et al.* found that nine series reported 5-year survivals for gastric lymphoma in 20–43 % of cases, with slightly poorer results for small and large intestine of 12–25 % [254]. All the survivors had radical surgery and a proportion were given postoperative orthovoltage irradiation. No conclusions on the value of radiation therapy could be made. Naqvi *et al.* in their large series of 162 cases found that regional node status had a significant impact on prognosis [255]. Gastric lymphoma without nodal disease had a 47 % 5-year survival, while regional node involvement lowered this to 27 % and more widespread abdominal disease decreased the results to 15 %. Similar observations were made for intestinal lesions. 82 % of these patients received adjuvant postoperative irradiation but its role was not defined. Support for postoperative irradiation came from Loehr *et al.* in 1969, who found that of 42 patients treated by definitive resection alone and followed for 5 years, 23 (55%) remained alive, while in a similar group of 13 patients given 3000–4000 rads following surgery, 11 (85%) remained alive [256]. Similar suggestive evidence in favor of adjuvant radiation was provided by Bush [260] who found that for disease localized to bowel or regional nodes, postoperative radiation increased 5-year survival from 15% to about 50%. Doses of 2500 rads in 4–6 weeks to the whole abdomen virtually eliminated subsequent abdominal relapse. However, patients with extensive abdominal involvement were incurable.

More recent series have failed to produce any more definitive evidence on the role of radiation in these diseases. In a series of 50 patients with gastric lymphoma, 38 were found to be resectable by total or subtotal gastrectomy, 36 survived the operation and of these, 67% were alive at 5 years [259]. Fewer than half of the resectable cases received radiation and only 2/13 with early disease (not penetrating serosa, without nodal involvement) were irradiated and yet more than 80% survived 5 years. At Stanford all stage IE GIT lymphomas receive radiation therapy following total tumor resection and for DHL the reported FFR is 85% [235]. Advanced nonresectable lesions continue to have a poor outcome. The NCI workers have found a poor response to combination chemotherapy in the DHL subtypes with a high incidence of perforation or hemorrhage following institution of chemotherapy for nonresected lesions [252, 261].

Bone: Extranodal NHL presenting in bone constitutes a well defined clinicopathologic entity first clearly delineated by Parker and Jackson in 1939 [262] and almost exclusively referred to as 'primary reticulum cell sarcoma of bone' [263–265]. The histologic spectrum encountered in other extranodal presentations is represented in these lesions [266], but detailed analyses are unavailable. Clinically the involvement is confined to one bone and in 2/3 of cases one of the long bones of the limbs is affected [263, 266]. A peculiarly long history prior to definitive diagnosis occurs commonly [265, 267] and lesions are usually massive with significant soft tissue swelling due to extra-osseous extension [265, 267]. Radiologically the appearances are osteolytic, but non-diagnostic [264, 265]. Pathologically, care must be taken to differentiate Ewing's sarcoma, eosinophilic granuloma and osteomyelitis from lymphoma [265].

A variety of therapeutic approaches have been directed against reticulum cell sarcoma of bone, including amputation [262, 263, 268]. Coley's toxins [268] and local irradiation [265–267]. Five year survivals have been reported to lie between 35% and 64% [263–268]. In terms of survival, there is no advantage for amputation [266] and therefore, limb sacrifice has no place in the management of this disease. Radiation therapy in doses >4500 rads achieves local control in more than 90% (Table 26) and remains the treatment of choice. Five-year survival following radiation alone is

Table 26. Local control of 'reticulum cell sarcoma' of bone with radiation therapy.

<4500 rads	≥4500 rads	Investigators
8/11	5/5	Wang *et al.*, 1968 [265]
1/2	11/11	Phillips *et al.*, 1969 [267]
6/10	8/10	Newell *et al.*, 1970 [233]
15/23 (65%)	24/26 (92%)	

50% [265–267], though unexpectedly a number of late relapses and deaths have been documented [267]. Irradiation should include the whole bone from one articular surface to the other and should encompass all soft tissue extension leaving a strip of skin unirradiated for lymphatic drainage. Patterns of relapse following irradiation are poorly defined and most series speak of 'disseminated metastases'. Regional lymph node disease is said to occur in about 20% of patients and it has been recommended that these be included on a prophylactic basis [265]. Whether this is really necessary cannot be stated. However, there is no reason to regard this disease entity any differently to the extranodal NHL in terms of the staging procedures necessary at diagnosis.

Skin: Cutaneous extranodal NHL typically presents as a solitary, reddish-purple skin nodule or, less frequently, as a cluster of small nodules localized to one site [269]. Growth tends to be rapid and ulceration supervenes. Most commonly, the skin of the forehead, cheek, scalp or interscapular area is involved [269, 270]. Multiple lesions in a variety of sites are best regarded as cutaneous manifestations of systemic disease. Pathologically the lesions have been classified as lymphosarcoma or reticulum cell sarcoma. Wide field skin irradiation is highly effective in controlling solitary lesions and of 19 cases in two series, no treatment failures were recorded and systemic disease did not develop in any patient with follow-up up to 10 years [269, 270]. Doses varying between 800 rads in one treatment and 3000 rads in 10 days were uniformly effective. However, a note of caution to the acceptance of all solitary cutaneous lymphomas as truly localized comes from a recent report where a patient with one cutaneous nodule on the nose was found to have occult abdominal disease at laparotomy [198].

CNS: With the advent of multi-agent chemotherapy and the lengthening of the median survival for advanced NHL patients, central nervous system (CNS) relapse has become a more common manifestation of NHL than primary 'reticulum cell sarcoma of the brain' [230, 271]. Nevertheless, primary CNS NHL is an important radiotherapeutic challenge since it often remains localized to the CNS and all too often proves recalcitrant to therapy.

The neuropathology of this disease is controversial and though most authorities report a histopathologic spectrum similar to that encountered in extraneural NHL [272–274], the terminology remains idiosyncratic with designations such as microglioma, reticulum cell sarcoma, and malignant reticuloendotheliosis which bear no clear relation to currently utilized lymphoma terminologies. The notion that these lesions arise from microglia has been challenged [273]. A number of pathologic facts are, however, crucial to a rational therapeutic approach. The disease is most common in the cerebrum (70% of cases), with a lower propensity for cerebellar and brain stem involvement (16% each); spinal cord presentations are very rare [273–275]. Macroscopically, the disease is multifocal in about 1/2 of the cases but at the microscopic level, multicentricity, especially in a perivascular distribution, is even higher [273]. Each nodule is poorly marginated with infiltration into surrounding brain substance. Spinal cord seeding certainly occurs and has been described in as many as six of 24 patients in one series [275], but was not detected in any of 83 cases in another series [273]. Perhaps the most striking fact is the rarity of extraneural disease even in those surviving for 3 years. Three series reporting a total of 126 patients found extraneural involvement in only 10 cases (8%) [273–275].

Therapeutic approaches to primary CNS lymphoma have included surgery or combined surgery with postoperative radiation [273, 274]. Since the disease is often multifocal and the individual lesions poorly marginated, surgery alone is inadequate. Unfortunately, the addition of radiation has failed to produce significant curative results and this disease has a prognosis reminiscent of glioblastoma multiforme. A literature review by Littman and Wang [274] could find only six patients surviving for 5 years out of 150 reported (4%). In their own experience with 19 cases, these authors had 15 deaths by 6 years, three were treated too recently for commont and only one was a survivor beyond the 6-year mark. Significantly, of the 15 deaths, neurologic deterioration occurred in 12 prior to death, suggesting either local recurrence or extension. Similar findings were reported by Sagerman et al. who attributed active intracranial neoplasm as the cause of death in 12 of 16 fatalities following radiation therapy [275]. The vast majority of reported cases, however, received less than 4500 rads and often only to 'the site of the lesion' [273–275]. These data clearly indicate the need for an aggressive radiation therapy approach to primary cerebral NHL. Whole brain irradiation to 5000 rads followed by cone-down boosts of 1000–1500 rads to involved foci seem appropriate. Prophylactic spinal irradiation has been recommended [275], though it is not clear whether all patients need this [273]. In lieu of spinal radiation, an argument can be made for adjuvant intrathecal chemotherapy and even perhaps for systemic treatment as an aid to local CNS control.

In relation to primary CNS lymphoma, the entity described as 'ocular reticulum cell sarcoma' needs brief mention. The disease presents as a chronic steroid-resistant uveitis and is usually diagnosed by biopsy after a prolonged and fruitless uveitis evaluation [276, 277]. Following diagnosis, radiation therapy to *both* eyes is indicated and the whole brain should be treated prophylactically.

Testis: NHL arising as an apparent primary lesion has been described in the ovary [278, 279] and testis [280, 281]. Testicular NHL has a particular relevance to radiation therapy in that this tumor is often approached in a manner analogous to the treatment of testicular seminoma [281–283], with inguinal orchiectomy, LAG-staging and para-aortic-pelvic node irradiation. While a small minority of patients managed this way to achieve long-term survival, the vast majority rapidly relapse and die within 2 years [279, 281, 282]. One recent series of 17 CS IE or IIE patients followed for more than 3 months (12 staged by LAG), reports relapse in 10, with a median time to relapse of 5 months [281]. Local-regional treatment was considered to have been curative in four patients. Another series on 21 CS IE and IIE patients reported 15 deaths with a median of 12 months and only two patients were alive and well at 6 and 47 months [279]. A high incidence of clinically occult disease accounts for this rapid failure pattern. At least 1/2 of the patients will have a positive LAG [279, 281] and one study documented liver involvement in two such patients subjected to laparotomy [279]. The same report also had three patients with negative LAG who were explored and all three had abdominal disease (liver involved in two).

In all series of testicular lymphoma, relapse patterns have been disseminated with failure in lung, liver, spleen and Waldeyer's ring being common. Clearly, testicular NHL is rarely localized at presentation and the majority of patients will be found to have widespread disease, well beyond the reach of curative radiation therapy. For those patients remaining in the truly localized category, it seems prudent to administer radiation in the same manner as used for localized germ cell tumors [281].

2.4.3. Pathologic Staging and Combined Modes. Compared to Hodgkin's disease, early stage NHL presents a more formidable therapeutic challenge – results have not reached levels where fine tuning of treatment approaches, with the hopes of minimizing complications and yet maintaining high cure rates, is a reality. A primary goal remains the definition of those treatment programs which will assure a high FFR. Approches aimed at achieving this goal have included extended field irradiation [192, 222], comprehansive sequential staging [42, 43, 45, 203, 215] and combined radiation-chemotherapy protocols [192, 212, 218]. Enthusiasm for high dose, large-volume irradiation in early NHL has been infrequent and the patterns of relapse following IF therapy (Tables 23 and 24) imply that relatively little would be gained by systematic prophylactic treatment beyond proximal uninvolved nodal areas.

The Stanford trial, addressing this question for PS I and II favorable histology (NLWD, NLPD, NM, DLWD) NHL, had too few patients followed for adequate times to draw firm conclusions, but there appeared to be no significant difference in outcome following IF or TNI irradiation [192]. Most investigators have relied upon the better definition of disease extent and/or the use of combined radiation-chemotherapy to improve treatment results.

The relatively prolonged natural history, with slow progression and late relapse hinders short-term evaluation of therapeutic approaches to favorable histology NHL (NLPD, NM, NLWD). Survival curves for early stages do not become parallel to a corresponding normal population curve for at least 6 years [28] and a decade of observation of any cohort of patients seems necessary to draw firm conclusions [192]. Accordingly, the results of recent studies are only tentative. Truly localized nodular NHL is rare but radiation is curative in about 60% of stage I cases [28]. However, there is little evidence that intensive staging better identifies these curable cases. The Milan series on PS I and II NHL reported a 5-year FFR in 55% of patients with nodular histology receiving IF radiation therapy [228]; the M.D. Anderson report on laparotomy staged I and II nodular NHL gave a 3-year FFR in about 35% [212]; the University of Chicago series on fully staged localized lymphocytic and mixed cellularity NHL (nodular and diffuse) had a 75% FFR at 6 years following radiation [15]. These results are entirely comparable to the earlier reports summarized in Table 20. The addition of adjuvant chemotherapy to the radiation treatment of localized nodular lymphoma also appears to have little effect on the ultimate outcome. In the Milan study there was no statistically significant difference between radiation therapy alone and radiation followed by CVP chemotherapy (5-year FFR 55% vs 63% respectively, P = 0.6) [212]. Similarly the preliminary report from M.D. Anderson on comparing radiation alone with radiation followed by CHOP-Bleo chemotherapy, found no difference [215].

These data do not support the routine use of adjuvant chemotherapy following irradiation for early stage nodular NHL. Radiation therapy remains the only available potentially curative modality for these patients. Sequential staging short of laparotomy will identify the majority of advanced cases and the use of laparotomy is controversial (section 2.3).

The unfavoragle histologies of NHL (DLPD, DHL, DM), having a short natural history, yield to short-term evaluation. In addition, advanced stages, especially DHL, are yielding to chemotherapy and the outlook, at least in principle, for effective adjuvant treatment in early stages is more realistic than for nodular variants. Adequate staging alone appears to improve the outlook for irradiated patients. The University of Chicago investigators reported on 20 laparotomy staged I and II DHL patients receiving radiation theapy (10 SNI, 6 TNI, 4 IF), with an FFR at 5 years of 78% (median follow-up about 27 months [203]. This result appears superior to previous reports on CS I and II DHL (Table 22). A recent update of this experience shows that none of the 14 PS I DHL patients relapsed with disease (median freedom from relapse 54 months), while 10 of 14 PS II patients have failed (median freedom from relapse 14 months) with successful chemotherapy salvage in only 25% of the failures [45]. Stanford has reported a 65% FFR at 5 years for PS I and II DHL receiving TNI, with an overal survival of 70% [192]. These results indicate that a careful staging work-up can delineate truly localized DHL amenable to curative radiation therapy. PS I DHL probably needs only local-regional radiation to achieve a high cure expectation. However, PS II DHL retains a high relapse rate especially with multiple sites of involvement [45, 203] or bulky disease [284].

Few reports on adjuvant chemotherapy in PS I and II unfavorable histology NHL have been published and follow-up in the three major studies has been short [192, 212, 228]. The Milan group report a statistically significant superior FFR at 5 years in diffuse PS I and II NHL treated with radiation therapy followed by six cycles of CVP chemotherapy [228]; this superiority in freedom from first relapse was not, however, translated into a superior survival when compared to radiation followed by salvage chemotherapy. It should be noted too, that only 3/4 of the patients in this study had laparotomy, the remainder were laparoscopy-staged. The 45% FFR at 5 years following irradiation alone is disappointingly low for PS I and II and may reflect inadequate staging. The M.D. Anderson study on PS I and II NHL could find no difference in FFR or survival between patients treated with radiation alone and patients receiving adjuvant CHOP-Bleo chemotherapy: in DHL, 3-years FFR was about 55% and survival 85% [212]. In this study, however, all patients were not randomized and those with mediastinal disease or lower torso presentations were directly assigned to both modalities. The Stanford study on early stage unfavorable NHL also failed to delineate any advantage in FFR or survival in the adjuvant chemotherapy arm [192]. They acheived a 65% FFR at 5 years with radiation alone (survival, 70%) and 45% FFR with both modalities ($P = 0.48$) (survival 65%).

These data indicate that the best chances for cure in early unfavorable histology NHL lie in a full staging work-up, including laparotomy, followed by local-regional radiation therapy. The chemotherapeutic advances in the treatment of advanced DHL have not yet been shown to clearly alter the outlook for early stage patients receiving radiation therapy. Chemotherapy alone in one uncontrolled study [285] produced surprisingly good results. This experience needs to be confirmed.

2.5. Advanced NHL: Stages III and IV

2.5.1. Advanced Nodular NHL. The relatively favorable nodular variants of NHL pose perplexing and paradoxic problems. The vast majority of patients with these histologies have advanced disease (section 2.3) and though remission induction is relatively easy with a number of different therapeutic approaches, the *durable* complete remission has proven to be elusive. Multi-agent chemotherapy is able to produce CR in 75–90% of advanced nodular NHL [215, 218, 286–288], but relapses occur with disconcerting frequency and median duration of remission is only about 24 months [196, 215, 286]. Single agent chemotherapy in one trial was found to be no less effective than multi-agent combinations or combined radiation-chemotherapy [287]. Moreover, advanced nodular NHL has proven to be an exception to the generally valid dictum that complete remission prolongs survival, since many patients with demonstrable disease continue to survive for prolonged periods without significant disability. A recent analysis from Stanford lends some support for a policy of masterly inactivity for asymptomatic advanced nodular NHL [219]. In a retrospective review of 44 patients with stages III or IV nodular NHL whose treatment was postponed until dictated by symptoms or disease progression, it was found that the median time to first treatment was 31 months. The median survival of these 44 patients was 10 years and compared to 67 similar asymptomatic patients who received treatment on diagnosis there were no differences either in response to treatment or ultimate survival [219]. There are advantages and disadvantages to withholding treatment [289] but some investigators have turned to radiation therapy as an alternative modality for advanced nodular NHL.

For stage III disease, TNI has proven to be surprisingly effective with FFR at 5 years in about one-half of patients (Table 27). This radiation therapy experience has also revealed a number of potentially significant therapeutic facts. Virtually all stage III nodular NHL patients receiving TNI achieve CR [205, 210, 290]. In the Stanford experience [207, 217], with a median follow-up of 80 months, 28/51 patients relapsed and of the 28 failures, 18 were confined to lymph nodes. Six nodal relapses were confined to epitrochlear or brachial nodes and these were salvaged by further radiation. Since all

Table 27. Results of TNI in stage III nodular NHL *.

Patients	FFR (5 year)	Survival (5 year)	Investigators
47	40%	65%	Jones *et al.*, 1973 [207]
51	43%	75%	Glatstein *et al.*, 1976 [217]
22	65%	90%	Cox, 1978 [205] **
120	40–65%	65–90%	

* CR following TNI occurred in 86/86 (100%) patients in 3 series [205, 217, 290].
** TNI and whole abdominal irradiation.

these relapses occurred in patients with ipsilateral axillary or bulky supra-clavicular lymphadenopathy, prophylactic epitrochlear irradiation seems indicated in such cases. The whole abdomen was irradiated only in eight patients and since 24% of NLPD and NM variants with initial subdiaphrag-matic disease relapse in the abdomen following inverted Y treatment [216], it was concluded that whole abdominal irradiation might have achieved a higher FFR. Cox [205] has provided evidence that doses lower than the traditional 4000 rads utilized at Stanford are equally as effective for nodular disease. Using four fields in sequence (Waldeyer's ring, mantle, abdomen, pelvis), each given 2500–3000 rads, an impressive 65% 5-year FFR was reported. Only three of 161 involved sites sustained a true recurrence (2%). This technique of extensive irradiation has been designated as comprehen-sive lymphatic irradiation – CLI [52]. Although further follow-up and more experience with this technique is necessary, it is possible that a proportion of those patients free from disease at 5 years are cured.

An alternative radiotherapeutic approach to advanced nodular NHL is fractionated total body irradiation (TBI). The renaissance of TBI owes much to the efforts of Johnson [290–294] whose encouraging results have prompted others to explore this modality. Historically the effectiveness of TBI is linked with 'lymphosarcoma' and this relationship is evident in current studies where most investigators report on the use of TBI for lymphocytic or mixed lymphocytic-histiocytic NHL of nodular or diffuse pattern. However, TBI produces only very short-term CR in DLPD and DM lymphoma with FFR at 3 years in fewer than 25% [292, 195–298]. In view of recent reports of high durable CR rates in DLPD and DM variants with multi-agent chemotherapy [215, 286], it seems unlikely that TBI will play a primary role in these subtypes. For nodular variants, on the other hand, TBI may have a role. TBI is usually delivered ar 15 rads mid-pelvic dose twice weekly to a total of 150 rads in 5 weeks [292, 295, 296, 298]. For stages III and IV nodular NHL, CR occurs in 84–95% of patients (Table 28). The evolution of CR is gradual, beginning with a softening of lymphadenopathy, followed by a slow regression often requiring 6–8 weeks to reach remission status [295]. The treatments have little if any symptomatic side effects and alopecia does not occur [295, 296, 298]. The major toxicity is thrombocyto-penia beginning usually midway through the course with nadir platelet counts usually at 2–4 weeks after completion [295, 296, 298]. Frequent blood counts are mandatory and treatment needs to be interrupted or curtailed in up to 1/3 of patients because of thrombocytopenia. Patients with splenome-galy and/or marrow involvement may be at greater risk for thrombocytope-nia and those with initially depressed platelet counts are not suitable for this treatment [295]. As non-toxic and acceptable as this treatment is, the long-term results are not altogether satisfactory. The median duration of remission is 24–34 months and the vast majority of patients relapse by 5

Table 28. Results of TBI in nodular NHL.

Patients	Remission	MEDIAN Duration CR (months)	FFR (3 year)	Investigators
22	19	24	38%	Johnson *et al.*, 1978 [292]
20	17	34	50% **	Thar *et al.*, 1979 [295]
43	41	24	38% ***	Carabell *et al.*, 1979 [298]
31	26	24	26%	Choi *et al.*, 1979 [296]
116	103 (89%)	24–34%	26–50%	

FFR (5 year)   *   <20%
                    **   35%
                  *** 25%

years [292, 295, 296, 298]. This result is no different to that achieved by chemotherapy and the NCI trials have shown equivalent therapeutic effects for TBI and multi-agent chemotherapy with considerable lesser toxicity with TBI [218, 292]. However, for stage III disease, CLI appears to achieve significantly better results than TBI. In one study, 30 stage III nodular NHL patients treated with TBI all achieved CR but this had a median duration of 26 months, a 5-year FFR of less than 20% and all patients relapsed by 68 months [295]. In all series TBI has emerged as a palliative maneuver, offering little, if any, prospects for long-term freedom from disease, quite unlike CLI which in stage III may be curative in a proportion of patients (Table 27). TBI has its major value in stage IV nodular NHL where it produces results comparable to chemotherapy with fewer complications.

Patients who fail to enter CR after one course of TBI or who relapse following CR are best treated by chemotherapy since repeat courses of TBI produce only short CR at best and appear to predispose to the development of acute non-lymphocytic leukemia [295, 298].

Although intensive therapies have thus far failed to produce FFR rates superior to those of less intense treatment for advanced nodular NHL, analysis of the patterns of relapse following chemotherapy reveals that initial sites of disease are also the first sites to relapse [227, 299]. In one study, 22/28 sites of nodal relapse were in regions involved prior to induction therapy and no patient initially relapsed in a previously uninvolved extranodal site [227]. This finding suggests that following chemotherapy remission induction, adjunctive radiation to areas of initial gross disease may be beneficial. This consolidation radiation approach (section 1.5) is being evaluated for advanced nodular NHL by the Eastern Cooperative Oncology Group (ECOG protocol 4477) [300]. In this study patients with NLPD,

NLWD and NM stage III or IV NHL are assigned to induction therapy with cyclophosphamide and prednisone and after eight cycles those patients achieving CR or PR are randomized to receive either four additional chemotherapy cycles or relatively low dose irradiation to areas of pre-chemotherapy involvement. Sites of complete remission (nodal and visceral) receive 1500–2000 rads and sites of residual disease receive 3000 rads. Results of this ongoing study are not available. The Stanford trial on advanced nodular NHL which compared single agent chemotherapy, CVP chemotherapy and split course CVP-TNI-CVP, showed no benefit to the combined modality approach [192, 287]. However, patients who relapsed from the split course CVP-TNI-CVP arm received significantly reduced doses of cyclophosphamide as a result of TNI-indused pancytopenia [287]. The Stanford group abandoned the split course schedule in favor of full induction with CVP followed by adjunctive radiation therapy. Whether such combined mode. radiation consolidation programs will succeed in eradicat-ing advanced nodular NHL remains to be seen.

2.5.2. Advanced Diffuse NHL. The role of radiation thearpy in advanced unfavorable histology NHL (DLPD, DHL, DM, DU) is poorly defined. Used alone, radiation is ineffective in producing extended disease-free survival. For stage III diffuse histology NHL treated with TNI a 5-year FFR of 28% with a survival of 39% has been reported [217]. Stage III DHL treated by TNI has a FFR of less than 10% at 2 years [207] and DLPD NHL achieves a 30% FFR at 3 years following TNI. TBI has been used in stages III and IV diffuse lymphocytic or mixed histiocytic variants with CR reported in 43–93% [295, 296, 298]. Median duration of remission, however, is about 12 months and eventually all patients relapse. DHL does not respond to TBI [291]. Both the volume and dose used inTNI or CLI techniques are close to maximal and it is unlikely that advances in radiation therapy *per se* will significantly alter the outcome for advanced diffuse NHL. The crucial problem is to define the role of radiation within a chemotherapy program and to optimally integrate the two modes [29]. The results of multi-agent chemotherapy serve to define problem areas that potentially might yield to such an integrated approach.

Multi-agent chemotherapy induces CR in 39–66% of adanced diffuse NHL patients [195, 197, 288, 301, 302]. The median survival of complete responders is in excess of 2 years and the majority seem to have permanent eradication of disease. In contrast, the 34–61% who fail to achieve a CR have very poor survival prospects with a median survival of 6 to 9 months and virtually none live beyond two years. Clearly the achievement of higher CR rates is an urgent goal. Failure to achieve CR appears to reflect two mechanisms: some patients have disease with a high growth rate with regrowth between successive chemotherapy cycles [195], others appear to have a good respose but residual disease is detected on systematic restaging at the end of therapy [195, 299]. A smaller proportion of patients develop disease extension to new areas during induction therapy [299]. The challenge for radiation oncology is to devise an irradiation program, integrated with chemotherapy, which does not reduce marrow tolerance to cytotoxic agents. For the patients with rapidly regrowing disease, the radiation would have to be interdigitated with cycles of chemothrapy and one might envisage a scheme similar to the 'ping-pong' technique developed at Stanford for advanced Hodgkin's disease (section 1.5). A variant of this approach has been explored by the Stanford investigators. Patients with advanced unfavorable histology NHL were randomized to receive chemotherapy alone (cytarabine, adriamycin, thioguanine) for DHL and CVP for others, or to receive the same chemotherapy for two or three cycles, followed by TNI and followed by additional chemotherapy [192]. The results were in favor of the combined modality approach with CR in 75%, compared to 45% and a survival at 4 years of 47% compared to 24% ($P = 0.05$). However, these are disappointing figures, especially since the FFR for the combined modes was only 24% at 5 years. In an attempt to improve hematologic tolerance and to maintain optimal drug doses, the Stanford group have reduced radiation to 3000 rads and alternate cycles of chemotherapy with cycles of radiation to the mantle, upper abdomen and pelvis [192]. Whether this proves more effective remains to be seen.

Another approach to enhancing the achievement of CR has been explored by the Northwest Oncology Group in Seattle [303]. In their three-Phase program for advanced diffuse NHL, Phase I consists of four cycles of CHOP-procarbazine chemotherapy, phase II consists of TBI to 150 rads in 5 weeks (a few patients received regional irradiation to 3500 rads only) in conjunction with prednisone, vincristine and bleomycin, and phase III has four further cycles of CHOP-procarbazine. This rather formidable approach proved to be relatively well tolerated and CR occurred in 38/46 patients (83%). Interestingly, 13 of the CR (including three histiocytic cases) were achieved during phase II. Actuarial FFR for the 36 patients assigned to TBI was 61% at 2 years.

The optimal method for combining radiation and chemotherapy in an attempt to improve CR for advanced diffuse NHL has not been defined. Which, if any, of the approaches outlined proves significantly beneficial awaits further investigation.

It is now recognized that a significant proportion of lymphoma patients in apparent complete clinical remission have residual disease detectable by systematic restaging at completion of chemotherapy [299]. The largest series addressing this problem found an 18% incidence of occult disease in advanced lymphoma patients in CR following chemotherapy [299]. Others have found such occult disease in 33% of complete clinical remissions [195].

Those patients with demonstrable occult residual disease fare little better than non-responders [195, 299]. In diffuse lymphoma, about 60% of such occult residual lesions are in sites originally known to have been involved [199]. Sites of original bulk disease also determine patterns of relapse. The group of true complete responders delineated by removing those with occult but demonstrable disease, tends to relapse in sites of previous involvement. In one series, 62% of relapses from CR occurred in sited of known prior involvement [299]. These patterns of disease suggest a role for relatively low dose consolidation radiation administered to sites of prior disease in patients achieving CR following chemotherapy. This approach, however, can only benefit the 40–66% of patents who achieve CR.

2.6. Pediatric NHL

Childhood NHL has undergone a profound change in prognosis over the past two decades with 2-year survival rates increasing from 15 to 30% during the 1960s [304–306] to 60–75% in the 1970s [306–308]. Relapses beyond two years are uncommon [305, 308]. This improved prognosis essentially reflects advances in combination chemotherapy and the role of radiation is becoming increasingly clouded, though most protocols continue to include an irradiation phase [306]. Treatment programs for childhood NHL have evolved from radiation alone [305], to radiation with single agent chemotherapy [309], to radiation with multiple agent chemotherapy [306, 309], to multiple agent chemotherapy with radiation [307, 310] and there has occurred a definite de-emphasis of radiation therapy with some questioning of its value in current programs [311].

The vast majority of children with NHL have systemic disease and unless successfully treated will pass into a leukemic phase with super added massive disseminated extramedullary disease, often including CNS involvement [304, 306, 308, 312]. This systematic dissemination has hindered the development of a useful staging system, though Ann Arbor stages I and II do define a small subgroup in whom regional treatment may play an important role. Even within the apparently localized group of childhood NHL, anatomic disease site influences prognosis.

Localized GIT NHL in children most commonly involving the ileocecal region [310, 313] is a common and relatively favorable presentation. Children with involvement limited to the bowel or with involvement limited to adjacent nodes only and having total resection followed by whole abdominal irradiation have a prolonged disease-free survival in 40–60% [309, 313]. Disease limited to the bowel without mesenteric involvement treated in the same way has resulted in an 85% long-term survival [313]. Surgery followed by no adjuvant treatment, or by single agent chemotherapy, or by localized irradiation results in a considerably poorer outcome than resection followed by whole abdominal treatment [309]. Post-operative doses of 2500–

3000 rads appear adequate [309, 313]. Leukemia or CNS involvement as first manifestations of relapse are extremely rare with these localized GIT presentations [306, 309].

Localized head and neck presentations are relatively common in childhood NHL and such disease in stage I has a relatively favorable outlook following regional radiation, with extended survival in 50–60% of cases [305, 312, 314]. However, in most reports some chemotherapy, usually single agent, was added and the only report using radiation alone had no long-term survivors among 11 children with extranodal head and neck disease [315]. Even in relatively favorable localized cases the need for adjuvant chemotherapy is strong. There is no reason, however, to dispense with radiation therapy in these early stages.

Unlike the relatively favorable presentations, apparently localized mediastinal disease in children and adolescents has a dismal prognosis when treated by local radiation alone. The vast majority of such lesions are classified as lymphoblastic lymphoma and almost invariably a leukemic phase supervenes (>90%) with CNS involvement in the majority [229, 304, 307, 312]. Extensive evaluation at presentation often fails to disclose the systemic nature of this disease, but apart from the occasional emergency indication to relieve mediastinal compression, definitive radiation has no place in the management of this disease [306, 312].

The Ann Arbor demarcation between stages II and III is not a useful division between localized (favorable) and advanced childhood NHL. Stage III is very rarely encountered in children [306] and many stage II presentations are distinctly unfavorable. Abdominal NHL in children is commonly extensive with massive disease involving para-aortic and mesenteric nodes [310, 313]. This pattern is as unfavorable for the child as it is for the adult. The best results have been achieved with the LSA_2-L_2 Memorial Sloan-Kettering protocol, with a 5-year FFR of about 75% [310]. This protocol employs a 10-drug-chemotherapy schedule and emphasizes total surgical removal of all abdominal disease either at initial laparotomy or at a subsequent laparotomy after about 20 days of induction chemotherapy [307, 310]. Abdominal irradiation is delayed beyond the second laparotommy and is given only to those with residual nonresectable disease. An attempt to deliver radiation therapy during the first few days of induction chemotherapy proved prohibitively toxic [310]. A number of other protocols are being currently evaluated [306] and each incorporates radiation at some phase, directed to areas of bulk disease. Recently, however, the value of such radiation therapy has been questioned. In a study where induction therapy consisted of cyclophosphamide, vincristine, prednisone and adriamycin, 21 children were randomized to further chemotherapy alone and 25 were given radiation in addition to chemotherapy [311]. 3000–3500 rads were given to sites of prior bulk disease. There was no difference in incidence of CR or survival between the two groups. FFR at 2 years for advanced stages (including bulky abdominal disease) was about 35% for both approaches [311]. Further controlled trials are clearly essential to elucidate the value of radiation therapy in advanced childhood NHL.

2.7.. Summary of Treatment Policies for Non-Hodgkin's Lymphoma

Deliberate, systematic, sequential staging as outlined in Table 19 is crucial for all patients with NHL. Extranodal presentations require the same work-up philosophy as nodal disease. Patients who remain CS I or II should have laparotomy staging unless contraindicated. Favorable histology (NLPD, NM, DLWD) cases that remain truly localized following comprehensive staging are potentially curable with radiation therapy and receive involved-field therapy to a dose of 3500–4000 rads at 150 rads per day. No firm policy for stage III and IV favorable histology NHL can be formulated. Stage III nodular lymphoma can be managed with CLI with perhaps some chance for cure in a proportion of cases. Stage IV modular NHL can be palliated by fractionated TBI; chemotherapy is thus far non-curative for this disease.

Localized (PS I and II) unfavorable histology NHL (nodal and extranodal) is managed by involved-field radiation therapy to a dose of 4500–5000 rads at 150 rads per day. The majority of PS I patients will be cured with this approach. The need for adjuvant chemotherapy in PS II diffuse NHL is recognized, but as yet no clear evidence as to its utility is available. Advanced unfavorable histology NHL is managed with multi-agent chemotherapy and the only defined role for radiation is in the palliation of relapsing or refractory disease.

REFERENCES

1. Pusey WA: Cases of sarcoma and of Hodgkin's disease treated by exposure to X-rays. J Am Med Assoc 38:166–169, 1902.
2. Gilbert R: Radiotherapy in Hodgkin's disease (malignant granulomatosis): anatomic and clinical foundations, governing principles, results. Am J Roentgenol 41:198–241, 1939.
3. Buschke F: Radiation therapy: the past, the present, the future. Am J Roentgenol 108:236–246, 1970.
4. Bowing HH: The value of radium and x-ray therapy in Hodgkin's disease. J Radiol 2:20–24, 1921.
5. Reed DM: On the pathological changes in Hodgkin's disease, with especial reference to its relation to tuberculosis. Johns Hopkins Hosp Rep 10:133–196, 1902.
6. Rappaport H, Winter WJ, Hicks EB: Follicular lymphoma. A re-evaluation of its position in the scheme of malignant lymphoma, based on a survey of 253 cases. Cancer 9:972–821, 1956.
7. Easson ED, Russell MH: The cure of Hodgkin's disease. BMJ 1:1704–1707, 1963.
8. Jackson H: Classification and prognosis of Hodgkin's disease and allied disorders. Surg Gynecol Obstet 64:465–467, 1937.

9. Leucutia T: Irradiation in lymphosarcoma, Hodgkin's disease and leukemia. Am J Med Sci 188:612–623, 1934.

10. Merner TB, Stenstrom KW: Roentgen therapy in Hodgkin's disease. J Radiol 48:355–368, 1947.

11. Peters MV: A study of survivals in Hodgkin's disease treated radiologically. Am J Roentgenol 63:299–311, 1950.

12. Peters MV, Middlemiss KCH: A study of Hodgkin's disease treated by irradiation. Am J Roentgenol 79:114–121, 1958.

13. Kaplan HS: The radical radiotherapy of regionally localized Hodgkin's disease. Radiology 78:553–561, 1962.

14. Kaplan HS, Rosenberg SA: Extended-field radical radiotherapy in advanced Hodgkin's disease: short-term results of 2 randomized clinical trials. Cancer Res 26:1268–1276, 1966.

15. Johnson RE, Cook PL: Hodgkin's disease: negative lymphogram in guiding radiotherapy. Am J Roentgenol 102:883–890, 1968.

16. Prosnitz LR, Hellman S, von Essen C, Kligerman MM: The clinical course of Hodgkin's disease and other malignant lymphomas treated with radical radiation therapy. Am J Roentgenol 105:668–628, 1969.

17. Rubin P, Keys H, Mayer E, Antmann R: Nodal recurrences following radical radiation therapy in Hodgkin's disease. Am J Roentgenol 120:536–548, 1974.

18. Kaplan HS: On the natural history, treatment and prognosis of Hodgkin's disease. The Harvey Lectures, series 64:215–259, 1968–1969.

19. Glatstein E, Guernsey JM, Rosenberg SA, Kaplan HS: The value of laparotomy and splenectomy in the staging of Hodgkin's disease. Cancer 24:709–718, 1969.

20. Kaplan HS, Dorfman RF, Nelson TS: Staging laparotomy and splenectomy in Hodgkin's disease: analysis of indications and patterns of involvement in 285 consecutive, unselected patients. Natl Cancer Inst Monogr 36:291–301, 1973.

21. Peters MV: The evolution of the radiotherapeutic concept in Hodgkin's disease. Ser Haematol 6:117–138, 1973.

22. Piro AJ, Hellman S: Laparotomy alters treatment in Hodgkin's disease. Natl Cancer Inst Monogr 36:307–311, 1973.

23. Andrews JR: The radiobiology of human radiotherapy. Baltimore: University Park Press, 1978.

24. Fletcher GH: Textbook of radiotherapy. Philadelphia: Lea & Febiger, 1980, pp 180–219.

25. Kaplan HS: Evidence for a tumoricidal dose in the radiotherapy of Hodgkin's disease. Cancer Res 26:1221–1224, 1966.

26. Friedman M, Pearlman AN, Turgeon L: Hodgkin's disease. Tumor lethal dose and iso-effect recovery curve. Am J Roentgenol 99:843–850, 1967.

27. Fletcher GH, Shukovsky LJ: The interplay of radiocurability and tolerance in the irradiation of human cancers. J Radiol Electrol 56:383–400, 1975.

28. Bush RS, Gospadarowicz M, Sturgeon J, Alison R: Radiation therapy of localized non-Hodgkin's lymphoma. Cancer Treat Rep 61:1129–1136.

29. Steel GG, Peckham MJ: Exploitable mechanisms in combined radiotherapy-chemotherapy: the concept of additivity. Int J Radiat Oncol Biol Phys 5:85–91, 1979.

30. Oates JA, Wilkinson GR: Principles of drug therapy. In: Harrison's principles of internal medicine, Isselbacher KJ, Adams RD, Braumwald E, Petersdorf RG, Wilson JD, eds. New York: McGraw-Hill, 1980, p 382.

31. Rubin P, Cooper R, Phillips TL: Radiation biology and radiation pathology syllabus (set R.T. 1: radiation oncology). Chicago: American College of Radiology, 1975.

32. Kaplan HS, Stewart JR: Complications of intensive megavoltage radiotherapy for Hodgkin's disease. Natl Cancer Inst Monogr 36:439–444, 1973.

33. Rubin P: Statement of the clinical oncologic problem. In: Clinical oncology for medical students and physicians. A multidisciplinary approach, Rubin P, Bakemeier RF, eds; Rochester, N. Y.: American Cancer Society, 1978, pp 1-10.
34. Spittle MF, Harmer CL, Cassady Jr, Kaplan HS: Analysis of primary relapses after radiotherapy in Hodgkin's disease. Natl Cancer Inst Monogr 36:497-508, 1973.
35. Kaplan HS, Rosenberg SA: Current status of clinical trials: Stanford experience, 1962-72. Natl Cancer Inst Monogr 36:363-371, 1973.
36. Gamble JF, Fuller LM, Martin RG, Sullivan MP, Jing B-S, Butler JJ, Shullenberger CC: Influence of staging celiotomy in localized presentations of Hodgkin's disease. Cancer 35:817-825, 1975.
37. Sweet DL, Kinnealey A, Ultmann JE: Hodgkin's disease: problems of staging. Cancer 42:957-970, 1978.
38. Kaplan HS, Bissinger PA: Survival and relapse rates in Hodgkin's disease: Stanford experience, 1961-71. Natl Cancer Inst Monogr 36:487-496, 1973.
39. Glatstein E: Radiotherapy in Hodgkin's disease. Past achievements and future progress. Cancer 39:837-841, 1977.
40. Peckham MJ, Ford HT, McElwain TJ, Harmer CL, Atkinson K, Austin DE: The results of radiotherapy for Hodgkin's disease. Br J Cancer 32:391-400, 1975.
41. Weller SA, Glatstein E, Castellino RA, Kaplan HS, Rosenberg SA: Initial relapse in previously treated Hodgkin's disease - II. Retrograde transdiaphragmatic extension. Int J Radiat Oncol Biol Phys 2:863-872, 1977.
42. Chabner BA, Johnson RE, Young RE, Canellos GP, Hubbard SP, Johnson SK, DeVita VT: Sequential nonsurgical and surgical staging of non-Hodkin's lymphoma. Ann Intern Med 85:149-154, 1976.
43. Goffinet DR, Warnke R, Dunnick NR, Castellino R, Glatstein E, Nelson TS, Dorfman RF, Rosenberg SA, Kaplan HS: Clinical and surgical (laparotomy) evaluation of patients with non-Hodgkin's lymphomas. Cancer Treat Rep 61:981-992, 1977.
44. Bonadonna G, Lattuada A, Banfi A: Recent trends in the treatment of non-Hodgkin's lymphomas. Eur J Cancer 12:661-673, 1976.
45. Sweet DL, Golomb HM: The treatment of histiocytic lymphoma. Semin Oncol 7:302-309, 1980.
46. Peters MV, Brown TC, Rideout DF: Prognostic influences and radiation therapy according to pattern of disease. JAMA 223:53-59, 1973.
47. Fuller LM, Madoc-Jones H, Hagemeister FB, Rodgers RW, North LB, Butler JJ, Martin RG, Gamble JR, Schullenberger CC: Further follow-up of results of treatment in 90 laparotomy-negative stage I and II Hodgkin's disease patients: significance of mediastinal and non-mediastinal presentations. Int J Radiat Oncol Biol Phys 6:499-808, 1980.
48. Hoppe RT, Coleman CN, Kaplan HS, Rosenberg SA: Hodgkin's disease, pathologic stage I-II. The prognostic importance of initial sites of disease and extent of mediastinal involvement. Proc Am Soc Clin Oncol 21:471, 1980.
49. Seydel HG, Bloedorn FG, Wizenberg MJ: Time-dose-volume relationship in Hodgkin's disease. Radiology 89:919-922, 1967.
50. Fischer JJ, Fischer DB: The determination of time-dose relationships from clinical data. Br J Radiol 44:785-792, 1971.
51. Ibrahim E, Fuller LM, Gamble JF, Jing B-S, Butler JJ, Gehan EA: Stage I Hodgkin's disease. Comparison of surgical staging with incidence of new manifestations in lymphogram and prelymphogram studied patients. Radiology 104:145-151, 1972.
52. Million RR: The lymphomatous disease. In: Textbook of radiotherapy, Fletcher GH, ed. Philadelphia: Lea & Febiger, 1980, pp 584-636.
53. Fazekas JT, Cox JD, Turner WM: Irradiation of stage I and II Hodgkin's disease. Am J Roentgenol 123:154-162, 1975.
54. Johnson RE, Ruhl U, Johnson SK, Glover M: Split-course radiotherapy of Hodgkin's

disease. Local tumor control and normal tissue reactions. Cancer 37:1713-1717, 1976.

55. Kaplan HS: Hodgkin's disease. Cambridge, Mass.: Harvard University Press, 1980.

56. Hall EJ: Radiobiology for the radiologist. Hagerstown, Md: Harper & Row, 1978.

57. Johnson RE: Clinical and technical aspects of total nodal irradiation for Hodgkin's disease. In: Textbook of radiotherapy, 2nd edn, Fletcher GH, ed. Philadelphia: Lea & Febiger, 1973, pp 527-544.

58. Johnson RE, Zimbler H, Berard CW, Herdt J, Brereton HD: Radiotherapy results for nodular sclerosing Hodgkin's disease after clinical staging. Cancer 39:1439-1444, 1977.

59. Stoffel TJ, Cox JD: Hodgkin's disease stage I and II. A comparison of two different treatment policies. Cancer 40:90-97, 1977.

60. Mauch P, Goodman R, Hellman S: The significance of mediastinal involvement in early stage Hodgkin's disease. Cancer 42:1039-1045, 1978.

61. van der Werf-Messing B: Morbus Hodgkin's disease, stages I and II: trial of the European Organization for Research on Treatment of cancer. Natl Cancer Inst Monogr 36:331-386, 1973.

62. Mill WB, Palmer-Hanes LA, Purdy JA, Tillack TW, Reinhard EH, Loeb V, Parnell DN, Penkoske MA, Franssila KO: Extended field radiation therapy in Hodgkin's disease. Analysis of failures. Cancer 40:2896-2904, 1977.

63. Levi JA, Wiernik PH, O'Connell MJ: Patterns of relapse in stages I, II and IIIA Hodgkin's disease: Influence of initial therapy and implications for the future. Int J radiat Oncol Biol Phys 2:853-862, 1977.

64. Mintz J, Miller JB, Golomb HM, Kinzie J, Sweet DL, Lester EP, Variakojis D, Roth NO, Blough RR, Ferguson DJ, Ultmann JE: Pathologic state I and II Hodgkin's disease 1968-1975. Relapses and results of retreatment. Cancer 44:72-79, 1979.

65. Prosnitz LR, Curtis AM, Knowlton AH, Peters LM, Farber LR: Supradiaphragmatic Hodgkin's disease: significance of large mediastinal masses. Int J Radiat Oncol Biol Phys 6:809-814, 1980.

66. Marks JE, Haus AG, Sutton HG, Griem ML: Localization error in the radiotherapy of Hodgkin's disease and malignant lymphoma with extended mantle fields. Cancer 34:83-90, 1974.

67. Prosnitz LR, Montalvo RL, Fischer DB, Silberstein AB, Berger DS: Treatment of stage IIIA Hodgkin's disease: is radiotherapy alone adequate? Int J Radiat Oncol Biol Phys 4:781-787, 1978.

68. Carmel RJ, Kaplan HS: Mantle irradiation in Hodkin's disease. An analysis of technique, tumor eradication, and complications. Cancer 37:2813-2825, 1976.

69. Thar TL, Million RR, Hasner RJ, McKetty MHB: Hodgkin's disease, stages I and II. Ralationship of recurrence tosize of disease, radiation dose, and number of sites involved. Cancer 43:1101-1105, 1979.

70. Mauch P, Goodman R, Rosenthal DS, Botnick L, Piro AJ, Hellman S: An evaluation of total nodal irradiation as treatment for stage IIIA Hodgkin's disease. Cancer 43:1255-1261, 1979.

71. Suit H, Lindberg R, Fletcher GH: Prognostic significance of extent of tumor regression at completion of radiation therapy. Radiology 84:1100-1107, 1975.

72. Prosnitz LR, Farber LR, Fischer JJ, Bertino JR, Fischer DB: Long term remissions with combined modality therapy for advanced Hodgkin's disease. Cancer 37:2826-2833, 1976.

73. Bonadonna G, Zucali R, DeLena M, Valagussa P: Combined chemotherapy (MOPP or ABVD) - radiotherapy approach in advanced Hodgkin's disease. Cancer Treat Rep 61:769-777, 1977.

74. Goodman R, Mauch P, Piro A, Rosenthal D, Goldstein M, Tullis J, Hellman S: Stages IIB and IIIB Hodgkin's disease. Results of combined modality treatment. Cancer 40:84-89, 1977.

75. Coltman CA, Montague E, Moon TE: Chemotherapy and total nodal radiotherapy in pathological stage IIB, IIIA and IIIB Hodgkin's disease. In: Adjuvant therapy of cancer, Salmon SE, Jones SE, eds. Amsterdam: Elsevier North-Holland Biomedical, 1977, pp 529-536.

76. Mauch P, Hellman S: Supradiaphragmatic Hodgkin's disease: is there a place for MOPP chemotherapy in patients with bulky mediastinal disease? Int J Radiat Oncol Biol Phys 6:947-950, 1980.

77. Fuller LM, Gamble JF, Valazquez WS, Rodgers RW, Butler JJ, North LB, Martin RG, Gehan EA, Shullenberger CC: Evaluation of the significance of prognostic factors in stage III Hodgkin's disease treated with MOPP and radiotherapy. Cancer 45:1352-1364, 1980.

78. Landbert T, Svahn-Tapper G, Wintzell K: Mantle treatment of Hodgkin's disease. Preliminary report of side effects and early results. Acta Radiol Ther Phys Biol 10:174-186, 1971.

79. Hellman S, Mauch P, Goodman RL, Rosenthal DS, Maloney WC: The place of radiation therapy in the treatment of Hodgkin's disease. Cancer 42:971-978, 1978.

80. Marks JE, Moran EM, Griem ML, Ultmann JE: Extended mantle radiotherapy in Hodgkin's disease and malignant lymphoma. Am J Roentgenol 121:772-788, 1974.

81. Page V, Gardner A, Karzmark CJ: Physical and dosimetric aspects of the radiotherapy of malignant lymphomas. I. The mantle technique. Radiology 96:609-626, 1970.

82. Page V, Gardner A, Karzmark CJ: Physical and dosimetric aspects of the radiotherapy of malignant lymphomas. II. The inverted-Y technique. Radiology 96:619-626, 1970.

83. Cundiff JH, Cunningham JR, Golden R, Lanzl LH, Meurk ML, Ovadia J, Page V, Pope RA, Sampiere VA, Saylor WL, Shalek RJ, Suntharalingham N: A method for the calculation of dose in the radiation treatment of Hodgkin's disease. Am J Roentgenol 117:30-44, 1973.

84. Weisenberger TH, Juillard GJF: Upper extremity lymphangiography in the radiation therapy of lymphomas and carcinoma of the breast. Radiology 122:227-230, 1977.

85. Nisce LZ, Gonzales ET, D'Angio GJ, Lee BJ: Hilar irradiation in early stage Hodgkin's disease. Clin Bull 7:135-139, 1977.

86. Palos B, Kaplan HS, Karzmark CJ: The use of thin lung shields to deliver limited whole-lung irradiation during mantle-field treatment of Hodgkin's disease. Radiology 101:441-442, 1971.

87. Desser RK, Golomb HM, Ultmann JE, Ferguson DJ, Moran EM, Griem ML, Vardiman J, Miller B, Oetzel N, Sweet D, Lester EP, Kinzie JJ, Blough R: Prognostic classification of Hodgkin's disease in pathologic stage III, based on anatomic considerations. Blood 49:883-893, 1977.

88. Stein RD, Golomb HM, Diggd HC, Mauch P, Hellman S, Wiernik PH, Ultmann JE, Rosenthal DS: Anatomic substages of stage IIIA Hodgkin's disease. A collaborative study. Ann Intern Med 92:159-164, 1980.

89. Gamble JF, Fuller LM, Loh KK, Martin RG, Jing B-S, Sinkovics JG, Shullenberger CC, Butler JJ: Hodgkin's disease and the non-Hodgkin's lymphomas. In: Cancer patient care at M.D. Anderson Hospital and Tumor Institute, Clark RL, Howe CD, eds. Chicago: Year Book Medical, 1976, pp 125-163.

90. Fuller LM, Madoc-Jones H, Gamble JF, Butler JJ, Sullivan MP, Fernandez CH, Gehan EA: New assessment of the prognostic significance of histopathology in Hodgkin's disease for laparotomy - negative I and stage II patients. Cancer 39:2174-2182, 1977.

91. Portlock CS, Rosenberg SA, Glatstein E, Kaplan HS: Impact of salvage treatment on initial relapses in patients with Hodgkin's disease, stage I-III. Blood 51:825-833, 1978.

92. Weller SA, Glatstein E, Kaplan HS, Rosenberg SA: Initial relapses in previously treated Hodgkin's disease. I. Results of second treatment. Cancer 37:2840-2846, 1976.

93. Tubiana M, van der Werf-Messing B, Langier A, Hayat M, Henry-Amar M, Attie E, Leroy

T: Survival after recurrence: prognostic factors and spread patterns in clinical stages I and II of Hodgkin's disease. Natl Cancer Inst Monogr 36:513–530, 1973.

94. Collaborative Study: Survival and complications of radiotherapy following involved and extended field therapy of Hodgkin's disease, stages I and II. Cancer 38:288–305, 1976.

95. Chan WC, Tan CTC, Martinez A, Exelby PR, Teft M, Middleman P, D'Angio GJ: Involved field radiation therapy for early stage Hodgkin's disease in children. Preliminary results. Cancer 37:1625–1632, 1976.

96. Miller JB, Moran EM, Desser RK, Griem ML, Ultmann JE: Results of involved field and extended field radiotherapy in patients with pathologic stage I and II Hodgkin's disease. Am J Roentgenol 127:833–839, 1976.

97. Peters V: The need for a new clinical classification in Hodgkin's disease. Cancer Res 31:1713–1722, 1971.

98. Ultmann JE, DeVita VT: Hodgkin's disease and other lymphomas. In: Harrison's principles of internal medicine, Isselbcher KJ, Adams RD, Braunwald E, Petersdorf RG, Wilson JE, eds. New York: McGraw-hill, 1980, pp 1633–1647.

99. Fuller LM, Gamble JF, Shullenberger CC, Butler JJ, Gehan EA: Prognostic factors in localized Hodgkin's disease treated with regional radiation. Radiology 98:641–654, 1971.

100. Tiber C, Conrad F, Gehan E: Laparotomy in stage I Hodgkin's. Proc Am Soc Clin Oncol 21:467, 1980.

101. Krikorian JG, Portlock CS, Rosenberg SA, Kaplan HS: Hodgkin's disease, stages I and II occurring below the diaphragm. Cancer 43:1866–1871, 1979.

102. Kaplan HS: Hodgkin's disease: unfolding concepts concerning its nature, management and prognosis. Cancer 45:2439–2474, 1980.

103. Smithers DW: Spread of Hodgkin's disease. Lancet 1:1262–1267, 1970.

104. Hoppe RT: Radiation therapy in the treatment of Hodgkin's disease. Semin Oncol 7:144–154, 1980.

105. Goodman RL, Piro AJ, Hellman S: Can pelvic irradiation be omitted in patients with pathologic stages IA and IIA Hodgkin's disease? Cancer 37:2834–2839, 1976.

106. Costello P, Mauch P: Radiographic features of recurrent intrathoracic Hodgkin's disease following radiation therapy. AJR 133:201–206, 1979.

107. Fuller LM, Gamble JF, Ibrahim E, Jing B-S, Butler JJ, Shullenberger CC: Stage II Hodgkin's disease. Significance of mediastinal and nonmediastinal presentations. Radiology 109:429–435, 1973.

108. Strum SB: The natural history, histopathology, staging, and mode of spread of Hodgkin's disease. Series Haematol 6:20–115, 1973.

109. Valentjas E, Barrett A, McElwain TJ, Peckham MJ: Mediastinal involvement in early-stage Hodgkin's disease. Response to treatment and pattern of relapse. Europ J Cancer 16:1065–1068, 1980.

110. Levi JA, Wiernik PH: Limited extranodal Hodgkin's disease. Unfavourable prognosis and therapeutic implications. Am J Med 63:365–372, 1977.

111. Carbone PP, Kaplan HS, Musshoff K, Smithers DW, Tubiana M: Report of the committee on Hodgkin's disease staging classification.Cancer Res 31:1860–1861, 1971.

112. Ewing J: Neoplastic diseases, 4th edn. Philadelphia: W.B. Saunders, 1940.

113. Thomson AD: The thymic origin of Hodgkin's disease. Br J Cancer 9:37–50, 1955.

114. Keller AR, Castleman B: Hodgkin's disease of the thymus gland. Cancer 33:1615–1623, 1974.

115. Filly R, Blank N, Castellino RA: Radiographic distribution of intrathoracic disease in previously untreated patients with Hodgkin's disease and non-Hodgkin's lymphoma. Radiology 120:277–281, 1976.

116. Peckham MJ: Lung involvement. In: Hodgkin's disease, Smithers D, ed. Edinburgh: Churchill Livingstone, 1973, pp 118–127.

117. Musshoff K: Prognostic and therapeutic implications of staging in extranodal Hodgkin's disease. Cancer Res 31:1814, 1971.
118. Rosenberg SA, Kaplan HS, Glatstein EJ, Portlock CS: Combined modality therapy of Hodgkin's disease. A report on the Stanford trials. Cancer 42:991-1000, 1978.
119. Rosenberg SA, Kaplan HS: The management of stages I, II, and III Hodgkin's disease with combined radiotherapy and chemotherapy. Cancer 35:55-63, 1975.
120. Coltman CA, Fuller LM, Fisher R, Frei E: Extended field radiotherapy versus involved field radiotherapy plus MOPP in stage I and II Hodgkin's disease. In: Adjuvant therapy of cancer, Jones SE, Salmon SE, eds. New York: Grune & Stratton, 1979.
121. Castellino RA, Glatstein E, Turbow MM, Rosenberg SA, Kaplan HS: Latent radiation injury of lungs or heart activated by steroid withdrawal. Ann Intern Med 80:593-599, 1974.
122. Gains RA: Complications of chemotherapy in the treatment of Hodgkin's disease. Semin Oncol 7:184-186, 1980.
123. DeVita VT, Simon RM, Hubbard SM, Young RC, Berard CW, Moxley JH, Frei E, Carbone PP, Canellos GP: Curability of advanced Hodgkin's disease with chemotherapy. Ann Intern Med 92:587-595, 1980.
124. Coltman CA: Chemotherapy of advanced Hodgkin's disease. Semin Oncol 7:155-173, 1980.
125. Frei E, Luce JK, Gamble JF, Coltman CA, Constanzi JJ, Talley RW, Monto RW, Wilson HE, Hewlett JS, Delaney FC, Gehan EA: Combination chemotherapy in advanced Hodgkin's disease. Induction and maintenance of remission. Ann Intern Med 79:376-382, 1973.
126. DeVita VT, Lewis BJ, Rozencweig M, Muggia FM: The chemotherapy of Hodgkin's disease. Past experiences and future directions. Cancer 42:979-990, 1978.
127. Olweny CLM, Katongole-Mbidde E, Kiire C, Lwanga SK, Magrath I, Ziegler JL: Childhood Hodgkin's disease in Uganda. A ten year experience. Cancer 42:787-792, 1978.
128. Jenkin RDT, Berry MP: Hodgkin's disease in children. Semin Oncol 7:202-211, 1980.
129. Jenkin RDT, Brown TC, Peters MV, Sonley MJ: Hodgkin's disease in children. A retrospective analysis: 1958-73. Cancer 35:979-990, 1975.
130. Hays DM: The staging of Hodgkin's disease in children reviewed. Cancer 35:973-978, 1975.
131. Hagemeister FB, Fuller LM, North LB: Combination radiotherapy and chemotherapy in mediastinal Hodgkin's disease. Proc Am Soc Clin Oncol 21:466, 1980.
132. Lee CKK, Bloomfield CD, Levitt S: Prophylactic whole lung irradiation for extensive mediastinal Hodgkin's disease. Proc Am Soc Clin Oncol 20:441, 1979.
133. Piro AJ, Weiss DR, Hellman S: Mediastinal Hodgkin's disease: a possible danger for intubation anesthesia. Int J Radiat Oncol Biol Phys 1:415-419, 1976.
134. British National Lymphoma Investigation: Initial treatment of stage IIIA Hodgkin's disease. Comparison of radiotherapy with combined chemotherapy. Lancet 2:991-995, 1976.
135. Rosenberg SA: The management of Hodgkin's disease. New Engl J Med 299:1246-1247, 1978.
136. Timothy AR, Sutcliffe SBJ, Lister TA, Wrigley PFM, Jones AE: The management of stage IIIA Hodgkin's disease. Int J Radiat Oncol Biol Phys 6:135-142, 1980.
137. Hoogstraten B, Glidwell O, Holland JF, Blom J, Stutzman L, Nissen NI, Perlberg HJ, Kramer S: Long term follow-up of combination chemotherapy-radiotherapy of stage III Hodgkin's disease. Cancer 43:1234-1244, 1979.
138. Levi JA, Wiernik PH: The therapeutic implications of splenic involvement in stage IIIA Hodgkin's disease. Cancer 39:2158-2165, 1977.
139. Aisenberg AD: Current concepts in cancer. The staging and treatment of Hodgkin's

disease. New Engl J Med 299:1228–1231, 1978.

140. DeVita VT: The role of combined modality therapy in the treatment of stage IIIA Hodgkin's disease. Int J Radiat Oncol Biol Phys 5:913, 1979.

141. Stein RS, Hilborn RM, Flexner JM, Bolin M, Stroup S, Reynolds V, Krautz S: Anatomic substages of stage III Hodgkin's disease. Implications for staging, therapy, and experimental design. Cancer 42:429–436, 1978.

142. Murthy AK, Hendrickson FR: Stage IIIA Hodgkin's disease – a heterogeneous group? Proc Am Soc Clin Oncol 21:463, 1980.

143. Shipley WU, Piro AJ,Hellman S: Radiation therapy of Hodgkin's disease: significance of splenic involvement. Cancer 34:223–229, 1974.

144. Shultz HP, Glatstein E, Kaplan HS: Management of presumptive or proven Hodgkin's disease of the liver: a new radiotherapy technique. Int J Radiat Oncol Biol Phys 1:1–8, 1975.

145. Ingold JA, Reed GB, Kaplan HS: Radiation heptatitis. Am J Roentgenol 93:200–208, 1965.

146. LeBourgeois JP, Meignan M, Parmentier C, Tubiana M: Renal consequences of irradiation of the spleen in lymphoma patients. Br J Radiology 52:56–60, 1979.

147. Dailey MO, Coleman CN, Kaplan HS: Radiation-induced splenic atrophy in patients with Hodgkin's disease and non-Hodgkin's lymphomas. N Engl J Med 302:215–217, 1980.

148. Kun LE, DeVita VT, Young RC, Johnson RE: Treatment of Hodgkin's disease using intensive chemotherapy followed by irradiation. Int J Radiat Oncol Biol Phys 1:619–626, 1976.

149. Hoppe RT, Portlock CS, Glatstein E, Rosenberg SA, Kaplan HS: Alternating chemotherapy and irradiation in the treatment of advanced Hodgkin's disease. Cancer 43:472–481, 1979.

150. Bergsagel D, Basco V, Bush R, Gillies J, Israels L, Whitelaw M, Miller A: Trial of MOPP alone versus MOPP and radiotherapy for advanced Hodgkin's disease. Proc Am Soc Clin Oncol 21:464, 1980.

151. Young RC, Canellos GP, Chabner BA, Hubbard SM, DeVita VT. Patterns of relapse in advanced Hogkin's disease treated with combination chemotherapy. Cancer 42:1001–1007, 1978.

152. Fisher RI, DeVita VT, Hubbard SP, Simon R, Young RC: Prolonged disease-free survival in Hodgkin's disease with MOPP reinduction after first relapse. Ann InternMed 90:761–763, 1979.

153. Prosnitz LR, Farber LR, Fischer JJ, Bertino JR: Low-dose radiation therapy and combination chemotherapy in the treatment of advanced Hodgkin's disease. Radiology 107:187–193, 1973.

154. Farber LR, Prosnitz LR, Cadman EC, Lutes R, Bertino JR, Fischer DB: Curative potential of combined modality therapy for advanced Hodgkin's disease. Cancer 46:1509–1517, 1980.

155. Eastern Cooperative Oncology Group – ECOG Protocol 1476 – Combined modality treatment protocol for advanced stage IIIB, IIISB and IV Hodgkin's disease, Glick JH, Study Chairman. Ecog Operations Office 905 University Avenue, Suite 415, Madison, WI 53715.

156. Seydel HG, Bloedorn FG, Wizenberg MJ: Results of radiotherapeutic treatment of relapsing Hodgkin's disease. Cancer 23:1033–1037, 1969.

157. Rybak ME, Weichselbaum R, Rosenthal D, Hellman S: The influence of initial pathological stage on the survival of patients who develop relapse from Hodgkin's disease. Proc Am Soc Clin Oncol 21:470, 1980.

158. Timothy AR, Sutcliffe SBJ, Wrigley PFM: Hodgkin's disease: combination chemotherapy for relapse following radical radiotherapy. Int J Radiat Oncol Biol Phys 5:165–169, 1979.

159. Sullivan MP, Fuller LM, Butler JJ: Hodgkin's disease in children. In: Clinical pediatric oncology, Sutow WW, Vietti TJ, Fernbach DJ, eds. St Louis: CV Mosby, 1977, pp 408–443.

160. Parker BR, Castellino RA, Kaplan HS: Pediatric Hodgkin's disease. I. Radiographic evaluation. Cancer 37:2430–2435, 1976.

161. Smith IE, Peckham MJ, McElwain TJ, Gazet JC, Ausin DE: Hodgkin's disease in children. Br J Cancer 36:120–129, 1977.

162. Botnick LE, Goodman R, Jaffe N, Filler R, Cassady JR: Stages I–III Hodgkin's disease in children. Results of staging and treatment. Cancer 39:599–603, 1977.

163. Fuller LM, Sullivan MP, Butler JJ: Results of regional radiotherapy in localized Hodgkin's disease in children. Cancer 32:640–645, 1973.

164. Dearth JC, Gilchrist GS, Bergert EO: Management of stage I, II and III Hodgkin's disease in children. Proc Am Soc Clin Oncol 19:391, 1978.

165. Donaldson SS, Glatstein E, Rosenberg SA, Kaplan HS: Pediatric Hodgkin's disease. II. Results of therapy. Cancer 37:2436–2447, 1976.

166. Probert JC, Parker BR, KaplanHS: Growth retardation in children after megavoltage irradiation of the spine. Cancer 32:634–639, 1973.

167. Armata J, Stopyrowa J, Depowski M, Strzesynski J, Borkowski W, Kaezor Z, Depowska T: MVPP chemotherapy combined with radiotherapy in the treatment of Hodgkin's disease in children. Acta Paediatr Scand 67:269–273, 1978.

168. Jenkin D, Freedman m, McClure P, Peters V, Saunders F, Sonley M: Hodgkin's disease in children: treatment with low-dose radiation and MOPP without staging laparotomy. A preliminary report. cancer 44:80–86, 1979.

169. Thar TL, Million RR: Complications of radiation treatment of Hodgkin's disease. Semin Oncol 7:174–183, 1980.

170. Kim YH, Fayos JV, Sissen JC: Thyroid function following neck irradiation for malignant lymphoma. Radiology 134:205–208, 1980.

171. Nelson DF, Reddy KV, O'Mara RE, Rubin P: Thyroid abnormalities following neck irradiation for Hodgkin's disease. Cancer 42:2553–2562, 1978.

172. Glatstein E, McHardy-Young S, Brast N, Eltringham JR, Kriss JP: Alterations in serum thyrotrophin (TSH) and thyroid function following radiotherapy in patients with malignant lymphoma. J Clin Endocrinol 32:833–841, 1971.

173. Speiser B, Rubin P, Casarett G: Aspermia following lower truncal irradiation in Hodgkin's disease. Cancer 32:692–698, 1973.

174. Salzman JR, Kaplan HS: Effects of splenectomy on hematological tolerance during total lymphoid radiotherapy of patients with Hodgkin's disease. Cancer 27:471–478, 1971.

175. Rubin P, Scarantino CW: The bone marrow organ: the critical structure in radiation–drug interaction. Int J Radiat Oncol Biol Phys 4:3–23, 1978.

176. Rubin P, Landman S, Mayer E, Keller B, Ciccio S: Bone marrow regeneration and extension after extended field irradiation in Hodgkin's disease. Cancer 32:699–711, 1973.

177. Sacks EL, Goris ML, Glatstein E, Gilbert E, Kaplan HS: Bone marrow regeneration following large field radiation. Influence of volume, age, dose and time. Cancer 42:1057–1065, 1978.

178. Steele HA, Lillicrap SC, Clink HM, Peckham MJ: The recovery of iron uptake in erythropoietic bone marrow following large field radiotherapy. Br J Radiol 52:61–66, 1979.

179. Gale RP: Autologous bone marrow transplantation in patients with cancer. JAMA 243:540–542, 1980.

180. Coleman CN, Williams CJ, Flint A, Glatstein EJ, Rosenberg SA, Kaplan HS: Hematologic neoplasia in patients treated for Hodgkin's disease. New Engl J Med 297:1249–1252, 1977.

181. Brody RS, Schottenfeld D, Reid A: Multiple primary cancer risk after therapy for Hodgkin's disease. Cancer 40:1917-1926, 1977.
182. Cadman EC, Capizzi RL, Bertino JR: Acute nonlymphocytic leukemia. A delayed complication of Hodgkin's disease therapy: analysis of 109 cases. Cancer 40:1280-1296, 1977.
183. Foucar K, McKenna RN, Bloomfield CD, Bowers TK, Brunning RD: Therapy-related leukemia. A panmyelosis. Cancer 43:1285-1296, 1979.
184. Brody RS, Schottenfeld D: Multiple primary cancers in Hodgkin's disease. Semin Oncol 7:187-201, 1980.
185. Rosenberg SA, Dorfman RF, Kaplan HS: A summary of the results of a review of 405 patients with non-Hodgkin's lymphoma at Stanford University. Br J Cancer 31 (supppl II):168-173, 1975.
186. Brown TC, Peters MV, Bergsagel DE, Reid J: A retrospective analysis of the clinical results in relation to the Rappaport histological classification. Br J Cancer 31 (Suppl II):174-186, 1975.
187. Nathwani BN: A critical analysis of the classifications of non-Hodgkin's lymphomas. Cancer 44:347-384, 1979.
188. Mathe G: Integration of modern data in W.H.O. categorization of lymphosarcomas. Its value for prognosis prediction and therapeutic adaptation to prognosis. Biomedicine 26:377-384, 1977.
189. Rosenberg SA, Kaplan HS: Clinical trials in the non-Hodgkin's lymphomata at Stanford University. Experimental design and preliminary results. Br J Cancer 31 (Suppl II):456-464, 1975.
190. Fuks Z, Kaplan HS: Recurrence rates following radiation therapy of nodular and diffuse malignant lymphomas. Radiology 108:675-684, 1973.
191. Reddy S, Saxena VS, Pellettiere EV, HendricksonFR: Early nodal and extra-nodal non-Hodgkin's lymphomas. Cancer 40:98-104, 1977.
192. Glatstein E, Donaldson SS, Rosenberg SA, Kaplan HS: Combined modality therapy in malignant lymphomas. Cancer Treat Rep 61:1199-1207, 1977.
193. Chen MG, Prosintz LR, Gonzaler-Serva A, Fischer DB: Results of radiotherapy in control of state I and II non-Hodgkin's lymphoma. Cancer 43:1245-1254, 1979.
194. Rudders RA, Kaddis M, LeLellis RA, Casey H: Nodular non-Hodgkin's lymphoma (NHL). Factors influencing prognosis and indications for aggressive treatment. Cancer 43:1643-1651, 1979.
195. Schein PS, DeVita VT, Hubbard S, Chabner BA, Canellos GP, Berard C, Young RC: Bleomycin, adriamycin, cyclophosphamide, vincristine, and prednisone (BACOP) combination chemotherapy in the treatment of advanced diffuse histiocytic lymphoma. Ann Intern Med 85:417-422, 1976.
196. McKelvey EM, Moon TE: Curability of non-Hodgkin's lymphomas. Cancer Treat Rep 1:1185-1190, 1977.
197. Sweet DL, Golomb HM, Ultmann JE, Miller BJ, Stein RS, Lester EP, Mintz U, Bitran JD, Streuli RA, Daly K, Roth NO: Cyclophosphamide, vincristine, methotrexate with leucovorin rescue, and cytarabine (COMLA) combination chemotherapy for advanced diffuse histiocytic lymphoma. Ann Intern Med 92:785-790, 1980.
198. Heifetz LJ, Fuller LM, Rodgers RW, Martin RG, Butler JJ, North LB, Gamble JF, Shullenberger CC: Laparotomy findings in lymphangiogram - staged I and II non-Hodgkin's lymphomas. Cancer 45:2778-2786, 1980.
199. Peters MV: The contribution of radiation therapy in the control of early lymphomas. Am J Roentgenol 90:956-967, 1960.
200. Newall J, Friedman M: Reticulum-cell sarcoma. Part II: Radiation dosage for each type. Radiology 94:643-647, 1970.
201. Seydel HG, Bloedorn FG, Wizenberg M, Berk S: Time-dose relationships in radiation

therapy of lymphosarcoma and giant follicle lymphoma. Radiology 98:411–418, 1971.
202. Cox JD, Koehl RH, Turner WM, King FM: Irradiation in the local control of malignant lymphoreticular tumors (non-Hodgkin's malignant lymphoma). Radiology 112:179–185, 1974.
203. Bitran JD, Kinzie J, Sweet DL, Variakojis D, Griem ML, Golomb HM, Mille JB, Oetzel N. Ultmann JE: Survival of patients with localized histiocytic lymphoma. Cancer 39:342–346, 1977.
204. Hoppe RT, Burke JS, Glatstein E, Kaplan HS: Non-Hodgkin's lymphoma. Involvement of Waldeyer's ring. Cancer 42:1096–1104, 1978.
205. Cox JD: Central lymphatic irradiation to low-dose for advanced nodular lymphoreticular tumors (non-Hodgkin's lymphoma). Radiology 126:767–772, 1978.
206. Fraser RW, Chism SE, Stern R, Fu KK, Buschke F: Clinical course of early extranodal non-Hodgkin's lymphomas. Int J Radiat Oncol Biol Phys 5:177–183, 1979.
207. Jones SE, Fuks Z, Kaplan HS, Rosenberg SA: Non-Hodgkin's lymphomas. V. Results of radiotherapy. Cancer 32:682–691, 1973.
208. Banfi A, Bonadonna G, Ricci SB, Milani F, Molinari R, Monfardini S, Zucali R: Malignant lymphomas of Waldeyer's ring: Natural history and survival after radiotherapy. Br Med J 3:140–143, 1972.
209. Hellman S, Chaffey JT, Rosenthal DS, Moloney WC, Canellos GP, Skarin AT: The place of radiation therapy in the treatment of non-Hodgkin's lymphomas. Cancer 39:843–851, 1977.
210. Peckham MJ, Guay J-P, Hamlin IME, Lukes RJ: Survival in localized nodal and extranodal non-Hodgkin's lymphomata. Br J Cancer 32 (Suppl II):413–424, 1975.
211. Musshoff K, Schmidt-Vollmer H: Prognostic significance of primary site after radiotherapy in non-Hodgkin's lymphomata. Br J Cancer 31 (Suppl II):425–434, 1975.
212. Toonkel LM, Fuller LM, Gamble JF, Butler JJ, Martin RG, Shullenberger CC: Laparotomy staged I and II non-Hodgkin's lymphomas. Preliminary results of radiotherapy and adjunctive chemotherapy. Cancer 45:249–260, 1980.
213. Fuller LM: Results of large volume irradiation in the management of Hodgkin's disease and malignant lymphomas originating in the abdomen. Radiology 87:1058–1064, 1966.
214. Fuller LM, Banker FL, Butler JJ, Gamble JF, Sullivan MP: The natural history of non-Hodgkin's lymphomata stages I and II. Br J Cancer 31 (Suppl II):270–285, 1975.
215. Bitran JD Golomb HM, Ultmann JE, Sweet DL, Lester EP, Stein RS, Miller JB, Moran EM, Kinnealey AE, Vardiman JE, Kinzie J, Roth NO: Non-Hodgkin's lymphoma, poorly differentiated lymphocytic and mixed cell types. Results of sequential staging procedures, response to therapy, and survival of 100 patients. Cancer 42:88–95, 1978.
216. Goffinet DR, Glatstein E, Fuks Z, Kaplan HS: Abdominal irradiation in non-Hodgkin's lymphomas. Cancer 37:2797–2806, 1976.
217. Glatstein E, Fuks Z, Goffinet DR, Kaplan HS: Non-Hodgkin's lymphomas of stage III extent. Is total lymphoid irradiation appropriate treatment? Cancer 37:2806–2812, 1976.
218. Young RC, Johnson RE, Canellos GP, Chabner BA, Brereton HD, Berard CW, DeVita VT: Advanced lymphocytic lymphoma: randomized comparisons of chemotherapy and radiotherapy, alone or in combinations. Cancer Treat Rep 61:1153–11569, 1977.
219. Portlock CS, Rosenberg SA: No initial therapy for stage III and IV non-Hodgkin's lymphomas of favourable histologic types. Ann Intern Med 90:10-13, 1979.
220. Johnson RE, Chretien PB, O'Conor GT, DeVita VT, Thomas LB: Radiotherapeutic implications of prospective staging in non-Hodgkin's lymphoma. Radiology 110:655–657, 1974.
221. Fuks Z, Glatstein E, Kaplan HS: Patterns of presentation and relapse in the non-Hodgkin's lymphomata. Br J Cancer 31 (Suppl II):286–297, 1975.
222. Levitt SH, Bloomfield CD, Lee CKK, Nesbit ME, McKenna W: Extended field radiother-

apy in non-Hodgkin's lymphoma. Radiology 118:457–459, 1976.

223. Tubiana M, Pouillart P, Hayat M, Schlienger M, Gerard-Marchuat R, Schlumberger J, Brugere J, Amiel J-L, Mathe G: Results of radiotherapy in stages I and II of non-Hodgkin's lymphoma. Br J Cancer 31 (Suppl II):402–412, 1975.

224. Mill WB, Lee FA, Franssila KO: Radiation therapy treatment of stage I and II extranodal non-Hodgkin's lymphoma of the head and neck. Cancer 45:653–661, 1980.

225. Risdall R, Hoppe RT, Warnke R: Non-Hodgkin's lymphoma. A study of the evolution of the disease based upon 92 autopsied cases. Cancer 44:529–542, 1979.

226. Glatstein E: Alice in lymphoma-land. Int J Radiat Oncol Biol Phys 1:561–563, 1976.

227. Schein PS, Chabner BA, Canellos GP, Young RC, DeVIta VT: Non-Hodgkin's lymphoma: Patterns of relapse from complete remission after combination chemotherapy. Cancer 35:354–357, 1975.

228. Manfardini S, Banfi A, Bonadona G, Rilke F, Milani F, Valagussa P, Lattuada A: Improved five year survival after combined radiotherapy–chemotherapy for stage I-II non-Hodgkin's lymphoma. Int J Radiat Oncol Biol Phys 6:125–134, 1980.

229. Nathwani BN, Kim H, Rappaport H: Malignant lymphoma, lymphoblastic. Cancer 38:964–983, 1976.

230. Herman TS, Hammond N, Jones SE, Butler JJ, Byrne GE, McKelvey EM: Involvement of the central nervous system by non-Hodgkin's lymphoma. The Southwest Oncology Group Experience. Cancer 43:390–397, 1979.

231. Rosenberg SA, Diamond HD, Jaslowitz B, Craver LF: Lymphosarcoma: a review of 1269 cases. Medicine 40:31–84, 1961.

232. Freeman C, Berg JW, Cutler SJ: Occurrence and prognosis of extranodal lymphomas. Cancer 29:252–260, 1972.

233. Newall J, Friedman M, de Narvaez F: Extra-lymph-node reticulum-cell sarcoma. Radiology 91:708–712, 1968.

234. Cox JD: Prognostic factors in malignant lymphoreticular tumors of the small bowel and ileocecal region: a review of 50 case histories. Int J Radiat Oncol Biol Phys 5:185–190, 1979.

235. Rosenfelt F, Rosenberg SA: Diffuse histiocytic lymphoma presenting with gastrointestinal tract lesions. The Stanford experience Cancer 45:2188–2193, 1980.

236. Brugere J, Schienger M, Gerard-Marchant R, Tubiana M, Pouillart P, Cactim Y: Non-Hodgkin's malignant lymphomata of upper disgestive and respiratory tract: natural history and results of radiotherapy. Br J Cancer 31 (Suppl II) 435–440, 1975.

237. Wang DS, Fuller LM, Butler JJ, Shullenberger CC: Extranodal non-Hodgkin's lymphomas of the head and neck. Am J Roentgenol 123:471–481, 1975.

238. Wang CC: Malignant lymphoma of Waldeyer's ring. Radiology 92:1335–1339, 1969.

239. Terz JJ, Farr HN: Primary lymphosarcoma of the tonsil. Surgery 65:772–776, 1969.

240. Wang CC: Primary malignant lymphoma of the oral cavity and paranasal sinuses. Radiology 100:151–153, 1971.

241. Sofferman RA, Cummings CW: Malignant lymphoma of the paranasal sinuses. Arch Otolaryngol 101:287–292, 1975.

242. Woolner LB, McConatrey WM, Beatirs OH, Black BM: Primary malignant lymphoma of the thyroid. A review of forty-six cases. Am J Surg 111:502–523, 1966.

243. Ragfield EJ, Nishiyama RH, Sisson JC: Small cell tumors of the thyroid. A clinicopathologic study. Cancer 28:1023–1030, 1971.

244. Burke JS, Butler JJ, Fuller LM: Malignant lymphomas of the thyroid. A clinical pathologic study of 35 patients including ultrastructural observations. Cancer 39:1587–1602, 1977.

245. Williams ED: The pathology of thyroid malignancy. Br J Surg 62:757–759, 1975.

246. Cameron RG, Seemayer TA, Wang N-S, Ahmed MN, Tabath EJ: Small cell malignant tumors of the thyroid. A light and electron microscopic study. Human Pathology 6:731–740, 1975.

247. Halnan KE: The non-surgical treatment of thyroid cancer. Br J Surg 62:769–771, 1975.

248. Kim YH, Fayos JV: Primary orbital lymphoma: a radiotherapeutic experience. Int J Radiat Oncol Biol Phys 1:1099–1105, 1976.

249. Isaacson P, Wright DH, Judd MA, Mepam BL: Primary gastrointestinal lymphomas. A classification of 66 cases. Cancer 43:1805–1819, 1979.

250. Lewin KJ, Rauchod M, Dorfman RF: Lymphomas of the gastrointestinal tract. A study of 117 cases presenting with gastrointestinal disease. Cancer 42:693–707, 1978.

251. Freeman HJ, Weinstein WM, Shmitka TK, Piercy JRA, Wensel RH: Primary abdominal lymphoma. Presenting manifestation of celiac sprue or complicating dermatitis herpetiformis. Am J Med 63:585–594, 1977.

252. Hande KR, Fisher RI, DeVita VT, Chabner BA, Young RC: Diffuse histiocytic lymphoma involving the gastrointesinal tract. Cancer 41:1984–1989, 1978.

253. Dawson IMP, Cornes JS, Morson BC: Primary malignant lymphoid tumors of the intestinal tract. Report of 37 cases with a study of factors influencing prognosis. Br J Surg 49:80–89, 1961.

254. Nicoloff DM, Haynes LB, Wangensteeen OH: Primary lymphosarcoma of the gastrointestinal tract. Surg Gynecol Obstet 117:433–437, 1963.

255. Naqvi MS, Burrows L, Kark AE: Lymphoma of the gastrointestinal tract. Prognostic guides based on 162 cases. Ann Surg 170:221–231, 1969.

256. Loehr WJ, Miyahead Z, Zahn FD, Gray GF, Thorbjarnarson T: Primary lymphoma of the gastrointestinal tract: a review of 100 cases. Ann Surg 170:232–238, 1969.

257. Kahn LB, Selzer G, Kaschula ROC: Primary gastrointestinal lymphoma. A clinicopathologic study of fifty-seven cases. Am J Dig Dis 17:219–232, 1972.

258. Freund H, Lavi A, Pfeffermann R, Durst AL: Primary neoplasms of the small bowel. Am J Surg 135:757–759, 1978.

259. Lim FE, Hartman AS, Tan EGC, Cady B, Meissner WA: Factors in the prognosis of gastric lymphoma. Cancer 39:1715–1720, 1977.

260. Bush RS, Ash CL: Primary lymphoma of the gastrointestinal tract. Radiology 92:1349–1354, 1969.

261. Fisher RI, DeVita VT, Johnson BL, Simon R, Young RC: Prognostic factors for advanced diffuse histiocytic lymphoma following treatment with combination chemotherapy. Am J Med 63:177–182, 1977.

262. Parker F, Jackson H: Primary reticulum cell sarcoma of bone. Surg Gynecol Obstet 68:45–53, 1939.

263. Francis KC, Higinbotham NL, Coley Bl: Primary reticulum cell sarcoma of bone. Report of 44 cases. Surg Gynecol Obstet 99:142–146, 1954.

264. Donal PA: Reticulum cell sarcoma of bone. Am J Roentgenol 87:121–127, 1962.

265. Wang CC, Fleischli DJ: Primary reticulum cell sarcoma of bone. With emphasis on radiation therapy. Cancer 22:994–998, 1968.

266. Dahlin DC: Is it worthwhile to differentiate Ewing's sarcoma and primary lymphoma of bone? Seventh National Cancer Conference Proceedings. Philadelphia: JB Lippincott, 1973, pp 941–945.

267. Phillips TL, Sheline GE: Radiation therapy of malignant bone tumors. Radiology 92:1537–1545, 1969.

268. Miller TR, Nicholson JT: End results in reticulum cell sarcoma of bone treated by bacterial toxin therapy alone or combined with surgery and/or radiotherapy (47 cases) or with concurrent infection (5 cases). Cancer 27:524–548, 1971.

269. Ribeiro GG: Primary lymphosarcoma and reticulum cell sarcoma of skin. A review of thirty-two cases. Clin Radiol 23:279–285, 1972.

270. Kim R, Winkelmann RF, Dockerty M: Reticulum cell sarcoma of the skin. Cancer 16:646–655, 1963.

271. Levitt JL, Dawson DM, Rosenthal DS, Moloney WC: CNS involvement in the non-

Hodgkin's lymphomas. Cancer 45:454-552, 1980.

272. Shawnburg HH, Plank CR, Adams RD: The reticulum cell sarcoma – microglioma group of brain tumors. Brain 95:199-212, 1972.

273. Henry JM, Heffner RR, Dillard SH, Earle KM, Dewis RL: Primary malignant lymphoma of the central nervous system. Cancer 34:1293-1302, 1974.

274. Littman P, Wang CC: Reticulum cell sarcoma of the brain. A review of the literature and a study of 19 cases. Cancer 35:1412-1420, 1975.

275. Sagerman RH, Cassady JR, Chang CH: Radiation therapy for intracranial lymphoma. Radiology 88:552-554, 1967.

276. Klingele TG, Hogan MJ: Ocular reticulum cell sarcoma. Am J Ophthalmol 79:39-47, 1975.

277. Margolis L, Fraser R, Lichter A, Char DH: The role of radiation therapy in the management of ocular reticulum cell sarcoma. Cancer 45:688-269, 1980.

278. Chorlton I, Norris HJ, King FM: Malignant reticuloendotheial disease involving the ovary as a primary manifestation. A series of 19 lymphomas and 1 granulocytic sarcoma. Cancer 34:397-407, 1974.

279. Paladuga RR, Bearman RM, Rappaport H: Malignant lymphoma with primary manifestation in the gonad. A clinicopathologic study of 38 patients. Cancer 45:561-571, 1980.

280. Mostofi FK: Testicular tumors. Epidemiologic, etologic and pathologic features. Cancer 32:1186-1201, 1973.

281. Duncan PR, Checa F, Gowing NFC, McElwain TJ, Peckham MJ: Extranodal non-Hodgkin's lymphoma presenting in the testicle. A clinical and pathologic study of 24 cases. Cancer 45:1578-1584, 1980.

282. Sussman EB, Hajdu SI, Lieberman PH, Whitmore WR: Malignant lymphoma of the testis: a clinicopathologic study of 37 cases. J Urol 118:1004-1007, 1977.

283. Talerman: Primary malignant lymphoma of the testis. J Urol 118:783-786, 1977.

284. Kushlan P, Coleman CN, Glatstein EJ, Rosenberg SA, Kaplan HS: Prognostic factors in stage II diffuse histiocytic lymphoma. ASCO Abstracts C-122, 1978, p 337.

285. Miller TP, Jones SE: Chemotherapy of localized histiocytic lymphoma. Lancet 1:358-360, 1979.

286. Skarin AT, Rosenthal DS, Moloney WC, Frei E: Combination chemotherapy of advanced non-Hodgkin's lymphomas with bleomycin, adriamycin, cyclophosphamide, vincristine, and prednisone (BACOP). Blood 49:759-770, 1977.

287. Portlock CS, Rosenberg SA, Glatstein E, Kaplan HS: Treatment of advanced non-Hodgkin's lymphomas with favourable histiologies: Preliminary results of a prospective trial. Blood 47:474-756, 1976.

288. Rodriguez V, Cabarillas F, Burgess MA, McKelvey EM, Valdivesio M, Bodey GP, Freireich EJ: Combination chemotherapy ('CHOP-Bleo') in advanced (non-Hodgkin) malignant lymphoma. Blood 49:325-333, 1977.

289. Chabner BA: Nodular non Hogkin's lymphoma: the case for watchful waiting. Ann Int Med 90:115-117, 179.

290. Johnson RE: Management of generalized malignant lymphomata with 'systemic' radiotherapy. Br J Cancer 31 (Suppl II):450-455, 1975.

291. Johnson ER, O'Conor, T, Levin D: Primary management of advanced lymphosarcoma with radiotherapy. Cancer 25:787-791, 1970.

292. Johnson RE, Canellos GP, Young RC, Chabner BA, DeVita VT: Chemotherapy (cyclophosphamide, vincristine, and prednisone) versus radiotherapy (total body irradiation) for stage III-IV poorly differentiated lymphocytic lymphoma. Cancer Treat Rep 62:321-325, 1978.

293. Johnson RE: Evaluation of fractionated total body irradiation in patients with leukemia and disseminated lymphomas. Radiology 86:185-189, 1966.

294. Johnson RE: Total body irradiation (TBI) as primary therapy for advanced lymphosarco-

ma. Cancer 35:242-245, 1975.

295. Thar TL, Million RR, Noyes WD: Total body irradiation in non-Hodgkin's lymphoma. Int J Radiat Oncol Biol Phys 5:171-176, 1979.

296. Choi NC, Timothy AR, Kaufman SD, Carey RW, Aisenberg AC: Low dose fractionated whole body irradiation in the treatment of advanced non-Hodgkin's lymphoma. Cancer 43:1636-1642, 1979.

297. Chaffey JT, Rosenthal DS, Moloney WC, Hellman S: Total body irradiation as treatment for lymphosarcoma. Int J Radiat Oncol Biol Phys 1:399-405, 1976.

298. Caravell SC, Chaffey JT, Rosenthal DS, Moloney, WC, Hellman S: Results of total body irradiation in the treatment of advanced non-Hodgkin's lymphomas. Cancer 43:994-1000, 1979.

299. Herman TS, Jones SE: Systematic re-staging in the management of non-Hodgkin's lymphomas. Cancer Treat REP 61:1009-1015, 1977.

300. Eastern Cooperative Oncology Group - ECOG Protocol 4477 - Combined modality treatment protocol for stages III and IV favorable (nodular) histologic subtypes of non-Hodgkin's lymphoma. Glick JH, Study Chairman. ECOG Operations Office, 905 University Avenue, Suite 415, Madison, WI 53715.

301. Elias L, Portlack CS, Rosenberg SA: Combination chemotherapy of diffuse histiocytic lymphoma with cyclophosphamide, adriamycin, vincristine and prednisone (CHOP). Cancer 42:1705-1710, 1978.

302. Jones SE, Grozea PN, Metz EN, Haut A, Stephens RL, Morrison FS, Butler JJ, Byrne GE, Moon TE, Fisher R, Haskins CL, Coltman CA: Superiority of adriamycin-containing combination chemotherapy in the treatment of diffuse lymphoma. A Southwest Oncology Group Study. Cancer 43:417-425, 1979.

303. Harrison DT, Neiman PE, Sullivan K, Hafermann M, Rudolph BH, Einstein EB: Combined modality therapy for advanced diffuse lymphocytic and histiocytic lymphomas. Cancer 42:1697-1704, 1978.

304. Pinkel D, Johnson W, Aur RJA: Non-Hodgkin's lymphoma in children. Br J Cancer 31 (Suppl II):298-323, 1975.

305. Lemerle M, Gerard-Marchant R, Sancho H, Schweizguth O: Natural history of non-Hodgkin's malignant lymphomata in children. A retrospective study of 190 cases. Br J Cancer 31 (Suppl II):324-331, 1975.

306. Murphy SB: Management of childhood Non-Hodgkin's lymphoma. Cancer Treat Rep 61:1161-11783, 1977.

307. Wollner N, Lieberman P, Exelby P, D'Angio G, Burchenl J, Fang S, Murphy ML: Non-Hodgkin's lymphoma in children: results of treatment with LSA$_2$-L$_2$ protocol. Br J Cancer 31 (Suppl II):337-342, 1975.

308. Murphy SB: Classification staging and end results of treatment of childhood non-Hodgkin's lymphomas: Dissimilarities from lymphomas in adults. Semin Oncol 7:332-339, 1980.

309. Nelson DF, Cassady JR, Traggis D, Baez-Giangreco A, Vawater GF, Jaffe N, Filler RM: The role of radiation therapy in localized resectable intestinal non-Hodgkin's lymphoma in children. Cancer 39:89-97, 1977.

310. Wollner N, Wachtel AE, Exelby PE, Centore D: Improved prognosis in children with intra-abdominal non-Hodgkin's lymphoma following LSA$_2$L$_2$ protocol chemotherapy. Cancer 45:3034-3039, 1980.

311. Murphy SB, Hustu HO: A randomized trial of combined modality therapy of childhood non-Hodgkin's lymphoma. Cancer 45:630-637, 1980.

312. Carabell SC, Cassady JR, Weinstein HJ, Jaffe N: The role of radiation therapy in the treatment of pediatric non-Hodgkin's lymphomas. Cancer 42:2193-2205, 1978.

313. Jenkins RDT, Souley MJ, Stephens CA, Darte JMM, Peters MV: Primary gastrointestinal tract lymphoma in childhood. Radiology 92:763-767, 1969.

314. Traggis D, Jaffe N, Vawater G, Baez-Giangreco A: Non-Hodgkin's lymphoma of the head and neck in childhood. J Pediatr 87:933–936, 1975.
315. Jenkin RDT: The management of malignant lymphoma in childhood. In: Modern radiotherapy-malignant disease in children, Dealey TJ, ed. London: Butterworths, 1974, pp 341–359.

5. Chemotherapy of Hodgkin's and Non-Hodgkin's Lymphomas *

JOHN H. GLICK

The management of patients with Hodgkin's and non-Hodgkin's lymphoma has improved significantly over the past two decades. It is now possible to offer potentially curative therapy to all newly diagnosed patients with disseminated Hodgkin's disease and to demonstrate a clear survival advantage for chemotherapy responders in the non-Hodgkin's lymphomas. However, the management of an individual patient is frequently controversial. The proliferation of clinical studies utilizing a bewildering array of chemotherapy combinations, often in conjunction with radiotherapy, has led to new recommendations being proposed before they are compared to standard practice. Interpretation of promising results must be viewed with caution in the absence of controlled trials, because of differences in patient selection, sites of disease, and prognostic factors. Careful consideration of the toxicity-benefit ratio for each chemotherapy or combined modality program is the responsibility of all physicians caring for these patients. The optimal management and greatest opportunity for improved disease-free survival in the lymphomas depends on collaborative, well-designed clinical trials. This chapter will review the important role of chemotherapy in the management of both advanced and localized Hodgkin's and non-Hodgkin's lymphoma in adults. Emphasis will be placed on evaluation of ongoing clinical investigations in comparison to what has become accepted as standard therapy. A list of abbreviations and acronyms of the various chemotherapy regimes is given in the Appendix at the end of this chapter [1].

* Supported in Part by USPHS Grants No. CA-15488 and CA-16520.

1.   HODGKIN'S DISEASE

1.1. Single Agent Chemotherapy

The treatment of advanced Hodgkin's disease with chemotherapy began in the early 1940s with the demonstration that nitrogen mustard could produce dramatic clinical responses. The early studies of Goodman et al. [2] were confirmed and extended by Karnofsky et al. [3] and Zanes et al. [4], and provided the cornerstone on which future successful combination chemotherapy programs could be built. Carter and Livingston [5] have reviewed the collective literature of single agent chemotherapy generated through 1970. They reported that objective responses may be expected in approximately 65% of patients treated with nitrogen mustard. These responses were noted to occur quite rapidly, frequently within a few days after the initial injection, but the median duration of response was less than 3 months. There were sufficient data to report a composite complete response (CR) rate of 13% in 95 evaluable patients [5]. These retrospective data were confirmed in a prospective trial of single agent nitrogen mustard conducted by Huguley et al. [6] in 47 patients with a complete response rate of 13%.

Other alkylating agents were also evaluated during the 1960s with similar overall and complete response rates (Table 1). Comparative trials of nitrogen mustard and cyclophosphamide have noted a slightly higher, but not statistically significant, response rate and median survival for patients treated with nitrogen mustard [5]. Chlorambucil also has equivalent single agent

Table 1. Single agent chemotherapy in advanced Hodgkin's disease.

Drug	No. of evaluable cases	% overall response	No. of cases evaluable for complete response	% complete response	References
Nitrogen mustard	843	62	142	13	5, 6
Cyclophosphamide	469	54	227	12	5, 7
Chlorambucil	305	60	57	16	5, 8
Vinblastine	682	68	293	30	5, 9
Vincristine	115	58	28	36	5, 8
Procarbazine	366	69	138	38	5, 10
Prednisone	105	61	–	0	5, 8
Carmustine (BCNU)	213	44	94	5	11, 12, 13
Lomustine (CCNU)	84	48	57	12	13, 14
Bleomycin	198	38	91	6	15–17
Adriamycin	116	30	98	5	18–20
Dimethyl-triazeno-imidazole carboxamide (DTIC)	18	56	18	6	21

activity in advanced Hodgkin's disease and offers the advantage of oral administration and less toxicity. It has frequently been used as maintenance chemotherapy once remissions had been induced with other alkylating agent regimens.

The vinca alkaloids, vinblastine and vincristine, were identified during the 1960s as having single agent effectiveness against advanced Hodgkin's disease. Vinblastine was noted to have a complete response rate of 30% in the compiled series reported by Carter and Livingston, while the complete response rate with vincristine was an impressive 36% in a small number of patients [5]. In a randomized trial reported by Carbone et al. [7], previously untreated patients were randomized to vinblastine (CR 27%, overall response rate 75%) or cyclophosphamide (CR 18%, overall response rate 54%). However, no significant difference in survival of the two groups was noted. Stutzman et al. [9] also confirmed the superiority of vinblastine over cyclophosphamide, but obtained similar response rates when nitrogen mustard was used as the alkylating agent in a direct comparison with vinblastine.

The methlhydrazine derivative, procarbazine, was introduced for the treatment of Hodgkin's disease in the early 1960s and demonstrated impressive single agent activity (compiled complete response rate of 38% [5, 10]). More importantly, patients exhibited no cross-resistance to this drug relative to prior treatment with alkylating agents or vinca alkaloids.

Data on the efficacy of glucocorticoids is controversial, because steroids frequently produce subjective improvement that is difficult to differentiate from true objective responses. An overall response rate of 61% has been reported, with no complete responses being observed with steroids alone [5, 8].

With the advent of modern combination chemotherapy for Hodgkin's disease, it has been increasingly difficult to evaluate the efficacy of newer single agents. The poor prognosis of previously treated patients, with prior myelosuppression, frequently necessitates significant downward dose modification of experimental agents. Nonetheless, the nitrosoureas BCNU and CCNU have both been reported to have demonstrated single agent activity in far-advanced Hodgkin's disease resistant to alkylating agents, the vinca derivatives, and combination chemotherapy. Overall response rates have been noted to approach 50% for both these nitrosoureas; however, the complete remission rates are disappointing [11–13]. CCNU has been shown to be superior to BCNU in a controlled trial [14], and has the advantage of oral administration. Table 1 also summarizes the single agent activity of bleomycin, adriamycin, and DTIC [15–21]. Although these recently developed agents have been evaluated in a relatively small series of Phase II trials, they have been incorporated into combination chemotherapy programs, particularly as part of salvage regimens.

Thus, a wide variety of single agents with different mechanisms of action and non-overlapping toxicities have been identified as being active in advanced Hodgkin's disease. However, the duration of single agent responses was short, and even the complete remissions lasted an average of three months. The impact on survival was not dramatic because the frequency of complete remissions did not approach 50%, and the survival of complete responders was rarely separated from the median survival of all patients [22].

1.2. Combination Chemotherapy – the Early Trials

Lacher and Durant [23] were the first to explore the use of a two-drug combination of vinblastine and chlorambucil in 16 patients with advanced Hodgkin's disease, almost all of whom had prior radiotherapy and chemotherapy. Their complete response rate of 63% was impressively better than that which had been achieved in previously reported studies with single agents. Not only were these agents administered with safety, the average response duration was 7.5 months.

The National Cancer Institute group pioneered the use of quadruple-drug combination therapy in 1963. Their treatment program included cyclophosphamide, vincristine, methotrexate, and prednisone, and was known as the MOMP regimen [24]. An 80% complete response (CR) rate was achieved in 14 patients, 12 of whom were previously untreated. Nine patients with localized disease received this combination of drugs in conjunction with radiotherapy to all involved sites, while five stage III patients were treated with chemotherapy alone. The complete responses were prompt, generally occurring within the first cycle of therapy. However, the duration of responses was generally brief because the initial MOMP trial had been developed as only a $2\frac{1}{2}$ month treatment program based on current conventions at that time [24]. Interestingly, three of the original patients treated with MOMP were alive and disease-free at 7 and 8 years [25].

Preliminary combination chemotherapy studies were also investigated in the cooperative group setting. Luce et al. [26] explored the use of a three-drug regimen, cyclophosphamide, vincristine and prednisone (COP) in 107 patients with advanced Hodgkin's disease. Thirty-six percent of patients achieved complete remission with a median duration of unmaintained response in previously untreated patients of 19 weeks. Lenhard [27] also investigated the COP combination and compared it to vinblastine alone. While the overall response rates were similar in the vinblastine and combination arms, the COP regimen achieved a higher complete remission rate (38%), but again the median response duration was brief (6.2 months with the combination).

These preliminary efforts in multiple agent chemotherapy for Hodgkin's disease clearly established that drugs could be used safely in combination with predictable toxicity and apparently higher complete response rates than had previously been documented. The stage was clearly established for the development of the MOPP program.

1.3. MOPP as Primary Treatment

1.3.1 The National Cancer Institute Experience. The combination of nitrogen mustard, vincristine, procarbazine, and prednisone into the MOPP program was initiated in 1964 by DeVita and associates at the National Cancer Institute (NCI) [28]. Forty-three consecutive, previously untreated patients with advanced Hodgkin's disease were treated with a minimum of six cycles of the MOPP regimen. A complete remission rate of 81% was achieved and, at the time of their original report, the median response duration had not yet been reached with a minimum follow-up of 32 months. Seventeen of the 35 patients obtaining complete remission were still free of disease as of 1970, and the median survival of the 35 patients achieving complete response had not been reached. This complete remission rate represented at least a three-fold improvement over what had previously been obtainable with single agent chemotherapy.

The high complete response rate and dramatic improvement in relapse-free survival of patients with advanced Hodgkin's disease treated with MOPP represented the first evidence that Hodgkin's disease was indeed potentially curable. The data from the NCI have recently been updated by DeVita *et al.* [29] and amply confirmed their initial observations. A total of 198 patients have been treated with the MOPP program. Three groups of patients have been part of the NCI prospective trials. Eighty-four patients were treated with MOPP until complete remission was obtained after which time all therapy was discontinued. Eighty-six additional patients were treated with MOPP as their remission induction program; 57 of the complete responders in this group were then randomized to one of three therapeutic options to test the efficacy of maintenance drug treatment versus observation alone on remission duration and survival. A third group of 28 patients with clinical stage IIIB Hodgkin's disease were treated with MOPP as induction therapy followed by total nodal irradiation. Results of treatment in all these three groups have been combined by DeVita *et al.* for purposes of their most recent analysis. Only 23 of the 198 patients (10.6%) were asymptomatic, and only 5% were stage II. Thus, the vast majority of these patients had stage IIIB or IV Hodgkin's disease and all had received no prior chemotherapy. Complete remission was obtained in 80% of patients (159/198), with a median of three cycles needed to achieve complete remission. Although the initial study [28] called for a fixed induction scheme of six cycles, the NCI group actually utilized a flexible treatment policy as to the number of cycles of MOPP that should be administered to an individual patient. The total duration of MOPP chemotherapy was adjusted to the speed of response. All patients were given a minimum of six cycles or as many cycles as needed to achieve a complete remission plus two additional cycles. Twenty-five percent of the patient who obtained complete remission required more than six cycles of MOPP [30].

Although a dose-modification table was included in the original 1970 report by DeVita *et al.* [28], the NCI group did not emphasize until recently their general treatment policy concerning the individualization of drug dose depending on that particular patient's bone marrow tolerance. If the blood counts had not returned to normal by the 28th day of the previous cycle, but ar least 50% of the myelosuppressive drugs (nitrogen mustard and procarbazine) could be given according to the dose modification schedule, NCI physicians proceeded with the next cycle of MOPP at the reduced dose level to preserve the timing of sequential cycles while still giving some of all the agents. If the peripheral blood counts were reduced to a level that would require more than a 50% decrease of nitrogen mustard and procarbazine or omission of any drug from the combination, an additional week off chemotherapy was allowed between cycles to facilitate further recovery of the blood counts [29]. This enabled NCI investigators to administer higher doses of the MOPP regimen than are frequently given in conventional practice. Nausea and vomiting was rarely considered an indication to decrease the dose of nitrogen mustard, and paresthesias did not result in dose reduction for vincristine. Patients were highly motivated by their physicians to continue this toxic and difficult chemotherapy, because the importance of obtaining a complete remission was emphasized. Young and DeVita [31] appropriately stress that any comparative trial of MOPP or an alternative combination should provide data on the intensity with which the investigators adhere to the planned regimen. Without such information, dose modifications alone may account for different results with MOPP or alternative chemotherapy programs.

Even more important than the impressive complete remission rate obtained by DeVita *et al.* was the ability of the MOPP regimen to produce durable disease-free remissions [29]. Sixty-eight percent of patients achieving complete remission at risk for five years or more have remained disease-free. Thus, 55% of all patients have remained free of recurrent Hodgkin's disease at five years. Only three relapses have occurred more than 42 months from the end of MOPP chemotherapy. With 79 patients at risk at least 10 years from the institution of MOPP chemotherapy, the relapse-free survival of patients who achieved complete remission at 10 years is 63.4% (Figure 1). These impressive survival data, with ample follow-up time, documented that advanced Hodgkin's disease is indeed curable by combination chemotherapy. Only a retrospective comparison of survival from the era of single agent or two-drug combination chemotherapy, in which fewer than 10% of patients with advanced disease survived five years and only an exceptional

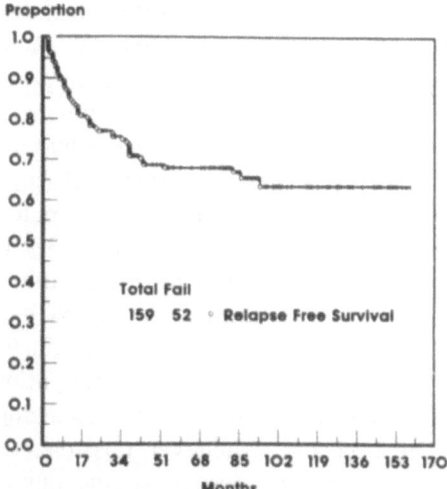

Figure 1. Relapse-free survival of the 159 patients who achieved complete remission with MOPP treatment. (Reprinted, by permission, from DeVita *et al.* [29].)

patient survived beyond the five-year point relapse-free, allows us to appreciate the importance of the MOPP program.

The updated data reported by DeVita *et al.* [29] remain the benchmark against which all current and future treatment programs for advanced Hodgkin's disease must be measured. It is no longer sufficient to gauge the

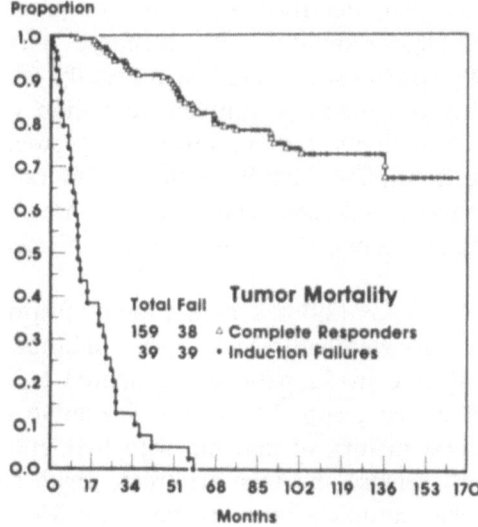

Figure 2. Survival of complete responders and patients who failed to achieve complete remission after MOPP. (Reprinted, by permission, from DeVita *et al.* [29].)

success of any alternative regimen by its ability to induce a high complete remission rate. Rather, relapse-free survival after all therapy is discontinued remains the goal of any therapeutic program. The importance of obtaining a complete remission is emphasized in the NCI series by the fact that the 39 patients who failed to achieve complete remission had a median survival of 11 months, and none of these patients survived beyond five years. In contrast, the probability of surviving beyond five years for patients achieving complete remission is 82%, and for 10 years it is 73% (Figure 2).

The importance of extensive restaging procedures after the attainment of a clinical complete remission was emphasized by the NCI group. All radiologic and biopsy procedures that yielded a positive result during the pretreatment staging workup were repeated at the time of restaging in order to document a pathologic complete remission. Tomography, lymphangiography, CAT scans, all had to return to normal and, whenever possible, the original sites of extra-nodal involvement were re-biopsied to rule out occult disease. The latter usually involved repeat percutaneous bone marrow biopsies and frequently peritoneoscopy-directed liver biopsies. Herman and Jones [32] confirmed the importance of systematic restaging for advanced Hodgkin's disease. Their study from the Southwest Oncology Group noted that 12% of patients in clinical complete remission had occult residual disease identified by the above restaging procedures. Without this restaging information it is difficult to interpret the efficacy of alternative chemotherapy programs when compared with DeVita's data on the MOPP regimen, because the failure to detect occult residual disease at the completion of initial induction treatment obviously has a major effect on relapse-free survival.

DeVita et al. [29] also identified a number of prognostic factors that influenced the complete remission rate, response duration, and overall survival. The only prognostic factor significantly associated with an increased probability of obtaining complete remission was the absence of B-symptoms. All 23 patients without fever, night sweats, or weight loss obtained complete remission compared to a CR rate of 78% in the symptomatic patients ($P = 0.025$). The favorable prognostic impact of A symptoms on complete response rates has been confirmed by other investigators [6, 33, 34].

Interestingly, DeVita et al. [29] observed a trend toward a higher complete response rate in patients who had received prior radiotherapy before MOPP treatment (94% CR rate in 32 patients) compared to the 78% CR with MOPP in the unirradiated group ($P = 0.065$). The authors speculate that the more indolent natural history of patients who first present with localized disease, subsequently relapse and then are treated with chemotherapy, may account for the higher complete response rate with MOPP in patients who have failed previous radiotherapy. The degree of myelosuppression and percentage of ideal chemotherapy dose per cycle did not differ in the groups who had received prior radiotherapy and the previously untreated patients [35]. This observation that major prior radiotherapy does not seriously compromise the response rate to subsequent chemotherapy has been confirmed by other investigators with the MOPP regimen and with alternative combinations [33, 36–39]. Prior radiotherapy has been reported to have no influence [33, 36], a negative influence [37], and a positive effect [38] on the response duration to MOPP chemotherapy.

However, the complete response rate of patients receiving MOPP after failing to respond to either single agent or combination chemotherapy has been disappointing. Lowenbraum *et al.* [40] reported a 50% complete response rate with MOPP in a small series of patients who had received prior radiotherapy and chemotherapy, but an 87% CR rate among those with prior radiotherapy alone. This observation, that prior chemotherapy seriously compromises not only the complete remission rate but also relapse-free and overall survival, has also been amply confirmed [36, 38, 39, 41].

When DeVita *et al.* [29] analyzed their data for the important characteristics affecting relapse-free survival, the most important single factor was again B-symptoms. Patients with B-symptoms had a significantly shorter disease-free period than the asymptomatic group ($P<0.002$). In addition, patients with nodular sclerosing Hodgkin's disease had a significantly shorter disease-free interval than did patients with mixed cellularity Hodgkin's disease ($P<0.02$) or lymphocyte-depleted Hodgkin's disease ($P<0.02$). The negative effect of nodular sclerosis on response duration has been confirmed by one group [42], but not by others [33, 34].

1.3.2. Confirmatory Studies with MOPP. The promise of the MOPP regimen was promptly confirmed. Ziegler *et al.* [43] initially described a 100% complete response rate in 24 African children treated with six cycles of MOPP. Since radiotherapy was not available in Uganda, seven of these 24 patients had localized disease. In a 10-year follow-up of the African study reported by Olweny *et al.* [44], 48 children with all stages of Hodgkin's disease have been treated with MOPP. Eighty-eight percent have achieved a complete remission, with a 74% disease-free survival at 10 years and a 67% overall survival.

Moore *et al.* [37] reported the initial Stanford experience in 81 patients treated with MOPP with a 74% complete response rate. The median duration of complete remission was estimated to be 26 months. Patients with no prior radiotherapy had a similar response rate to that reported by DeVita *et al.* [29], but the median response duration was only 11 months. Moore *et al.* [37] attributed this to the larger number of patients in their series with stage IV disease, age greater than 45 years, and bone marrow involvement. The Stanford observation, that initial bone marrow involvement signifies a high risk of subsequent relapse after MOPP therapy, is not supported by the

NCI results, in which the durability of complete remission for patients with marrow involvement is similar to that of patients with other extranodal sites.

Additional confirmation came from both the early trials of the cooperative groups and from larger single institutions. Frei *et al.* [36] treated 178 patients with advanced Hodgkin's disease with a MOPP regimen similar to the NCI program except that patients received only 10 rather than 14 days of procarbazine and prednisone. The overall complete response rate was 66%, but rose to 80% in the 93 patients with no prior therapy. Since a fixed induction program of six cycles of MOPP was employed and pathologic restaging was not mandatory, patients in clinical complete remission were difficult to compare to the NCI patients. Frei *et al.* did report that 55% of the patients who received six months of MOPP, obtained complete remission and did not receive maintenance chemotherapy, remained disease-free two years from the end of treatment. A follow-up trial by the Southwest Oncology Group reported a 62% complete response rate with MOPP in 206 patients with advanced Hodgkin's disease [45]. Subsequent studies by the cooperative groups have revealed complete remission rates with MOPP ranging from 61 to 75% [1, 6, 41, 46, 47]. While various factors such as age and stage [34, 37, 38] appear to relate to the complete remission rate, the two most important prognostic factors in both the cooperative group and single institution studies is whether the patient has had major prior chemotherapy and whether a complete response is obtained. Nixon and Aisenberg [48] reported a 91% complete response rate in 35 advanced Hodgkin's disease patients with no prior treatment, of whom 66% remained disease-free with a median remission duration exceeding 22 months. In their patients with prior treatment, complete responses were noted in 71%, of whom only 47% remained disease-free. Complete response rates with MOPP-like regimens in patients with prior chemotherapy are even lower in the experience of most cooperative groups, with a range of 28–50% [34, 36, 38, 39].

These confirmatory studies clearly support the data of DeVita *et al.* [28, 29] and represent the standard by which all alternative combination chemotherapy programs or combined modality treatment plans must be judged.

1.4. The Search for an Alternative Regimen to MOPP

Although the initial data of DeVita and associates with the MOPP regimen for previously untreated patients were truly impressive, the lack of a concurrent control group made it difficult for some investigators to accept the superiority of MOPP over intensive single agent chemotherapy or alternative combination chemotherapy programs. Table 2 summarizes a series of nine randomized prospective clinical trials comparing MOPP with other regimens. The purpose of these trials was to confirm the superiority of

Table 2. Randomized trials comparing MOPP with alternative regimens for advanced Hodgkin's disease.

Author	Regimen	No. of evaluable patients	% CR	Disease-free survival (%/yr)	Overall survival (%/yr)	Comment
Huguley *et al.* [6]	MOPP vs	61	48	40/3	55/3	MOPP OS significantly better
	HN₂	47	13	23/3	35/3	because of higher CR
British *et al.* [49]	MOPP vs	49	80	–	No significant	Prednisone in all cycles;
	MOP	41	44	–	difference	increased toxicity with MOPP
Jacobs *et al.* [50]	MOPP vs	157	82	64/6	No significant	Retrospective analysis
	MOP	54	78	60/4	difference	
Stutzman *et al.* [52]	MOPP vs	81	61	50/2	–	MOPP more toxic
	VPBCPr * vs	89	61	25/2	–	
	VPBCPr +	77	49	20/2	–	
Nissen *et al.* [42]	MOPP vs	104	62	62/4	62/4	Lack of plateau in
	BOPP vs	103	67	54/4	55/4	survival curves;
	OPP vs	112	42	50/4	40/4	BOPP less toxic than MOPP
	BOP	107	40	30/4	30/4	
Cooper *et al.* [53]	MOPP vs	138	57	57/4	45/4	CCNU most significant
	MVPP vs	125	66	45/4	43/4	determinant of prolonged CR
	CCNU-OPP vs	132	65	59/4	41/4	
	CCNU-VPP	137	69	71/4	56/4	
Bakemeier *et al.* [34]	MOPP vs	152	73	49/5	64/5	BCVPP significantly
	BCVPP	154	77	62/5	64/5	less toxic
Coltman *et al.* [1, 47]	MOPP vs	44	70	62/3	62/3	Borderline advantage in CR
	MOPP-LDB	118	84	64/3	78/3	and OS for MOPP-LDB
	MOPP-HDB	38	76	53/3	65/3	
Bonadonna *et al.* [77]	MOPP vs	29	66	–	–	All CR received
	ABVD	26	69	–	–	consolidation XRT

Abbreviations: * Simultaneous; + Sequential; CR = Complete Response; OS = Overall Survival.

MOPP, to identify a program equivalent to or better than MOPP, and to find an alternative regimen with less toxicity than MOPP. It is frequently difficult to compare one trial with another because of multiple prognostic and treatment factors that differ in the patient populations studied (e.g., differences in patient selection, amount of previous therapy, extent of restaging to determine complete response, variable length of the initial treatment period with MOPP or the alternative regimen, the difference in maintenance treatment programs versus unmaintained remissions, lack of information on the intensity of the drug programs administered, and short follow-up period).

Huguley *et al.* [6] initiated a randomized trial in 1967 in the Southeastern Group designed to compare six cycles of MOPP versus single agent nitrogen mustard administered to tolerance for an equivalent time period. The complete remission rate of 48 % with MOPP was significantly better than the 12 % CR with nitrogen mustard. Although the complete remissions with MOPP lasted a median of 15 months, which was not significantly different from the 12-month relapse-free survival after nitrogen mustard, 40 % of the patients treated with MOPP were disease-free at three years. Most importantly, there was a significant difference in overall survival with a median of 38 months for MOPP versus 13 months for the nitrogen mustard treated patients. This significant difference in overall survival was due almost entirely to the fact that a much higher percentage of patients treated with MOPP achieved a complete remission. This trial unequivocally demonstrated the superiority of MOPP over an active single agent given to tolerance levels.

The inclusion of corticosteroids as part of the MOPP regimen by the NCI group has been the subject of controversy. As previously decribed, corticosteroids alone are relatively ineffective as single agents in inducing objective remissions. Corticosteroids produce margination of granulocytes from the bone marrow pool, thus potentially allowing higher doses of the myelosuppressive agents to be administered because the blood counts are artificially higher on day 8 of the MOPP cycle. The British National Lymphoma Investigation [49] randomized patients to receive MOPP with prednisone given at a dose of 25 mg/m^2 daily for 14 days in each cycle versus the same drugs without prednisone (MOP). There was a highly significant difference in the complete remission rates in favor of MOPP (80 % CR) compared with MOP (44 % CR). Unfortunately, the British study did not provide information on the amount of myelosuppressive drugs actually given in the two treatment groups. Information on disease-free survival was also not provided, but there was no significant difference in the overall survival. Three deaths were associated with bone marrow depression in the 40 patients treated with MOPP, compared with no hematologic deaths in the MOP group.

These results, however, have not been confirmed by the Stanford group. Jacobs et al. [50] retrospectively reviewed 157 patients treated with MOPP and compared them to 54 patients treated with MOP. They found no differences in either the complete remission rate or length of remission between patients who received prednisone in cycles one and four, those who received no prednisone, and those who received some prednisone. The impetus for deleting prednisone at Stanford came from an observation by Castellino et al. [51] who described seven patients with prior mantle irradiation who developed pneumonitis or pericarditis shortly after completing either cycle one or four of the MOPP program with prednisone. It was thought that subclinical radiation injury to the lungs or heart might be activated by rapid withdrawal of high-dose steroids. Subsequent treatment policy at Stanford was to eliminate prednisone from the MOPP regimen in those patients who had previously received mediastinal irradiation. As noted previously by DeVita et al. [29], patients who have had prior radiotherapy, then relapse and are treated with MOPP, have a higher CR rate and a favorable prognosis. Since the only reason that prednisone was omitted from MOPP at Stanford was because of previous mantle irradiation, this may account for the excellent 78% complete response rate and the disease-free survival of 60% at 6 years reported for those patients receiving MOP without prednisone. Certainly, in an individual patient who demonstrates corticosteroid intolerance, prednisone can be deleted without significantly compromising prognosis. However, there does not seem to be any demonstrated efficacy of including prednisone in every MOPP cycle.

The MOPP program is also associated with significant nausea, vomiting, neurological, and psychologic complications. These toxic reactions frequently result in difficulties with both patient and physician compliance, leading to compromised drug doses or deletion of an active agent from the MOPP regimen. Stutzman and Glidewell [52] reporting for the CALGB found that both hematologic and neurologic toxicity were at least twice as severe with MOPP as compared with a five-drug program of vincristine, vinblastine, chlorambucil, prednisone, and procarbazine (VPBCPr) given simultaneously or in sequence. Although the complete response rates in previously untreated patients were identical at 61% for the MOPP and the simultaneous VPBCPr arms, the disease-free survival for MOPP was 50% at 2 years compared with 25% and 20% in patients with no prior therapy on the simultaneous and sequential regimens. The improvement in disease-free survival with MOPP more than compensated for its increased toxicity. Nissen et al. [42] recently updated the results of a second CALGB trial begun in 1969 in which a new combination BOPP, derived by substitution of BCNU for nitrogen mustard in the regimen, was compared to MOPP and two 3-drug regimens, derived by removing the procarbazine in BOPP or removing the alkylating agent. The 4-drug programs gave significantly higher complete remission rates than the 3-drug programs, with significantly longer disease-free and overall survival. Although BOPP had a therapeutic activity equal to MOPP, it was accompanied by significantly less hematologic toxicity. However, interpretation of the results of this study are complicated by the fact that all patients received maintenance chemotherapy for 3 years. The lack of a plateau in survival curves and the continued incidence of relapse is disturbing.

Since CCNU was established as the most active nitrosourea single agent when compared with BCNU in a randomized Phase II study [14], CCNU has also been substituted for nitrogen mustard in the MOPP regimen, Cooper et al. [53] prospectively randomized 566 patients with stage III and IV Hodgkin's disease to test whether CCNU and/or vinblastine were more effective than nitrogen mustard and/or vincristine with procarbazine and prednisone. The combination of CCNU, vinblastine, procarbazine, and prednisone (CCNU-VPP) was shown to be a highly effective program with a complete response rate of 69% compared to 57% for those treated with MOPP. This difference is mostly attributable to patients who had no prior therapy and to those who had radiation therapy without prior chemotherapy. The use of CCNU as part of the induction program was shown to be the most significant determinant of prolonged remissions. In patients without prior therapy, those regimens containing vinblastine had significantly higher complete response rates than those receiving regimens containing vincristine (the CR rate of 73% for the MVPP regimen is noteworthy). Reduced vomiting and neurotoxicity, as well as the oral administration were the chief advantages of the CCNU-VPP program as compared with MOPP. These factors resulted in improved patient and physician compliance. However, a significantly higher frequency of fatal hematologic toxicity was observed in those regimens containing vinblastine when compared to the vincristine arms. This higher frequency of fatal hematopoietic toxicity was almost exclusively seen in the elderly or in patients previously treated with both chemotherapy or radiotherapy. The CALGB experience with MOPP (57–62% CR in three trials) is less than what has been reported by both DeVita et al. [29] and Moore et al. [37]. These discrepancies are undoubtedly due to differences in patient selection, extent of prior therapy, flexible duration of induction treatment, and the difficulties associated with large multi-center trials involving various degrees of experience of the cooperating physicians. Because relapse-free and overall survival must be considered the most important endpoints in any study of advanced Hodgkin's disease, it is interesting to note that 71% of the complete responders treated with CCNU-VPP remain in remission compared with the 57% disease-free survival in the MOPP group as reported by Cooper et al. [53]. However, there is no difference in overall survival among the four induction regimens.

MOPP has also been directly compared to other nitrosourea-containing

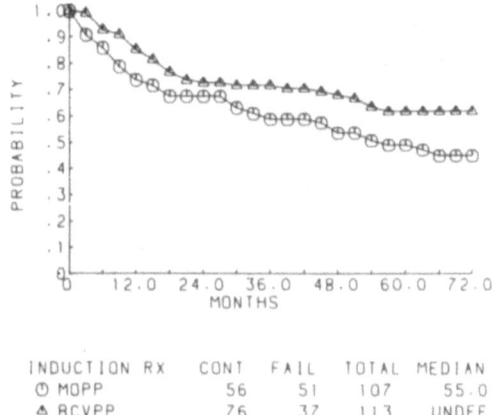

INDUCTION RX	CONT	FAIL	TOTAL	MEDIAN
☉ MOPP	56	51	107	55.0
▲ BCVPP	76	37	113	UNDEF

Figure 3. Relapse-free survival of patients attaining complete remission with MOPP compared with BCVPP induction chemotherapy.

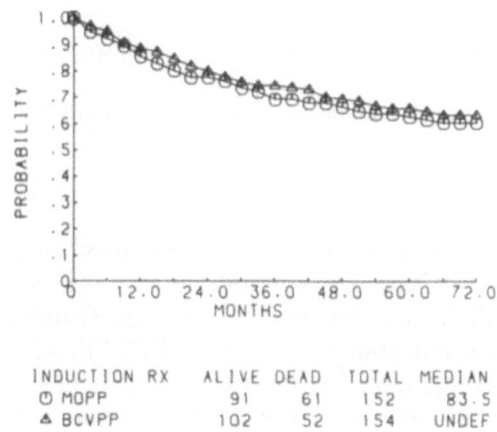

INDUCTION RX	ALIVE	DEAD	TOTAL	MEDIAN
☉ MOPP	91	61	152	83.5
▲ BCVPP	102	52	154	UNDEF

Figure 4. Survival of all patients from initiation of treatment according to induction chemotherapy regimen.

regimens. Bakemeier *et al.* [34] have recently updated the Eastern Cooperative Oncology (ECOG) experience in 306 patients with stage III-IV Hodgkin's disease who were randomized to an induction chemotherapy program comparing MOPP versus BCVPP (BCNU, cyclophosphamide, vinblastine, procarbazine, and prednisone). The complete response rate was 73% with MOPP and 77% with BCVPP, which was not significantly different. However, patients receiving BCVPP induction chemotherapy had a significantly longer complete response duration (62% at five years) than did MOPP

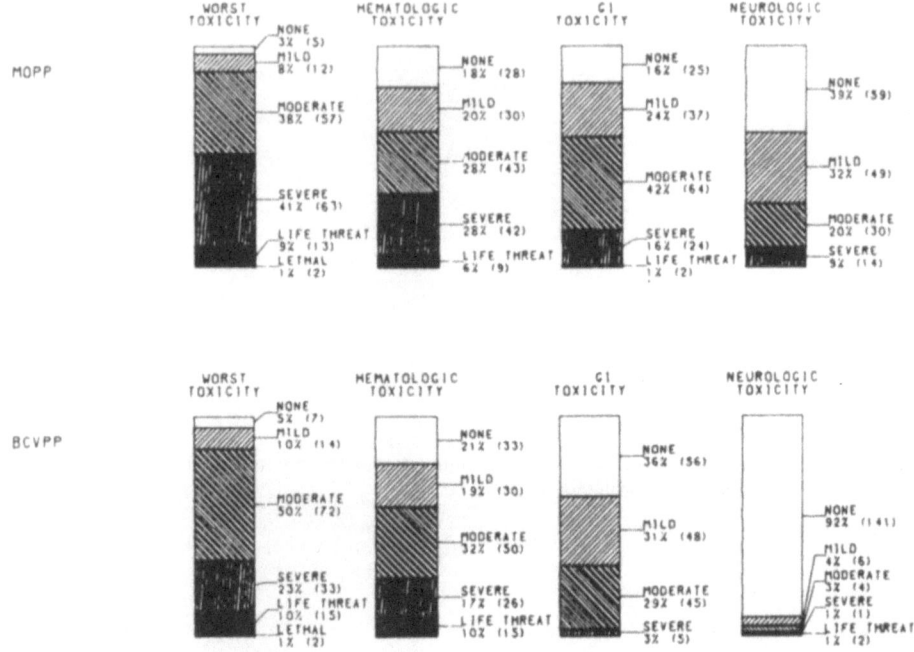

Figure 5. Toxicity of induction chemotherapy with MOPP compared with BCVPP.

(Figure 3). To date, no differences in survival between the induction arms have been observed (Figure 4), with an overall 5-year survival of 64%. An important observation was that MOPP produced significantly more serious neurologic and gastrointestinal toxicity than BCVPP, although bone marrow suppression was comparable for the two regimens (Figure 5). Although an additional 2–4 years follow-up are required for more definitive relapse-free and overall survival results to become available in order to compare the ECOG trial and the NCI data, BCVPP appears to be an entirely acceptable alternative to MOPP. The lower toxicity and ease of administration of BCVPP (it only requires a once monthly outpatient visit) are attractive both to patients and physicians.

Durant *et al.* [54] also utilized the BCVPP regimen, but in a non-randomized trial of 324 evaluable patients studied by the Southeastern Cancer Group (see Table 3 for summary of trials with alternative regimens to MOPP). Of 180 patients with either no or minimal prior therapy, a 68% complete response rate with BCVPP was noted. Durant *et al.* concluded that although platelet and neurologic toxicity were less with BCVPP when retrospectively compared to the widely reported results with MOPP, no improvement in the duration of remission or survival was observed.

Table 3. Alternative combination chemotherapy regimens for advanced Hodgkin's disease.

Author	Regimen	No. of evaluable patients	% CR	Disease-free survival (%/yr)	Overall survival (%/yr)
Durant *et al.* [54]	BCVPP	324	68	70/4	—
Morgenfeld *et al.* [55]	CVPP vs	157	71	50/3	80% of CR/4
	CCNU-CVPP	141	78	64/3	80% of CR/4
Bloomfield *et al.* [56]	CVPP	38	74	57/4	63/5
Diggs *et al.* [57]	CVPP	50	62	50/3	—
McElwain *et al.* [58]	ChlVPP	70	76	—	—
Sutcliffe *et al.* [38]	MVPP	91	82	75/5	65/5 No prior therapy 85/5 Prior XRT
Jones *et al.* [62]	MOP-BAP vs	165	76	90/2	—
	MOPP-LDB	123	64	74/2	—

CR = Complete Response; XRT = Radiotherapy.

Although the randomized trials of Cooper *et al.* [53] and Bakemeier *et al.* [34] provide a clue of the importance of including a nitrosourea in an alternative regimen to MOPP, a prospective study reported by Morgenfeld *et al.* [55] did not confirm the benefit of adding CCNU to a four-drug program containing cyclophosphamide, vinblastine, procarbazine, and prednisone (CVPP). The complete response rates of 71% (CVPP) and 78% (CCNU-CVPP) are not significantly different, nor are the 3-year disease-free survivals of 50% and 64%. The survival of complete responders for both treatment regimens was 80% at 4 years. Since all patients received maintenance chemotherapy for 3 years, it was difficult to interpret disease-free survival.

Two non-randomized trials have also evaluated the CVPP regimen. Bloomfield *et al.* [56] reported a 74% complete response rate in 38 patients, with no difference noted in those who had previously received radiotherapy and in the untreated group. All patients who obtained complete remission were given maintenance therapy with the same drugs every 2–4 months. Maintenance chemotherapy was discontinued after a median time of 34 months. Of the 28 complete responders, 11 have relapsed and one patient died of sepsis while on maintenance chemotherapy. Thus, 16 of 28 (57%) are in continuous complete remission greater than 4 years [33]. Eighty-two percent of patients achieving complete remission have survived 5 years, and the overall survival for all 38 patients at 5 years was 63%.

Diggs *et al.* [57] also evaluated the CVPP program and reported a 62% CR in 50 patients. This complete remission rate was somewhat lower than the previous studies summarized above, but complete remission status was documented by extensive restaging procedures. Diggs *et al.* noted that patients who received more than six courses of induction therapy have had significantly fewer relapses and longer remissions than those patients who received six courses or less of induction treatment. This also suggested that a flexible induction scheme designed to individualize the number of monthly courses of chemotherapy required to achieve complete remission was more important than a fixed 6-month induction program. Both Bloomfield *et al.* [56] and Diggs [57] noted decreased gastrointestinal and neurologic toxicity when compared with their previous experience using MOPP, but these were not controlled trials.

McElwain *et al.* [58] have also modified the MOPP regimen by substituting chlorambucil for nitrogen mustard and vinblastine for vincristine in order to avoid the severe nausea and vomiting and neurotoxicity seen with MOPP. McElwain's ChlVPP program also took advantage of Lacher and Durant's observation that vinblastine in combination with chlorambucil produced a 63% complete remission rate in advanced Hodgkin's disease [23]. In a non-randomized trial, McElwain *et al.* [58] treated 70 patients with the ChlVPP regimen and obtained a complete remission rate of 76% with remarkably little bone marrow, neurologic or gastrointestinal toxicity. Actual doses of drug administered as a percentage of the calculated ideal doses exceeded 95% for all four agents in the regimen. Although this is an attractive alternative to MOPP, McElwain *et al.* did not present long-term disease-free or overall survival data.

Nicholson *et al.* [59] were the first to modify the MOPP program by substituting velban for vincristine, lengthening the time interval between courses from a 2-week to 4-week rest period, and giving corticosteroids in each cycle. Complete remissions were obtained initially in six out of seven patients (86%) who had previously received no treatment, in 15 of 19 (79%) who had only prior radiotherapy, and in nine of 26 (35%) who had previously been given chemotherapy with or without prior radiotherapy. The long-term results of this MVPP combination have recently been reported by Sutcliffe *et al.* [38]. Complete responses were documented in 76% of the 49 previously untreated patients and in 90% of 42 patients who had relapsed after prior radiotherapy. The corresponding 5-year survival rates were 65% and 86% respectively. They estimated that 75% of patients who had previously received no prior treatment or irradiation and achieved complete remission were expected to continue in their initial remission beyond 5 years. These results are certainly not superior in response rate, duration or survival to that of the original MOPP regimen. However, the substitution of vinblastine for vincristine resulted in no appreciable neurotoxicity and the lengthening of the interval between cycles did not appear to jeopardize the potential long-term disease-free survival of complete responders.

The alternative regimens discussed above are based on the principle of substituting either a different alkylating agent (cyclophosphamide or chlorambucil for nitrogen mustard) and/or a different vinca alkaloid (vinblastine for vincristine) into the MOPP regimen. The expansion of the four-drug program to a five-drug regimen including a nitrosourea has been accomplished without undue toxicity and a suggestion of prolonged remission duration, but no conclusive evidence exists that any alternative chemotherapy program is better than MOPP alone in the management of advanced Hodgkin's disease.

The addition of another active single agent to MOPP was evaluated by the Southwest Oncology Group (SWOG) as an alternative approach to improving induction therapy. Coltman et al. [1, 47] reported the results of trials in which the relatively non-myelosuppressive antibiotic bleomycin was added to MOPP (Table 2). Two different dose levels of bleomycin were utilized. In the low-dose regimen, 2 units/m^2 of bleomycin were administered on days 1 and 8 of the first six cycles of MOPP. Ten units/m^2 of bleomycyin were given in the high-dose arm, but this was discontinued early in the trial because of increased myelosuppression, with three cases of irreversible bone marrow failure attributed to the high dosages of bleomycin. The complete response rates in the initial SWOG study were 70% for MOPP alone compared with 84% for MOPP plus low-dose bleomycin. It is difficult to interpret disease-free or overall survival from this trial because all patients were entered into maintenance chemotherapy or consolidation studies with radiotherapy. In addition, pathologic restaging of clinical remissions was not mandatory in the earlier bleomycin-MOPP trials. Interestingly, a subsequent SWOG protocal utilizing the identical low-dose bleomycin-MOPP regimen demonstrated a significantly lower complete response rate of 54%. This lower complete response frequency was carefully analyzed, and was attributed to a higher proportion of marrow-positive and a lower proportion of asymptomatic patients in the second trial in spite of randomization. Long-term follow-up of the initial SWOG trial suggested evidence that low-dose bleomycin-MOPP appeared to improve survival with more than 50% of patients alive at 7 years. This approaches but does not yet reach statistical significance when compared to MOPP alone. Preliminary data from an Eastern Cooperative Oncology Group trial of an identical low-dose bleomycin-MOPP induction program do not confirm a higher complete response rate when compared to the ECOG experience with MOPP alone [60]. Thus, there is no conclusive evidence that the addition of bleomycin to MOPP should be accepted as standard therapy in the treatment of advanced Hodgkin's disease. Bleomycin in low doses has also been added to the nitrosourea-containing regimen BCVPP. The preliminary data from this trial by Gams et al. [61], reporting for the Southeastern Cancer Study Group, noted a 78% complete remission rate in 41 patients with a significant improvement in complete response duration and survival over their previous BCVPP protocol. However, the follow-up period was only 40 months at the time of their initial report.

With the introduction of adriamycin as an active single agent in the management of refractory Hodgkin's disease, Jones et al. [62] initiated a SWOG study to determine if the addition of adriamycin to the low-dose bleomycin-MOPP regimen would improve the complete response rate and survival. This study differed significantly from previous SWOG trials in that systematic restaging was required in order to determine the completeness of the patient's response. The six-drug program incorporating both adriamycin and bleomycin (MOP-BAP) was compared to low-dose bleomycin-MOPP. Although there was a significantly higher complete response rate of 76% in the 165 evaluable patients treated with MOP-BAP compared with 64% CR in the 123 patients on MOPP-Bleo, there were no significant differences in CR duration or overall survival. Jones et al. [62] noted that the apparent therapeutic advantage of the MOP-BAP regimen was limited particularly to asymptomatic patients, who achieved a 94% complete response rate with the adriamycin-containing regimen. To put this in perspective, one must recall that DeVita et al. [29] reported a 100% complete remission rate in 23 patients with advanced Hodgkin's disease who were asymptomatic. Thus, one cannot accept the introduction of adriamycin into the MOPP regimen with or without bleomycin as being superior to MOPP alone. No alternative regimen has as yet proven conclusively to be superior to MOPP given differences in patient selection, restaging evaluation, and adequate follow-up.

1.5. Maintenance Chemotherapy

Although 65–80% of patients with advanced Hodgkin's disease attain a complete remission with combination chemotherapy, approximately one-third of these patients ultimately relapse, most often within 2 years. A variety of maintenance chemotherapy regimens have been investigated to see if this relapse rate can be decreased. However, overall survival is the critically important endpoint to be evaluated in any trial of the value of maintenance chemotherapy. It is also important to separate those clinical trials that utilize pathologic restaging to document complete remission prior to the institution of maintenance chemotherapy from those studies employing a fixed induction schedule with all patients going on to maintenance regimens.

Carbone et al. [7], in an early single-agent study, provided some insight into the evaluation of maintenance chemotherapy. Patients were randomized initially either to vinblastine or cyclophosphamide induction, and then were rerandomized to continue oral cyclophosphamide as maintenance or to receive no further therapy. Remission duration was prolonged with contin-

Author	Induction regimen	Restaged CR	Maintenance regimen	Duration of maintenance	Effect on relapse-free survival	Effect on overall survival
Young et al. [30]	MOPP (variable No. of cycles to CR)	Yes	MOP vs BCNU vs No therapy	15 mos	None	None
Coltman et al. [63]	MOPP (6 cycles)	No	MOPP vs No therapy	18 mos	None	None
Durant et al. [54]	BCVPP (6 cycles)	No	MOPP vs BCVPP vs No therapy	6 mos	None	None
Bakemeier et al. [34]	MOPP vs BCVPP (6 cycles)	No	BCVPP vs BCG vs No therapy	6 mos	None	None
Morgenfeld et al. [55]	CVPP vs CCNU-CVPP (6 cycles)	No	CVPP vs CCNU-CVPP	36 mos	None	None
Nissen et al. [42]	MOPP vs BOPP vs BOP vs OPP (6 cycles)	No (Both CR and PR randomized to maintenance)	Vinblastine vs CLB vs CLB + vinblastine + Prednisone	36 mos	None	None
Cooper et al. [53]	MOPP vs MVPP vs. CCNU-OPP vs CCNU-VPP (6 cycles)	No (Both CR and PR randomized to maintenace)	Vinblastine continuously vs Reinforcement with same induction	24 mos	No significant difference	None
Sutcliffe et al. [38]	MVPP	Yes	MVPP vs Vinblastine + Procarbazine	Not stated	None	None
Diggs et al. [57]	CVPP (variable No. of cycles to CR)	Yes	CCNU + Vinblastine vs No therapy	>24 mos	None	None

CR = Complete Response.

ued maintenance chemotherapy, but no difference was noted in overall survival. They noted that patients who received no maintenance chemotherapy were easily re-treated with the same drug that initially produced the response, while those on continued maintenance chemotherapy were no longer responsive. The initial report by DeVita *et al.* [28] on MOPP utilized a fixed induction shedule of six cycles to obtain their 81 % complete response rate. Their general treatment policy was subsequently modified to give all patients a minimum of six cycles of MOPP or as many cycles as were needed to achieve a complete remission plus two additional cycles. Thus, 25 % of the NCI patients required more than six cycles of MOPP in order to document complete response [22].

Table 4 reviews nine trials in which maintenance chemotherapy was continued beyond complete response. Utilizing the principle of a flexible number of MOPP cycles as induction chemotherapy, Young *et al.* [30] randomized 57 restaged complete responders to either no further therapy, intermittent MOPP given as two cycles every 3 months for 15 months, or intermittent treatment with BCNU administered every 3 months for a total of 15 months. They demonstrated no difference in the duration of either relapse-free or overall survival. However, those patients receiving maintenance chemotherapy were noted to have a significant increase in toxicity, including myelosuppression and infectious complications.

A subsequent study reported by Frei *et al.* [36] for the Southwest Oncology Group initially indicated that maintenance chemotherapy was of value. After a fixed six cycles of induction chemotherapy with MOPP, patients were randomized to observation versus nine cycles of MOPP maintenance given every 2 months. At the time of the initial report, patients randomized to MOPP maintenance had a significantly longer disease-free survival than the unmaintained group. However, no significant difference in overall survival was noted at that time. Extensive restaging was not utilized in that trial. An updated analysis of these data with a follow-up period of over 7 years demonstrated that differences in remission duration had disappeared, and there was no significant difference in relapse-free or overall survival between the maintained and unmaintained patients [1, 63]. In a subsequent SWOG trial, all patients who achieved a complete response after six cycles of induction MOPP were randomly assigned to single-agent actinomycin-D, methotrexate, or vinblastine at varying intervals for 18 months. There was no significant difference in remission duration or overall survival between the three single agents. When these three maintenance arms were combined and retrospectively compared to the unmaintained response duration of the previous SWOG trial, there was no advantage of single-agent maintenance chemotherapy over unmaintained remissions [1].

Durant *et al.* [64] were also initially encouraged that maintenance, with six monthly cycles of either MOPP or BCVPP, was of value in the previously

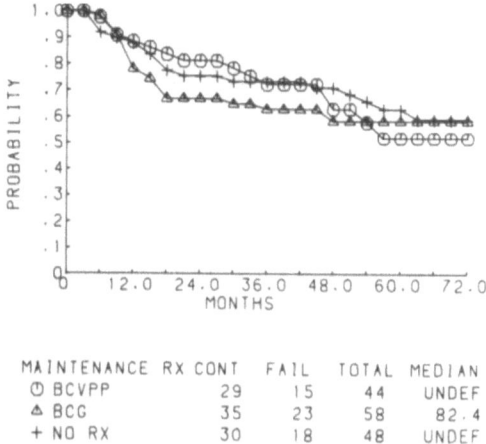

Figure 6. Relapse-free survival of patients attaining complete remission with either MOPP or BCVPP, analyzed according to subsequent maintenance therapy.

untreated patient who gained a complete remission after a fixed six cycles of BCVPP induction. Subsequent analysis [54] demonstrated that failure to prospectively stratify according to age and histologic subtype probably resulted in an erroneous initial conclusion because a greater number of younger patients with nodular sclerosis were randomized to maintenance chemotherapy. When multivariate regression analysis was performed, no influence of maintenance chemotherapy on the duration of complete remission or survival was noted. These results indicate how careful investigators must be in the design of future studies. Particular attention must be focused on the important prognostic factors that not only influence the complete response rate, but also response duration and overall survival.

The Eastern Cooperative Oncology Group also evaluated BCVPP maintenance chemotherapy for six monthly cycles after attainment of complete remission with a fixed induction program of either MOPP or BCVPP. One hundred and fifty patients in CR were randomized to either BCVPP, BCG immunotherapy, or to no treatment. As seen in Figures 6 and 7, there is no difference in disease-free survival or in overall survival of patients obtaining complete remission with MOPP or BCVPP according to subsequent maintenance therapy [34]. Morgenfeld *et al.* [55] also evaluated a nitrosourea-containing regimen CCNU-CVPP as maintenance therapy for 3 years and compared this regimen to the same drugs without CCNU. Again, no significant difference in disease-free or overall survival was noted.

Other trials of maintenance chemotherapy beyond induction of CR have also demonstrated no advantage to continuing chemotherapy. Nissen *et*

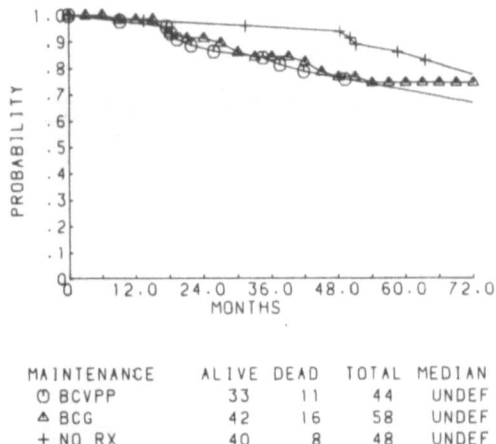

Figure 7. Survival of patients attaining complete remission with either MOPP or BCVPP, analyzed according to subsequent maintenance therapy.

al. [42] randomized complete and partial responders to maintenance treatment with either vinblastine, chlorambucil, or chlorambucil plus monthly vincristine and prednisone. No significant difference in relapse rates between the regimens was noted, nor could a reinforcement phase late in the maintenance program be shown to be of benefit. Cooper *et al.* [53] also randomized both complete and partial responders after six courses of induction therapy to one of two maintenance programs for two years. Although the remission durations maintained by vinblastine with periodic reinforcement were longer when compared with vinblastine maintenance alone, this was not statistically significant, and there was no corresponding increase in survival. No assessment for complete response was required after six induction courses of chemotherapy and, thus, the influence of maintenance is difficult to interpret. Sutcliffe *et al.* [38] failed to demonstrate a significant difference in disease-free or overall survival in patients induced into complete remission with MVPP who were subsequently randomized to receive vinblastine and procarbazine maintenance versus continued MVPP.

Diggs *et al.* [57] randomized patients attaining a complete response with CVPP to either alternating CCNU and vinblastine or to no further treatment. Although the numbers of patients were small, there was no significant difference in response duration or survival. However, patients who received more than six courses of induction therapy have had significantly fewer relapses and longer remissions than those patients who received only six courses of CVPP induction. This confirmed the observation of Young *et al.* [31] that a flexible approach to induction with continuing chemotherapy to the documentation of a restaged complete response, rather than a fixed treatment schedule of six cycles, was the most important factor in procuding prolonged disease-free survival.

On the basis of the information presented above, one must conclude that in patients documented to be in complete remission by extensive restaging, there is no significant advantage to maintenance chemotherapy.

1.6. Salvage Chemotherapy of MOPP Failures

Although the results of DeVita *et al.* [29] with MOPP as initial therapy for advanced Hodgkin's disease are truly impressive, it must be remembered that 20–30% of these patients will not achieve an initial complete remission. Since a partial remission or no remission almost inevitably will lead to the patient's demise, these patients are a difficult management problem and are candidates for non-cross-resistant combination chemotherapy programs. Furthermore, of the 70–80% of patients who achieve a complete response on MOPP, one-third will subsequently relapse, frequently within two years from the end of therapy. As discussed above, maintenance chemotherapy has not been successful in preventing these relapses. Frei *et al.* [36] noted that patients who received only six cycles of MOPP, obtained complete remission, and subsequently relapsed during the observation phase, had a 77% chance of obtaining a second complete remission on retreatment with MOPP. Those patients who received MOPP maintenance chemotherapy and relapsed while on treatment were no longer responsive to reinduction with additional MOPP therapy.

Fisher *et al.* [65] reviewed the NCI experience with 32 Hodgkin's patients who relapsed after a first complete remission induced by MOPP. These patients were subsequently treated with MOPP reinduction and 59% achieved a second complete remission. Patients successfully retreated with MOPP often received intermittent MOPP maintenance therapy on an every-other or every-third-month schedule for an additional one or two years in constrast to the NCI policy of unmaintained initial complete remissions. The median duration of the second complete remission was 21 months. Fourteen of fifteen (93%) patients whose first complete remission was longer than 12 months achieved a second complete response, in contrast to five of 17 (29%) patients whose initial complete remission lasted less than 12 months ($P<0.001$). The median survival of this entire group of 32 patients who were retreated with MOPP exceeded four years following their first relapse. The median survival of those achieving a second complete remission has not been reached, but will exceed 5 years after their first relapse. However, in the Stanford experience second remissions induced with MOPP have not been sustained, and all patients have ultimately relapsed [66]. The report by Fisher *et al.* [65] is, thus, more optimistic and demonstrates that patients who relapse after a first complete remission induced by MOPP are

Table 5. Salvage chemotherapy of MOPP failures.

Author	Regimen	No. of evaluable patients	% CR	Disease-free survival	Overall survival
Frei et al. [36]	MOPP	17	77	—	—
Fisher et al. [65]	MOPP	32	59	21 mos	4+ years
Goldman et al. [67]	CCNU-Vlb-Bleo	39	26	—	—
Lokich et al [68]	B-DOPA	15	60	14+ mos	—
Vinciguerra et al. [69]	BVDS	10	30	—	—
Levi et al. [70]	SCAB	17	35	8+ mos	16+ mos
Porzig et al. [71]	B-CAVe	22	50	35+ mos	17 mos
Rogers et al. [72]	ABDIC	29	35	28+ mos	9.5 mos
Bonadonna et al. [80]	ABVD	46	52	38% at 5 yrs	CRs = 44 mos; Non-CRs = 9.5 mos
Case et al. [75]	ABVD	24	4	—	—
Krikorian et al. [76]	ABVD	27	22	—	—

CR = Complete Response.

not necessarily resistant to further MOPP chemotherapy and can achieve long-term survival. There is a clear prognostic difference between those patients who relapse more than one year after obtaining their initial complete remission from that of patients who have progressive disease while on initial MOPP therapy or who relapse shortly following the end of remission induction (less than 6 months). Salvage chemotherapy of the latter two groups of patients should be attempted with a combination program composed primarily of drugs not included in the MOPP regimen.

This has led to the search for non-cross-resistant combinations. Table 5 lists 11 different trials involving such combinations. Most of these studies have, unfortunately, included small numbers with a mixture of MOPP-resistant and MOPP-relapsed patients, and a limited period of follow-up. Goldman and Dawson [67] reported a 26% complete response rate with CCNU, vinblastine, and bleomycin in 39 MOPP or MVPP failures, who appeared to be primarily resistant to their their induction therapy. Their regimen was said to be well tolerated and without significant toxicity. Lokich et al. [68] reported the results of the B-DOPA regimen in which bleomycin, imidazole carboxamide (DTIC), vincristine, prednisone and adriamycin were used to treat 20 patients, of whom 15 were evaluable for determination of response. In six patients who had not entered CR on initial MOPP or who relapsed within 6 months of discontinuing MOPP, five (83%) achieved a complete response with B-DOPA. However, of nine patients who relapsed in unmaintained MOPP remission after more than 6 months off therapy, only four (44%) achieved complete remission with this combination. The median response duration of both the complete and partial responders was 14+ months. Additional trials with B-DOPA in clearly MOPP-resistant patients are required to determine the value of this combination in ultimately salvaging this poor prognostic group.

Vinciguerra et al. [69] combined bleomycin, vinblastine, adriamycin and stretozotocin into the BVDS regimen. Three complete remissions were obtained in 10 patients and all three were alive at 18–27 months at the time of their initial report. Levi et al. [70] obtained a 35% complete remission rate cofirmed by restaging in 17 patients on a regimen of streptozotocin, CCNU, adriamycin and bleomycin (SCAB). Patients appeared to be truly MOPP-resistant, and no maintenance chemotherapy was administered so that response duration can be evaluated. The median response duration for the complete responders was 8+ months, with a corresponding median survival of 16+ months. However, the toxicity was substantial. Porzig et al. [71] also evaluated CCNU, adriamycin, and bleomycin, but utilized vinblastine in their combination (B-CAVe) for 22 patients with extensive prior MOPP chemotherapy and disease progression. Fifty percent clinical complete responses were noted with a median survival of 24 months. Median relapse-free survival for complete responders has not been reached at 35+ months while that for partial responders was only 14 months. Significant adriamycin cardiac toxicity was encountered in two patients. Although there were no life-threatening bacterial infections following B-CAVe administration, two patients died of *Pneumocystis carinii* several months after the end of treatment. Rogers *et al.* [72] administered adriamycin, bleomycin, DTIC, CCNU, and prednisone (ABDIC) to 29 evaluable MOPP-resistant patients with a 35% CR rate. Median survival and relapse-free survival for CR exceeded 28 months.

It remains to be determined if this or any of the combinations mentioned above would produce longer survival than single-agent chemotherapy. For example, Warren *et al.* [73] reported that palliative chemotherapy with vinblastine was capable of inducing complete remissions in 7% of patients and partial responses in 55%. It is our experience in MOPP-resistant patients that occasional long-term clinical complete remissions may be obtained with vinblastine initially administered weekly and then every other week with minimal toxicity. A comparative trial of non-cross-resistant combination chemotherapy with the same drugs used single and in sequence is clearly warranted.

The most extensive and exciting information on non-cross resistant chemotherapy is available for the ABVD regimen reported by Santoro and Bonadonna [74]. These four agents, adriamycin, bleomycin, vinblastine and DTIC induced an objective complete response of 62% in 21 patients who were resistant to MOPP as manifested by progressive disease either during induction chemotherapy or within 6 months from the end of MOPP. These data have now been updated in 46 evaluable patients with longer follow-up [80]. ABVD was given for a minimum of six cycles or to CR plus two additional cycles. No maintenance treatment was administered once CR was achieved. Complete response was documented in 24/46 (52%). More specifically, CR were noted in 70% of patients with nodal and 35% of extranodal ± nodal disease. There was no difference in the incidence of CR with ABVD between primary MOPP failures or those who relapsed soon after MOPP. The actuarial 5-year disease-free survival for CR was 38%, while the median survival of CRs was 44 months compared to 9.5 months for non-CRs. Unfortunately, the ABVD regimen has been evaluated by two other groups with lower complete response rates ranging from 4 to 22% [75, 76], and with brief response durations. This discrepancy may relate to patient selection, different sites of relapse or intensity of drug administration. At the present time ABVD is the most promising regimen for MOPP-resistant patients, but further clinical trials are clearly indicated.

1.7. Alternating Sequential Induction Chemotherapy

Although these attempts to salvage patients who relapse after primary drug therapy are important, the clinical research effort in advanced Hodgkin's disease must be directed at the prevention of relapse from induction chemotherapy. The failure of maintenance chemotherapy to improve response duration once compete remission has been obtained has refocused efforts to intensify initial induction programs in order to increase complete remission rates, and more importantly, to improve relapse-free and overall survival. Although the role of ABVD in MOPP-resistant Hodgkin's disease remains controversial, Bonadonna et al. [77] conducted a prospective randomized trial in previously untreated patients with Stage IIB-IVB disease comparing six cycles of MOPP versus ABVD. With extensive restaging, MOPP produced a complete response rate of 66% in 29 patients which was equivalent to the 69% CR rate in 26 patients treated with ABVD. Unfortunately, because patients obtaining a complete remission on either induction regimen received moderate-dose radiotherapy to extended field or total nodal sites, the remission duration and overall survival achieved by ABVD alone cannot be determined.

The next trial from the Milan group built upon this observation that ABVD induced a similar complete response rate as MOPP in previously untreated patients. Santoro et al. [78] randomized 77 patients with pathologic stage IV disease to receive either MOPP alone for 12 monthly cycles or one cycle of MOPP alternating monthly with one cycle of ABVD for a total of 12 cycles to test the hypothesis that sequential non-cross-resistant combinations would increase the complete response and cure rate. A total of 65 patients were evaluable at the time of the initial presentation. Sixty-seven percent of the 33 patients on MOPP alone achieved complete remission documented by extensive restaging procedures performed one month after the completion of 12 cycles, versus a complete response rate of 87.5% in the 32 patients receiving MOPP+ABVD ($P<0.05$). No patient demonstrated progressive disease during the MOPP+ABVD program, while 27% of the MOPP alone patients progressed during the initial 12 months of therapy. The alternating treatment (MOPP+ABVD) was also significantly superior to MOPP alone in the duration of both complete response (96% vs 66% at 4 years) and overall survival (86% vs 54% at 4 Years). The difference in favor of MOPP+ABVD versus MOPP alone was particularly striking in the subgroup of patients with systemic symptoms. Toxicity was considered acceptable, but nausea, vomiting, and hair loss were more frequent and severe after sequential chemotherapy. These extremely encouraging results obviously require longer follow-up and confirmation before MOPP+ABVD can be accepted as the recommended treatment for stage IV Hodgkin's disease, even in the presence of systemic symptoms.

Straus et al. [79] have recently updated the Memorial experience with alternating monthly cycles of MOPP and ABVD, in which chemotherapy was interrupted during the fifth month for low-dose radiotherapy delivered to initial areas of bulky nodal disease. Alternating cycles of MOPP and

ABVD at monthly intervals were then continued for 4 months following the completion of radiotherapy and for an additional 14 months on an every-other-month basis. This regimen achieved complete remission rates of 80% in the 49 previously untreated stage IIB-IVB patients, 65% in the 17 patients with prior radiotherapy and/or minimal prior chemotherapy, and 50% of patients with heavy prior chemotherapy. The complete remission rate for the 66 patients with stage IIB-IIIA-IIIB-IV disease and either no prior treatment or prior radiotherapy/minimal prior chemotherapy was 76% (for the 42 IIIB-IV patients, CR was 79%). This is certainly not different from the 80% complete response rate reported by DeVita *et al.* [29] in a similar group of patients treated with MOPP alone. Among the 49 previously untreated patients (all stages), there were no primary treatment failures, an observation similar to that made by Santoro *et al.* [78]. Straus *et al.* [79] observed an estimated 2-year relapse rate of 9% among the previously untreated patients achieving complete response. Additional follow-up time is obviously required before definitive conclusions can be drawn as to the potential increase in relapse-free and overall survival from this combined modality approach. If the therapeutic effectiveness of this program is eventually demonstrated, the design of this trial will not allow us to conclude whether the benefit is due to either or both the two non-cross-resistant drug combinations and/or the low-dose adjuvant radiotherapy to initial sites of bulky disease. It should be noted that the toxicity of this combined modality approach was considerable. Intolerable nausea and vomiting affected the investigators' ability to administer the entire protocol. Forty percent of patients had nitrogen mustard changed to either cyclophosphamide or thiotepa. Despite the substitutions, 12% of patients were unable to tolerate induction and 29% did not complete 23 months of maintenance chemotherapy, usually because of this side effect. The amount of myelosuppression noted with this combined modality program was felt to be similar to that reported for MOPP, but of course this was not a controlled trial. There were no cases of adriamycin-related cardiac toxicity and little pulmonary toxicity was noted. One case of acute leukemia (1%) was reported, but it is possible that additional cases may occur with longer follow-up.

Additional controlled trials have been initiated to test the hypothesis of alternating non-cross-resistant chemotherapy regimens. The NCI is comparing MOPP alone with an alternating regimen of MOPP-SCAB (streptozotocin, CCNU, adriamycin, bleomycin) in carefully staged patients with III$_2$A-IVB disease. A flexible induction scheme is utilized after which time patients will be followed off of all therapy. There are no preliminary results from this study. The Southeastern Cancer Group reported the preliminary results of its trial which compares low-dose bleomycin plus BCVPP to the same regimen alternating monthly with adriamyvin, DTIC and bleomycin. A 6-month induction scheme is utilized with complete responders receiving 4 additional months of treatment. At the time of their preliminary report in 1979, Gams *et al.* [61] noted a complete response of 78% for the continuous Bleo + BCVPP regimen and a 66% CR for the alternating program. These rates were not significantly different from each other nor from the previous SEG study with BCVPP [54]. The alternating group experienced more hematologic, gastrointestinal, skin and hair toxicity, but in both groups, the rate of life-threatening toxicity was low. Longer follow-up is required before making any definitive conclusions about the efficacy of the alternating non-cross resistant chemotherapy approach. Young and DeVita [31] have commented that the contribution, if any, of alternating sequential chemotherapy will be much more easily evaluated in protocols where radiotherapy is not included.

1.8. The Role of Combined Modality Therapy

1.8.1. Advanced Disease. Although the results with MOPP chemotherapy for advanced Hodgkin's disease have resulted in potential cure of 55% of patients, it is quite obvious that there is room for improvement. Knowledge of the initial sites of relapse in patients with advanced disease provides a clue to the design of clinical trials which, hopefully, should improve both disease-free and overall survival. It has been well documented that patients with stage IIIB disease treated with total lymphoid irradiation alone usually relapse initially in extranodal sites [37, 81]. Conversely, patients treated with MOPP chemotherapy alone have their initial manifestations of relapse in sites of pretreatment involvement, particularly in areas of bulky lymph node disease [36, 82]. These results strongly suggest that combining radiation therapy and chemotherapy in the treatment of advanced Hodgkin's disease is a rational approach to improve the complete remission rate and, as importantly, to decrease the relapse rate from either modality. The integration of these two modalities presents many challenges and questions: 1) Which modality should be given first? 2) Is there any benefit to 'sandwich' radiotherapy between courses of combination chemotherapy? 3) Should full doses of radiation be employed or should lower doses be investigated with potential lower toxicity? 4) What is the acute and chronic toxicity of this combined modality approach, particularly with respect to the induction of acute leukemia and second neoplasms?

It is clear from the Stanford clinical trials for pathologic stage IIIB disease that the results of total nodal radiotherapy (TNI) alone are unacceptable. Rosenberg *et al.* [83] reported the 10-year actuarial survival of 46 IIIB patients randomized to TNI or to TNI plus six cycles of MOPP. Although 37% of the TNI group were alive at 10 years, only 9% were disease-free. However, the relapse-free survival for patients treated by both modalitiies (50% disease-free at 10 years) appears no better than the similar group of patients treated by DeVita *et al.* [29] with MOPP alone. In addition, the

Table 6. Combined modality trials in advanced Hodgkin's disease.

Author	Regimen	Stage	No. of evaluable patients	% CR	Disease-free survival (%/yr)	Overall survival (%/yr)
Rosenberg et al. [83]	TNI vs	IIIB–III₅B	24	–	9/10	37/10
	TNI+MOPP		22	–	50/10	63/10
DeLena et al. [84]	MABOP+XRT	IIB–IIIB	27	89	–	–
Kun et al. [85]	MOPP+TNI	II_EA–IIIB	28	96	61/4	–
Rosenberg et al. [86]	MOPP×6+TNI vs	IV	18	–	67/7	59/7
	MOPP×8		15	–	58/7	43/7
Farber et al. [88]	MVVPP+ low-dose XRT+MVVPP	IIIB–IV	124	84	74/5	80/5
Bonadonna et al. [89]	MOPP+moderate-dose XRT	IIB–IV	41	71	84/3	–
	vs ABVD+moderate-dose XRT		35	80	91/3	–
Straus et al. [79]	Alternating MOPP-ABVD with 'sandwich' low-dose XRT	IIB–IV	66	76	10% relapse rate at 2 yrs for CR	–
Hoppe et al. [91]	MOPP or PAVe alternating with 'sandwich' full-dose XRT	IIIB–III₅B	25	88	79/3.5	84/3.5
Goodman et al. [92]	MOPP×3+TNI+MOPP×3	IIIB	19	100	89/4	79/4
Santoro et al. [93]	MOPP×3+XRT+MOPP×3 vs	IIIB	N.S.	79	79/4	–
	ABVD×3+XRT+ABVD×3			96	95/4	–

CR = Complete Response; N.S. = Not Stated; TNI = Total nodal irradiation; XRT = Radiotherapy.

Stanford investigators noted that when the planned chemotherapy immediately followed total lymphoid irradiation, it was particularly difficult to administer full doses of drugs. An appreciable number of patients required delays in the administration of the later cycles of MOPP due to prolonged myelosuppression [66]. Table 6 summarizes 10 trials which have investigated the role of combined modality therapy in advanced Hodgkin's disease.

In an effort to provide full chemotherapy doses to these patients, several investigators have administered six cycles of chemotherapy followed by full-dose irradiation. DeLena *et al.* [84] used a five-drug combination (nitrogen mustard, adriamycin, bleomycin, vincristine and prednisone) followed by radiotherapy in stage IIB-IIIB disease. They reported a CR rate of 64% for IIB patients with a median duration of remission exceeding 24 months. Interestingly, those patients with stage III disease had a CR of 89% with a median duration of 17+ months. Unfortunately, the number of patients were small and these data have not been updated. The radiation therapy was not well tolerated by approximately half the stage III patients because of prolonged severe leukopenia and/or thrombocytopenia. A similar study was conducted at the NCI by Kun *et al.* [85] in 28 patients with stages II$_E$A-III disease (19 of whom had IIIB). Utilizing six cycles of MOPP followed by total nodal radiation, 96% of patients achieved a complete remission with a 61% 4-year disease-free survival. Although this was not a randomized trial, these results were virtually identical to what DeVita *et al.* [29] have reported for MOPP alone. However, serious treatment-related morbidity was observed by Kun *et al.* [85] in 54% of the patients; four of the complications resulted in death with no residual Hodgkin's identified at autopsy. Rosenberg *et al.* [86] reported similar results in 33 stage IV patients who were randomized to six cycles of MOPP followed by total nodal radiotherapy versus eight cycles of MOPP alone. There were no significant differences in either disease-free or overall survival. Thus, the sequence of MOPP chemotherapy followed by full-dose total lymphoid irradiation does not seem warranted, particularly in view of the severe hematologic toxicity.

An alternative approach has been to administer full schedule and doses of chemotherapy followed by less extensive and lower-dose radiotherapy. Prosnitz *et al.* [87] were the first to utilize low-dose radiotherapy in conjunction with chemotherapy. Sixty-three previously untreated patients with stage IIIB-IV and 61 patients who had relapsed following prior radiotherapy were evaluated by the Yale group on a program that consisted of 6 months of nitrogen mustard, vincristine, vinblastine, procarbazine, and prednisone followed by 1500–2500 rads to all sites of clinically detectable tumor present prior to the start of chemotherapy with the exception of bone marrow. The use of low-dose radiotherapy was predicated on the rationale that even in the presence of complete response, 10^4–10^5 viable tumor cells may still be present, especially in nodal areas of previous bulk disease, and low–moderate doses of radiation can sterilize residual lymphoma. Following irradiation, two additional drug cycles of the above chemotherapy were administered. Farber et al. [88] have updated the data from the Yale trial and reported that 102 patients (84%) entered complete remission, 92 of whom remain disease-free with a median follow-up of 5 years. Ten patients have relapsed, and acute leukemia has developed in two. The cumulative survival rate for all 124 patients is 80% at 5 years; the relapse-free survival is 74%. This very low relapse rate among the complete responders (10%) and excellent disease-free survival of 74% appear to be superior to the results reported with chemotherapy alone, in which a 32% relapse rate and a 5-year disease-free survival of 55% can be expected [29]. If confirmed in a randomized trial against MOPP alone, the data from Yale could represent a significant improvement in the treatment of advanced Hodgkin's disease. Farber et al. [88] also identified two subgroups of patients for whom the prognosis was worse: patients over the age of 40 and those with multiple extranodal sites of involvement both had a five-year survival rate of less than 50%. The low-dose irradiation was well tolerated following chemotherapy, with a minimum of serious side-effects directly related to the radiation.

Bonadonna et al. [89] also evaluated this combined modality approach in 55 patients with stage IIB-III$_s$A-IIIB and IV disease who were previously untreated and in 21 patients who were in first relapse following primary radiotherapy. Combination chemotherapy consisted of six cycles of either MOPP or ABVD. Four to six weeks from the end of chemotherapy, complete plus good partial responders ($\geq 75\%$) received subtotal or total nodal irradiation (3000–3500 rads). In patients with extranodal disease, 2000–2500 rads were delivered to all nodal and extranodal sites of pretreatment involvement except the bone marrow. Restaged complete remission rates were similar in both treatment groups after chemotherapy (MOPP 63%, ABVD 71.5%). A total of 10 complete responders after chemotherapy did not receive the planned irradiation (seven patient refusals; one suicide; one hepatitis; one cerebrovascular accident). The restaged CR rate after the combined modality treatment was 93% in patients initially receiving MOPP and 96% in the ABVD group. No difference was observed between patients with prior or no prior radiotherapy, presence or absence of systemic symptoms, nodal or extranodal extension. However, to put these complete response rates in perspective, the overall CR rate for all untreated patients, including the 20% that did not receive the planned irradiation, was 76%. This does not differ from what has been previously reported by DeVita et al. [29]. Bonadonna et al. [89] noted that at 4 years from the end of treatment, 87% of all complete responders remained alive and continuously disease-free with no difference in the untreated patients between MOPP and ABVD. Overall survival at 5 years from the initiation of combined treatment was 89% for complete responders. The tolerance to the combined modality treatment was better than might be expected. More than 85% of the planned dose for each drug could be administered in both regimens during six cycles and the radiotherapy was administered on schedule. Two fatalities attributed to the treatment program have occurred, one in each group (irreversible pneumonitis after pulmonary radiation; one case of acute non-lymphocytic leukemia).

Straus et al. [79] also observed a relapse rate of 9% in their patients achieving a complete remission with alternating sequential cycles of MOPP-ABVD plus low-dose irradiation to sites of pretreatment involvement followed by maintenance chemotherapy. Unfortunately, it is impossible to conclude whether the lower relapse rate was attributable to the use of two non-cross resistant combinations or the low-dose radiotherapy. Although the lower relapse-rates in the combined modality trials reported by Bonadonna et al. [89] and Farber et al. [88] are promising, it is difficult to compare these trials since chemotherapy regimens and schedules were different, and Bonadonna's study included radiotherapy to clinically uninvolved nodal areas with higher tissue doses in previously untreated stage IIB-IIIB patients. Neither trial included a chemotherapy alone control group. The preliminary results of the National Cancer Institute of Canada study in IIIB and IV Hodgkin's disease utilizing such a control arm have recently been reported by Bergsagel et al. [90]. All patients received three courses of MOPP. Patients in complete remission or with adequate control at 3 months were then randomized to receive 2000–3000 rads in 2–4 weeks to the total abdomen and upper mantle or to continue with three more courses of MOPP. Radiotherapy had no effect on the actuarial risk of extranodal relapse but did significantly reduce the risk of relapsing in nodal sites. Data were not presented on disease-free survival but the overall survival of both groups was similar.

Rather than compromise on the dose of radiotherapy, Hoppe et al. [91] investigated the possibility that a more flexible scheduling sequence of radiotherapy and chemotherapy might be less toxic and more effective. Thus, the Stanford group treated 25 patients with pathologic stage IIIB or III_sB disease with total lymphoid irradiation (4000–4400 rads) in a split course or alternating approach with the drug cycles sequenced in two to three cycle blocks around a specific radiotherapy field. When the total lymphoid fields were divided into three regions, treatment to each was alternated with two cycles of chemotherapy until the entire program was complete. The duration of the combined modality therapy ranged from 9 to 18 months. Patients in the split course group received an average of 65% of the calculated drug doses and those in the alternating group received an average of 77%. The primary complications were hematologic, with mean lowest recorded WBC of 2200/mm^3 and platelet count of 101,000/mm^3. Twenty-two of the 25 patients achieved an initial complete remission and 20 remained free of disease with a median follow-up interval of 28 months. Actuarial survival for the entire group, including a patient who died prior to the institution of therapy, was 84%, while for those who achieved a complete remission it was 100%. Disease-free survival in the same groups was 79% and 90% respectively. Hoppe *et al.* [91] compared these results with a retrospective group of patients from Stanford who received sequential total lymphoid irradiation followed by MOPP chemotherapy for IIIB disease. These patients achieved a 62% overall survival and 50% disease-free survival, which was felt to be inferior to the split course or alternating technique described above. Goodman *et al.* [92] reported an 89% 4-year disease-free survival in 19 IIIB patients with a similar combined modality plan.

Santoro *et al.* [93] also utilized a 'sandwich' approach with either MOPP or ABVD before and after 3000–3500 rads administered to both involved fields and adjacent uninvolved sites. Of the MOPP treated IIIB patients, 79% achieved a complete response compared to 96% for patients receiving ABVD. Actuarial relapse-free survival appeared better for the ABVD group but this was not significantly different at 4 years. The median duration of remission has not yet been reached for either group. There was no substantial difference in the incidence of severe myelosuppression during or after combined treatment. No cardiomyopathy or lung fibrosis has been noted in the ABVD + radiotherapy arm; and one MOPP-patient developed diffuse histiocytic lymphoma. Azospermia was significantly less in the ABVD group (16.5%) versus 100% with MOPP.

The combined modalities studies for advanced disease described in this section are certainly encouraging, but longer follow-up is clearly required before concluding that radiotherapy is an integral component for all patients with either IIIB or IV disease. The data of Farber *et al.* [88], Bonadonna *et al.* [89], Straus *et al.* [79], and Hoppe *et al.* [91] are encouraging in that the relapse rate from their combined modality programs ranges from 9 to 20%. However, none of these combined modality approaches has been compared directly to MOPP given in an optimal fashion. In addition, the morbidity of these chemotherapy–radiotherapy approaches must be weighed in the equation. It is particularly important to remember that approximately 5% of patients treated with both modalities will develop acute non-lymphocytic leukemia [94], and thus, eventual overall survival figures for chemotherapy–radiotherapy trials may be lower with additional observation. Since the trials above were not randomized, it is difficult to arbitrarily choose which radiotherapy schedule and dose is most appropriate if combined modality therapy is to be used for advanced disease. Most importantly, recent studies by Santoro *et al.* [78] with alternating non-cross-resistant chemotherapy regimens (MOPP–ABVD) have demonstrated an 87.5% complete remission rate with 96% of the CR remaining disease-free at 4 years. Certainly, these impressive results with chemotherapy alone require confirmation and must be compared to the combined modality programs noted above. Ultimately, any one of these new approaches to the treatment of Hodgkin's disease offers the potential for improving the cure rate of advanced disease.

1.8.2. Stage IIIA. Although only 15–20% of patients who undergo laparotomy and splenectomy are pathologically stage IIIA or III$_s$A, the optimal treatment of this stage is controversial. The dilemma for the clinician remains: (1) What relapse rate after radiotherapy will we accept in order to justify a policy of watchful waiting without the addition of chemotherapy? (2) What is the salvage rate with chemotherapy administered at the time of relapse after radiotherapy alone? (3) Is there a subgroup of stage IIIA patients that does so poorly as to warrant adjuvant drug therapy? (4) Is chemotherapy alone acceptable treatment for this stage? (5) Are the potential complications of combined modality therapy a deterrent for any subgroups of IIIA patients?

Treatment of stage IIIA Hodgkin's disease with total nodal irradiation (TNI) has resulted in a definite improvement in both remission duration and survival compared to less aggressive forms of radiotherapy alone [66]. Nonetheless, a significant proportion of these patients continue to relapse, primarily at extranodal sites. Prosnitz et al. [95] reported that only 35% of their 48 pathologically stage IIIA patients treated with TNI alone were relapse-free at 5 years, with a median follow-up of approximately 3 years. However, few of these patients were at risk beyond the 3-year point, and the ultimate percentage of relapse-free patients may change significantly with time. Of note is their observation that recurrence within the treated field was observed in 17 of 48 patients. The data of other investigators appear less pessimistic with a range of 49–74% disease-free survival in laparotomy-staged patients initially treated with TNI alone [96–100]. Overall survival of those patients initially treated with TNI is excellent and exceeds 75% in all series because of the demonstrated efficacy of salvage chemotherapy. Fifty percent of patients treated with MOPP after failing primary radiotherapy achieve long-term disease-free status [35, 101].

DeVita [102] has suggested that combination chemotherapy alone be utilized in the treatment of IIIA disease. These conclusions are based on a small series of 23 patients with stage IIIA and IVA disease (only five of whom actually had clinical stage IIIA). All 23 of these patients obtained a complete response with MOPP. Their 5-year disease-free survival is 94%, with an overall survival at 10 years of 94%. Nixon et al. [48] also utilized MOPP alone in eight patients with stage IIIA disease and obtained 100% complete responses with no relapses but the follow-up was brief (8–32

Table 7. Stage IIIA Hodgkin's disease – is combined modality therapy required?

Author	Laparotomy staged	Anatomically substaged	Total patients	Regimen	% CR	Disease-free survival (%/yr)	Overall survival (%/yr)	Comments
BNLI [96]	Yes	No	42 / 39	TNI vs MOPP	95 / 74	74/4, 46/4	92/4, 90/4	DFS significantly better for TNI but no difference in OS
	No	No	18 / 18	TNI vs MOPP	78 / 67	71/2, 53/2	76/2, 86/2	No significant difference
Timothy et al. [99]	Yes	NO	20 / 20	TNI vs MVPP	100 / 100	74/5, 87/5	88/5, 95/5	No significant difference
Prosnitz et al. [95]	Yes	III_1 / III_2	18 / 30	TNI	96	56/5, 33/5	80/5	Adverse effect of splenic involvement & age <20
Stein et al. [98]	Yes	III_1	48 / 26	TNI / TNI+MOPP*	Not stated	63/5, 96/5	91/5, 100/5	DFS significantly better for TNI+MOPP, but OS similar
		III_2	37 / 19	TNI / TNI+MOPP*		32/5, 76/5	56/5, 84/5	Both DFS & OS better for TNI+MOPP
Hoppe et al. [100]	Yes	III_1	46 / 46	TNI** / TNI+MOPP or PAVe	Not Stated	64/5, 96/5	90/5, 88/5	DFS significantly better with TNI+chemotherapy, but no differences in overall survival
		III_2	40 / 39	TNI** / TNI+MOPP or PAVe		69/5, 75/5	88/5, 91/5	
Santoro et al. [93]	Yes	No	Not stated	MOPP×3+XRT+ MOPP×3 vs ABVD×3+XRT+ ABVD×3	100 / 92	56/3, 100/3	100/3, 92/3	No significant difference
Coltman et al. [1]	Yes	No	69	MOPP×3-6+TNI	90	–	–	All patients received XRT
Nixon et al. [48]	Yes	No	8	MOPP	100	100/8–32 mos	100/8–32 mos	
DeVita et al. [29]	No	No	5 IIIA / 18 IVA	MOPP	100	94/5	94/10	
Grozea et al. [104]	Yes	No	80 (includes IIIA, IIIB)	MOPP-Bleo×10 / MOPP-Bleo×3+TNI	71 / 80	91/2, 73/2	90/2, 96/2	No significant difference between IIIA vs IIIB

* Collaborative, retrospective analysis (some patients received COPP or CVPP).

CR = Complete response; TNI = Total Nodal Irradiation; TNI ** = TNI included prophylactic whole lung XRT if hilum involved and prophylactic liver XRT if spleen positive; XRT = Radiotherapy; DFS = Disease-Free Survival; OS = Overall Survival.

months). However, not all investigators report such impressive complete response rates and relapse-free survival for this group of patients. Two consecutive trials by the Southwest Oncology Group utilizing MOPP chemotherapy alone for stage IIIA-IVA disease have noted that only 42 of 55 (76%) patients achieved a complete remission, and 16/55 (29%) have died [103]. If just the 27 patients in the SWOG series with pathologic stage IIIA disease who were treated with MOPP are examined, only 19/27 (70%) achieved a complete remission. These data are more consistent with those achieved by the British National Lymphoma study (described below) than those reported by DeVita. Grozea et al. [104] recently reported a 71% complete remission rate with MOPP plus low-dose Bleomycin in patients with IIIA and IIIB disease. Their disease-free survival of 91% and overall survival of 90% are impressive but the follow-up is short (2 years). These investigators noted no significant difference between the chemotherapy alone arm and the same drug combination administered for three cycles followed by TNI.

Table 7 summarizes the results of 10 clinical trials for stage IIIA disease. The British National Lymphoma Investigation [96] directly compared TNI versus MOPP in a randomized clinical trial initiated in 1970. Their data were separately analyzed for the 81 patients pathologically staged by laparotomy and for the 36 patients in whom laparotomy was not performed. In the former group, a 95% complete response rate was noted in the 42 patients treated with TNI versus a 74% CR in the 39 patients treated with MOPP. Disease-free survival was significantly better for the TNI group (74% at 4 years) as compared to MOPP (46% DFS), but there was no difference in overall survival at the time of their initial report. In the group whose staging did not include laparotomy (clinical stage IIIA), there were no significant differences in the complete response rate, relapse-free or overall survival. It has been commented on that these results may differ from those observed in the laparotomy-staged group, because of the inclusion of patients with advanced occult extra-nodal disease in both treatment arms of the non-laparotomized study. Such occult stage IV sites would remain untreated in the patients receiving TNI alone, but would be expected to be responsive to systemic MOPP chemotherapy. Thus, this portion of the study carries a bias in favor of MOPP chemotherapy in patients staged without laparotomy and splenectomy [66]. Unfortunately, the observation period is short, and a further decline in both the relapse-free and overall survival can be expected. Information was not provided in the British study as to multiple prognostic factors, including histologic subtype, influence of splenic involvement, or anatomical substaging. Timothy et al. [99] also compared TNI to chemotherapy alone (MVPP) and reported a 100% complete response rate in 40 laparotomized patients, half of whom were treated with each modality. There were no significant differences in disease-free or overall survival between the radiotherapy alone and chemotherapy alone groups. These two trials continue to support the conclusion that radiotherapy alone is an acceptable alternative for stage IIIA disease.

However, determining a single optimal therapy for all patients with stage IIIA disease may be impossible because of multiple prognostic factors, the most important of which appears to be anatomical substage. Desser *et al.* [105] reported that patients with disease limited to the spleen and/or splenic, celiac, or portal nodes (anatomic substage III_1) had a more favorable 5-year survival than did patients with involvement of para-aortic, iliac, or mesenteric nodes (anatomic substage III_2). They further observed that the addition of combination chemotherapy to total nodal irradiation was associated with improved survival of patients in stage III_2, but not those in stage III_1.

Stein *et al.* [98] pooled the raw data from three institutions which had published studies of substage in IIIA disease [105–107] and from a fourth series which had not considered substage [108]. Patients were eligible for review if they had undergone pathologic staging including laparotomy before therapy was instituted. On the basis of the definitions above, patients were separated into anatomical substage III_1A and III_2A. Eighty-five patients received radiotherapy alone, 78 of whom were treated with TNI. Forty-five patients received combined modality treatment; 34 underwent TNI plus chemotherapy and 11 (all III_1) received mantle and para-aortic irradiation followed by chemotherapy. The combination chemotherapy employed was either standard MOPP or a minimal variant (cyclophosphamide substituted for nitrogen mustard or vinblastine for vincristine). Although most patients received chemotherapy after radiation was completed, seven patients received three to four cycles of chemotherapy before radiotherapy. For the entire series of 130 patients, both disease.free survival (89% vs 49%, $P<0.001$) and overall survival (89% vs 76%, $P<0.02$) were better in patients receiving combined modality treatment (median follow-up of 58 months). However, this difference in survival was limited to the stage III_2A groups. In patients with stage III_1A, disease-free survival was superior in the combined modality group (96% vs 63%, $P<0.002$); but with the use of salvage chemotherapy, there was no significant difference in overall survival. In stage III_2A patients, both disease-free survival and overall survival were significantly better in patients receiving combined modality therapy. No influence of histologic subtype or splenic involvement was noted.

Thus, it would appear from the collaborative report by Stein *et al.* [98] that total nodal irradiation alone is acceptable initial treatment for those patients with III_1A disease. By utilizing TNI alone in this more favorable subgroup, a significant proportion of patients can be spared the short and long-term complications of combination chemotherapy, including an increased risk of second neoplasms. Of those who relapsed, at least 50% may be salvaged with MOPP or more aggressive treatment programs. The presence of splenic involvement alone (PS III$_s$A) in a patient with clinical stage I, IIA disease did not necessarily confer an unfavorable prognosis. The studies of Desser *et al.* [105] demonstrated greater than 70% 5-year relapse-free survival with TNI alone in patients with disease limited to the spleen. The small series of Levi and Wiernik [106] confirmed the favorable relapse-free survival of patients with splenic involvement when treated with even less irradiation, i.e. extended field radiotherapy alone.

Hoppe *et al.* [100] retrospectively reviewed the Stanford data and have been unable to confirm the observation that anatomic substage was an important prognostic parameter in 171 previously untreated patients with pathologic stage IIIA disease. Eighty-six patients were treated with TNI and 85 with TNI followed by adjuvant chemotherapy either with MOP (without prednisone) or with PAVe (procarbazine, Alkeran, and vinblastine). Five-year survival rates were not significantly different in the two groups; however, the 5-year disease-free survival was significantly better in the combined modality group (66% vs 86%, $P<0.003$). Because of the success with MOP in the salvage therapy of patients who had relapsed after treatment with irradiation alone, the 5-year freedom from second relapse rates in the two groups were not significantly different. Analysis of a large number of possible prognostic factors failed to identify any subgroup of patients whose survival was significantly improved by the use of adjuvant chemotherapy, including patients with anatomic stage III$_2$, clinical stage III, unfavorable histology, older age or sex. Among patients treated with irradiation alone, the 5-year freedom from relapse rates are nearly identical for anatomical stages III$_1$ and III$_2$. The most important prognostic factors in the Stanford series, indicating a benefit from adjuvant chemotherapy on survival, were extensive splenic involvement (more than four nodules detected in the splenectomy specimen), and $\geq$ five sites of initial involvement including those above and below the diaphragm. However, neither of these two factors was statistically significant. The difference in the results reported by Hoppe *et al.* [100] from those reported by Stein *et al.* [98] may reflect differences in treatment techniques. Particular nuances of the Stanford radiotherapy techniques include: higher standard dose (4400 rads); routine treatment of the uninvolved pulmonary hila (4400 rads), and policy of prophylactic whole lung irradiation (1500 rads) in the presence of hilar involvement; and prophylactic irradiation of the liver (2200 rads) in the presence of splenic involvement.

Thus, the treatment of stage IIIA Hodgkin's disease remains controversial. Clearly, it would be premature for radiation therapists to abandon TNI for patients with clinical stage I, IIA disease who were found to have microscopic involvement in the spleen or upper abdominal nodes at the time of laparotomy (PS IIIA; Desser III$_1$A). In this favorable subgroup, only those who relapse after primary radiation should receive chemotherapy, thus sparing the majority of patients the risks of combined modality therapy. For the patient with CSIIIA/PSIIIA disease (equivalent to Desser's III$_2$A), acceptable treatment alternatives include: total nodal irradiation utilizing the Stanford techniques (including prophylactic liver irradiation when the spleen is involved); combined modality therapy with total nodal or subtotal nodal (omitting the pelvis) radiotherapy plus MOPP; initial chemotherapy followed by low-dose irradiation to sites of pretreatment involvement as advocated by Prosnitz [95] for stages IIIB and IV; or chemotherapy alone. The goal in patients with unfavorable prognostic factors and an unacceptably high relapse rate should be to determine how to best prevent relapse in the first place.

1.8.3. Localized Disease. There is no stage of Hodgkin's disease for which our current therapy is invariably successful. Studies at Stanford initiated in 1968 were designed to evaluate the role of adjuvant chemotherapy in combination with radiation in the management of Hodgkin's disease. These studies have been described in detail [66, 109–110]. Patients, staged by laparotomy and splenectomy, were then randomized to radiotherapy alone or to radiotherapy followed by six cycles of MOPP chemotherapy. Although the initial relapse-free survival is significantly better in the I-IIA patients on the combined modality arm, overall survival at 10 years is not significantly different [110]. This effect appears to be due to the ability of MOPP treatment to salvage radiotherapy failures in approximately 50% of the cases. It is interesting to note that chemotherapy did not improve disease-free survival for patients with IB and IIB disease. Patients with B symptoms and stage I-II disease treated with total nodal irradiation alone had an 80% disease-free survival at 10 years and an 87% survival overall. This latter point is an extremely important observation, and strongly argues against the use of adjuvant chemotherapy for this subgroup, an all too common situation in clinical practice.

A second series of trials was initiated by the Stanford group in 1974 for stage I-IIA disease, randomizing patients to subtotal nodal irradiation versus involved field irradiation plus adjuvant MOPP (prednisone deleted for patients receiving mediastinal irradiation). Although the results are preliminary, there are no differences in freedom from relapse or overall survival between the two groups [111]. While MOPP chemotherapy appeared as efficacious as radiation in the treatment of clinically occult disease, its failure to control such involvement in two patients, who relapsed in unirradiated nodes contiguous with previous sites of involvement, suggests that MOPP alone may be inadequate as the sole treatment for patients with PS I-IIA disease.

The Southwest Oncology Group also conducted a trial of subtotal nodal radiotherapy versus involved field radiotherapy plus MOPP in pathologically staged I and II (A + B) Hodgkin's disease. Coltman *et al.* [112] reported that although there was a relapse-free survival advantage to the combined modality arm for all patients, as well as those with B symptoms, mediastinal involvement, stage II and IIE disease, there was no overall survival advantage in any category. These results confirmed the Stanford experience, and similar results were also obtained by Wiernik *et al.* [113]. Thus, in patients with localized disease, adjuvant combination chemotherapy can effectively substitute for 'prophylactic' radiotherapy of apparently uninvolved sites [66].

However, a combined modality program not only prolongs the period of initial treatment, but is fraught with both acute and possible long-term toxicity. Acute toxicity includes increased nausea and vomiting, bone marrow depression, increased risk of serious infections, and sterility in virtually all male patients. The most disturbing and significant of all possible long-term complications is the appparent increase in incidence of second malignancies in patients treated with both modalities [94, 114, 115]. Acute non-lymphocytic leukemia [94] and diffuse undifferentiated, or histiocytic, non-Hodgkin's lymphoma [116] are invariably fatal complications which may be seen in as high as 5% of patients at risk 10 years following combined modality therapy. This high-risk of second malignancies, and the success of salvage MOPP chemotherapy, strongly argue for the use of radiotherapy alone in patients with localized disease.

Although there is not a clear justification for the uniform use of radiotherapy plus chemotherapy for the overwhelming majority of patients with pathologically staged I or II Hodgkin's disease, there are certain subsets for whom a combined modality approach may be indicated. The presence of large mediastinal involvement has been associated with an increased risk of relapse as compared to patients with mediastinal masses measuring less than one-third of the chest diameter or those who have no mediastinal disease at presentation. In the initial report from Mauch *et al.* [117], 50% of such patients with large mediastinal masses relapsed following primary treatment with radiation therapy alone, compared with a disease-free survival of 92% in patients with lesser or no mediastinal disease. The majority of relapses have been intrathoracic, manifested as either mediastinal recurrences within the treated field, recurrences at the margin of treatment, and diffuse pulmonary involvement. Hoppe *et al.* [118] have reviewed the Stanford data in 102 patients with mediastinal Hodgkin's disease. In patients treated with radiotherapy alone, those with a mediastinal mass/thoracic ratio ≥ 0.3 had a significantly worse disease-free survival and a borderline worse overall survival than those with smaller mediastinal masses.

The long-term survival of patients with large mediastinal Hodgkin's disease who relapse and then receive chemotherapy is currently unknown. Mauch and Hellman [119] compiled data from three series and noted that

18/28 patients with large mediastinal masses who relapsed after radiotherapy were disease-free with salvage chemotherapy. An alternative approach has been to utilize chemotherapy plus involved field irradiation as initial treatment. Coltman *et al.* [120] and Levi *et al.* [121] reported a decreased risk of intrathoracic relapse using this combined modality approach. The question remains, if MOPP can effectively salvage patients with large mediastinal masses who relapse, then there is no overall survival advantage in using chemotherapy initially. Mauch and Hellman [119] favor the use of radiation therapy alone in patients with mediastinal masses if a substantial portion of the heart and lung can be shielded during treatment. They argue that when extranodal lung or pericardial disease is present, shielding of these vital organs during radiation is more technically difficult and may justify the combined use of chemotherapy and involved field radiation, both to reduce the risk of relapse and the risk of radiation pneumonitis or pericarditis.

Therefore, the approach to any patient with localized Hodgkin's disease and a large mediastinal mass must be individualized. The treatment plan for such a patient must be on the basis of close consultation between the radiation therapist and medical oncologist. The enthusiasm for adding chemotherapy to the initial treatment program for patients with large mediastinal masses must be tempered by the knowledge of both increased second neoplasms and sterility from this combined modality approach. The use of chemotherapy alone in the treatment of these patients has not been well-evaluated. However, Young *et al.* [82] reported a 61% relapse rate in the mediastinum in advanced Hodgkin's disease patients with large mediastinal masses who were treated with chemotherapy alone. This would again argue against the use of chemotherapy alone for any subset of stage I or II Hodgkin's disease outside of a well-designed controlled clinical trial.

1.9. Summary

The past decade has witnessed a dramatic improvement in the prognosis of patients with advanced Hodgkin's disease resulting from the development of curative combination chemotherapy. MOPP represents the standard against which all alternative chemotherapy programs or combined modality approaches must be judged. The landmark studies of DeVita demonstrated that more than 50% of all patients with advanced Hodgkin's disease were potentially cured with chemotherapy alone, and have been confirmed both at single institutions and by the cooperative groups. No alternative chemotherapy regimen has proven conclusively superior to MOPP given differences in patient selection, prognostic factors, restaging evaluation, and adequate follow-up. However, comparable results to MOPP have been achieved with a variety of alternative chemotherapy combinations which may offer significantly less toxicity than MOPP. Combinations that contain cyclophosphamide or chlorambucil instead of nitrogen mustard, vinblastine in place of vincristine, and/or the addition of a nitrosourea (e.g. ChlVPP or BCVPP) appear to be as efficacious as MOPP in producing durable complete responses, but are subtantially less toxic and better tolerated. It has been amply demonstrated that maintenance chemotherapy beyond documentation of restaged complete remission is of no advantage in improving either disease-free or overall survival.

Although patients who relapse after definitive irradiation for early stage disease are often salvaged and cured with MOPP chemotherapy, those patients who relapse after chemotherapy present a difficult therapeutic challenge. Patients who achieve an initial complete remission with MOPP, have a disease-free interval greater than 6 months from the end of treatment, and then relapse should be re-treated with the same induction chemotherapy regimen. However, patients who are truly MOPP-resistant should be placed on non-cross-resistant combinations. Unfortunately, the compete response rates to the second-line regimens are low and, except for ABVD, there are no reports of durable complete remissions in adequate numbers of patients. However, the identification of an active non-cross-resistant combination in the relapsed patient has led to the investigation of sequential alternating chemotherapy regimens (e.g., monthly cycles of MOPP–ABVD) as primary induction therapy. The objective is to increase complete remission rates above what has been demonstrated with MOPP and, more importantly, to improve relapse-free and overall survival. This approach shows considerable promise, but longer follow-up will be required before adopting this strategy as standard practice for advanced Hodgkin's disease.

An alternative approach has been to integrate radiotherapy into a combined modality treatment plan for advanced stages of Hodgkin's disease. By administering either conventional or low-dose radiotherapy to areas of major pretreatment involvement, the goal is to reduce the 34% recurrence rate seen following chemotherapy alone. The preliminary results of this combined modality strategy are extremely encouraging, but the results of confirmatory trials are not available at this time. Ultimately, either alternating sequential non-cross-resistant induction chemotherapy or a combined modality approach offers the potential for improving the cure rate of advanced disease. These leads are systematically being investigated in well-designed ongoing clinical trials.

The treatment of stage IIIA Hodgkin's disease also remains controversial. Retrospective studies have concentrated on identifying prognostic subgroups in which there is an unacceptably low disease-free survival with radiotherapy alone. At the present time, it would be premature for radiation therapists to abandon total nodal irradiation for prognostically favorable IIIA patients, i.e. those with clinical stage I, IIA, who are found to have microscopic involvement in the spleen or upper abdominal nodes at the time of laparotomy (Desser III$_1$A). In this favorable subgroup, only those who

relapse after primary radiotherapy should receive combination chemotherapy. Thus, the majority of IIIA patients will be spared the acute and long-term
treatment morbidity of a combined modality approach. For the patient with
clinical stage IIIA/pathologic stage IIIA disease (Desser III$_2$A), no one
management strategy has proven superior. Acceptable treatment alternatives
for this subgroup include: total nodal irradiation utilizing the Stanford
technique (including prophylactic liver radiation when the spleen is
involved); combined modality therapy with total nodal or subtotal nodal
radiotherapy plus MOPP; initial chemotherapy followed by low-dose irradiation to sites of pretreatment involvement; or chemotherapy alone.

There is also active debate as to whether chemotherapy alone or as an
adjuvant to radiotherapy should be utilized for patients with localized
Hodgkin's disease and unfavorable prognostic parameters. Adjuvant chemotherapy can effectively substitute for prophylactic irradiation of apparently
uninvolved sites, but to date, there is no clear justification for the routine use
of a combined modality approach for the overwhelming majority of patients
with pathologically staged I or II disease. However, there are certain subsets
for whom combined modality treatment may be indicated because of an
unacceptably high relapse rate (e.g. patients with large mediastinal masses).
Any potential survival advantage seen after combined modality therapy for
localized disease must be balanced by the potential risk of late complications,
particularly second malignancies. With dramatically improved treatment
results, the challenge facing physicians and investigators caring for patients
with all stages of Hodgkin's disease must be to carefully weigh the toxicity-
benefit ratio for each new recommended regimen.

2. NON-HODGKIN'S LYMPHOMA

The management of an individual patient with advanced non-Hodgkin's
lymphoma remains controversial. Since this is a heterogenous group of
lymphoreticular disorders, treatment is selected primarily on the basis of
histologic subtype. Unfortunately, new histopathologic classifications
abound, leading to problems in defining histologic subgroups with meaningful clinical correlation. This becomes even more frustrating for the individual physician when he realizes that there is lack of concordance between an
institutional pathologic diagnosis and review by a group of referee lympho-
pathologists in approximately 40% of cases [122, 123]. This frustration is
compounded by the realization that the non-Hodgkin's lymphomas are a
clinically diverse group of malignant diseases ranging from the very aggressive and rapidly fatal to among the most favorable and indolent neoplasms [124].

At the present time, the Rappaport classification remains the most widely used histopathologic system. Its wide acceptance is based on its useful clinico-pathologic correlations. As described elsewhere in this volume, the Rappaport classification allows patients with non-Hodgkin's lymphomas to be separated into two prognostic groups. A 'favorable' prognostic category consists of patients with nodular histologies and with relatively small lymphoid cells. These patients have a median survival in excess of 5–7 years, in contrast to the median survival of less than 2 years for patients with 'unfavorable' histologies (diffuse patterns and large lymphoid cells). At the present time, treatment selection is primarily on the basis of placing an individual patient into one of these two broad prognostic categories.

Since the vast majority of patients with non-Hodgkin's lymphomas have stage III or IV disease at the time of diagnosis, chemotherapy remains the mainstay of the therapeutic approach to these patients. In contrast to Hodgkin's disease, where a curative strategy is possible for all stages and histologic subtypes and for whom survival has improved significantly over the past decade, the treatment of non-Hodgkin's lymphomas remains a challenge in terms of our ability to cure an individual patient.

2.1. Favorable Prognosis Histology

The 'favorable' non-Hodgkin's lymphomas are primarily a group of B-cell lymphoid malignancies characterized by disseminated disease at presentation, an indolent natural history with long median survival, and are extremely responsive to a wide range of systemic therapies. According to the Rappaport classification, diseases in this category include: nodular lymphocytic, poorly differentiated lymphoma (NLPD); nodular mixed lymphocytic-histiocytic lymphoma (NM); and diffuse lymphocytic well-differentiated lymphoma (DLWD). According to the Lukes and Collins classification, follicular center cell lymphoma (FCC) of small cleaved cells or larged cleaved cells, small lymphocytic lymphoma, and plasmacytoid lymphocytic disease would be included in this favorable prognostic group. A variety of approaches have been utilized in the treatment of these patients including single alkylating agents, aggressive combination chemotherapy, whole-body irradiation and combined modality therapy. Although any one of these treatment options are extremely effective in achieving a high-rate of complete response, prolonged relapse-free survival is a goal that has generally eluded this group of patients.

2.1.1. Single-Agent Chemotherapy and the CVP Combination.

Almost all the known chemotherapeutic agents have single-agent activity in these favorable histologic subtypes, yielding some objective evidence of tumor regression in 20–80% [125]. Gold et al. [126] first demonstrated in 1963 that single alkylating agents were active in the treatment of lymphosarcoma. Early comparative studies reported by Carbone et al. [7] noted that cyclophos-

phamide-treated patients with lymphosarcoma had a consistently higher
remission induction rate when compared with those receiving vinca alkaloids. These studies were conducted prior to the widespread use of the
Rappaport histopathologic classification and in patients who previously had
been treated.

Jones et al. [127] retrospectively reviewed the Stanford experience with
single-agent chemotherapy and reported a complete response rate of 28–48%
for those patients with any degree of nodularity. The highest CR rate of 48%
was noted in patients with NLPD, who exhibited a median survival of 60+
months from the initiation of a single alkylating agent therapy. Cyclophosphamide and chlorambucil were found to be interchangeable without loss of
effectiveness in a small number of patients when one or the other agent was
not well tolerated. For patients who achieved complete remission with either
cyclophosphamide or chlorambucil, the median time from initiation of
treatment to clinical CR was 2 months. However, some patients required
almost 2 years of treatment before their apparent complete response was
documented. Jones et al. were unable to demonstrate any significant difference in response rate or survival from the initiation of alkylating agents in
those patients whose first treatment modality was chemotherapy compared
to those patients treated post-radiotherapy. Three recent trials have also
documented the ability of either oral chlorambucil or cyclophosphamide to
achieve complete response rates ranging from 13 to 65% [128–130]. The
median disease-free survival ranged in these three studies from 12 months to
more than 36 months, with a range of overall survival from 30 to more than
60 months.

Vincristine alone produced an overall objective response rate of 46% (9%
CR) in one series, with a median remission duration maintained by
alkylating agents of 3 months [7]. Corticosteroids are known lympholytic
agents and their use in the treatment of non-Hodgkin's lymphomas is based
on older series reporting objective tumor responses in 58–67% of patients
(0–12% CR) [131–133]. The median response duration on daily maintenance
prednisone was 5 months, with rapid relapse when steroids were discontinued even in apparent clinical complete responders [133].

Although most patients will experience an objective response with single
alkylating agents and many will achieve a complete remission, a pattern of
continuous relapse is observed, and this therapeutic approach is clearly not
curative. The initial report by Hoogstraten [134] was the first trial comparing
single-agent cyclophosphamide with both a high- and low-dose combination
of cyclophosphamide, vincristine, and prednisone (CVP). Although the older
term lymphosarcoma was used, both CVP combinations significantly
increased the percentage of remissions when compared to cyclophosphamide
alone. The 100% complete and partial remission rate obtained with the
high-dose CVP combination was better than any previously reported in the

Table 8. Chemotherapy for advanced favorable histology non-Hodgkin's lymphoma.

Author	Histology	Regimen	No. of evaluable patients	% CR	Disease-free survival (median in months)	Overall survival (median in months)	Comment
Luce et al. [135]	Lymphosarcoma	CVP	35	63	No maintenance = 5 Maintenance = 12	N.R.	Adverse effect of major prior radiotherapy
Coltman et al. [136]	NLPD	CVP	17	53	N.R.	36+	Survival of CR significantly longer than PR
Anderson et al. [138]	NLPD	CVP	49	67	16	83	
Portlock et al. [128]	Favorable	CVP vs CTX or CLB vs CVP-TNI	20 23 20	83 65 70	50 52 52	70% at 7 yrs for all arms	No significant differences according to histology
Lister et al. [129]	Favorable	CVP vs CLB	35 31	37 13	12 12	48+ 48+	No difference in remission duration between CR and 'good' PR
Kennedy et al. [130]	Nodular	CVP vs Sequential C-V-P	16 13	81 46	37+ 25+	50+ 30	No significant difference
Bitran et al. [139]	NLPD, NM	COPP	29	41	74% at 2 yrs	48	DFS curve demonstrated continuous pattern of relapse
Benjamin et al. [140]	NLPD	CVP vs MOPP	8 5	75 60	8/9 pts. in original CR	85% alive at 3 yrs	MOPP more toxic
Coltman et al. [136]	NLPD	MOPP	14	43	N.R.	31	No advantage to addition of Bleo; Similar survival of CR & PR
Portlock et al. [142]	NLPD	CVP ± Bleo	24	41	–	90% alive at 2 yrs	
Durant et al. [144]	Favorable	CVP vs BCVP	28 27	42 36	17 13	– –	No advantage to addition of BCNU
Edinli et al. [141]	Favorable	COPP vs BCVP vs CP	87 114 125	69 59 58	43 25 36	73% at 2 yrs 73% at 2 yrs 88% at 2 yrs	CP associated with significantly longer survival
McKelvey et al. [147]	NLPD, NLWD	CHOP vs HOP	57 54	79 67	88% at 1 yr	85% at 2 yrs	Short follow-up; no significant differences
Rodriguez et al. [148]	NLPD	CHOP-Bleo	13	62	48+	48+	
Skarin et al. [149]	Nodular	CHOP-Bleo (BACOP)	9	89	14+	25+	
Bodey et al. [150]	NLPD	CHOP-Bleo vs CHOP-Bleo+PEPA	8 9	50 77	Only 1/11 CR has relapsed	–	No advantage to dose escalation with PEPA
Jones et al. [143]	Nodular	COP-Bleo vs CHOP-Bleo vs. CHOP-BCG	75 66 65	71 67 67	25 29 29	78% at 2 yrs 85% at 2 yrs 97% at 2 yrs	BCG improved survival although CR rate and DFS unaffected

CR = Complete Response; PR = Partial Response; N.R. = Not Reached; DFS = Disease-Free Survival; PEPA = Protected Environment, Prophylactic Antibiotics with Dose Escalation.

literature. However, the 6-week duration of induction therapy did not allow adequate evaluation of the cyclophosphamide alone arm, since it has been subsequently documented that patients treated with single alkylating agent therapy may require up to 2 years to achieve their maximal response.

Table 8 summarizes the results of 17 chemotherapy trials in advanced favorable non-Hodgkin's lymphoma. Luce *et al.* [135] utilized a more aggressive CVP combination in 2-week cycles with the treatment aim of producing a complete remission. Patients in CR after ten courses of treatment were randomly allocated to either no further treatment or continued maintenance CVP until relapse. They obtained 63% complete remissions in 35 previously untreated patients with lymphosarcoma. A median remission duration of 5 months without maintenance drug treatment and 12 months with maintenance drug treatment was reported. Survival of all patients at 1 year was 81%, and for complete responders, it was 90%. A more protracted treatment program utilizing the same drugs in 4-week cycles was instituted in 1968 by the Southwest Oncology Group. They reported a 53% complete response rate in 17 patients with NLPD and a median survival in excess of 3 years [136].

Bagley *et al.* [137] at the NCI pioneered the use of a more aggressive CVP combination utilizing cylcophosphamide 400 mg/m^2 per day orally for 5 days of a 21-day cycle. This combination was administered every 3 weeks until a pathologically documented complete remission was obtained, after which time chemotherapy was stopped. A minimum of 6 months of CVP was administered to 35 patients with advanced lymphosarcoma (32 previously untreated) with a complete response rate of 57%. Twenty-five of these patients were subsequently noted to have nodular lymphocytic poorly differentiated lymphoma. A very rapid response rate was observed with the median time to clinical complete remission being 2 months. As initally reported by Bagley *et al.*, the duration of complete response (89% at 1 year) appeared significantly better than that previously reported. These results led to the widespread adoption of CVP as the 'standard' therapy in the early 1970s for favorable histologies, particularly NLPD.

Anderson *et al.* [138] reported the updated NCI results in 49 patients with NLPD treated with this same CVP program. Thirty-three patients (67%) achieved a restaged CR. The median duration of remission was 16 months with 21 (64%) having relapsed. The median survival of CR patients was 95 months compared to 35 months for those patients achieving only a partial response or not responding. This difference was highly significant ($P < 0.001$). The median survival for the entire group of NLPD patients was 83 months. A pattern of continuous late relapse was again documented for this histology, but these patients could be retreated with the same chemotherapy when they relapsed, producing the excellent overall median survival.

Three recent trials have prospectively compared single alkylating agent therapy to the CVP combination. Portlock *et al.* [128] randomized 63 stage IV patients with favorable histologies (48 of whom had NLPD) to either CVP, split course CVP plus total nodal irradiation, or to daily oral cyclophosphamide or chlorambucil. The CVP regimen utilized in the Stanford trial was the same as the NCI regimen, but maintenance chemotherapy was administered for 2 years after the documentation of complete remission. There was no difference in the pathologically restaged complete remission rates between the three arms. However, patients receiving oral alkylating agents alone required significantly more time to achieve a complete remission (median 2 years) than did those patients receiving combination chemotherapy. An updated analysis of these data was recently reported by Portlock [125], and continued to demonstrate a pattern of continuous relapse in patients achieving complete remission. The median disease-free survival was similar in all three treatment arms (approximately 50 months), and the overall actuarial survival was identical for all three treatment groups (70% at 7 years). Portlock concluded that single-agent chemotherapy, given continuously, was capable of inducing a high percentage of pathologically documented complete remissions, with an overall survival similar to that achieved with more aggressive treatment programs.

Lister *et al.* [129] compared a fixed 6-month regimen program of CVP with 14 weeks of oral chlorambucil in 66 previously untreated patients with advanced stage III and IV favorable histologies (30 NLPD, 11 NM, 12 DLWD, and 13 DLPD-intermediate). No maintenance treatment was given to those who achieved either a complete remission or good partial remission. Although more patients achieved CR with CVP (37%) than with the single alkylating agent (13%), the median duration of remission and overall survival were not significantly different. The lower complete response rates and shorter duration of remission noted by Lister *et al.* [129] may be accounted for by the fixed and limited duration of initial induction chemotherapy. The only factor shown to influence overall survival was the response to treatment, with responders surviving significantly longer than nonresponders. However, there were no differences in survival between those patients who achieved a complete remission and those with good partial remission. This may reflect the lack of pathologic restaging in the CR group. The CVP combination also has been prospectively compared with the same drugs used sequentially as single agents in maximal doses starting with cyclophosphamide. Kennedy *et al.* [130] reported the results of their randomized trial in 29 patients with nodular histologies. The CR rate with the CVP combination was 81% versus 46% on the sequential single agent arm. Although the disease-free and overall survival were better for patients receiving the CVP combination, there were no statistically significant differences between these two regimens.

Thus, three randomized trials provide no evidence that combination chemotherapy with CVP is superior to the use of oral alkylating agent therapy given in an optimal manner. If the goal of chemotherapy in the disseminated favorable non-Hodgkin's lymphomas is complete remission, a prolonged period of induction chemotherapy may be required to achieve a pathologically restaged complete response. However, the duration of remission is short and a pattern of continuous late relapse is reported in all studies, with no plateau being observed in the disease-free survival curves. Combination chemotherapy, however, induces a more rapid tumor regression, and this may be important in an individual patient with symptomatic disease or more serious organ dysfucnction (e.g. ureteral obstruction or airway compromise).

2.1.2 Alternative Combination Chemotherapy Regimens. Given the numerous single agents active in the treatment of nodular lymphomas, it is not surprising that many investigators have attempted to develop more aggressive combination chemotherapy programs than CVP (Table 8). The addition of procarbazine to the CVP regimen either as COPP or MOPP (as for Hodgkin's disease) has shown no benefit in four trials in the NLPD histologic subtype [136, 139–141]. Similarly, the addition of bleomycin to the CVP program has not significantly improved the complete remission rate or altered the pattern of continuous relapse [142, 143]. The same is true for the addition of BCNU to CVP [141, 144].

Ezdinli *et al.* [141] recently reported the preliminary results of an ECOG trial randomizing 326 patients with favorable histologies to induction chemotherapy with 8–16 cycles of BCVP (BCNU+CVP), COPP, or to a non-aggressive arm of cyclophosphamide-prednisone (CP). Complete responders were then randomized to maintenance BCVP or to no treatment. As initially published, the CR rates for all three induction arms were similar, as were the response durations (the median for the entire group was 31.6 months) [145]. However, the incidence of severe and life-threatening hematologic toxicity was significantly higher with BCVP and COPP as compared to CP. This may account for the significantly longer survival observed with CP as compared to either BCVP or COPP. Since approximately 75% of patients remain alive, these survival results must be regarded as preliminary, but provide additional evidence for non-aggressive chemotherapy regimens in favorable histologies.

The ECOG has also reviewed the influence on survival of the degree of nodularity and the quality of the response. Three hundred and twenty-two patients with NLPD and 101 patients with NM entered on ECOG protocols active from 1972 to 1978 were analyzed by Ezdinli *et al.* [146]. The median survival of 75.4 months in the 268 patients with a pure nodular pattern (*N*-LPD) was significantly better than the 43.6 month median survival of 54 patients with both nodular and diffuse pattern (*ND*-LPD). The same survival difference was also noted in 68 patients with pure nodular mixed (*N*-M median of 56.3 months) versus 33 patients with *ND*-M (median 25.5 months). These differences in survival were not due to differences in complete response rates, which were similar for these four histologic patterns. Multivariate analysis revealed the survival of all NLPD patients to be significantly better than NM, and the nodular pattern to have superior survival over the nodular and diffuse group. A proportional hazard model showed the death risk to increase two-fold for partial responders and five-fold for non-responders when compared to complete reponders for all subtypes. Ezdinli *et al.* concluded by noting that the subdivision of nodular pattern lymphomas into pure nodular versus nodular and diffuse categories increased the prognostic accuracy of the Rappaport classification. Pure *N*-LPD remained the most favorable subtype, but still gained a two-fold survival advantage when CR over PR was obtained [146]. These retrospective ECOG results confirm the report of Anderson *et al.* [138], which noted a significant survival advantage for CR over PR in both NLPD and NM histologies.

Attempts to develop even more aggressive combination chemotherapy programs for these histologies have included the addition of adriamycin to the CVP regimen with little benefit. McKelvey *et al.* [147] compared the cyclophosphamide, adriamycin, vincristine, prednisone (CHOP) combination to adriamycin, vincristine, and prednisone (HOP) in 111 patients with NLPD and NLWD. Their complete remission rate was 79% for CHOP and 67% for HOP, but there were no significant differences in disease-free or overall survival with short follow-up. Eighty-eight percent of the patients remained in complete remission at 1 year which was not different from what has been reported for single agent or CVP chemotherapy. Similarly, the 2-year overall survival reported by McKelvey *et al.* of 85% was virtually identical to a variety of less aggressive combinations.

The addition of bleomycin to the CHOP regimen was separately investigated by Rodriguez *et al.* [148], Skarin *et al.* [149], Bodey *et al.* [150] and Jones *et al.* [143], with restaged CR rates ranging from 50 to 89%. All four trials were in previously untreated patients, the vast majority of whom had the NLPD subtype. Interestingly, the trial by Bodey *et al.* [150] involved randomization of patients to either CHOP-Bleo or the same regimen plus protected environment, prophylactic antibiotics (PEPA) and dose escalation to tolerance. Although the numbers are small, there did not seem to be any advantage to dose escalation and the PEPA program. Further evidence against the concept of adriamycin combination chemotherapy in the favorable histologies was demonstrated in the recent SWOG trial reported by Jones *et al.* [143, 151]. Two hundred and six evaluable patients with nodular histologies were randomized to CVP plus bleomycin versus CHOP plus bleomycin versus CHOP plus BCG immunotherapy. The complete remission rates and median disease-free survival among the three arms were virtually identical. The most interesting observation in this trial was that the overall survival of patients with nodular lymphoma who received CHOP plus BCG immunotherapy was better than that achieved with CHOP plus bleomycin ($P = 0.08$) and superior to that achieved with COP plus bleomcyin ($P = 0.02$). However, the follow-up time was short (approximately 2 years), and it was difficult to explain the improved survival with BCG since it did not appear to improve either the compete response rate or remission duration. Because of the results of this trial, the SWOG initiated a further investigation of immunotherapy in the non-Hodgkin's lymphomas, randomizing patients to either CHOP alone, CHOP plus levamisole, or CHOP plus levamisole plus BCG. To date, there are no results from this trial.

Thus, there are no data from randomized trials defending the use of more intensive induction chemotherapy in nodular lymphocytic poorly differentiated lymphoma. High complete remission rates can be achieved either with single alkylating agents, non-aggressive combination regimens, and more intensive chemotherapy programs. Once chemotherapy is initiated, the goal should be the achievement of complete remission which appears to confer a significant survival advantage. However, with any of these therapeutic options a pattern of continuous late relapse is noted, yet overall survival remains excellent.

2.1.3 No Initial Therapy. An alternative strategy for stage III and IV favorable histologies has been advocated by Portlock and Rosenberg [152]. They observed that most patients with disseminated favorable lymphomas were clinically asymptomatic at diagnosis and the size or location of their lymphadenopathy presented no major organ dysfunction. Since many of these patients were elderly, as well as asymptomatic, the Stanford group retrospectively reviewed a series of 44 selected patients in whom initial therapy was not instituted until serious symptoms developed. The major reason for requiring treatment was bulky lymphadenopathy. The median time before the initiation of treatment was 31 months for all 44 patients, 32 months for the 21 patients with NLPD and 8+ years for the eight patients with DLWD. A significantly shorter time to requiring treatment was observed in the eight patients with NM histology (median 8 months). For all patients, the median survival was 10 years with no significant differences observed among the histologic subtypes. When these 44 patients were compared to 112 patients entered on the randomized Stanford clinical trials for favorable histologies, there were no differences in actuarial survival between the group which was initially observed with no treatment and the protocol patients, all of whom received initial chemotherapy, radiotherapy, or both [152]. An important additional observation was that seven of the 44 patients, who were in the initial no treatment group, were noted to have spontaneous tumor regressions with observation alone (3 CR and 4 PR) [153]. The histologic sybtypes included 3 NLPD, 2 NM, and 2 DLWD. These spontaneous remissions were frequently of long duration, ranging from 21 + to 60+ months in the CR group and 6–34 months for the PR patients. Gattiker *et al.* [154] also observed spontaneous complete, partial or minor regressions in 18/140 cases of nodular lymphoma. In seven of their cases with spontaneous CR or PR, the duration of spontaneous regression lasted more than one year.

These unique series require confirmation but argue strongly for a palliative approach in patients with disseminated NLPD and DLWD, but not for nodular mixed histology. This approach should be reserved for those NLPD and DLWD patients who are asymptomatic and without significant organ dysfunction. Close observation is required, with particular attention to the tempo of the individual patient's tumor progression, bone marrow funtion, systemic symptoms, and threat of serious problems. Careful observation of the patient's clinical status and lymph node size over a period of months and even years provides valuable information about the natural history of that patient's tumor. If the disease progresses and/or if the patient is anxious because of the visible lymphadenopathy, continuous or intermittent oral single alkylating agent therapy is a satisfactory, well-tolerated alternative. Local radiotherapy may be utilized in a palliative approach without the addition of chemotherapy if warranted by the clinical situation. If the patient rapidly becomes symptomatic and/or develops compromise of organ function, combination chemotherapy to induce a rapid remission may be employed. This palliative approach chooses between the toxicity and morbidity of intensive combination chemotherapy, which to date has not produced evidence of long-term cure in NLPD and DLWD, and the existing data which strongly suggest adequate control by single-agent therapy or non-aggressive combinations (e.g. cyclophosphamide-prednisone) in those patients requiring treatment.

2.1.4 Strategies to Prevent Relapse

Maintenance chemotherapy: Different therapeutic strategies have been advocated to prevent relapse following induction of restaged complete remissions. No significant advantage for extended maintenance chemotherapy has been documented with either oral alkylating agents, CVP, or more aggressive combinations [128–130, 151, 155–157]. The Eastern Cooperative Oncology Group [157] evaluated patients with favorable histologies who achieved complete remission after induction chemotherapy with BCVP, COPP or CP. Patients in complete remission were randomized on the maintenance phase between observation and BCVP chemotherapy until relapse. One hundred and thirty-eight patients were randomized to maintenance, 89 of whom were of the NLPD subtype, 24 NM and 17 DLWD.

Although BCVP maintenance produced an increase in the duration of complete remission; once the disease reappeared, patients who received BCVP maintenance tended to die sooner than those who received no maintenance treatment. Overall survival times from entry to maintenance were not significantly different between the two groups. This trial confirmed the observation that once a patient with favorable histology non-Hodgkin's lymphoma obtains a complete response, chemotherapy can be stopped and the patient closely followed.

Histologic conversion: When patients with indolent lymphomas relapse, rebiopsy of accessible lymph nodes is strongly recommended to document the presence of either the same histology or transformation to a more unfavorable histologic subtype. If a similar favorable histologic pattern is documented, then the same induction chemotherapy regimen can be re-instituted with the expectation of good control. However, histologic transformation is frequently observed. Jones *et al.* [158] have reported the NCI experience in 118 patients with all histologies of non-Hodgkin's lymphomas who were re-biopsied more than 3 months following their initial diagnostic biopsy. Forty-four (37%) exhibited histologic changes with 80% of the latter biopsies demonstrating progression from nodular to diffuse pattern, greater cytologic immaturity, or both. The median survival from histologic change of nodular lymphoma patients who subsequently converted to any diffuse histology was only 8 months. Following conversion to a diffuse histology, 7/22 patients achieved a complete remission with a median post-conversion survival of 32+ months. The 15 patients who failed to achieve a CR had a post-conversion median survival of 4 months with none still alive. These data had been supported by a recent autopsy series reported by Risdal *et al.* [159], in which only 25% of patients with NLPD and 17% with NM had their original histology at autopsy. The remaining patients progressed to one of the diffuse unfavorable histologies.

DeVita *et al.* [160] have initiated a randomized trial in stage IV NLPD and DLWD to observe the true incidence of histologic conversion. Patients are randomized to no initial treatment versus aggressive combination chemotherapy. This protocol will test the concept that no treatment, unless necessitated by clinical or histologic evolution, may be superior to the immediate institution of intense chemotherapy. DeVita *et al.* paradoxically have proposed that, by allowing conversion to histologically unfavorable subtypes (e.g. diffuse histiocytic lymphoma, DH), more patients might be cured. This is based on data in DH where long-term disease-free survival has been noted in more than 50% of complete responders following combination chemotherapy.

Combined modality trials: The studies of Schein *et al.* [161] and Fuks *et al.* [162] noted that relapses after chemotherapy for patients with nodular lympomas most frequently occurred in sites of pretreatment involvement.

Table 9. Combined modality trials in advanced favorable histology non-Hodgkin's lymphomas.

Author	Histology	Regimen	No. of evaluable patients	% CR	Disease-free survival (%/yr)	Overall survival (%/yr)	Comments
Portlock et al. [128]	Favorable	CVP vs CTX or CLB vs CVP-TNI-CVP	20 23 20	83 65 70	45/5 52/5 45/5	69/7 72/7 69/7	No significant differences in DFS or OS; Prolonged myelosuppression after CVP-TNI
Hoppe et al. [163]	Favorable	CVP vs CTX or CLB vs TBI (+Boost to involved regions)	17 17 17	88 76 71	31/3 33/3 30/3	88/3 94/3 100/3	No significant difference
Young et al. [164]	NLPD, NM	CVP or C-MOPP vs TBI	42 33	62 85	24/4 24/4	85/4 82/4	CR rate higher with TBI but repeat liver biopsies not performed in 49% of CRs on TBI arm
Brereton et al. [165]	NLPD, NM	CVP or C-MOPP vs TBI+CVP or C-MOPP	17 16	82 75	73/1.5 58/1.5	100/2 100/2	No significant difference; increased hematologic toxicity with TBI+chemo

CR = Complete Response; DFS = Disease-Free Survival; OS = Overall Survival; TNI = Total Nodal Irradiation; TBI = Total Body Irradiation.

Furthermore, two-thirds of these relapses occurred in lymph nodes. This suggested that adjunctive radiation therapy might be of benefit in preventing the pattern of continuous relapse. Table 9 summarizes the results of four randomized trials comparing chemotherapy alone to radiotherapy alone or radiotherapy plus chemotherapy. The studies reported by Portlock et al. [128] and Hoppe et al. [163] present the consecutive Stanford protocol experience. Although the majority of the patients in these two studies had NLPD, patients with NM and DLWD were also eligible. In the initial trial reported by Portlock et al. [128], only patients with pathologic stage IV were entered. There were no significant differences in disease-free or overall survival between patients receiving single-alkylating agent chemotherapy, CVP, or CVP sandwiched around total nodal irradiation. The combined modality arm was the most toxic with persistent cytopenias in five patients. The administration of chemotherapy after TNI was compromised by the previous radiation. The second Stanford trial was recently reported by Hoppe et al. [163], and compared the same single-agent chemoeherapy to CVP and to total body irradiation (TBI) 150 rads over 5 weeks. The TBI was followed by boost irradiation to all involved lymphoid regions (2000 rads/2 weeks) by conventional fields. There were again no significant differences in complete response rates, median disease-free survival or overall survival.

Young et al. [164] reported the NCI results in 75 previously untreated patients with stage III and IV nodular lymphomas who were randomized to combination chemotherapy or total body irradiation delivered by a wide variety of techniques (including TNI in a small number of patients). Patients randomized to chemotherapy who had NLPD histology received CVP and those with NM received C-MOPP. Although the complete remission rate of 85% was higher in the radiotherapy arm, 19 of the TBI patients achieving CR had initial liver involvement which was not reassessed by biopsy. At 4 years, only 24% of the complete responders on both arms remained relapse-free, but the overall survival exceeded 80% and was identical for both treatment options. Young et al. reported that TBI was more easily tolerated than CVP as initial therapy. Late complications consisted of two TBI patients who developed a myeloproliferative disorder and two CVP patients who experienced persistent disabling neurotoxic reactions. One patient died from Candida sepsis following the first cycle of CVP.

A second trial from the NCI was recently reported by Brereton et al. [165]. This trial randomized 33 patients with NLPD and NM to either CVP or C-MOPP versus TBI 100 rads in ten fractions over 12 days plus the same combination chemotherapy regimen. The complete remission rates, response duration, and overall survival were comparable for both treatment groups. However, there was increased hematologic toxicity noted in the radiotherapy plus the chemotherapy arm. They concluded that the use of both treatment modalities had no therapeutic benefit.

The role of adjuvant CVP chemotherapy after definitive radiotherapy for localized nodular histologies has been investigated by Bonadonna *et al.* [166]. Patients with pathologic stage I-II disease were randomized to radiotherapy alone (involved field plus proximal uninvolved lymph node regions) or to radiotherapy followed by six cycles of CVP. The adjuvant chemotherapy failed to significantly influence either the relapse-free or overall survival. A continuous pattern of relapse over time irrespective of treatment was observed, similar to what has been reported for stage III and IV disease.

Thus, there does not seem to be an advantage for combined modality therapy of localized or advanced favorable histologies of non-Hodgkin's lymphomas. Single alkylating agent therapy or combination chemotherapy provide equivalent complete remission rates and overall survival as does an initial combined modality approach, but with significantly less hematologic toxicity and without the increased leukemogenic potential. One investigational approach that is currently being explored is the use of low-dose radiotherapy to all sites of pretreatment involvement after documentation of complete remission with chemotherapy. This strategy has been employed in advanced Hodgkin's disease with promising results, but it is premature to recommend this approach for any patient with non-Hodgkin's lymphoma.

2.1.5 Selected Controversies in the Favorable Histologies

Nodular mixed lymphoma – is it curable?: In the retrospective review of previously untreated patients with non-Hodgkin's lymphomas referred to Stanford University between 1960 and 1971, Jones *et al.* [167] observed that the actuarial survival for 74 patients with all stages of nodular mixed lymphoma was similar to 69 patients with NLPD. Median survival for both groups was 7 years and a pattern of continuous late relapse was observed. Other investigators have also noted that the survival of NM is as good as that observed with NLPD histology [147, 168]. Table 10 summarizes the results of six chemotherapy trials in advanced NM lymphoma. Anderson *et al.* [138], reporting for the NCI group, have argued that patients with disseminated NM are potentially curable. They based this conclusion on a series of 31 previously untreated NM patients with stage III or IV disease treated with combination chemotherapy. Twenty-four of these patients received the C-MOPP regimen. This consists of substituting cyclophosphamide for nitrogen mustard in the MOPP combination after it was recognized that cyclophosphamide had a higher response rate as a single agent. Six of the NCI patients received CVP and one the BACOP combination, because initially their biopsies were reported as another histologic subtype but were eventually reclassified as NM. Only one patient received maintenance CVP therapy after achieving a restaged complete remission. Twenty-four of the 31 patients (77%) with NM achieved a CR. Since only four patients had

Table 10. Chemotherapy for advanced nodular mixed lymphoma.

Author	Regimen	No. of evaluable patients	% CR	Disease-free survival (%/yr)	Overall survival (%/yr)	Comment
Jones et al. [167]	CTX or CLB	16	31	median 17+ months	47/2	
Anderson et al. [138]	C-MOPP (24) CVP (6) BACOP (1)	31	77	79/4	70/5	CR survived significantly longer than PR or non-responders
Lister et al. [129]	CVP or CLB	11	91 (includes CR and 'good' PR)	65/2	—	Only one patient at risk beyond 3 years
McKelvey et al. [147]	CHOP vs HOP	9 11	78 64	71/1	88/1	Sharp fall-off in overall survival at 2 years
Ezdinli et al. [170]	Various	80	45	58/2	59/2	CR survived significantly longer than PR
Glick [169]	COPP vs BCVP vs CP	18 14 20	61 50 65	For COPP: median DFS = 32 months with only 33% relapse-free at 3 yrs	70/2 70/2 94/2	Pattern of continuous relapse observed; no significant differences between 3 arms

CR = Complete Response; PR = Partial Response.

relapsed at the time of the last publication in 1977, the median duration of remission had not yet been reached. Seventy-nine percent of patients were still in their original CR, but it was important to note that only 10 patients were at risk beyond 2.5 years. Thus, the plateau in the relapse-free survival curve must be regarded with caution because of the limited follow-up and well-known tendency of nodular mixed patients to relapse with time. Without further data on the duration of disease-free survival in this limited series, it would be premature to accept that the NM subtype is indeed curable.

The Eastern Cooperative Oncology Group failed to confirm the NCI observation utilizing a virtually identical cyclophosphamide, vincristine, procarbazine, prednisone (COPP) combination in 18 patients with this histology [169]. A complete remission rate of 61% with COPP was observed, with only 3/11 complete responders remaining in their initial remission. The median response duration of the CRs was 31.7 months. Median survival of the entire group was 40.8 months with only 8/18 still alive. When the COPP regimen for NM was compared in this randomized trial to the BCVP and CP regimens, no significant differences in complete response rates, disease-free or overall survival were noted. A pattern of continuous relapse was observed for all three induction regimens with this histology.

An investigation of the adriamycin-containing combinations CHOP and HOP was conducted by the Southwest Oncology Group. McKelvey *et al.* [147] reported the SWOG results in 20 patients with nodular mixed lymphoma. A 78% CR rate was observed with CHOP as compared to 64% CR with HOP. The disease-free survival of complete responders was only 71% at 1 year. The overall survival at 1 year for all 20 patients was 88%, but a sharp fall-off in the actuarial survival curve at 2 years was noted. Obviously, longer follow-up is required for the SWOG data to be meaningful, but preliminary analysis does not seem to confirm the report of Anderson *et al.* [138] of long-term relapse-free survival.

Ezdinli *et al.* [170] have retrospectively reviewed 80 patients with nodular mixed lymphoma entered on four different ECOG protocols active between 1972 and 1978. They were compared with 249 patients with NLPD who were treated on the same studies. Ninety percent of the previously untreated NLPD, but only 59% of the comparable group of NM, survived 2 years ($P<0.001$). Patients with NM in whom the pattern was reported as both nodular and diffuse had a significantly shorter 2-year survival than did patients with a pure nodular pattern. In addition, patients with NM who achieved a complete response survived significantly longer than did partial responders.

Thus, the optimal treatment for nodular mixed lymphocytic-histiocytic lymphoma remains controversial. Portlock and Rosenberg [152] did not recommend deferring initial treatment for this histology. In their small group eight NM patients who were initially observed, little was gained by withholding initial treatment. The median time to treatment was 8 months, and all but one patient required therapy within 2 years. Since the NM group may occupy an intermediate position between the clearly favorable NLPD histologic subtype and diffuse histiocytic lymphoma, it then becomes important to ask what is the optimal chemotherapy program. Clearly the more aggressive C-MOPP regimen has produced the best results, but these have not been confirmed in one small prospective series. Because complete responders survive significantly longer than partial responders, the goal for NM patients should be the attainment of a complete remission. At the present time, moderate chemotherapy with cyclophosphamide-prednisone appears to be as effective as more aggressive combination regimens. However, a search for more effective induction chemotherapy programs is necessary in order to improve the complete response rate, and thus to improve overall survival for this histology.

Diffuse, lymphocytic well-differentiated lymphoma – an intermediate prognostic category?: Diffuse, lymphocytic well-differentiated lymphoma (DLWD) is generally classified as a prognostically favorable type of lymphoma with prolonged survival. It is frequently difficult to differentiate DLWD from chronic lymphocytic leukemia (CLL). The latter diagnosis is frequently made when the peripheral lymphocyte count is greater than $4000/mm^3$. Pangalis et al. [171] retrospectively reviewed 108 patients originally diagnosed as DLWD on the basis of lymph node biopsies. In 41 patients neither absolute lymphocytosis nor monoclonal gammopathy was evident. Of the 41, 11 had no bone marrow involvement at the time of lymph node biopsy and 35 never developed lymphocytosis over follow-up periods ranging from 24 to 150 months. The median survival of this group was 124 months on a variety of therapies. Pangalis et al. concluded that malignant lymphoma of the well-differentiated lymphocytic type may be a tissue manifestation of CLL, but may also exist as a distinct form of non-Hodgkin's lymphoma.

Evans et al. [172] retrospectively reviewed 84 cases of DLWD on the basis of lymph node biopsy. Seventeen patients presented without monoclonal gammopathy or CLL. Median survival for this group was 68 months. They observed that patients with high mitotic rates in excess of 30 or more mitoses per 20 high power fields showed a significantly decreased survival. They concluded that malignant lymphoma of small lymphocytic type is a definite clinico-pathologic entity which may or may not exhibit monoclonal gammopathy or CLL. Evans et al. proposed that the term 'intermediate lymphocytic lymphoma' be applied only to those cases showing histopathologic chararteristics of small lymphocytic lymphoma at a mitotic rate of 30 or more mitoses per 20 high power fields.

Icli et al. [173] concluded that DLWD was a less favorable lymphoma type than NLPD and should be treated with aggressive chemotherapy since the achievement of a complete response appeared to favorably improve survival. They based this conclusion on an analysis of 34 patients with a lymph node biopsy diagnosis of DLWD confirmed by a group of referee pathologists. These patients were entered on a single ECOG protocol, and were randomized to induction chemotherapy with either BCNU-prednisone or cyclophosphamide-prednisone. Responders were re-randomized to mainrenance with either BCNU + CVP (BCVP) or oral chlorambucil every 2 weeks. A complete response rate of 32% was reported, but this rose to 45% in previously untreated patients. This study also demonstrated that the survival in DLWD was favorably influenced by chemotherapy responsiveness. The estimated 2-year survival of CR was 89%, PR 65%, and for progressive disease 44%. Median survival for the entire group of 34 patients from the time of diagnosis was 39+ months. The presence of lymphocytosis over 4000/mm^3 had little effect on response rates or survival. Comparison with NLPD patients entered on the same protocol demonstrated a 2-year survival of 83% for NLPD and 67% for DLWD ($P<0.05$).

More aggressive combination chemotherapy programs have been reported for this histology in small clinical trials (Table 11). Anderson et al. [138] treated 11 patients with the CVP regimen and reported a 64% complete remission rate. The median disease-free survival was only 23 months, yet the overall survival was excellent (median 78 months). McKelvey et al. [147] randomized 45 patients to the adriamycin-containing regimens CHOP or HOP. The CR rates were 61% and 55% on the two arms respectively, and 85% of complete responders remained disease-free at 1 year. Yet, the overall survival was 53% at 2 years. These data must be regarded with caution since their follow-up period was extremely short. Ezdinli et al. [170] randomized 39 patients with DLWD to COPP versus BCVP versus non-aggressive therapy with cyclophosphamide-prednisone (CP). Although there were no significant differences in the CR rates between the three arms, the CP regimen had the highest CR rate of 60%. Again, the follow-up is short with the median disease-free and overall survival not yet being reached. Ezdinli et al. did observe that the 1-year survival rate for DLWD of 75% was inferior to the 97% survival rate for NM and 90% for NLPD patients entered on the same protocol.

The retrospective and prospective trials in DLWD summarized above do not provide a clear answer as to how favorable the prognosis for patients with this histology is. Portlock and Rosenberg [152], in a small series of eight patients with DLWD in whom initial therapy was deferred, noted that the median time to initiation of treatment for DLWD was in excess of 8 years. The 5-year survival of these eight patients was 75%. Thus, each patient with this histology must be approached individually. Deferring initial treatment is a reasonable alternative if the patient is asymptomatic and without organ

Table 11. Chemotherapy for diffuse lymphocytic well-differentiated lymphoma.

Author	Regimen	No. of evaluable patients	% CR	Disease-free survival (median in months)	Overall survival (median in months)
Pangalis *et al.* [171]	Various	41	NS	NS	124
Evans *et al.* [172]	Various	17	NS	NS	68
Icli *et al.* [173]	BCNU-Pred vs CP induction (Maintenance BCVP vs CLB)	34	32 (45% CR in previously untreated group)	20+	39+ (median not reached)
Lister *et al.* [129]	CVP or CLB	12	58 (CR and 'good' PR)	15	NS
Anderson *et al.* [138]	CVP	11	64	23	78
McKelvey *et al.* [147]	CHOP vs HOP	23 22	61 55	85% at 1 yr	53% at 2 yrs
Ezdinli *et al.* [170]	COPP vs BCVP vs CP	39	51 40 60	59% at 1 yr (median not reached)	75% at 1 yr (median not reached)

CR = Complete Response; NS = Not Stated.

dysfunction. At the time of disease progression, chemotherapy can be instituted with the reasonable expectation that more than 50 % of patients will achieve a complete remission. There is no evidence to date that aggressive chemotherapy offers a higher complete response rate or disease-free survival than does a conservative approach. Clearly, there is a need for additional clinical trials in this histologic subtype.

2.1.6. Summary. The treatment of disseminated favorable histology non-Hodgkin's lymphomas remains a challenge in terms of our ability to demonstrate significantly improved survival over the past decade. The management of an individual patient is controversial and is based not only on the specific histologic subtype, but also on sites of involvement, tempo of tumor progression, symptoms (both local and systemic), threat of serious organ dysfunction, and general medical condition. No single management approach has been shown to be significantly better in terms of complete response rate, duration of response, or overall survival.

For asymptomatic patients with NLPD and DLWD histology whose disease is not progressing rapidly, deferral of initial therapy is recommended. Careful observation of the patient's clinical status and lymph node size over a period of months and even years provides valuable information about the natural history of that patient's tumor. Spontaneous tumor regression with observation alone has been observed. If the disease slowly progresses, mild symptoms develop, or if the patient desires therapy for psychological reasons, continuous or intermittent oral alkylating agent therapy alone is a satisfactory, well-tolerated alternative. There is no evidence that combination chemotherapy with the CVP regimen is superior to the use of oral alkylating agents given in an optimal manner. However, combination chemotherapy induces a more rapid remission than does the alkylating agent approach. There is no evidence that the addition of adriamycin, bleomycin, procarbazine or BCNU to the CVP regimen has significantly improved the complete response rate, remission duration or overall survival. A pattern of continuous late relapse from complete remission has been observed in all these regimens for NLPD and DLWD histologies. One group has reported prolonged disease-free survival with the C-MOPP regimen in patients with nodular mixed lymphoma, but this has not been confirmed by other investigators. However, the NM subtype may occupy an intermediate prognostic category, as patients with this histology appear to have a shorter median survival than do similarly treated patients with NLPD. Deferral of initial treatment for NM patients is not generally recommended, except in the elderly asymptomatic individual. Once chemotherapy is initiated for all favorable histologies, the goal should be the achievement of a restaged complete remission since there appears to be a significant survival advantage for CR over PR.

However, despite documenting complete remission status, a pattern of continuous relapse is noted, usually at the rate of 10–15 % per year year after the end of treatment. Different therapeutic strategies have been proposed to prevent relapse, but there is no significant benefit for either maintenance chemotherapy or adjuvant radiation. Combined modality programs do not offer an advantage over single alkylating agents or combination chemotherapy.

Thus, although the favorable histology non-Hodgkin's lymphomas are highly responsive to therapy, a curative strategy still eludes this group of patients. However, survival is excellent with currently available management. Future well-designed clinical trials are clearly needed. Because of the indolent and heterogenous natural history of this group of tumors, we cannot adopt an aggressive investigational approach, with the risks of greater acute and chronic toxicity, unless significant benefit can be demonstrated in terms of improved survival when compared to standard palliative treatment.

2.2. Unfavorable Prognosis Histology

The 'unfavorable' non-Hodgkin's lymphomas are associated with an overall poorer prognosis and significantly shorter median survival than their nodular counterparts. According to the Rappaport classification, diseases in this unfavorable category include: diffuse histiocytic lymphoma (DH); diffuse mixed histiocytic-lymphocytic lymphoma (DM); diffuse lymphocytic, poorly differientiated lymphoma (DLPD); diffuse undifferentiated or stem cell (DU); and Burkitt's lymphoma. In addition, it is now accepted that the nodular histiocytic (NH) group should be included in this category. Despite a median survival of approximately 1 year for the diffuse histologies, it is possible to achieve prolonged relapse-free survival, tantamount to cure, for a significant number of these patients, in contrast to the favorable histologies. An aggressive combination chemotherapy program is always indicated at diagnosis for patients with stage III and IV unfavorable histologies and, as will be discussed, for stage II disease as well. The goal of treating these patients must be a pathologically documented complete remission; there is no role for deferring initial treatment or adopting a palliative strategy for this group of patients.

2.2.1. Diffuse Histiocytic Lymphoma.

Although it is recognized that the term 'histiocytic' does not reflect that the majority of histiocytic lymphomas are diseases of large transformed B-lymphocytes, the use of the DH category has been associated with a significant improvement in survival over the past decade. It is possible that within the heterogeneous group of diseases currently labeled histiocytic lymphoma there are distinct clinical entities that can be separated out on the basis of clinical factors, immunologic typing, and histopathologic patterns. In the future we may recommend different treatment strategies for particular subgroups if the newer proposed classifications are adopted. However, for the pupuses of this review, we will continue to view the category histiocytic lymphoma as a single clinicopathologic entity since the advances of the past 10 years are based on this description.

Single-agent chemotherapy has no role in the treatment of diffuse histiocytic lymphoma. Although the same chemotherapeutic agents have single-agent activity in both the favorable and unfavorable histologic subtypes, single drug programs achieve only 5–10% complete remissions in DH. Relapse is rapid and median survival of less than 1 year is the rule [127]. As opposed to the wide discrepancy between disease-free and overall survival in the favorable histologies, relapse and death are closely associated in DH. The goal of any therapeutic program must be the achievement of a restaged complete remission, because the survival of patients with partial responses closely parallels that of non-responding patients and is significantly inferior to that seen in the CR group. Since relapses usually occur within 6–12 months from the end of therapy, and relapses beyond 2 years are distinctly uncommon, it is reasonable to choose the 2-year disease-free survival point as the most meaningful assessment of the value of any chemotherapy program. Although the complete response rates with combination chemotherapy have significantly improved in recent years, overall survival has not changed. Median survival data may be misleading because the plateau of the survival curve is just below the 50% level in most studies. Thus, the goal in treating diffuse histiocytic lymphoma must be to improve the complete remission rate, since it is only this subgroup which may possibly be cured.

The CVP regimen, which was so widely used in the early 1970s for favorable histologies, was also investigated in diffuse histiocytic lymphoma (Table 12). Coltman et al. [136] summarized the consecutive Southwest Oncology Group studies with the cyclophosphamide, vincristine, prednisone combination which they labeled COP. The complete response rate varied from a low of 23% in the COP 1 study, in which cyclophosphamide and vincristine were administered intravenously on day 1 of an every-2-week cycle, to 49% CR in COP 2 when cyclophosphamide was administered orally for 14 days and vincristine given intravenously on days 1 and 8 of an every 4-week cycle. In the COP 3 program, there were no significant differences in the complete response rates with or without the addition of cytosine arabinoside (Ara-C). Most interestingly, this latter protocol produced the longest disease-free survival (46 months), but was considered unsatisfactory because of the relatively low complete remission rate. Thus, CVP (or COP) offered an increased CR rate over what had historically been reported with single agents, and there was evidence of a plateau in the survival curve beyond 2 years at approximately 20% in the SWOG studies [136]. However, the CVP regimen as originally proposed by the NCI group was evaluated in 13 DH patients at Stanford with a disappointingly low 15% complete responses [142].

Table 12. Chemotherapy of advanced diffuse histiocytic lymphoma – the early trials.

Author	Regimen	No. of evaluable patients	% CR	Disease-free survival (median in months)	% All patients in CR at 2 years*
Portlock et al. [142]	CVP	13	15	NR	15
Coltman et al. [136]	COP 1	53	23	–	–
	COP 2	49	49	14	–
	COP 3 ± Ara-C	65	34	46	–
	COP+Bleo	16	63	25	40
DeVita et al. [174]	C-MOPP or MOPP	27	41	NR	38
Coltman et al. [136]	MOPP	36	29	26.5	–
Stein et al. [175]	COPP	16	16	NR	16
Durant et al. [176]	BCVP	28	50	8.5	21
Durant et al. [144]	BCVP vs	29	34	NR	24
	CVP	23	13	4	–

* Figures are estimated from graphs in some studies as this specific information is not available for all regimens.
CR = Complete Response; NR = Not Reached.

The dramatic results achieved with MOPP chemotherapy for advanced Hodgkin's disease led to this regimen being evaluated in diffuse histiocytic lymphoma. Utilizing MOPP or C-MOPP (cyclophosphamide substituted for nitrogen mustard), DeVita *et al.* were the first to demonstrate in 1975 that advanced DH was potentially curable [174]. These regimens produced a complete remission rate of 41% in 27 patients with advanced DH, but more importantly, 10 of the 11 complete responders remained disease-free 26–105 months from the end of treatment. The one patient who relapsed after achieving a complete remission did so at 5 months from the end of treatment and died 24 months from the time of diagnosis. All 16 patients who failed to achieve a complete response expired with a median survival time of 5 months. A life-table analysis of the entire population revealed a plateau in the survival curve at 38% with all patients at risk at least 32 months from the onset of therapy.

Although these results with MOPP or C-MOPP are truly impressive, there is a paucity of confirmatory data. Coltman *et al.* [136] treated 36 patients with MOPP, but reported only a 29% complete response rate with a median disease-free survival of 26.5 months and an overall survival of 9.5 months. A plateau in the survival curve was noted with 20% of patients surviving beyond 3 years. Stein *et al.* [175] treated 16 DH patients with COPP but achieved only a 16% CR rate. Both of Stein's complete responders remained disease-free at 2 years. Thus, these regimens are capable of producing from 16 to 38% prolonged disease-free survival in advanced diffuse histiocytic lymphoma. However, no randomized trials comparing C-MOPP to the newer adriamycin-bleomycin containing combinations have been reported.

At the same time, other investigators presented similar results with the addition of BCNU to the CVP regimen (BCVP) (Table 12). Durant *et al.* [176] noted a 50% CR rate in 28 patients with little or no prior therapy, compared to 24% CR in 21 heavily pretreated patients. The median survival for previously untreated patients who achieved a complete remission was nearly 2 years, and 6/14 remained in their initial unmaintained remission. Twenty-one percent of all evaluable patients were disease-free at 2 years. These preliminary results led the Southeastern Oncology Group to conduct a randomized trial comparing BCVP to CVP [144]. Complete response was assessed at 6 months from the initiation of therapy, but pathologic restaging was not mandatory. The 34% complete response rate with BCVP was superior to CVP (13% CR), and this advantage carried over in duration of remission. Survival was improved only in those patients achieving complete response. Although 7/9 complete responders with BCVP remained in CR at 2 years, this translated into only a 24% 2-year disease-free survival for all patients treated with BCVP. The BCVP program was also evaluated by the Eastern Cooperative Oncology Group, although the dose of BCNU was lower than employed by Durant *et al.* [144]. Lenhard *et al.* [177] reported the results of the ECOG trial in which BCVP was compared with CVP and with the non-aggressive cyclophosphamide-prednisone (CP) regimen. Pathologic restaging was not employed, but the clinical complete response rates were still considered inadequate with a total of 28% of the 65 DH patients achieving CR. Only 32% of the entire group were alive at 1 year. Although both the BCVP and CVP regimens achieved higher complete response rates than did CP, the longest survival was seen in the CVP arm. The authors concluded that all three drug combinations were inadequate in diffuse histiocytic lymphoma.

The demonstration that adriamycin had impressive activity in malignant lymphoma, even among patients refractory to alkylating agents and combination chemotherapy, led to the integration of adriamycin into regimens with already established drugs [178]. Table 13 summarizes 11 trials with adriamycin combinations. McKelvey et al. [147] reported that two adriamycin-containing regimens CHOP (cyclophosphamide, adriamycin, vincristine, and predisone) and HOP (adriamycin, vincristine and prednisone) were able to achieve the highest complete remission rates reported at that time. Two-thirds of the patients obtained CR, although pathologic restaging was not mandatory in that SWOG study. Sixty-eight percent of the complete responders remained disease-free at 1 year, and the median relapse-free survival has not been reached. Forty-six percent of all patients entered into this study remained in CR at 2 years. There were no significant differences between CHOP and HOP regimens. All patients received maintenance chemotherapy, either with CVP or with vincristine, Ara-C, and prednisone; but there were no differences in the duration of complete response on either maintenance arm. The CHOP regimen was subsequently evaluated at Stanford by Elias et al. [179]. A lower complete response rate of 39% was observed in 23 patients with an actuarial disease-free survival of 75% at 2 years. Eighty-eight percent of the complete responders remained alive at 2 years, whereas the median survival of partial responders and non-responders was less than 15 months. Patients with stage III disease had a significantly higher complete response rate (88%) compared to stage IV disease (13%).

At this time bleomycin was reported to also have a single-agent activity in far-advanced refractory malignant lymphomas [16]. Because of its lack of myelosuppression, bleomycin was incorporated into the CVP (COP) regimen by the SWOG. Coltman et al. [136] reported a 63% CR in a small series of 16 patients with the COP + Bleo program. Although the median relapse-free survival was 25 months, 7 patients (40%) were alive at greater than 2 years. This observation led the Southwest Oncology Group to launch a randomized trial comparing COP + Bleo versus CHOP versus CHOP + BCG immunotherapy. The study design emphasized systematic restaging to define complete remission and no maintenance chemotherapy, although complete responders were re-randomized to BCG immunotherapy or observation. For

Table 13. Chemotherapy of advanced diffuse histiocytic lymphoma – recent investigations.

Author	Regimen	No. of evaluable patients	% CR	Disease-free survival (%/yr)	% All patients in CR at 2 years *
McKelvey et al. [147]	CHOP vs	53	68	68/1	46
	HOP	62	66		
Elias et al. [179]	CHOP	23	39	75/2	30
Jones et al. [143]	† COP-Bleo vs	59	46	38/1	–
	CHOP-Bleo vs	90	48	58/1	–
	CHOP-BCG	92	54	67/1	–
				Median DFS (months)	
Johnson et al. [180]	COPA vs	31	47	11.5	–
	CPOB (day 15 VCR, Bleo) vs	22	55	22	–
	COPB (day 1 VCR, Bleo) vs	24	25	6	–
	BCVP	13	31	3	–
Schein et al. [181]	BACOP	25	48	100/1	48
Skarin et al. [149]	BACOP	18	56	60/2	32
Rodriguez et al. [148]	CHOP-Bleo	26	69	83/1	58
Canetta et al. [182]	CVP-ABP	37	49	–	32
Garrett et al. [184]	CTX-L2	30	23	86/1	20
Cadman et al. [188]	COMA	30	40	50/5	20
Sweet et al. [189]	COMLA	42	55	87/2	48
Fisher et al. [191]	† ProMACE-MOPP	27	63	82/1	52
Skarin et al. [192]	M-BACOD	56	80	–	63

* Figures are estimated from graphs in some studies as this specific information is not available for all regimens.
† All diffuse histologies, not limited to histiocytic lymphoma.
CR = Complete Response.

patients with diffuse lymphomas (all histologies), the CR rate was higher
with the CHOP programs than with COP-Bleo $(P = 0.10)$ [143, 151]. In
diffuse histiocytic lymphoma, both CHOP regimens were noted to produce a
complete response rate of 61 % versus 48 % with COP + Bleo. There were no
significant differences in response duration for the two CHOP programs. A
plateau in the disease-free survival curve was noted for all three arms
(particularly for those treated with adriamycin chemotherapy), and approximately 40 % of all patients appeared to achieve prolonged relapse-free status.
Survival of patients treated with the two adriamycin-containing regimens
was superior to that achieved with COP + Bleo for patients with diffuse
lymphoma, although this was not specifically broken down for the specific
diffuse histologic subtypes. Although survival was not significantly different
for patients receiving CHOP + BCG compared to COP + bleomycin, the
divergence of the survival curves after the first year is of interest, but the
follow-up period is short [143].

The COP + Bleo regimen chosen by the SWOG involved the administration of oral cyclophosphamide daily for 14 days, while vincristine and
bleomycin were given on days 1 and 8 of an every-28-day cycle [151]. The
Eastern Cooperative Oncology Group also investigated the relative roles of
adriamycin, bleomycin, or BCNU as additions to the CVP combination [180]. Ninety patients with stage III or IV diffuse histiocytic lymphoma
were randomized to receive COPA (with the only difference between this
program and CHOP being a higher dose of cyclophosphamide in the latter),
BCNU + CVP (BCVP), or one of two CVP + bleomycin regimens. The only
difference in the two bleomycin-containing combinations was the timing of
the bleomycin and vincristine. In the CPOB arm, vincristine and bleomycin
were both administered on day 15 of a 21-day cycle, whereas in the COPB
arm all drugs were administered on day 1. All patients were treated with
eight cycles of chemotherapy and were pathologically restaged. Complete
responders were randomized to no further therapy or BCVP maintenance
therapy every 6 weeks for 13 cycles (Table 13). The complete response rates
with BCVP and with the day 1 COPB regimen were 31 % and 25 %
respectively. These were significantly lower than the CR rates with the day
15 CPOB regimen (55 % CR) and with the adriamycin-containing COPA
program (47 % CR). The median duration of CR was significantly shorter
with BCVP (3.3 months) and COPB (5.7 months) than with CPOB (22
months) or COPA (11.5 Months). Fifty percent of the CPOB treated patients
remain in complete remission up to 59 months. The median survival of all
patients treated with COPB (29.4 months) was significantly greater than
COPB (11.0 months) or BCVP (10.7 months) but not COPA (13.1 months).
The longer survival with CPOB could not be attributed to more favorable
pre-treatment parameters, the effect of maintenance chemotherapy, or to
treatment following relapse. This study demonstrated the schedule depen-

dancy of bleomycin and vincristine in the treatment of diffuse histiocytic lymphoma [180]. The non-adriamycin-containing CPOB, with bleomycin and vincristine administered on day 15 of an every-21-day cycle, was as effective as COPA, and compared favorably with the published results of CHOP [147]. These data are in contrast to the report of Jones et al. [151], who observed that adriamycin-containing regimens were superior to COP + bleomycin. However, in the study by Jones et al., the vincristine and bleomycin were given on days 1 and 8 of an every-28-day cycle and this may account for the different results.

Four additional studies employing the same five drugs (reported as either BACOP or CHOP + Bleo) have been published (Table 13). The NCI group was the first to report on this 5-drug combination in 25 patients with advanced previoiusly untreated diffuse histiocytic lymphoma (although three of their patients had diffuse mixed histology). Schein et al. [181] reported the preliminary results with BACOP employing a schedule where the two non-myelosuppressive agents bleomycin and prednisone were administered during the second two weeks of each 28-day cycle. This was in an attempt to retard the regrowth of tumor while allowing for full bone marrow recovery. Forty-eight percent of their patients achieved a complete remission as determined by extensive restaging procedures 1 month after discontinuation of treatment. The median CR duration after completion of therapy was in excess of 1 year and no patient had relapsed at the time of their initial report. Six of the nine patients classified as partial responses had no clinical evidence of disease after six cycles of BACOP. However, the lymphoma was only suppressed by this chemotherapy, and their failure to achieve CR was demonstrated by restaging procedures. These 9 patients classified as partial responders would almost certainly have been designated as having a clinical complete response in other reports. Most importantly, all but one of the nine partial responders have subsequently died of recurrent lymphoma, with a median survival of only 9 months from the start of treatment. This observation emphasizes that an apparent clinical complete response, while a patient is receiving chemotherapy for DH, is not an accurate estimate of the ability of a specific program to eliminate all evidence of lymphoma. The BACOP regimen was well-tolerated in terms of hematologic toxicity with only 7/25 patients having a WBC less than $1500/mm^3$ and only four patients having platelet counts below $100,000/mm^3$ but never less than $50,000/mm^3$. With their original dose of bleomycin of 15 units/m^2, 4/16 patients developed clinically severe respiratory toxicity with one treatment-related death. No pulmonary toxicity was observed in 9 patients treated at the lower bleomycin dose of 5 units/m^2.

The BACOP regimen has also been investigated by Rodriguez et al. [148] in 26 DH patients. Sixty-nine percent achieved a complete response and only 3/18 of the CR have relapsed. The projected median duration of response for these patients was calculated to be greater than 2 years. Although the follow-up was still short, the survival curve became flat at 70 weeks. The dose schedule of Rodriguez *et al.* varies slightly from that reported by Schein *et al.* [181], in that all drugs were given at the beginning of an every-28-day cycle. Skarin *et al.* [149] also utilized a 5-drug BACOP program in a slightly different dose schedule. Their complete response rate of 56% in 18 patients is consistent with the above studies; 67% of the CRs were alive at 2 years.

Thus, four studies with CHOP-Bleo (or BACOP) all demonstrated complete response rates ranging from 48% to 69% (depending on the extensiveness of pathologic restaging), with approximately two-thirds of the complete responders remaining disease-free at 2 years. The 2-year relapse-free survival for all patients entering on this 5-drug regimen ranges from 32 to 58%. To put this in perspective, one must remember that 38% of the patients treated with C-MOPP by DeVita *et al.* [174] were disease-free at greater than 2 years. Any additional toxicity related to adriamycin and bleomycin must be carefully weighed, as the results of BACOP and C-MOPP from the NCI and the results of the COPA and day-15 CPOB regimens from ECOG are not significantly different.

Since only patients who achieve a documented complete remission with histiocytic lymphoma have the potential for cure, newer investigational approaches have been designed to increase the CR rate. Bodey *et al.* [150] randomized 32 patients to reveive either CHOP-Bleo or the same drugs with dose escalation to tolerance in a protected environment, prophylactic antibiotic (PEPA) program. Although the CR rate for both arms was excellent (78%), there were no significant differences in CR or response duration between the two arms. However, for patients in either group who received dose escalation, remission duration and survival were significantly improved. Although the major infection complication rate was reduced by PEPA (7% vs 29%), there did not seem to be any major advantage from the time-consuming and expensive PEPA program.

An alternative approach to improving both the complete response rates and disease-free survival in advanced Hodgkin's disease has been to use sequential non-cross-resistant chemotherapy regimens. This strategy has also been investigated in non-Hodgkin's lymphoma in a non-randomized study by Canetta *et al.* [182]. They alternated every 3-week cycles of CVP with a regimen containing adriamycin, bleomycin, prednisone (ABP). The latter regimen produced a 40% CR rate alone in a previous trial reported by Bonadonna *et al.* [183]. Thirty-seven patients with disseminated DH were entered on the sequential CVP-ABP program with CR being assessed through pathologic restaging after a minimum of six cycles [182]. In complete responders, six consolidation cycles were given. A 49% complete response rate was noted with 32% of all patients entered on this trial relapse-free at 4 years. These results do not appear to offer an advantage over the chemotherapy regimens discussed above.

Garrett *et al.* [184] treated 30 advanced DH patients with a complicated program known as the cyclophosphamide-L2 protocol modeled after an acute leukemia regimen. This protocol employed alkylating agents, vincristine, antimetabolites, prednisone, nitrosourea, and intrathecal methotrecate or cytosine arabinoside. Their CR rate of 23% (median duration of response exceeded 20 months) was unacceptably low, Because of this low CR rate, excessive toxicity (two deaths during periods of neutropenia), and the need for prolonged hospitalization, this approach cannot be recommended. Lister *et al.* [185] investigated another acute leukemia chemotherapy program consisting of vincristine, prednisone, adriamycin, and L-asparaginase (OPAL) with an overall complete response rate of 60%. However, patients with stage IV disease had a CR of only 39%.

In 1972 and 1975, Levitt *et al.* [186] and Berd *et al.* [187] retrospectively analyzed eight DH patients treated with a sequential chemotherapy program (COMA) consisting of cyclophosphamide, vincristine, moderately high doses of methotrexate with leucovorin rescue, and cytosine arabinoside. These data were based on the mouse leukemia L1210 model in which improved survival rates were achieved with sequential chemotherapy utilizing these agents. These initial reports noted that 6/8 patients achieved complete remission and only one of the six relapsed at 7 months and died 2 months later. The other five patients were alive and in continued unmaintained remission for 55–65 months. The Yale group extended their observations with COMA in 1977 to include 30 patients with DH, some of whom were treated with minor modifications of the COMA program [188] (Table 13). A 40% CR rate was documented in these 30 patients. Of the 12 complete responders, three relapsed during the weekly methotrexate-Ara-C phase of the protocol and three relapsed after treatment was completed. One of the six long-term complete responders relapsed after being in CR for 56 months. However, only 5/30 (17%) of all patients entered onto the COMA regimen achieved durable complete remissions, a figure that appears lower than reported by other investigators with less complicated regimens.

Sweet *et al.* [189] recently reported their results with the COMLA program (the same doses and schedule as Berd *et al.* [187], but with a different acronym). Twenty-three patients (55%) achieved a complete remission with COMLA as determined by strict restaging criteria. The median survival for the complete responders will be greater than 33 months, and only one of the 23 CRs has relapsed and died. The median survival of the eight partial responders is longer than 21 months, but the 11 non-responders had a median survival of only 5 months. All patients were observed in unmaintained remission. None of the responders relapsed in the central nervous system. There were no differences in response rates between patients with stage III or IV disease or between asymptomatic and symptomatic patients. Toxicity was acceptable with three episodes of sepsis during periods of leukopenia, but no significant hemorrhagic problems and no drug-related deaths. Although the COMLA regimen does not yield more superior complete response rates than the adriamycin-containing programs CHOP or BACOP, it does not contain the potentially toxic agents adriamycin or bleomycin. However, COMLA is a complicated program, and contains methotrexate, which may be extremely toxic if renal abnormalities are present. COMLA also requires expensive weekly treatments, a high degree of patient cooperation and physician expertise. Interestingly, COMLA does not appear to be efficacious in non-histiocytic lymphomas [186].

Stein et al. [190] applied the Lukes-Collins classification to 48 patients who received COMLA as initial chemotherapy for diffuse histiocytic lymphoma. Among the 40 B-cell lymphomas, 65% obtained a complete response, compared with 3/8 (38%) of the non-B-cell patients. The median CR duration was significantly better in B-cell than in non-B-cell lymphomas (60+ vs 11 months), as was median survival (60+ vs 9 months respectively). They concluded that the Lukes-Collins classification identified patients with DH in whom newer therapies were required for initial treatment. These results need to be confirmed.

Two recent reports have investigated the role of higher doses of methotrexate with leucovorin rescue in combination with the aggressive use of conventional chemotherapeutic agents. Fisher et al. [191] reported on the use of the ProMACE-MOPP regimen in 27 evaluable patients with diffuse unfavorable histologies of all subtypes. This regimen involved the administration of cyclophosphamide, adriamycin, and VP-16 by vein on days 1 and 8; prednisone by mouth daily for 14 days; and methotrexate 1.5 g/m^2 IV on day 14 followed by leucovorin rescue. The cycle was repeated every 28 days until the rate of tumor response decreased or until one cycle after clinically evident tumor disappeared. An identical number of MOPP consolidation cycles in standard doses was then administered. Late intensification with ProMACE completed therapy. Patients were also randomized to standard nutrition or total parenteral nutrition during ProMACE cycles. Restaged complete remissions were documented in 17/27 (63%), with no differences between those receiving standard or total parenteral nutrition. Of the 17 complete responders, three (18%) have relapsed. Median survival for all patients had not been reached at the time of the preliminary report but exceeded 19 months. This regimen was extremely toxic with myelosuppression being dose-limiting and septic deaths reported in 5/30 (17%). The excessive toxicity and complete response rate of 63% does not appear to justify the use of this extremely complicated program.

Skarin et al. [192] administered methotrexate 3 g/m^2 (with leucovorin) given midcycle between bleomycin, adriamycin, cyclophosphamide, vincristine, and dexamethasone (M-BACOD) every 3 weeks for 10 cycles to 56 patients with either diffuse histiocytic (50 patients) or diffuse undifferentitated (6 patients) lymphoma. Forty-five patients (80%) achieved a CR. Of this group, one died after six cycles with pancreatitis and had necrotic tumor at autopsy, while two developed central nervous system (CNS) lymphoma during the tenth cycle. The remaining 42 patients with CR have been followed for a median of 21+ months, and seven have relapsed from 1–7 months after completion of M-BACOD. Only one of these relapses occurred in the CNS. Thus, 35 (62.5%) patients originally entered onto this chemotherapy program remain in CR for a median disease-free survival of 20+ months. Although the follow-up time is short, both the complete response rate and percentage of patients in complete remission approaching 2 years is impressive. M-BACOD had acceptable toxicity with a median leukocyte count of $1800/mm^3$, which was not effected by methotrexate with leucovorin rescue administered at mid-cycle.

There are currently six combination chemotherapy regimens effective in treating and potentially curing approximately 50% of patients with advanced diffuse histiocytic lymphoma: C-MOPP, BACOP, CHOP, CPOB, COMLA, and M-BACOD. It is difficult to compare one regimen with the other in view of differences in patient selection, prognostic factors, and the variable use of maintenance therapy. Most of these programs have employed strict pathologic documentation of complete remission. No one regimen can be regarded as significantly superior in terms of complete remission rate, disease-free or overall survival. Few prospective randomized clinical trials have initiated to compare these effective regimens with each other. All investigators do agree on the importance of achieving a carefully restaged complete remission, as partial responders rarely survive 2 years, are not cured of their disease, and are poorly responsive to alternative regimens. There is no conventional salvage chemotherapy program for induction failures. Although patients with microscopic residual disease may benefit from additional induction chemotherapy in an attempt to achieve a complete response, there is no evidence that maintenance therapy is useful for those patients achieving a complete remission [144, 147, 148, 157, 175].

2.2.2. Prognostic Factors in Advanced Histiocytic Lymphoma. It is difficult to compare response rates and survival with various induction chemotherapy programs in histiocytic lymphoma because this histologic subtype is a heterogeneous clinical and immunologic entity. Response rates between different institutions may vary greatly because of patient selection, small numbers of patients entered into each trial, and most importantly, favorable or unfavorable prognostic factors. The NCI group originally reviewed 56 DH patients and reported that stage IV disease, bone marrow or gastrointestinal involvement, and a tumor mass greater than 10 cm in diameter were all poor prognostic indicators [193]. Fisher *et al.* [194] updated these results by reviewing the records of 151 cases of DH, DM, and diffuse undifferentiated lymphoma to determine clinical or pathologic features that influence survival. Patients of all stages were considered in their analysis. Radiation was the initial treatment for 25%, combination chemotherapy the primary treatment for 60%, and the remainder received either single agents or combined modality therapy. The treatment parameters which were associated with a significantly lower complete response rate included: tumor in the bone marrow, a mass greater than 10 cm in diameter involving the gastrointestinal tract, elevated lactic acid dehydrogenase (LDH), constitutional symptoms, or liver involvement. Increasing stage was inversely correlated with survival, except that the survival of stage III patients was greater than stage II; a fact attributed to the presence of patients with greater than 10 cm gastrointestinal masses in stage II. There were no significant differences in the survival curves for DM, DH, and DU patients according to histologic subtype. All DH cases were also classified according to the pathologic system proposed by Strauchen *et al.* [195], but these categories did not significantly correlate the with survival in the analysis by Fisher *et al.* [194].

MacKintosh *et al.* [196] reviewed the records of 240 consecutive patients with stage II_E, III, or IV histiocytic (33 Nodular, 207 diffuse) lymphoma seen at Stanford from 1968 to 1978. The probability of CR was decreased by bone marrow involvement, higher stage, diffuse histology, and was increased by treatment programs incorporating both adriamycin and cyclophosphamide. Pretreatment variables which decreased survival included bone marrow involvement or mediastinal involvement, diffuse histology, and age greater than 45 years. Attainment of complete response significantly improved survival, and for the 117 complete responders, no pretreatment variable predicted for relapse. Sweet *et al.* [189], in their COMLA trial, noted no difference in complete response rate between stage III and IV DH patients, nor between the asymptomatic and symptomatic groups. A decreased complete response rate was noted in the 14 patients who had received prior chemotherapy, radiation, or both. Only 2/14 achieved CR, but both are alive and disease-free 12 and 15 months since the end of COMLA therapy. Schein *et al.* [181] also noted that only 3/11 previously treated patients achieved a complete response with BACOP, and two of these relapsed promptly. Koziner *et al.* [197] confirmed that prior chemotherapy significantly decreased the complete remission rate. In their retrospective review of 66 DH cases treated at Memorial, an elevated LDH above 500 U/L correlated with a significantly decreased CR rate, but sex, age, B-symptoms, prior radiotherapy, and stage III versus IV were not found to influence chemotherapy responsiveness.

These results demonstrate that clinical factors, not pathologic subclassification, appear to influence the complete response rates and long-term survival in patients with histiocytic lymphoma. Bone marrow involvement at the time of diagnosis is a uniformly agreed upon poor prognostic factor, as is prior chemotherapy. Controversy exists as to whether stage IV extranodal sites other than bone marrow have a poorer prognosis than stage III, but this is influenced by the variability in staging workup between institutions. An elevated LDH in two studies correlated with significantly lower rates of complete response, but this needs to be confirmed. Although Stanford [196] and the Southwest Oncology Group [151] observed improved actuarial relapse-free survival for induction chemotherapy programs containing adriamycin, the results with C-MOPP, COMLA, and the schedule dependent CPOB combination from ECOG all demonstrate comparable CR rates and prolonged disease-free survival with non-adriamycin-containing programs. Despite these controversies, future clinical trials must prospectively stratify for these important prognostic factors in order to make the results of comparison between different forms of therapy more meaningful.

2.2.3. Localized Diffuse Lymphomas – Is There a Role for Chemotherapy?
Traditionally, definitive radiation has been regarded as the standard treatment for stage I and II diffuse histologies. Since 25–30% of patients with diffuse histiocytic lymphoma may present with localized disease, it is important to determine whether treatment with radiation alone will achieve long-term disease-free survival as in Hodgkin's disease. This discussion of localized disease is directed primarily toward diffuse histiocytic lymphoma, as it is the histologic subtype most likely to be localized at the time of presentation. Other diffuse histologies and localized nodular histiocytic lymphoma should probably be treated in the same manner.

The preceding chapter by Zagars and Rubin has reviewed the efficacy of radiotherapy for localized disease. The best results of radiotherapy have been reported in patients with stage I or I_E in which 50–90% of patients are disease-free 2 years from the end of therapy [198–200]. When DHL recurs after the end of treatment, over 90% of all the recurrences will become apparent within the first year. Thus, freedom from relapse at 2 years can be used for comparison of the curative potential of alternate regimens. Sweet *et al.* [201] have recently updated the University of Chicago experience with laparotomy-staged localized DH. Fourteen patients were pathologic stage I or I_E and 13 remain disease-free, with a median relapse-free survival greater than 43 months. One patient died from the complications of emphysema, but was counted as a relapse because an autopsy was not performed. In contrast, 10 of 15 patients with PS II or II_E DH have relapsed after primary radiotherapy, with a median disease-free survival of 14 months and a median overall survival of 18 months. The difference between stage I and II was highly significant ($P = 0.006$). The authors concluded that PS I disease, especially supradiaphragmatic presentations, is highly curable with radiation therapy alone, but strongly recommended chemotherapy for all stage II patients. Of the 10 stage II patients in the Chicago series who relapsed, only two responded to COMLA chemotherapy and are alive. Thus, it does not appear from this series that chemotherapy salvage of radiotherapy failures is as effective in localized diffuse histiocytic lymphoma as it is in Hodgkin's disease.

This failure to salvage patients who relapse after radiotherapy was also confirmed by Monfardini et al. [202].They randomized 66 patients with pathologic stage I and II diffuse lymphomas (all histologies) to primary radiotherapy alone or radiotherapy plus CVP adjuvant chemotherapy administered according to the original dose schedule of Bagley et al. [137]. In nine patients the disease progressed during radiotherapy and prior to actual randomization. This observation, that approximately 10% of patients develop progressive disease while receiving radiotherapy, has also been noted by Landberg et al. [203]. Kushlan et al. [204] reported an even higher failure rate in 27 stage II DH patients treated with extended field radiotherapy; 15 failed during the initial local radiation, thus preventing them from completing TNI.

In the Milan trial reported by Monfardini et al. [202], only six of 11 PS I diffuse lymphomas were relapse-free after radiotherapy, compared to all 11 patients remaining disease-free in the radiotherapy plus CVP group. For all PS stage I and II diffuse lymphomas, there was a highly significant difference in relapse-free survival between patients receiving combined modality therapy (76% at five years) when compared to radiotherapy alone (45% at five years). The difference in overall survival (80% vs 52% respectively) approaches but has not yet reached statistical significance ($P = 0.09$). Thus, the combined treatment program was felt to be of benefit for both stage I and II localized diffuse histologies. These results have been confirmed by Landberg et al. [203], who utilized a different CVP dose schedule following extended field radiotherapy for a similar patient population. They reported no relapses in 10 patients with DH who received adjuvant CVP compared with 5/10 relapses in those randomized to receive radiotherapy alone.

However, the Stanford group did not report an improved 5-year disease-free or overall survival in PS I-II patients with unfavorable histologies who received adjuvant chemotherapy [205]. Patients older than 65 were excluded from the Stanford trial, but included in the study reported by Monfardini et al. [202]. Miller and Jones [206] observed that 25% of their DH patients were over 65 years at diagnosis and, thus, would be excluded from laparotomy staging. The Stanford trial utilized total nodal irradiation including whole-abdominal radiotherapy and, therefore, most patients did not actually begin chemotherapy until 3–4 months after diagnosis. The chemotherapy regimen utilized at Stanford included cytosine arabinoside, adriamycin, and 6-thioguanine (CAT), which has a relatively low complete response rate in advanced disease [128]. This may also explain why this study failed to demonstrate any benefit from adjuvant chemotherapy, with 65% of both groups free of disease at 2 years [205].

A third approach to the treatment of patients with localized diffuse lymphomas has been the use of initial aggressive combination chemotherapy. Miller and Jones [207] administered adriamycin-containing chemotherapy (CHOP) to 31 patients with clinical stage I and II disease after a staging workup that did not include laparotomy. Only seven patients had stage I or I_E disease. Fifteen of the 31 patients had gastrointestinal tract involvement or bulky disease, and 11 patients were older than 60 years of age. Nineteen patients received chemotherapy alone, consisting of eight courses of CHOP followed by careful restaging for residual disease. Sixteen (84%) of these patients remain relapse-free at the time of their most recent report (Figure 8). Twelve additional patients received initial CHOP chemotherapy followed by involved field radiotherapy (minimum dose 4500 rads), and all 12 remain continuously free of disease. Currently, 30 of 31 (97%) of these patients are alive.

These results have been confirmed by Cabanillas et al. [208]. They investigated the role of chemotherapy alone (CVP – six patients, CHOP – 24 patients) in 30 patients with clinical stage I-II unfavorable histologies. Diffuse histiocytic lymphoma was present in 22 and nodular histiocytic in four. Bulky tumor (defined as either a palpable abdominal mass producing displacement of intra-abdominal organs, or a mediastinal mass) was present in 47%; 33% were older than 60 years of age. Five patients with diffuse histiocytic lymphoma had been rendered disease-free at the time of excisional biopsy and could not be considered for evaluation of chemotherapy

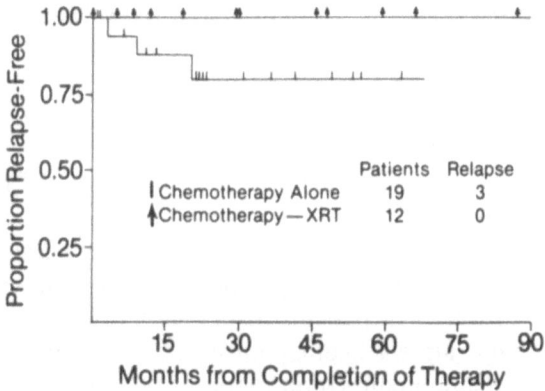

Figure 8. Relapse-free survival from completion of therapy for patients with localized diffuse lymphomas treated with initial CHOP chemotherapy. (Reprinted, by permission, from Miller and Jones [207].)

response. They were included in the evaluation of relapse-free survival. Of the 25 remaining patients with measurable disease, 22 (88%) achieved a complete remission. Of the 27 patients who achieved complete remission, 23 (85%) remain relapse-free. All eight patients with stage I and 15 of the 19 patients with stage II remain disease-free. No deaths have occurred in the group of eight patients with stage I disease treated with chemotherapy alone, but four patients with stage II have died.

The use of primary chemotherapy for localized diffuse lymphomas is an attractive approach because it avoids the necessity for strict initial pathologic staging which may be hazardous in the elderly patient. In addition, a significant proportion of patients (at least 10%) develop progressive disease outside of radiotherapy ports while undergoing initial treatment with this modality. The data from Miller and Jones [206, 207] and from Cabanillas et al. [208], employing adriamycin-containing regimens of proven efficacy in advanced stages, indicates that localized diffuse lymphomas may be cured with chemotherapy alone. Patients with stage II disease, irrespective of the staging evaluation utilized, should be treated with initial systemic chemotherapy. The role of adjuvant radiotherapy for the treatment of bulky disease sites remains to be defined, but clinical trials are in progress. Localized stage I disease probably should be treated by initial radiotherapy alone, with chemotherapy reserved for the small percentage who relapse. However, stage I patients with unfavorable prognostic factors may benefit from the use of adjuvant chemotherapy following definitive radiation or from initial chemotherapy followed by adjuvant radiotherapy.

2.2.4. Nodular Histiocytic Lymphoma. The natural history of nodular histiocytic (NH) lymphoma is not well-defined because of its relative rarity (less than 5% of all non-Hodgkin's lymphomas). Yet in 1973, Jones *et al.* [167] reported that patients with NH had a significantly shorter survival (median 28 months) than did patients with NLPD and NM. Recently, Osborne *et al.* [209] reviewed the NCI experience with 16 NH patients, 13 of whom had stage III or IV disease. A median survival of 31 months was reported with this histology, which was intermediate between NLPD (median survival of 78 months), NM (55 months), and DHL (10 months). Osborne *et al.* also noted that 11/16 NH patients received combination chemotherapy with eight complete remissions. Only one of these eight patients has relapsed, demonstrating the potential for long-term disease-free survival for this histology in patients achieving a documented CR.

The Eastern Cooperative Oncology Group retrospectively reviewed their non-Hodgkin's population entered on randomized studies between 1972 and 1978. Twenty-five patients with nodular histiocytic lymphoma and referee pathologic review were available for analysis [210]. Median survival for the entire group was 47 months and this represented the best reported survival for this histologic subtype. Forty-four percent entered CR with a median survival of 51.5 months versus 29.6 months for the 40% obtaining a PR. The six patients treated with the intentionally less aggressive chemotherapy regimen cyclophosphamide-prednisone survived shorter (median 18 months) than did the 19 patients treated with more aggressive combination chemotherapy programs (median 51 months). Four of the original complete responders remain disease-free of treatment and potentially may be cured. In contrast to what has been reported for NLPD and NM histologic subtypes, no significant difference in survival between NH patients with both nodular and diffuse histology and those classified as a pure nodular pattern was noted. This confirmed the observation reported by Osborne *et al.* [209].

Thus, the nodular histiocytic subtype should be classified as an unfavorable histology and should be treated with similar aggressive combination chemotherapy regimens as are used for diffuse histiocytic lymphoma. The goal for these patients should be the induction of a restaged complete remission, as the potential for long-term relapse-free survival exists. Adriamycin-containing combinations need to be systematically evaluated in this histology.

2.2.5. Diffuse Mixed Histiocytic-Lymphocytic Lymphoma. Diffuse mixed histiocytic-lymphocytic (DM) lymphoma is also a relatively uncommon histologic subtype accounting for 5–10% of all non-Hodgkin's lymphomas. Jones *et al.* [167] retrospectively reviewed the Stanford experience in 43 patients with all stages of this histology and reported a median survival of less than 2 years. Patients with DM and DLPD lymphomas had virtually identical survival. Few studies in the literature actually separate out the DM subgroup and, therefore it is difficult to report complete response rates and disease-free survival for these patients. Anderson *et al.* [138] treated 10 DM patients with three different chemotherapy combinations and reported only one complete response. That patient remained disease-free at 30+ months. McKelvey *et al.* [147] noted a 71% CR rate in 14 patients treated with CHOP and 50% CR in 12 patients treated with HOP. Sixty percent of all complete responders were disease-free at years. Canetta *et al.* [182] reported a 65% CR rate in 20 DM patients treated with every 3-week cycles of alternating CVP and ABP. Forty-four percent of the complete responders were projected to be alive at 4 years, with an estimated 4-year overall survival of 26% for all DM patients entered on this non-randomized study. With the lack of specific information available concerning the chemotherapeutic management of this histology, it appears reasonable to treat DM patients with the same aggressive combination chemotherapy regimens available for diffuse histiocytic lymphoma. Future clinical trials should report their specific results for this histology and not lump these patients with other unfavorable diffuse histologic subtypes.

2.2.6. Diffuse Lymphocytic Poorly Differentiated Lymphoma. In 1973, Jones *et al.* [167] reported on the natural history of 44 patients with diffuse lymphocytic poorly differentiated lymphoma. Median survival was approximately 2 years and was virtually identical for patients with diffuse mixed histiocytic-lymphocytic lymphoma. Until recently, the DLPD subtype was regarded as having an aggressive course and an unfavorable prognosis. DLPD has been shown to have a worse prognosis than NLPD and a significantly inferior survival [167, 211, 212]. Ezdinli *et al.* [211] commented that the difference in survivorship between DLPD and NLPD was so striking as to suggest the existence of two separate entities. The estimated 2-year survival in NLPD of 83% was almost double the 47% for the DLPD group.

However, recent studies of Bloomfield *et al.* [213] and Stein *et al.* [214] have shown that the B-cell subset of DLPD has a survival pattern similar to that of NLPD, a known B-cell neoplasm. Thus, the term DLPD does not account for the wide spectrum of differentiation and variable prognosis of what appeared to be a uniform histology. Although limited by small numbers, the report by Stein *et al.* [214] suggests that both nodular and diffuse forms of cleaved-cell lymphomas (B-cell subtypes of follicular center-cell origin) behave in a similar fashion with statistically insignificant differences in actuarial survival. Because the patients with diffuse cleaved-cell lymphoma received various forms of therapy, they could not conclude that their natural histology was indolent, as has been demonstrated for NLPD. In addition to the favorable B-cell subset, the DLPD category also has included the T-cell lymphoblastic lymphomas which have a very different natural history and an extremely poor prognosis. Neiman *et al.* [215] recently reviewed the Eastern Cooperative Oncology Group experience with DLPD on file in the Lymphoma Pathology Panel Repository. Although immunologic studies were not available, Neiman *et al.* found that the lymphoblastic category was the most common histologic subtype of DLPD. Including these patients in clinical trials of DLPD may be responsible for the poor prognosis often attributed to this category in past studies.

Table 14 reviews 12 studies utilizing chemotherapy for advanced stages of DLPD. These trials did not take into account that DLPD is a heterogenous subtype, and generally included patients with lymphoblastic lymphoma. Both single-agent chemotherapy [127] and the CVP combination [130, 138, 216] achieved low complete remission rates and short relapse-free survival. The median overall survival in these early studies was disappointingly low (less than 2 years). Ezdinli *et al.* [211] reported the largest series with this histology, but achieved only a 25% complete response rate in 77 patients with the non-aggressive combinations of either BCNU-prednisone or cyclophosphamide-prednisone induction followed by BCVP or chlorambucil maintenance. Only 36% of the complete responders were

Table 14. Chemotherapy for advanced diffuse lymphocytic poorly differentiated lymphoma.

Author	Regimen	No. of evaluable patients	% CR	Disease-free survival (median in months)	Overall survival (median in months)
Jones et al. [127]	CTX or CLB	9	22	13–17	4
Skarin et al. [216]	CVP	14	14	—	7
Anderson et al. [138]	CVP	25	32	8	23
Kennedy et al. [130]	CVP vs	12	50	9	25
	sequential C-V-P	12	50		
Ezdinli et al. [211]	BP vs CP induction	77	25	36% at 1 yr	23
	BCVP vs CLB maintenance				
Bitran et al. [139]	COPP, COPA	11	81	87% at 1 yr	60% at 4 yrs
McKelvey et al. [147]	CHOP vs	38	68	60% at 2 yrs	75% at 1 yr
	HOP	38	55		
Skarin et al. [149]	BACOP	15	80	18	38
Canetta et al. [182]	CVP alternating	34	65	56% at 4 yrs (projected)	51% at 4 yrs (projected)
	with ABP				
Garrett et al. [184]	CTX-L2	14	50	NR (6/7 still in remission)	60% at 2 yrs (projected)
Young et al. [164]	CVP vs	8	13	9	30
	TBI	16	69	17	36
Harrison et al. [218]	CHOP(P)+TBI	28	82	56% at 2 yrs	—

CR = Complete Response; NR = Not Reached.

disease-free at 1 year. However, 84% of the complete responders were alive at 2 years, and they concluded that the achievement of complete remission was a significant determinant for improved survival. In a small series from the University of Chicago, which excluded lymphoblastic lymphomas from the DLPD group, Bitran et al. [139] reported on 11 patients (two of whom had diffuse mixed) treated with COPP (eight patients) or COPA (three patients). An 81% CR rate was noted with 87% of these patients disease-free at 3 years. Interestingly, 60% of all patients were alive at 4 years.

The more aggressive adriamycin-containing combinations have also been evaluated in this subtype. McKelvey et al. [147] randomized patients to either CHOP or HOP. Although the follow-up was short, both regimens were associated with improved CR group. However, these authors noted no significant diminution of the rate of relapse with time [217]. The remission duration curve for DLPD patients entered in SWOG studies demonstrated a higher rate of relapse earlier in the course of treatment. However, there was an indication of a gradual concave arc in the remission-duration curve, suggesting an impending plateau and possible cure in a small fraction of these patients. This projection must be confirmed by a longer period of observation.

Skarin et al. [149] evaluated the bleomycin-containing BACOP regimen in 15 patients with an impressive 80% complete response. Although the median duration of CR was 18 months, a plateau on the survival curve was observed. Median survival for the entire group was 38 months (58% of patients alive at 2 years), whereas 83% of complete responders survived 2 years from the initiation of treatment. Canetta et al. [182] investigated alternating 3-week course of CVP and ABP (adriamycin, bleomycin, prednisone) in 34 stage IV DLPD patients. Although their 65% CR rate is no better than has been previously noted, 56% of all patients were projected to be relapse-free at 4 years. Garrett et al. [184] treated 14 patients with a regimen used for acute lymphoblastic leukemia, the Memorial cyclophosphamide-L2 protocol. Fifty percent achieved a complete response with 6/7 of the CR group still free of disease with short follow-up. These authors did not specify whether any of their patients had the lymphoblastic subtype.

An alternative approach utilizing systemic total body irradiation (TBI) has been reported by Young et al. [164]. They randomized previously untreated stage III and IV DLPD patients to either CVP chemotherapy (eight patients) or to TBI (16 patients). The CR rate with chemotherapy was a disappointing 13% compared with 69% CR on the radiotherapy arm. However, 7/11 of the TBI-induced CR had pretreatment liver involvement which was not reassessed by repeat biopsy. Relapse-free survival was not impressive (median 17 months) and at 4 years after initial treatment, only 13% of the patients treated with radiotherapy remained in continuous unmaintained complete remission. The median survival for all patients treated with radiotherapy was

36 months, and there were no significant differences in either disease-free or overall survival between patients on the CVP or TBI arms.

More impressive results utilizing TBI have been reported by Harrison *et al.* [218] in a combined modality program for 28 patients with this histology. Four cycles of CHOP plus procarbazine were administered and 54% achieved a complete response after this phase of the study. Complete responders and good partial responders were then treated with TBI (150 rads given 10 rads 3 times weekly), plus concurrent non-myelosuppressive drugs (prednisone, vincristine, and bleomycin). At the end of this second radiotherapy-chemotherapy phase, 82% of patients were found to be in complete remission. However, the relapse-free survival of 56% at 2 years is no better than what has been projected by McKelvey *et al.* [147] or Canetta *et al.* [182] with chemotherapy alone. The occurrence of three CNS relapses during the first 6 months of treatment in stage IV patients with positive bone marrows raised the issue of prophylactic CNS treatment in future protocols. At the present time there does not seem to be a defined role for systemic or adjuvant radiotherapy in patients with DLPD.

2.2.7. Lymphoblastic Lymphoma. Lymphoblastic lymphoma is a recently defined distinct clinicopathologic entity characterized by immature lymphoid cells which are morphologically indistinguishable from the blast cells of acute lymphoblastic leukemia [219]. Predominantly a T-cell disease, it occurs primarily in adolescent males, but a recent retrospective review by Nathwani *et al.* [220] observed that lymphoblastic lymphoma occurred in all age groups (almost 50% of the 95 patients were more than 30 years old). Bone marrow involvement is noted at the time of presentation in 25–30% of patients and in 80% of cases during the course of the disease. Central nervous system relapses are frequently observed. Although complete responses to a variety of lymphoma-like chemotherapy regimens are common, relaspse, within 1 year is typical and overal survival is dismal. Recently, systemic chemotherapy programs of the type used for prognostically unfavorable childhood or adult acute lymphocytic leukemia have been proposed to treat adults with lymphoblastic lymphoma. Coleman *et al.* [221] in a Stanford pilot treated 14 adult patients with lymphoblastic lymphoma (median age 22) with an intensive chemotherapy program consisting of induction with cyclophosphamide, adriamycin, vincristine and prednisone (modified CHOP); consolidation and central nervous system prophylaxis with methotrexate intrathecally and by high-dose intravenous injection plus leucovorin rescue, and L-asparaginase. Reinforcement chemotherapy with CHOP was then administered followed by maintenance with 6-mercaptopurine and methotrexate. The overall treatment duration was 1 year. All patients had a rapid clinical complete response. Of the 13 patients without initial CNS disease, four have relapsed (three with primary CNS relapse and one with a recurrent abdominal mass). Four patients have died – two from drug toxicity, one from CNS relapse and one from chronic myelogenous leukemia which was diagnosed simultaneously with the lymphoblastic lymphoma. With a median follow-up of 17 months, the actuarial survival at 2 years is 67% and the relapse-free survival is 55%. This represented a marked improvement over the previous Stanford experience with pulse lymphoma-like chemotherapy in which almost 100% of the patients died during a similar period of follow-up. These results compare favorably to what has been observed from four pediatric groups [222–225]. However, it is difficult to draw precise comparisons between these non-randomized studies since the childhood non-Hodgkin's lymphomas are a heterogeneous group of histologies and presentations. The pilot study of Coleman et al. [221] demonstrates that an aggressive acute lymphocytic leukemia-like protocol may be successful in treating adult lymphoblastic lymphoma. Because high-dose methotrexate with leucovorin rescue failed to prevent CNS relapse in 3/13 patients, the Stanford investigators are now using early CNS prophylaxis with cranial irradiation and intrathecal methotrexate, while omitting high-dose systemic methotrexate. There is a clear need for additional clinical trials in this histology for the adult population utilizing an acute leukemia approach. The limited numbers of patients available for study, and the large number of unresolved questions (how best to prevent CNS relapse, role of radiotherapy for mediastinal masses, intensity of consolidation and maintenance regimens) mandate innovative clinical trials.

2.2.9. Central Nervous System Involvement. It is well-known that non-Hodgkin's lymphomas of diffuse histologies may involve the central nervous system (CNS) at initial diagnosis or, more commonly, during progression of the disease. Recently the question has been raised whether some form of CNS prophylactic therapy is required for those patients with unfavorable histologies who achieve a complete remission or, alternatively have unfavorable prognostic features placing them at higher risk for CNS relapse. However, lymphomatous involvement of the CNS is rare in the nodular lymphomas, and is also relatively uncommon in large retrospective reviews of the diffuse lymphomas. Johnson et al. [226] reviewed the ECOG experience in 289 patients with stage III and IV unfavorable histologies entered in two consecutive ECOG trials from 1974 to 1980. All patients were treated with aggressive combination chemotherapy regimens. CNS involvement occurred in 7/159 patients with DH, 5/70 DLPD, and 3/11 diffuse undifferentiated lymphomas. The overall incidence of CNS lymphoma was 5.5%. Bone marrow involvement was present at diagnosis in 85 patients, but only five of these eventually developed CNS lymphoma. Conversely, 5/16 patients who developed CNS lymphoma had initial bone marrow involvement, but none of these patients achieved a complete remission with chemotherapy.

Although some investigators have reported a rate of CNS involvement as high as 28% [149], Sweet et al. [200] found an incidence of 8.4% in a collection of 514 DH patients reported in the literature. This also confirmed the Stanford experience [227], in which only 7% of DH patients had CNS disease at any time in their course. All investigators noted that CNS lymphoma occurs predominantly in patients with systemic progression or relapse during therapy, and that CNS involvement as a sole site of relapse is distinctly uncommon. Failure to achieve complete remission with systemic chemotherapy is the major risk factor for CNS disease, but bone marrow involvement at the time of diagnosis has also been recognized as an unfavorable feature [228, 229].

Recently, attempts have been made to design systemic combination chemotherapy regimens including high-dose methotrexate or cytosine arabinoside since both these agents penetrate the blood brain barrier. Herman et al. [230] administered maintenance chemotherapy to patients with all histologic subtypes of non-Hodgkin's lymphomas who achieved a complete remission with induction chemotherapy. They noted that maintenance with vincristine, prednisone, and parenteral cytosine arabinoside appeared to substantially reduce the incidence of late CNS relapse compared to maintenance treatment with oral cyclophosphamide in place of cytosine arabinoside. Sweet et al. [189] observed only one relapse in 42 DH patients receiving COMLA. They attributed this low rate of CNS relapse to the use of both methotrexate and Ara-C. However, the numbers of patients are small, and only six had bone marrow or bone involvement and were at high risk for this complication.

Skarin et al. [231] evaluated high-dose methotrexate ($1-7.5 \text{ g/m}^2$) with leucovorin rescue in six patients with CNS relapse with five responses (three had complete disappearance of CNS disease and one remained in remission 14+ months). These investigators then incorporated a 3 g/m^2 dose of methotrexate into the M-BACOD regimen for advanced stages of diffuse histiocytic or diffuse undifferentiated lymphoma [192]. Although an 80% complete response rate with the M-BACOD regimen was reported, two patients developed CNS lymphoma during the tenth cycle of therapy and one additional patient relapsed in the CNS. Thus, the incidence of CNS disease in this study is 6% with limited follow-up, and the conclusion that high-dose methotrexae may reduce CNS relapse appears unwarranted at present.

Prophylactic CNS therapy does not appear indicated for all patients with histologies of the non-Hodgkin's lymphomas. As has been discussed, it is certainly indicated as part of the initial management for patients with lymphoblastic lymphoma. In other unfavorable histologies the role of CNS therapy needs to be carefully evaluated only in those patients in whom control of their peripheral disease has been achieved with induction chemotherapy. Those patients with advanced diffuse lymphoma who have initial bone marrow involvement and achieve complete remission of their systemic disease are at higher risk for CNS involvement. It is in these patients that a controlled trial of CNS prophylaxis is clearly indicated.

2.2.9. Summary. Although the unfavorable histology non-Hodgkin's lymphomas have a poorer prognosis than their nodular counterparts, recent advances in chemotherapy have made it possible to achieve prolonged relapse-free survival for a significant number of these patients. The goal of any therapeutic program must be the achievement of a restaged complete remission, because the survival of patients with partial responses closely parallels that of non-responding patients and is significantly inferior to that seen in the CR group. The strategy in treating the diffuse histologies must be to improve the complete remission rate, since it is only this subgroup which is offered the possibility of cure.

There are six combination chemotherapy regimens which are capable of attaining complete remissions in 50–80% of patients with advanced diffuse histiocytic lymphoma: C-MOPP, CHOP, BACOP, CPOB, COMLA, and M-BACOD. Each of these combinations is capable of potentially curing approximately 50% of DH patients. No one regimen can be regarded as significantly superior in terms of complete remission rates, disease-free or overall survival given differences in patient selection and prognostic factors. Few prospective clinical trials have been initiated to compare these effective regimens with each other. Although adriamycin is an extremely active agent, three of these regimens (C-MOPP, CPOB, and COMLA) do not contain adriamycin, yet appear equally effective for DH. The comparison of these clinical studies has been hindered by the fact that histologic and immunologic subsets of histiocytic lymphoma may respond very differently to therapy. Future clinical trials must stratify patients not only by important clinical prognostic parameters such as bone marrow involvement, but also by immunologic and morphologic subgroups.

The recent advances in the chemotherapeutic management of patients with advanced histiocytic lymphoma has led to the application of chemotherapy for localized diffuse lymphomas as well. The use of primary chemotherapy for stage I and II diffuse lymphomas is an attractive approach because it avoids the necessity for strict pathologic staging which may be hazardous in the elderly patient. In addition, a significant proportion of patients develop progressive disease outside of radiotherapy ports while undergoing initial treatment with this modality, Thus, patients with stage II disease should be treated with initial systemic chemotherapy. Localized stage I disease probably should be treated by initial radiotherapy alone, with chemotherapy reserved for the small percentage of patients who relapse. However, stage I patients with unfavorable prognostic factors may benefit from the use of adjuvant chemotherapy following definitive radiation or from initial chemo-therapy followed by adjuvant radiotherapy.

Although there is a paucity of data concerning the mangement of patients with nodular histiocytic or diffuse mixed histiocytic-lymphocytic lylphoma, these histologic subtypes should be treated with similar aggressive combination chemotherapy regimens as are used for diffuse histiocytic lymphoma. The goal for these patients should be the induction of a restaged complete remission, as the potential for long-term relapse-free survival exists.

Until recently, patients with diffuse lymphocytic poorly differentiated lymphoma were regarded as having an aggressive histology and an unfavorable prognosis. Current studies have demonstrated that the B-cell subset of DLPD may have a survival pattern similar to that of NLPD. The term DLPD does not account for the wide spectrum of differentiation and variable prognosis of this heterogeneous subtype, which has also included in the past the T-cell lymphoblastic lymphomas. Aggressive adriamycin-containing combinations are definitely indicated for DLPD patients with non-B-cell disorders. There is a clear need for a controlled trial of aggressive versus non-aggressive chemotherapy for patients with diffuse cleaved cell lymphomas of B-cell origin. Lymphoblastic lymphoma is a discrete clinicopathologic entity and should be treated utilizing a similar approach as for prognostically unfavorable childhood acute lymphocytic leukemia. Early central nervous system prophylaxis and intensive induction, consolidation, and maintenance chemotherapy offer the potential for prolonged relapse-free survival in adult lymphoblastic lymphoma.

Prophylactic central nervous system therapy does not appear indicated for all patients with unfavorable histologies. Those patients with advanced diffuse lymphoma who have initial bone marrow involvement and achieve complete remission of their systemic disease are at higher risk for CNS involvement. However, CNS relapse as the sole site of failure is distinctly uncommon. The role of prophylactic CNS therapy needs to be carefully evaluated only in those patients in whom control of their peripheral disease has been achieved with induction chemotherpay.

Thus, although the unfavorable histology non-Hodgkin's lymphomas are considered to have a poorer prognosis and a short median survival, a curative strategy is possible for a significant portion of these patients.

APPENDIX: ABBREVIATIONS AND ACRONYMS OF DRUG COMBINATIONS

ABDIC: adriamycin, bleomycin, DTIC, CCNU, and prednisone
ABVD: adriamycin, bleomycin, vinblastine, and DTIC
BACOP: bleomycin, adriamycin, cyclophosphamide, vincristine, and prednisone
B-CAVe: bleomycin, CCNU, adriamycin, and vinblastine
BCG: Bacillus Calmette-Guérin
BCNU: 1,3-bis(2-chloroethyl)-1-nitrosourea

BCVP: BCNU, cyclophosphamide, vincristine, and prednisone
BCVPP: BCNU, cyclophosphamide, vinblastine, procarbazine and prednisone
B-DOPA: bleomycin, DTIC, vincristine, prednisone, and adiamycin
BOP: BCNU, vincristine, and prednisone
BOPP: BCNU, vincristine, procarbazine, and prednisone
BVDS: bleomycin, vinblastine, adriamycin, and streptozotocin
BVPP: BCNU, vincristine, procarbazine, and prednisone
CCNU: 1-(2-chloroethyl)-3-cyclohexyl-1-nitrosourea
CCNU-CVPP: CCNU, cyclophosphamide, vinblastine, procarbazine, and prednisone
CCNU-OPP: CCNU, vincristine, procarbazine, and prednisone
CCNU-VPP: CCNU, vinblastine, procarbazine, and prednisone
CHOP: cyclophosphamide, adriamycin, vincristine, and prednisone
CHOP-Bleo: cyclophosphamide, adriamycin, vincristine, prednisone, and bleomycin
CHOP(P): cyclophosphamide, adriamycin, vincristine, prednisone, and procarbazine
CLB: chlorambucil
CHlVPP: chlorambucil, vinblastine, procarbazine, and prednisone
CP: cyclophosphamide and prednisone
COMLA (COMA): cyclophosphamide, vincristine, methotrexate with leucovorin, and cytosine
    arabinoside
COP-Bleo: cyclophosphamide, vincristine, prednisone, and bleomycin
COPP (C-MOPP): cyclophosphamide, vincristine, procarbazine and prednisone
COPB: cyclophosphamide, vincristine, prednisone, and bleomycin
CPOB: cyclophosphamide, prednisone and day 15 vincristine and bleomycin
CTX: cyclophosphamide
CVP(COP): cyclophosphamide, vincristine, and prednisone
CVPP: cyclophosphamide, vinblastine, procarbazine and prednisone
DTIC: 5-(3,5-dimethyl-1-triazino) imidazole-4-carboxamide
HOP: adriamycin, vincristine, and prednisone
HN_2: nitrogen mustard
MABOP: nitrogen mustard, adriamycin, bleomycin, vincristine, and prednisone
M-BACOD: high-dose methotrexate with leucovorin, bleomycin, adriamycin, cyclophospham-
    ide, vincristine, and dexamethasone
MOP: nitrogen mustard, vincristine, and procarbazine
MOPP: nitrogen mustard, vincristine, procarbazine, and prednisone
MOPP-HDB: nitrogen mustard, vincristine, procarbazine, prednisone, and high-dose bleomy-
    cin
MOPP-LDB: nitrogen mustard, vincristine, procarbazine, prednisone, and low-dose bleomy-
    cin
MVPP: nitrogen mustard, vinblastine, procarbazine and prednisone
MVVPP: nitrogen mustard, vinblastine, vincristine, procarbazine, and prednisone
OPP: vincristine, procarbazine, and prednisone
PAVe: procarbazine, phenylalanine mustard, and vinblastine
ProMACE: cyclophosphamide, adriamycin, VP-16, prednisone, and high-dose methotrexate
    with leucovorin
SCAB: streptozotocin, CCNU, adriamycin, and bleomycin
VPBCPr: vincristine, prednisone, vinblastine, chlorambucil, and procarbazine

ACKNOWLEDGEMENTS

The author acknowledges the permission of Charles A. Coltman, JR.,
M.D. to use the format at the tables from his review in Seminars in Oncology

7: 155–173, 1980. The invaluable secretarial assistance of Deborah Altieri is gratefully acknowledged.

REFERENCES

1. Coltman CA: Chemotherapy of advanced Hodgkin's disease. Semin Oncol 7:155–173, 1980.
2. Goodman LS, Wintrobe MM, Dameshek W, et al.: Nitrogen mustard therapy. JAMA 132:126–132, 1946.
3. Karnofsky DA, Craver LF, Rhoads CP, Abels JC: An evaluation of methyl-bis-(B-chloroethyl)amine hydrochloride and tris-(B-chloroethyl)amine hydrochloride (nitrogen mustards) in the treatment of lymphomas, leukemia, and allied diseases. In: Approaches to tumor chemotherapy. Washington, DC: Am Assoc for the Advancement of Science, 1947, pp 319–337.
4. Zanes RP, Doan CA, Hoster HA: Studies in Hodgkin's syndrome. VII. Nitrogen mustard therapy. J Lab Clin Med 33:1002–1018, 1948.
5. Carter SK, Livingston RB: Single-agent therapy for Hodgkin's disease. Arch Intern Med 131:377–387, 1973.
6. Huguley CM JR, Durant JR, Moores RR, et al.: A comparison of nitrogen mustard, vincristine, procarbazine and prednisone (MOPP) vs nitrogen mustard in advanced Hodgkin's disease. Cancer 36:1227–1240, 1975.
7. Carbone PP, Spurr C, Schneiderman M, et al.: Management of patients with malignant lymphoma: a comparative study with cyclophosphamide and vinca alkaloids. Cancer Res 28:811–822, 1968.
8. Desser RK, Ultmann JE: The sensitivity of Hodgkin's disease to chemotherapeutic agents administered singly. Ser Haematol 6:152–181, 1973.
9. Stutzman L, Ezdinli EZ, Stutzman MA: Vinblastine sulfate versus cyclophosphamide in the therapy for lymphoma. JAMA 195:173–178, 1966.
10. Stolinsky J, Pugh RP, Stevens AR, et al.: Clinical experience with procarbazine in Hodgkin's disease, reticulum cell sarcoma, and lymphosarcoma. Cancer 26:984–990, 1970.
11. Lessner HE: BCNU 1,3-bis(2-chloroethyl)-1-nitrosourea: effects on advanced Hodgkin's disease and other neoplasia. Cancer 22:451–456, 1968.
12. Young RC, DeVita VT Jr, Serpick AA, Canellos GP: Treatment of advanced Hodgkin's disease with 1,3 bis(2-chloroethyl)-1-nitrosourea) BCNU. NEJM 285:475–479, 1971.
13. Katz ME, Glick JH: Nitrosoureas: a reappraisal of clinical trials. Cancer Clin Trials 2:297–316, 1979.
14. Selarwy OS, Hansen HH: Superiority of CCNU (1-(2-chlorethyl)-3-cyclohexyl-1-nitrosourea; NSC 79037) over BCNU 1,3-bis (2-chloroethyl)-1-nitrosourea; NSC 409962) in treatment of advanced Hodgkin's disease. Proc AACR 13:46, 1972.
15. Blum RH, Carter SK, Agre K: A clinical review of bleomycin: a new antineoplastic agent. Cancer 31:903–914, 1972.
16. Haas CD, Coltman CA Jr, Gottlieb JA, et al.: Phase II evaluation of bleomycin. Cancer 38:8–12, 1976.
17. Yagoda A, Mukherji B, Young C, et al.: Bleomycin: an antitumor antibiotic. Ann Intern Med 77:861–870, 1972.
18. Blum RH, Carter SK: Adriamycin: a new anticancer drug with significant clinical activity. Ann Intern Med 80:249–259, 1974.
19. Gottlieb JA, Gutterman JV, McCreedie KB, et al.: Chemotherapy of malignant lymphoma with adriamycin. Cancer Res 33:3224–3228, 1973.

20. Luce JK: Personal communication, 1980.
21. Frei E III, Luce JK, Talley RW, Vaitkevicius VK, Wilson HE: 5-(3,3-dimethyl-1-triazeno) immidazole-4-carboxamide (NSC-45388) in the treatment of lymphoma. Cancer Chemother Rep, Part I 56:667-670, 1972.
22. DeVita VT Jr, Lewis BJ, Rozencweig M, Muggia FM: The chemotherapy of Hodgkin's disease: past experience and future directions. Cancer 42:979-990, 1978.
23. Lacher MU, Durant JR: Combined vinblastine and chlorambucil therapy of Hodgkin's disease. Ann Intern Med 62:468-476, 1965.
24. Moxley JH, DeVita VT, Brace K, et al.: Intensive combination chemotherapy and x-irradiation in Hodgkin's disease. Cancer Res 27:1258-1263, 1967.
25. DeVita VT, Canellos GP, Moxley JH: A decade of combination chemotherapy of advanced Hodgkin's disease. Cancer 30:1495-1504, 1972.
26. Luce JK, Gamble JF, Wilson HE, et al.: Combined cyclophosphamide, vincristine, and prednisone therapy of malignant lymphoma. Cancer 28:307-317, 1971.
27. Lenhard RE: Eastern Cooperative Oncology Group Studies. Arch Intern Med 131:418-420, 1973.
28. DeVita VT Jr, Serpick AA, Carbone PP: Combination chemotherapy in the treatment of advanced Hodgkin's disease. Ann Intern Med 73:881-895, 1970.
29. DeVita VT Jr, Simon RM, Hubbard SM, Young RC, Berard CW, Moxley JH, Frei E III, Carbone PP, Canellos GP: Curability of advanced Hodgkin's disease with chemotherapy. Ann Intern Med 92:587-595, 1980.
30. Young RC, Canellos GP, Chabner BA, et al.: Maintenance chemotherapy for advanced Hodgkin's disease in remission. Lancet 2:1339-1343, 1973.
31. Young RC, DeVita VT: Chemotherapy of Hodgkin's disease. Clin Haematol 8:625-644, 1979.
32. Herman TA, Jones SE: Systematic restaging in patients with Hodgkin's disease. Cancer 42:1976-1982, 1978.
33. Gibbs G, Bloomfield CD, Peterson BA, et al.: Therapy of Hodgkin's disease with cyclophosphamide, vinblastine, procarbazine, prednisone: 5-year follow-up. Proc AACR 20:101, 1979.
34. Bakemeier R: Personal communication, 1980.
35. Canellos GP, Young RC, DeVita VT: Combination chemotherapy for advanced Hodgkin's disease in relapse following extensive radiotherapy. Clin Pharm Therap 13:750-754, 1972.
36. Frei E III, Luce JK, Gamble JF, et al.: Combination chemotherapy in advanced Hodgkin's disease: induction and maintenance of remission. Ann Intern Med 79:376-382, 1973.
37. Moore MR, Jones SE, Bull JM, et al.: MOPP chemotherapy for advanced Hodgkin's disease: prognostic factors in 81 patients. Cancer 32:52-60, 1973.
38. Sutcliffe SB, Wrigley PRM, Peto J, et al.: MVPP chemotherapy regimen for advanced Hodgkin's disease. Br Med J 1:679-683, 1978.
39. Durant JR, Gams RA, Velez-Garcia E, et al.: BCNU, velban, cyclophosphamide, procarbazine and prednisone (BVCPP) in advanced Hodgkin's disease. Cancer 42:2101-2110, 1978.
40. Lowenbraum S, DeVita VT, Serpick AA: Combination chemotherapy with nitrogen mustard, vincristine, procarbazine, and prednisone in previously treated patients with Hodgkin's disease. Blood 36:704-717, 1970.
41. Bakemaier RF, Costello WG, Horton J, et al.: Chemoimmunotherapy of Hodgkin's disease. Proc ASCO 20:392, 1979.
42. Nissen NI, Pajak TF, Glidewell O, et al.: A comparative study of a BCNU containing 4-drug versus MOPP versus 3-drug combinations in advanced Hodgkin's disease: a cooperative study by the Cancer and Leukemia Group B. Cancer 43:31-40, 1979.
43. Ziegler JL, Bluming AZ, Fass L, et al.: Chemotherapy of childhood Hodgkin's disease in

Uganda. Lancet 2:679–680, 1972.

44. Olweny CLM, Katongole-Mbidde E, Kiire C, Lwanga SK, Magrath I, Ziegler JL: Childhood Hodgkin's disease in Uganda: a ten-year experience. Cancer 42: 787–792, 1978.

45. Coltman CA Jr, Frei E III, Delaney FC: Effectiveness of actinomycin, methotrexate and vinblastine in prolonging the duration of combination chemotherapy (MOPP) induced remission in advanced Hodgkin's disease. Proc ASCO 9:78, 1973.

46. Nissen NI, Stutzman L, Holland JF, et al.: Chemotherapy of Hodgkin's disease in studies by Acute Leukemia Group B. Arch Intern Med 13:396–401, 1973.

47. Coltman CA JR, Jones SE, Grozea PN, et al.: Bleomycin in combination with MOPP for the management of Hodgkin's disease: Southwest Oncology Group experience. In: Bleomycins – current status and new developments, Carter SK, Crooke ST, Umezawa H, eds. New York: Academic, 1978, pp227–242.

48. Nixon DW, Aisenberg AC: Combination chemotherapy of Hodgkin's disease. Cancer 33:1499–1504, 1974.

49. British National Lymphoma Investigation: Value of prednisone in combination chemotherapy of stage IV Hodgkin's disease. Br Med J 3:413–414, 1975.

50. Jacobs C, Portlock CS, Rosenberg: Prednisone in MOPP chemotherapy for Hodgkin's disease. Br Med J 2:1469–1471, 1976.

51. Castellino RA, Glatstein E, Turbow MM, et al.: Latent radiation injury of lungs or heart activated by steroid withdrawal. Ann Intern Med 80:593–599, 1974.

52. Stutzman L, Glidewell O: Multiple chemotherapeutic agents for Hodgkin's disease. Comparison of three routines: a cooperative study by Acute Leukemia Group B. JAMA 225:1202–1211, 1973.

53. Cooper RM, Pagak TF, Nissen NI, et al.: A new effective four-drug combination of CCNU, vinblastine, prednisone, and procarbazine for the treatment of advanced Hodgkin's disease. Cancer 46:654–662, 1980.

54. Durant JR, Gams RA, Velez-Garcia E, et al.: BCNU, Velban, cyclophosphamide, procarbazine, and prednisone (BCVPP) in advanced Hodgkin's disease. Cancer 42:2101–2110, 1978.

55. Morgenfeld M, Somoza N, Magnasco J, et al.: Combined chemotherapy cyclophosphamide, vinblastine, procarbazine and prednisone (CVPP) vs CVPP plus CCNU (CCVPP) in Hodgkin's disease. Cancer 43:1579–1586, 1979.

56. Bloomfield CD, Weiss, RB, Fortuny I et al.: Combined chemotherapy with cyclophosphamide, vinblastine, procarbazine and prednisone (CVPP) for patients with advanced Hodgkin's disease. Cancer 38:42–48, 1976.

57. Diggs CH, Wiernik PH, Levi JA, Kvols LK: Cyclophosphamide, vinblastine, procarbazine and prednisone with CCNU and vinblastine maintenance for advanced Hodgkin's disease. Cancer 39:1949–1954, 1977.

58. McElwain TJ, Toy J, Smith E, et al.: A combination of chlorambucil, vinblastine, procarbazine and prednisone for treatment of Hodgkin's disease. Br J Cancer 36:276–280, 1977.

59. Nicholson WM, Beard MEV, Crowther D, et al.: Combination chemotherapy in generalized Hodgkin's disease. Br Med J 3:7–10, 1970.

60. Glick JH: Personal communication, 1980.

61. Gams RA, Durant JR, Omura GA, Bartolucci AA: Remission duration and survival in advanced Hodgkin's disease: the influence of bleomycin and alternating non-cross-resistant combination chemotherapy. Blood (Suppl 1) 54:187A, 1979.

62. Jones SE, Fisher RJ, Jones J, Coltman CA: Improved remission induction chemotherapy for patients with advanced Hodgkin's disease: a Southwest Oncology Group study. Proc ASCO 21:464, 1980.

63. Coltman CA Jr, Frei E III, Moon RE: MOPP maintenance (MM) vs (VMR) for MOPP

induced complete remission (CR) of advanced Hodgkin's disease (HD). Proc ASCO 17:300, 1976.

64. Durant JR, Bartolucci A, Gams RA, Dorfman RF, Velez-Garcia E: Southeastern cancer study group trials with nitrosoureas in Hodgkin's disease. Cancer Treat Rep 60:781-787, 1976.

65. Fisher RI, DeVita VT, Hubbard SP, Simon R, Young RC: Prolonged disease-free survival in Hodgkin's disease with MOPP reinduction after first relapse. Ann Intern Med 90:761-763, 1979.

66. Kaplan HS: Hodgkin's disease, 2nd edn. Cambridge, Mass.: Harvard University Press, 1980.

67. Goldman JM, Dawson AA: Combination therapy for advanced resistant Hodgkin's disease. Lancet 2:1225-1227, 1975.

68. Lokich JJ, Frei E III, Jaffe N, Tullis J: New multiple agent chemotherapy (B-DOPA) for advanced Hodgkin's disease. Cancer 38:667-671, 1976.

69. Vinciguerra V, Coleman M, Jarowski CI, et al.: A new combination chemotherapy for resistant Hodgkin's disease. JAMA 237:33-36, 1977.

70. Levi JA, Wiernik PH, Diggs CH: Combination chemotherapy of advanced previously treated Hodgkin's disease with streptozotocin, CCNU, adriamycin and bleomycin. Med Pediat Oncol 3:33-40, 1977.

71. Porzig KJ, Portlock CS, Robertson A, et al.: Treatment of advanced Hodgkin's disease with B-Cave following MOPP failure. Cancer 41:1670-1675, 1978.

72. Rodgers RW, Gamble JF, Loh KK, Shullenberger CC: Adriamycin, bleomycin, DIC, CCNU, and prednisone(ABDIC) chemotherapy in MOPP-resistant Hodgkin's disease. Cancer 46:2349-2355, 1980.

73. Warren RD, Bender RA, Norton L, Young RC: The treatment of combination chemotherapy-resistant Hodgkin's disease with single-agent vinblastine. Am J Hematol 4:47-55, 1978.

74. Santoto A, Bonadonna G: Prolonged disease-free survival in MOPP-resistant Hodgkin's disease after treatment with adriamycin, bleomycin, vinblastine and dacarbazine (ABVD). Cancer chemother Pharmacol 2:101-105, 1979.

75. Case DC Jr, Young CW, Lee BJ III: Combination chemotherapy of MOPP-resistant Hodgkin's disease with adriamycin, bleomycin, dacarbazine and vinblastine (ABVD). Cancer 39:1382-1386, 1977.

76. Krikorian JG, Portlock CS, Rosenberg SA: Treatment of advanced Hodgkin's disease with adriamycin, bleomycin, vinblastine and imidazole carboxamide (ABVD) after failure of MOPP therapy. Cancer 41:2107-2111, 1978.

77. Bonadonna G, Zucali R, Monfardino S, et al.: Combination chemotherapy of Hodgkin's disease with adriamycin, bleomycin, vinblastine and imidazole carboxamide versus MOPP. Cancer 36:252-259, 1975.

78. Santoro A, Bonadonna G, Bonfante V, Valagussa P: Non-cross-resistant regimens (MOPP and ABVD) vs MOPP alone in stage IV Hodgkin's disease. Proc ASCO 21:470, 1980.

79. Straus DJ, Myers J, Pass S et al.: The eight-drug/radiation therapy program (MOPP/ABDV/RT) for advanced Hodgkin's disease: a follow-up report. Cancer 46:233-240, 1980.

80. Bonadonna G, Santoro A, Bonfante V: Salvage chemotherapy with ABVD in MOPP-resistant Hodgkin's disease. Proc ASCO 22:522, 1981.

81. Johnson RE, Thomas LB, Schneiderman M, et al.: Preliminary experience with total nodal irradiation in Hodgkin's disease. Radiology 96:603-608, 1970.

82. Young RC, Canellos GP, Chabner BA, et al.: Patterns of relapse in advanced Hodgkin's disease treated with combination chemotherapy. Cancer 42:1001-1007, 1978.

83. Rosenberg SA, Kaplan HS, Brown BW Jr: The role of adjuvant MOPP in the therapy of Hodgkin's disease: an analysis after ten years. In: Adjuvant therapy of cancer II, Jones SE,

Samon SE, eds. New York: Grune & Stratton, 1979, pp 119–127.

84. De Lena M, Monfardini S, Beretta G, et al.: Clinical trials with intensive chemotherapy and radiotherapy and radiotherapy in Hodgkin's disease. International Symposium on Hodgkin's disease. NCI Monogr 36:403–420, 1972.

85. Kun LE, DeVita VT, Young RC, Johnson RE: Treatment of Hodgkin's disease using intensive chemotherapy followed by irradiation. Int J Radiat Oncol Biol Phys 1:619–626, 1976.

86. Rosenberg SA, Kaplan HS, Glatstein EJ, Portlock CS: Combined modality therapy of Hodgkin's disease: a report on the Stanford trials. Cancer 42:991–1000, 1978.

87. Prosnitz LR, Farber LR, Fisher JJ,: Long-term remission with combined modality therapy for advanced Hodgkin's disease. Cancer 37: 2826–2833, 1976.

88. Farber FR, Prosnitz LR, Cadman ED, et al.: Curative potential of combined modality therapy for advanced Hodgkin's disease. Cancer 46:1509–1517, 1980.

89. Bonadonna G, Santoro A, Zucali R, Valagussa P: Improved 5-year survival in advanced Hodgkin's disease by combined modality approach. Cancer Clin Trials 2:217–226, 1979.

90. Bergsagel D, Basco V, Bush R, et al.: Trial of MOPP alone versus MOPP and radiotherapy for advanced Hodgkin's disease. Proc ASCO 21:464, 1980.

91. Hoppe RT, Portlock CS, GlatsteinE, et al.: Alternating chemotherapy and irradiation in the treatment of advanced Hodgkin's disease. Cancer 43:472–481, 1979.

92. Goodman R, Mauch P, Piro A, et al.: Stages IIB and IIIB Hodgkin's Disease, results of combined modality treatment, Cancer 90:84–89, 1977.

93. Santoro A, Bonadonna G, Zucali R et al.: Therapeutic and toxicologic effects of MOPP vs ABVD when combined with RT in Hodgkin's disease. Proc ASCO 22:522, 1981.

94. Coleman CN, Williams CJ, Flint A, et al.: Hematologic neoplasia in patients treated for Hodgkin's disease. NEJM 297:1249–1252, 1977.

95. Prosnitz LR, Montalvo RL, Fischer DB: Treatment of stage IIIA Hodgkin's disease: is radiotherapy alone adequate? Int J Radiat Oncol Biol Phys 4:781–787, 1978.

96. British National Lymphoma Investigation: Initial treatment of stage IIIA Hodgkin's disease: comparison of radiotherapy with combined chemotherapy. Lancet 2:991–995, 1976.

97. Mauch P, Goodman R, Rosenthal DS, et al.: An evaluation of total nodal irradiation as treatment for stage IIIA Hodgkin's disease. Cancer 43:1255–1261, 1979.

98. Stein RS, Golomb HM, Diggs CH, et al.: Anatomic substages of stage IIIA Hodgkin's disease: a collaborative study. Ann Intern Med 92:159–165, 1980.

99. Timothy AR, Sutcliffe SBJ, Lister A, et al.: The management of stage IIIA Hodgkin's disease. Int J Radiat Oncol Biol Phys 6:135–142, 1980.

100. Hoppe RT, Rosenberg SA, Kaplan HS, Cox RS: Prognostic factors in pathological stage IIIA Hodgkin's disease. Cancer 46:1240–1246, 1980.

101. Portlock CS, Rosenberg SA, Glatstein E, Kaplan HS: Impact of salvage treatment on initial relapses in patients with Hodgkin's disease, stage I–III. Blood 51:825–833, 1978.

102. DeVita VT: The role of combined modality therapy in the treatment of stage IIIA Hodgkin's disease. Int J Radiat Oncol Biol Phys 5:913–914 (letter), 1979.

103. Glick JH: The role of combined modality therapy in the treatment of stage IIIA Hodgkin's disease. Int J Radiat Oncol Biol Phys 5:914 (letter), 1979.

104. Grozea PN, DePersio EJ, Fisher RJ, et al.: Chemotherapy versus chemotherapy plus radiotherapy for stage III Hodgkin's disease. Proc AACR 20:119, 1979.

105. Desser RK, Golomb HM, Ultmann JE, et al.: Prognostic classification of Hodgkin disease in pathologic stage III, based on anatomic considerations. Blood 49:883–893, 1977.

106. Levi JA, Wiernik PH: The therapeutic implications of splenic involvement in stage IIIA Hodgkin's disease. Cancer 39:2158–2165, 1977.

107. Stein RS, Hilborn RM, Glexner JM, et al.: Anatomical substages of stage III Hodgkin's

disease. Cancer 42:429–436, 1978.

108. Hellman S, Mauch P, Goodman RL, *et al.*: The place of radiation therapy in the treatment of Hodgkin's disease. Cancer 42:971–978, 1978.

109. Moore MR, Bull JM, Jones SE, *et al.*: Sequential radiotherapy and chemotherapy in the treatment of Hodgkin's disease: a progress report. Ann Intern Med 77:1–9, 1972.

110. Rosenberg SA, Kaplan HS, Brown BW: The role of adjuvant MOPP in the therapy of Hodgkin's disease: an analysis after ten years. In: Adjuvant therapy of cancer II, Jones SE, Salmon SE, eds: New York: Grune & Stratton 1979, pp 109–117.

111. Hoppe RT, Rosenberg SA, Kaplan HS, Glatstein E: The treatment of Hodgkin's disease stage I-IIA – subtotal lymphoid irradiation vs involved field irradiation plus adjuvant MOP(P). In: Adjuvant therapy of cancer II, Jones SE, Salmon SE, eds: New York: Grune & Stratton 1979, pp 137–144.

112. Coltman CA Jr, Fuller LA, Fisher R, Frei E: Extended field radiotherapy versus involved field radiotherapy plus MOPP in stage I and II Hodgkin's disease. In: Adjuvant therapy of cancer II, Jones SE, Salmon SE, eds. New York: Grune & Stratton, 1979, pp 129–136.

113. Wiernik PH, Gustafson J Schimpff SC, Diggs C: Combined modality treatment of Hodgkin's disease confined to lymph nodes: results eight years later. Am J Med 67:183–193, 1979.

114. Arseneau JC, Sponzo RW, Levin DL, Schnipper LR, Bonner H, Young RC, Canellos GP, Johnson RE, DeVita VT: Nonlymphomatous malignant tumors complicating Hodgkin's disease: possible association with intensive therapy. NEJM 287:1119–1122, 1972.

115. Toland DM, Coltman CA, Moon TE: Second malignancies complicating Hodgkin's disease: the Southwest Oncology Group experience. Cancer Clin Trials 1:27–33, 1978.

116. Krikorian JG, Burke JA, Rosenberg SA, Kaplan HS: Occurrence of non-Hodgkin's lymphoma after therapy for Hodgkin's disease. NEJM 300:452–458, 1979.

117. Mauch P, Goodman R, Hellman S: The significance of mediastinal involvement in early stage Hodgkin's disease. Cancer 42:1039–1045, 1978.

118. Hoppe RT, Coleman CN, Kaplan HS, Rosenberg SA: Hodgkin's disease pathologic stage I-II: the prognostic importance of initial sites of disease and extent of mediastinal involvement. Proc ASCO 21:471, 1980.

119. Mauch P, Hellman S: Supradiaphragmatic Hodgkin's disease: is there a role for MOPP chemotherapy in patients with bulky mediastinal disease? Int J Radiat Oncol Biol Phys 6:947–949, 1980.

120. Coltman CA Jr, Fuller LM: Patterns of relapse in localized (stage I and II) Hodgkin's disease (HD) following extended field radiotheraoy (EFXRT) vs involved field radiotherapy (IFXRT) plus MOPP. Blood 50:188, 1977.

121. Levi JA, Wiernik PH, O'Connell MJ: Patterns of relapse in stages I, II, and IIIA Hodgkin's disease: influence of initial therapy and implications for the future. Int J Radiat Oncol Biol Phys 2:853–862, 1977.

122. Jones SE, Butler JJ, Byrne GE JR, Coltman CA JR, Moon TE: Histopathologic review of Lymphoma cases from the Southwest Oncology Group. Cancer 39:1071–1076, 1977.

123. Ezdinli EZ, Costello W, Wasser LP, Lenhard RE, Berard CW, Hartsock R, Bennett JM, Carbone PP: Eastern Cooperative Oncology Group experience with the Rappaport classification of non-Hodgkin's lymphomas. Cancer 43:544–550, 1979.

124. Rosenberg SA: Non-Hodgkin's lymphoma – selection of treatment on the basis of histologic type. NEJM 301:924–928, 1979.

125. Portlock CS: Management of the indolent non-Hodgkin's lymphomas. Semin Oncol 7:292–301, 1980.

126. Gold G, Salvin LG, Shnider BI: A comparative study with 3 alkylating agents: mechloroethamine, cyclophosphamide, and uracil mustard. Cancer Chemother Rep 16:417–419, 1962.

127. Jones SE, Rosenberg SA, Kaplan ES, Kadin ME, Dorfman RF: Non-Hodgkin's lympho-

mas: single-agent chemotherapy. Cancer 30:31–38, 1972.

128. Portlock CS, Rosenberg SA: Chemotherapy of non-Hodgkin's lymphomas: the Stanford Experience. Cancer Treat Rep 61:1049–1055, 1977.

129. Lister TA, Cullen MH, Beard ME, Brearley RL, Whitehouse JM, Wrigley PF, Stansfeld AG, Sutcliffe SB, Malpas JS, Crowther D: Comparison of combined and single-agent chemotherapy in non-Hodgkin's lymphoma of favourable histological type. Br Med J 1:533–537, 1978.

130. Kennedy BJ, Bloomfield CD, Kiang DT, Vosika G, Peterson BA, Theologides A: Combination versus successive single agent chemotherapy in lymphocytic lymphoma. Cancer 41:23–28, 1978.

131. Kofman S, Perlin CP, Boesen E, et al.: The role of corticosteroids in the treatment of malignant lymphoma. Cancer 15:338–345, 1962.

132. Kyle RA, McParland CE, Dameshek W: Large doses of prednisone and prednisolone in the treatment of malignant lymphoproliferative disorders. Ann Intern Med 57:717–731, 1962.

133. Ezdinli EZ, Stutzman L, Aungst CW, et al.: Corticosteroid therapy for lymphomas and chronic lymphocytic leukemia. Cancer 23:900–909, 1968.

134. Hoogstraten B, Owens AH, Lenhard RE, et al.: Combination chemotherapy in lymphosarcoma and reticulum cell sarcoma. Blood 33:370–378, 1969.

135. Luce JK, Gamble JF, Wilson HE, et al.: Combined cyclophosphamide, vincristine and prednisone therapy of malignant lymphoma. Cancer. Cancer 38:306–317, 1971.

136. Coltman CA Jr, Luce JK, McKelvey EM, et al.: Chemotherapy of non-Hodgkin's lymphoma: 10 years' experience in Southwest Oncology Group. Cancer Treat Rep 61:1067–1078, 1977.

137. Bagley CM Jr. DeVita VT Jr, Berard CW, Canellos GP: Advanced lymphosarcoma: intensive cyclical combination chemotherapy with cyclophosphamide, vincristine and prednisone. Ann Intern Med 76:227–234, 1972.

138. Anderson T, Bender RA, Fisher RI, et al.: Combination chemotherapy in non-Hodgkin's lymphoma: results of long-term follow-up. Cancer Treat Rep 61:1057–1066, 1977.

139. Bitran JC, Golomb HM, Ultmann JE, et al.: Non-Hodgkin's lymphoma, poorly differentiated lymphocytic and mixed cell types: results of sequential staging procedures, response to therapy, and survival of 100 patients. Cancer 42:88–95, 1978.

140. Benjamin RS, Wiernik PH, O'Connell MJ, Chang P, Sutherland JC: A comparison of cyclophosphamide, vincristine and prednisone (COP) with nitrogen mustard, vincristine, procarbazine and prednisone (MOPP) in the treatment of nodular, poorly differentiated, lymphocytic lymphoma. Cancer 38:1896–1902, 1976.

141. Ezdinli EZ, Costello WG, Silverstein MN, et al.: Moderate versus intensive chemotherapy of prognostically favorable non-Hodgkin's lymphoma: a progress report. Cancer 46:29–33, 1980.

142. Portlock CS, Rosenberg SA: Combination chemotherapy with cyclophosphamide, vincristine and prednisone in advanced non-Hodgkin's lymphomas. Cancer 37: 1275–1282, 1976.

143. Jones SE, Salmon SE, Fisher R: Adjuvant immunotherapy with BCG in non-Hodgkin's lymphoma: a Southwest Oncology Group controlled clinical trial. In: Adjuvant therapy of cancer II, Jones SE, Salmon SE, eds. New York: Grune & Stratton, 1979, pp 163–171.

144. Durant JR, Gams RA, Bartolucci AA, Dorfman RF: BCNU with and without cyclophosphamide, vincristine, and prednisone (COP) and cycle-active therapy in non-Hodgkin's lymphoma. Cancer Treat Rep 61:1085–1096, 1977.

145. Costello WG, Orlow E, Jennison C: Technical Report No. 116E: analysis of Eastern Cooperative Oncology Group protocol EST 2474, March 1980 (personal communication William Costello).

146. Ezdinli EZ, Costello WG, Glick JH: Nodular non-Hodgkin's lymphomas: effect of

histologic pattern and response on survival. Proc ASCO 22:516, 1981.

147. McKelvey EM, Gottlieb JA, Wilson HE, *et al.*: Hydroxyldaunomycin (adriamycin) combination chemotherapy in malignant lymphoma. Cancer 38:1484–1493, 1976.

148. Rodriguez V, Cabanillas F, Burgess, *et al.*: Combination chemotherapy ('CHOP-BLEO') in advanced (non-Hodgkin) malignant lymphoma. Blood 49: 325–333, 1977.

149. Skarin AT, Rosenthal DS, Moloney WC, Frei E: Combination chemotherapy of advanced non-Hodgkin lymphoma with bleomycin, adriamycin, cyclophosphamide, vincristine, and prednisone (BACOP). Blood 49:759–768, 1977.

150. Bodey GP, Rodriquez V, Cabanillas F, Frereich EJ: Protected environment-prophylactic anti-biotic program for malignant lymphoma: randomized trial during chemotherapy to induce remission. Am J Med 66:74–81, 1979.

151. Jones SE, Grozea PN, Metz EN, *et al.*: Superiority of adriamycin-containing combination chemotherapy in the treatment of diffuse lymphoma: a Southwest Oncology Group study. Cancer 43:417–425, 1979.

152. Portlock CS, Rosenberg SA: No initial therapy for stage III and IV non-Hodgkin's lymphomas of favorable histologic types. Ann Intern Med 90:10-13, 1979.

153. Krikorian JH, Portlock CS, Cooney DP, Rosenberg SA: Spontaneous regression of non-Hodgkin's lymphoma: a report of nine cases. Cancer 46:2093–2099, 1980.

154. Gattiker HH, Wiltshaw E, Golton DAG: Spontaneous regression in non-Hodgkin's lymphoma. Cancer 45:2627–2632, 1980.

155. Kaufman JH, Ezdinli E, Aungst W, Stutzman L: Lymphosarcoma. Cancer 37: 1283–1292, 1976.

156. Ezdinli E, Pocock S, Berard CW, *et al.*: Comparison of intensive versus moderate chemotherapy of lymphomas: a progress report. Cancer 38:1060–1068, 1976.

157. Jennison C, Costello WG, Russell J: Technical Report No. 165E: analysis of maintenance phase of Eastern Cooperative Oncology Group Protocol EST 2474 and 3474, August, 1980 (personal communication William Costello).

158. Jones R, Young RC, Berard CW, *et al.*: Histologic progression in non-Hodgkin's lymphoma: implications for survival and clinical trials. Proc ASCO 20: 353, 1979.

159. Risdall R, Hoppe RT, Warnke R: Non-Hodgkin's lymphoma: a study of the evolution of the disease based upon 92 autopsied cases. Cancer 44:529–542, 1979.

160. DeVita VT, Glatstein EJ, Young RC, *et al.*: Changing concepts: the lymphomas. In: Adjuvant therapy of cancer II, Jones SE, Salmon SE, eds. New York: Grune & Stratton 1979, pp 173–190.

161. Schein PS, Chabner BA, Canellos GP, *et al.*: Non-Hodgkin's lymphoma: patterns of relapse from complete remission after combination chemotherapy. Cancer 35:354–357, 1975.

162. Fuks Z, Kaplan HS: Recurrence rates following radiation therapy of nodular and diffuse malignant lymphomas. Radiology 108:675–684, 1973.

163. Hoppe RT, Rosenberg SA, Kaplan HS: The treatment of stage III-IV non-Hodgkin's lymphoma of 'favorable' histologic type: a randomized comparison of whole body irradiation, combination chemotherapy, and single-agent chemotherapy. Int J Radiat Oncol 5 (suppl 2):164, 1979.

164. Young RC, Johnson RE, Canellos GP, *et al.*: Advanced lymphocytic lymphoma: randomized comparisons of chemotherapy and radiotherapy, alone or in combination. Cancer Treat Rep 61:1153–1159, 1977.

165. Brereton HD, Young RC, Longo DL, *et al.*: A comparison between combination chemotherapy and total body irradiation plus combination chemotherapy in non-Hodgkin's lymphoma. Cancer 43:2227–2231, 1979.

166. Bonadonna G, Lattuada A, Monfardini S, *et al.*: Combined radiotherapy-chemotherapy in localized non-Hodgkin's lymphomas: 5-year results of a randomized study. In: Adjuvant therapy of cancer II, Jones SE, Salmon SE, eds. New York: Grune & Stratton 1979, pp

145-153.

167. Jones SE, Fuks Z, Bull M, et al.: Non-Hodgkin's lymphomas IV: clinicopathologic correlation in 405 cases. Cancer 31:806-823, 1973.

168. Qazi R, Aisenberg AC, Long JC: The natural history of nodular lymphoma. Cancer 37:1923-1927, 1976.

169. Glick, JH: Personal communication, 1980.

170. Ezdinli EZ, Costello WG, Icli F, et al.: Nodular mixed lymphocytic-histiocytic lymphoma: response and survival. Cancer 45:261-267, 1980.

171. Pangalis GA, Nathwani BN, Rappaport H: Malignant lymphoma, well-differentiated lymphocytic: its relationship with chronic lymphocytic leukemia and macroglobulinemia of Waldenstrom. Cancer 39:999-1010, 1977.

172. Evans HL, Butler JJ, Youness EL: Malignant lymphoma, small lymphocytic type: a clinico-pathologic study of 84 cases with suggestive criteria for intermediate lymphocytic lymphoma. Cancer 41:1440-1455, 1978.

173. Icli F, Ezdinli EZ, Costello W, et al.: Diffuse well-differentiated lymphocytic lymphoma: response and survival. Cancer 42:1936-1942, 1978.

174. DeVita VT Jr, Canellos GP, Chabner B, et al.: Advanced diffuse histiocytic lymphoma, a potentially curable disease: results with combination chemotherapy. Lancet 1:248-250, 1975.

175. Stein RS, Moran EM, Desser RK, et al.: Combination chemotherapy of lymphomas other than Hodgkin's disease. Ann Intern Med 81:601-609, 1974.

176. Durant JR, Loeb V, Dorfman R, Chan YK: 1,3-bis(2-chloroethyl)-1-nitrosourea (BCNU), cyclophosphamide, vincristine and prednisone (BCOP): a new therapeutic regimen for diffuse histiocytic lymphoma. Cancer 36:1936-1944, 1975.

177. Lenhard RE, Ezdinli EZ, Costello W, et al.: Treatment of histiocytic and mixed lymphomas: a comparison of two, three and four drug chemotherapy. Cancer 42:41-52, 1978.

178. Gottlieb JA, Gutterman JU, McCredie KB, et al.: Chemotherapy of malignant lymphoma with adriamycin. Cancer Res 33:3024-3028, 1973.

179. Elias L, Portlock CS, Rosenberg SA: Combination chemotherapy of diffuse histiocytic lymphoma with cyclophosphamide, adriamycin, vincristine and prednisone (CHOP). Cancer 42:1705-1710, 1978.

180. Johnson GJ, Costello WB, Oken MM, et al.: Sequential cyclophosphamide-prednisone and vincristine-bleomycin: an effective schedule-dependent treatment for advanced diffuse histiocytic lymphoma. Proc ASCO 22:517, 1981.

181. Schein PS, DeVita VT, Hubbard S, et al.: Bleomycin, adriamycin, cyclophosphamide, vincristine, and prednisone (BACOP) combination chemotherapy in the treatment of advanced diffuse histiocytic lymphoma. Ann Intern Med 85:417-422, 1976.

182. Canetta R, Villa E, Musumeci R, et al.: Sequential non-cross-resistant regimens (CVP and ABP) in advanced non-Hodgkin lymphomas. Proc AACR 21:189, 1980.

183. Bonadonna G, Monfardini S, Villa E: Non-cross-resistant combinations in stage IV non-Hodgkin's lymphoma. Cancer Treat Rep 61:1117-1123, 1977.

184. Garrett TJ, Gee TS, Dowling MD, et al.: Cyclophosphamide-L2 protocol: a combination chemotherapeutic regimen for advanced non-Hodgkin's lymphoma. Cancer Treat Rep 61:7-16, 1977.

185. Lister TA, Cullen MH, Brearley RB, et al.: Combination chemotherapy for advanced non-Hodgkin's lymphoma of unfavorable histology. Cancer Chemother Pharmacol 1:107-112, 1978.

186. Levitt M, Marsh JC, DeConti RC, et al.: Combination sequential chemotherapy in advanced reticulum cell sarcoma. Cancer 29:630-636, 1972.

187. Berd D, Cornog J, DeConti RC, et al.: Long-term remission in diffuse histiocytic lymphoma treated with combination sequential chemotherapy. Cancer 35:1050-1054,

1975.
188. Cadman E, Farber L, Berd D, Bertino J: Combination therapy for diffuse histiocytic lymphoma that includes antimetabolites. Cancer Treat Rep 61:1109–1116, 1977.
189. Sweet DL, Golomb HM, Ultman JE, et al.: Cyclophosphamide, vincristine, methotrexate with leucovorin rescue, and cytarabine (COMLA): combination sequential chemotherapy for advanced diffuse histiocytic lymphoma. Ann Intern Med 92:785–790, 1980.
190. Stein RS, Collins RD, Ultmann JE: Diffuse histiocytic lymphoma: B-cell origin by Lukes-Collins criteria predicts favorable response to COMLA (cyclophosphamide, oncovin, methotrexate, leucovorin, cytosine arabinoside). Proc ASCO 21:469, 1980.
191. Fisher RI, DeVita VT, Hubbard SM, et al.: Pro MACE-MOPP combination chemotherapy: treatment of diffuse lymphomas. Proc ASCO 21:468, 1980.
192. Skarin A, Canellos G, Rosenthal D, et al.: Therapy of diffuse histiocytic and undifferentiated lymphoma with high-dose methotrexate and citrovorum factor rescue, bleomycin, adriamycin, cyclophosphamide, oncovin, and decadron (M-BACOD). Proc ASCO 21:463, 1980.
193. Fisher RI, DeVita VT, Johnson BL, et al.: Prognostic factors for advanced diffuse histiocytic lymphoma following treatment with combination chemotherapy. Am J Med 63:177–182, 1977.
194. Fisher RI, Hubbard SM, DeVita VT, et al.: Prognostic factors affecting the curability of diffuse mixed, diffuse histiocytic, and diffuse undifferentiated lymphoma. Proc AACR 21:162, 1980.
195. Strauchen JA, Young RC, DeVita VT, et al.: Clinical relevance of the histopathological subclassification of diffuse 'histiocytic' lymphoma. NEJM 299:1382–1387, 1978.
196. MacKintosh FR, O,Neil M, Rosenberg SA: Prognostic factors in advanced histiocytic lymphoma. Proc ASCO 21:465, 1980.
197. Koziner B, Little C, Passe S, et al.: Treatment of advanced diffuse histiocytic lymphoma: an analysis of prognostic variables. Proc AACR 21:145, 1980.
198. Chen MG, Prosnitz LR, Gonzalez-Serva A, Fischer DB: Results of radiotherapy in control of stage I and II non-Hodgkin's lymphoma. Cancer 43:1245–1254, 1979.
199. Jones SE, Fuks Z, Bull M, et al.: Non-Hodgkin's lymphomas V: Results of radiotherapy. Cancer 32:682–690, 1973.
200. Sweet DL, Golomb HM: The treatment of histiocytic lymphoma. Semin Oncol 7:302–309, 1980.
201. Sweet DL, Golomb HM, Kinzie J, et al.: Survival in localized diffuse histiocytic lymphoma. Proc ASCO 21:465, 1980.
202. Monfardini S, Banfi A, Bonadonna G, et al.: Improved five-year survival after combined radiotherapy-chemotherapy for stage II-II non-Hodgkin's lymphoma. Int J Radiat Oncol Biol Phys 6:125–134, 1980.
203. Landberg TG, Hakansson LG, Moller TR, et al.: CVP-remission CVP-remission-maintenance in stage I or II non-Hodgkin's lymphomas: preliminary results of a randomized study. Cancer 44:831–833, 1979.
204. Kushlan P, Coleman CN, Glatstein EJ, et al.: Prognostic factors in stage II diffuse histiocytic lymphoma. Proc ASCO 19:337, 1978.
205. Glatstein E, Portlock C, Rosenberg SA, Kaplan HS: Combined modality treatment in the malignant lymphomas. In: Adjuvant therapy of cancer I, Salmon SE, Jones SE, eds. New York: North Holland, 1977, pp 545–548.
206. Miller TP, Jones SE: Is there a role for radiotherapy in localized diffuse lymphomas? Cancer Chemother Pharmacol 4:67–70, 1980.
207. Miller TP, Jones SE: The management of localized diffuse lymphomas. Curr Concepts Oncol 3:6–9, 1981.
208. Cabanillas F, Bodey GP, Freireich EJ: Management with chemotherapy only of stage I and II malignant lymphoma of aggressive histologic types. Cancer 46:2356–2359, 1980.

209. Osborne CK, Norton L, Young RC, et al.: Nodular histiocytic lymphoma: an aggressive nodular lymphoma with potential for prolonged disease-free survival. Blood 56:98-103, 1980.
210. Glick JH, McFadden E, Costello W: Nodular histiocytic lymphoma: factors influencing prognosis and indications for aggressive chemotherapy. Proc AACR 21:142, 1980.
211. Ezdinli EZ, Costello W, Lenhard RE, et al.: Survival of nodular versus diffuse pattern lymphocytic poorly differentiated lymphoma. Cancer 41:1990-1996, 1978.
212. Schein PS, Chabner BA, Canellos GP, et al.: Potential for prolonged disease-free survival following combination chemotherapy of non-Hodgkin's lymphoma. Blood 43:181-189, 1974.
213. Bloomfield CD, Gajl-Peczalska KJ, Frizzera G, et al.: Clinical utility of lymphocyte surface markers combined with the Lukes-Collins histologic classification in adult lymphoma. N Engl J Med 301:512-518, 1979.
214. Stein RS, Cousar J, Flexner JM, et al.: Malignant lymphomas of follicular center cell origin in man: III. Prognostic features. Cancer 44:2236-2243, 1979.
215. Neiman RS, Kim H, Mann R, Rappaport H: Malignant lymphoma poorly differentiated type diffuse: a tumor of varying histologic subtypes. Proc Int Acad Pathol (submitted), 1981.
216. Skarin AT, Pinkus GS, Myerowitz RL, et al.: Combination chemotherapy of advanced lymphocytic lymphoma. Cancer 34:1023-1029, 1974.
217. McKelvey EM, Moon TE: Curability of non-Hodgkin's lymphoma. Cancer Treat Rep 61:1185-1190, 1977.
218. Harrison DT, Neiman PE, Sullivan K, et al.: Combined modality therapy for advanced, diffuse lymphocytic and histiocytic lymphomas. Cancer 42:1697-1704, 1978.
219. Nathwani BN, Kim H, Rappaport H: Malignant lymphoma, lymphoblastic: Cancer 38:964-983, 1976.
220. Nathwani BN, Diamond LW, Weinberg CD, et al.: Lymphoblastic lymphoma: a clinicopatholic study of 95 patients. Cancer, 1981, (in press).
221. Coleman CN, Cohen JR, Rosenberg SA: Adult lymphoblastic lymphoma - result of a pilot therapy protocol. Blood 57:679-684, 1981.
222. Brecher ML, Sinks LF, Thomas RRM, Freeman AI: Non-Hodgkin's lymphoma in children. Cancer 41:1997-2001, 1978.
223. Murphy SB and Hustu HO: A randomized trial of combined modality therapy of childhood non-Hodgkin's lymphoma. Cancer 45:630-637, 1980.
224. Weinstein HJ, Vance ZB, Jaffe N, et al.: Improved prognosis for patients with mediastinal lymphoblastic lymphoma. Blood 53:687-694, 1979.
225. Wollner N, Exelby PR, Lieberman PH: Non-Hodgkin's lymphoma in children: a progress report on the original patients treated with LSA-L2 protocol. Cancer 44:1990-1999, 1979.
226. Johnson GJ, Barnes JM, O'Connell MJ, et al.: Low incidence of central nervous system relapse following chemotherapy of unfavorable histology of non-Hodgkin's lymphoma. Proc AACR 22:195, 1981.
227. MacKintosh FR, Podolsky WJ, Rosenfelt FP, et al.: Central nervous system involvement in non-Hodgkin's lymphoma. Proc ASCO 20: 439, 1979.
228. Bunn PA, Schein PS, Banks PM, DeVita VT: Central nervous system complications in patients with diffuse histiocytic and undifferentiated lymphoma: leukemia revisited. Blood 47:3-10, 1976.
229. Young RC, Howser, DM, Anderson T, et al.: Central nervous system complications of non-Hodgkin's lymphoma: the potential role for prophylactic therapy. Am J Med 66:435-433, 1979.
230. Herman TS, Hammond N, Jones SE, et al.: Involvement of central nervous system by non-Hodgkin's lymphoma: the Southwest Oncology Group experience. Cancer 43:390-

397, 1979.

231. Skarin AT, Zuckerman KS, Pitman SW, *et al.*: High-dose methotrexate with folinic acid in the treatment of advanced non-Hodgkin lymphoma including CNS involvement. Blood 50:1039–1047, 1977.

Subject Index